The VITAMIN PUSHERS

Consumer Health Library®
Series Editor: Stephen Barrett, M.D.
Technical Editor: Manfred Kroger, Ph.D.

Other titles in this series:

A Consumer's Guide to "Alternative Medicine"
Kurt Butler, M.S.
"Alternative" Healthcare: A Comprehensive Guide
Jack Raso, M.S., R.D.
Examining Holistic Medicine
edited by Douglas Stalker, Ph.D., and Clark Glymour, Ph.D.
The Faith Healers
James Randi
Follies & Fallacies in Medicine
Petr Skrabanek, Ph.D., and James McCormick, M.D.
The Harvard Square Diet
Fredrick J. Stare, M.D., Ph.D., and Elizabeth M. Whelan, Sc.D., M.P.H.
Health or Hoax? The Truth about Health Foods and Diets
Arnold Bender
The Health Robbers: A Close Look at Quackery in America
Stephen Barrett, M.D., and William T. Jarvis, Ph.D.
The New Handbook of Health and Preventive Medicine
Kurt Butler, M.S., and Lynn Rayner, M.D.
Mystical Diets: Paranorma, Spiritual, and Occult Nutrition Practices
Jack Raso, M.S., R.D.
Panic in the Pantry: Facts & Fallacies about the Food You Buy
Elizabeth M. Whelan, Sc.D., M.P.H., and
Fredrick J. Stare, M.D., Ph.D.
The Smoke-Free Workplace
William Weis and Bruce Miller
Vitamin Politics
John Fried
Your Guide to Good Nutrition
Fredrick J. Stare, M.D., Ph.D., Virginia Aronson, M.S., R.D., and
Stephen Barrett, M.D.

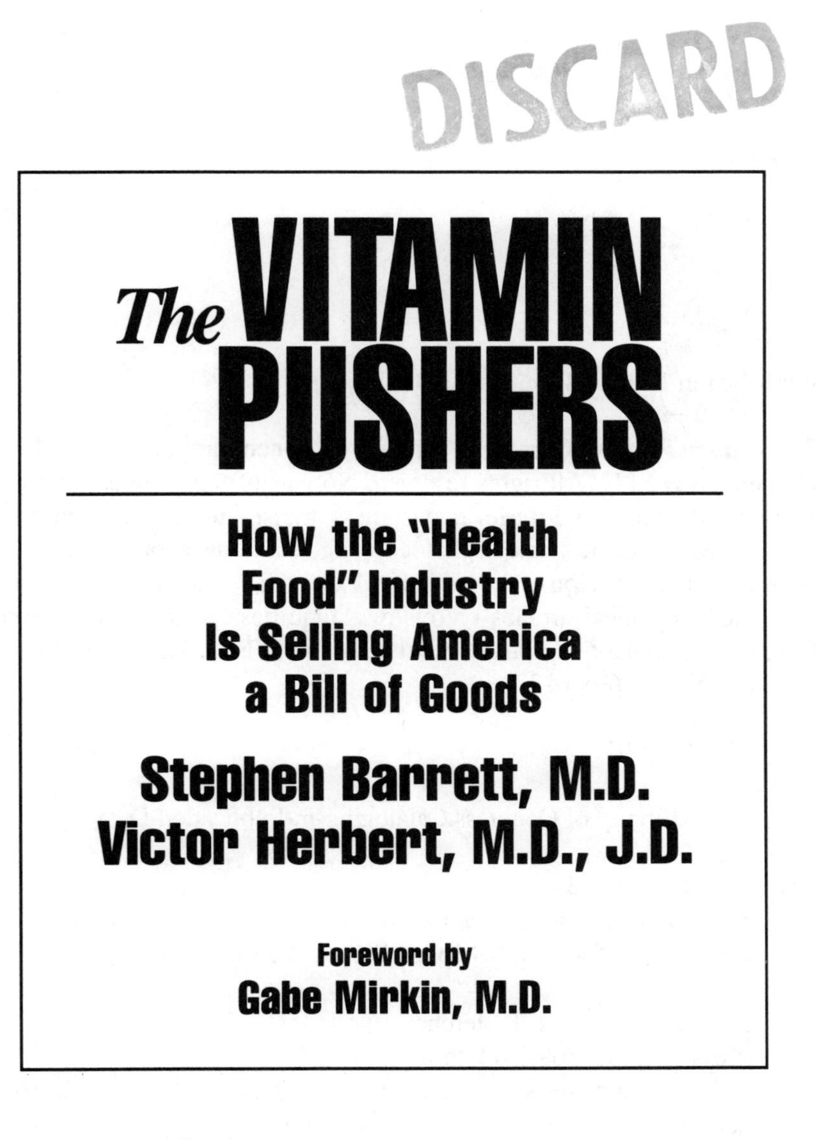

The VITAMIN PUSHERS

How the "Health Food" Industry Is Selling America a Bill of Goods

Stephen Barrett, M.D.
Victor Herbert, M.D., J.D.

Foreword by
Gabe Mirkin, M.D.

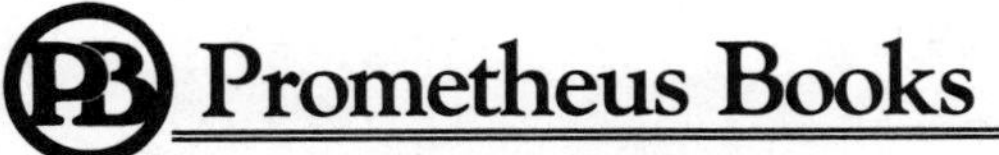

Prometheus Books
59 John Glenn Drive
Amherst, NewYork 14228-2197

Published in 1994 by Prometheus Books.

98 97 96 95 94 5 4 3 2

Library of Congress Cataloging-in-Publication Data

Barrett, Stephen, 1933–
The vitamin pushers : how the "health food" industry is selling America a bill of goods / Stephen Barrett. Victor Herbert.
p. cm.
Includes biographical references and index.
ISBN 0-87975-909-7 (cloth)
1. Quacks and quackery—United States. 2. Natural foods industry—United States. I. Herbert, Victor II. Title.
R730.B373 1994
363.19'2—dc20 94-21714
CIP

Printed in the United States on acid-free paper.

Contents

Foreword

Gabe Mirkin, M.D

Do you get angry when someone tries to hustle you? Would it bother you if someone promised you something and took your money, but gave you nothing in return? Do you think you have ever been hustled without realizing it?

What goes through your mind when you see an ad which suggests that a pill can help you lose weight permanently without dieting or exercising? If it doesn't strike you as phony, you don't know the facts. There is no such pill.

How about a magazine article which claims that a "dietary supplement" can make you a better athlete, help you live longer, or cure heart disease, diabetes, cancer, and a host of other ailments? If you think any such remedy exists, you had better read this book.

Do you take vitamin pills? Has it occurred to you to question whether you really need them? You should. Most of the hundred million or so Americans who take them are merely nourishing their toilets and making vitamin manufacturers rich.

But the issue is not simply one of wasted money. Each decision you make about your health must be based on an underlying judgment about whom to trust for advice. *If you cannot tell the difference between an expert and a hustler, you are likely to be misled.*

One of the factors that makes America great is our freedom of speech. To maintain this freedom, we must also run a risk. False prophets can get up on pedestals (such as radio and television talk shows) and tell you almost anything they please.

Such prophets abound in the field of nutrition. One reason they succeed is that too many people who know better are afraid to become involved in controversy.

The people who wrote this book *are* involved. Dr. Herbert has attacked nutrition frauds more forcefully than any other person in America. He has testified before legislators and in courts. He has spent his own money seeking justice. He is one of the most knowledgeable and respected nutrition scientists in the world—one to whom other experts turn frequently for advice. Dr. Barrett has investigated and written about quackery in more and different fields than any other living American.

This is one book you should not ignore. It is one of the most amazing investigative reports in the history of American journalism. It is likely to save you money. It can help you protect your health. It might even save your life!

Gabe Mirkin, M.D.

Preface

One lesson of the Watergate scandal during the Nixon Administration was that shady operations involving large sums of money are likely to create a "paper trail" of incriminating evidence. The "health food" industry—which has been selling its bill of goods for more than a century—is no exception. We regard this industry as a form of organized crime.

This book is based on more than twenty years of research. Like the Watergate story, it was inspired by "defectors" who provided information and documents that were not intended for public view. Our relentless investigation—aided by a network of reporters and other consumer advocates—has brought the whole seamy picture into focus.

The sale of unneeded and sometimes dangerous food supplements is a multibillion-dollar business. Political and intellectual harm are involved as well. This book explores four questions:

- How is the health-food industry organized?
- How do its salespeople learn their trade?
- How do its salespeople persuade the public to believe in false ideas?
- Most important, *how do they get away with what they are doing?*

Stephen Barrett, M.D.
Victor Herbert, M.D., J.D.

Acknowledgments

The authors are grateful to the following individuals for their many helpful suggestions during the preparation of the manuscript:

Project manager	Mark G. Hall, Managing Editor, Prometheus Books
Legal advisor	Michael Botts, Esq., Prescott, Wisconsin
Technical editor	Manfred Kroger, Ph.D., Professor of Food Science, The Pennsylvania State University
Consultant	William T. Jarvis, Ph.D., Professor of Health Promotion and Education, Loma Linda University

The authors also thank the many people who helped gather the thousands of source documents and other information used for this book.

About the Authors

• Stephen Barrett, M.D., a retired psychiatrist who practiced in Allentown, Pennsylvania, for more than twenty-five years, is a nationally renowned author, editor, and consumer advocate. He edited *Nutrition Forum Newsletter* for nine years and has contributed frequently to *Priorities Magazine, Healthline Newsletter,* and *Consumer Reports on Health.* He is a board member of the National Council Against Health Fraud and chairs its Task Force on Victim Redress. He is a scientific and editorial advisor to the American Council on Science and Health. His thirty-six books include *The Health Robbers: A Close Look at Quackery in America; Health Schemes, Scams, and Frauds*; *Vitamins and "Health" Foods: The Great American Hustle; Reader's Guide to "Alternative" Health Methods;* and four editions of the college textbook *Consumer Health—A Guide to Intelligent Decisions.* In 1984, he won the FDA Commissioner's Special Citation Award for Public Service in fighting nutrition quackery. In 1986, he was awarded honorary life membership in the American Dietetic Association. In 1987, he began teaching health education at The Pennsylvania State University.

• Victor Herbert, M.D., J.D., F.A.C.P., is professor of medicine at Mt. Sinai School of Medicine in New York City and chief of the Hematology and Nutrition Laboratory at the Sinai-affiliated Bronx V.A. Medical Center. He is a board member of the National Council Against Health Fraud and a member of the American Cancer Society's Committee on Questionable Methods. He has served on the Food and Nutrition Board of the National Academy of Sciences and its Recommended Dietary Allowances (RDA) Committee. He consults in nutrition to the World Health Organization (WHO), has been president of the American Society for Clinical Nutrition, and was chairman for five years of the American Bar Association's Committee on Life Sciences and the Law. He has received the FDA Commissioner's Special Citation Award for Public Service in fighting nutrition quackery and is an honorary life member of the American Dietetic Association. He has written more than seven hundred scientific articles and received seven national awards for his nutrition research. His books include *The Megaloblastic Anemias; Nutrition Cultism: Facts and Fictions; Vitamins and "Health" Foods: the Great American Hustle; The Mount Sinai School of Medicine Complete Book of Nutrition; Genetic Nutrition: Designing a Diet Based on Your Family Medical History;* and *Total Nutrition: The Only Guide You'll Ever Need.*

Important Definitions

- **"alternative" method:** a health-related method that is not generally accepted by the scientific medical community and lacks a plausible rationale
- **quackery:** the promotion of an unproven health product or service, usually for personal gain
- **drug:** any article (except a device) intended for use in the diagnosis, cure, mitigation, treatment, or prevention of disease; any article (other than food) intended to affect the structure or function of the body
- **intended use:** the real purpose of a product, as judged by the circumstances surrounding its sale
- **labeling (of a food or drug):** written, printed, graphic, or electronically recorded material that accompanies a product. Labeling must contain adequate directions for all intended uses.
- **new drug:** legal term for a drug not generally recognized as safe and effective by experts for its intended use
- **unapproved new drug:** a new drug that lacks FDA approval. Marketing an unapproved new drug in interstate commerce is a federal crime.
- **misbranded:** a product whose labeling lacks required information (such as adequate directions for use) or contains false or misleading information. Interstate marketing of a misbranded product is a federal crime.
- **disinformation:** misleading information intended to influence public opinion
- **health-food industry:** the network of quackery and disinformation promoters who greatly exaggerate the value of nutritional products or use scare tactics associated with a basic rejection of scientific facts
- **vitamin pusher:** anyone who promotes vitamins (or other "dietary supplements") with false or misleading claims
- **dietary supplement:** a term used by vitamin pushers to characterize vitamins, minerals, herbs, amino acids, and anything else people might consume "to increase total dietary intake of a substance." Consumer advocates would like the term restricted to essential nutrients that may be usefully added to the diet. This would make it illegal to market "supplement" products that are nutritionally useless or drugs in disguise.

1

Some Simple Truths about Nutrition

Most Americans who take vitamins don't need them. Could you be one of these people? Are you afraid that our food supply is lacking in nutrients?

Do you think that vitamin pills can give you extra energy? That extra vitamins should be taken in times of stress? That vitamin C can prevent colds? That vitamin E has been proven to prevent heart disease? That large doses of other nutrients can prevent or cure many other ailments? Or that methods labeled "alternative" offer something special?

Are you afraid there are "too many chemicals" in our food? Do you believe that foods labeled "natural" or "organic" are safer or more nutritious? Or that diet plays a major role in behavior? Or that most diseases are caused by improper eating?

Do you think that most nutrition advice in books, magazines, newsletters, and talk shows is reliable? Or that "alternative" health methods hold great promise? Or that the health marketplace is tightly regulated by government agencies?

If you have any of these fears or beliefs, you have plenty of company. But you have been misled!

America is in the midst of a vitamin craze. Health hustlers who spread false ideas have developed a huge public following. But nutrition is not a religion. It is a science—composed mainly of human biochemistry and physiology. What a nutrient can or cannot do in the body is determined by its specific chemical structure and the specific biochemical reactions in which that structure can become involved.

How can you tell what to believe? The answer to this question has two parts. First, you should know what is meant by "scientific truth." Then you must determine who is telling the truth.

How Do We Know What We "Know"?

How are medical facts determined? Humans have always been curious about disease and what causes it. The more we understand, of course, the better we can control illness. Down through the centuries, thousands of theories have been formulated to explain the reasons for both health and sickness. During the past century, however, speculation has been supplanted by reliable knowledge based on experimentation and sound clinical experience. Armed with this new knowledge, doctors have been able to prevent and cure many diseases in a way that seems almost miraculous.

As part of the process of scientific development, good methods have been developed to test whether theories are logical. The sum of these methods is known as the "experimental" or "scientific" method. This method is used to answer questions like: "If two things happen, one after the other, are they related?" For example, suppose you take a pill when you have a headache and the headache goes away one hour later. How can we tell whether the pill relieved you or whether the headache would have gone away by itself anyway? Throughout the world, hundreds of thousands of scientists are working continuously to determine the boundaries of scientific thought.

As mountains of information are collected, how can we tell which evidence is valid? "Valid" means honestly collected and properly interpreted—using valid techniques of analysis. One hallmark of a good experiment is that others can repeat it and get the same results.

This brings us to the question of who can best interpret experimental findings. Scientists are judging each other all the time. People with equal or superior training look for loopholes in each others' experimental techniques and design other experiments to test conclusions. Skilled reviewers also gather in groups whose levels of ability far exceed that of the average scientist. Such experts are not likely to be misled by poorly designed experiments. Among the reviewers are editors and editorial boards of scientific journals; these people carefully screen out invalid findings and enable significant ones to be published. (Most reliable journals that cover nutrition topics are listed in the *Index Medicus* of the National Library of Medicine.)

As good ideas are put to use, more reports are generated. When controversies arise, further research can be devised to settle them. Gradually a shared set of beliefs is developed that is felt to be scientifically accurate. Expert panels convened by government agencies, professional groups, voluntary health agencies, and other organizations also contribute to this effort. When we speak of the "scientific community," we refer to this overall process of separating what is truly fact from what is not.

Three basic questions are involved in evaluating whether a treatment method works:

1. Is it more effective than doing nothing, or than a placebo?
2. Is it as safe as doing nothing?
3. If there is a question about safety, does the potential for benefit exceed the likelihood of harm?

One of the central premises of science is that *no method should be regarded as proven until it is actually proven.*

Quacks, of course, operate outside of the scientific community. They do not use the scientific method to evaluate what they see. In fact, they seldom bother to experiment at all and ignore the three questions listed above. When scientists point out that they are wrong, quacks try to cover up their inadequacies by pointing out that the scientific community has made mistakes in the past. This, of course, is true but irrelevant. In recent years, the odds of major error by the scientific community have decreased greatly. So if you find someone referred to as a "scientist ahead of his time," he is probably a quack. Quacks may boast of "thousands of cases" in their files. But they won't tell you that none of these cases separates cause and effect from coincidence, suggestibility, or misdiagnosis. Nor do they ever keep score and reveal how many failures they have had for each "success."

Interpretation of experimental findings is not always simple. Consider antioxidants, for example. Certain recent studies have found a lower incidence of death from heart disease among people who take vitamin E supplements than among similar people who do not. Does this prove that taking high doses of vitamin E will reduce the risk of a heart attack? Does this prove that taking high doses of vitamin E will do more good than harm? Does this mean that everyone should take a vitamin E supplement?

The answer to each of these questions is no. The reduction in death rate among the vitamin E group may have resulted from other lifestyle characteristics of the group such as eating a more healthful diet. Studies to answer the first question are underway and may be completed within a few years. Even if the results are promising, however, they may not indicate which people should take a supplement, what dose would be optimal, or whether long-term administration of vitamin E will turn out to have a detrimental effect.

Basic Principles of Good Nutrition

Many people think that to achieve good health they must know what each nutrient does in the body. This is absolutely untrue! You don't need to know the biochemical properties of specific nutrients any more than you must know how the parts of a car work in order to be a good driver. Running the human machine, from a nutritional point of view, is quite simple. You need to recognize only three basic facts:

1. The basic principles of healthy eating are *moderation*, *variety*, and *balance*.
2. All the nutrients most people need can be obtained by eating a balanced variety of foods.
3. Body weight is a matter of arithmetic. If you eat more calories than you burn, you will gain weight. To lose weight, you must burn off more calories than you take in.

Moderation means not eating too much of any one food or nutrient because too much of anything is unhealthy. It also means that too little of any nutrient is unhealthy. Variety refers to eating foods from each of the five food groups—as well as different foods within each group—as described below. Balance, which automatically results from moderation and variety, requires an appropriate intake of essential nutrients, without too much of some and too little of others. It also refers to balancing caloric input and energy expenditure to maintain a healthy weight.

To help translate dietary standards into prudent food choices, scientists have classified foods into five groups according to their similarity in nutrient content. This enables consumers to select foods by group rather than by having to calculate the amount of each nutrient individually. Thus the fundamentals of food choice are simple: To get the amounts and kinds of nutrients your body needs, eat moderate amounts from each of the five food groups designated by the U.S. Department of Agriculture's Daily Food Guide. You should eat a wide variety within each group. Your daily average should include:

Bread, Cereal, Rice, & Pasta Group	6 to 11 servings
Vegetable Group	3 to 5 servings
Fruit Group	2 to 4 servings
Milk, Yogurt, & Cheese Group	2 to 3 servings
Meat, Poultry, Fish, Dry Beans, Eggs, & Nuts Group	2 to 3 servings

Except for the milk group, the number of recommended servings depends on the individual's age, gender, size, and activity level, with the lowest numbers for people needing about 1,600 calories daily and the highest ones for those needing about 2,800 calories. Food classifications, serving sizes, and general dietary guidelines are defined in literature published by the Agriculture Department and described in Appendix A of this book. This system provides adequate quantities of all vitamins, minerals, protein components, and dietary fiber. In fact, normal people eating a balanced variety of foods are likely to consume *more* nutrients than they need. Of course, health hucksters won't tell you this because their income depends upon pushing products.

Vegetarian Eating

Vegetarians are individuals who restrict or eliminate foods of animal origin (meat, poultry, fish, eggs, milk) from their diet. "Strict" vegetarians (vegans) eat no animal products at all. Lactovegetarians eat milk and cheese products in addition to vegetables. Lacto-ovo-vegetarians eat no meat, poultry, or fish but do include eggs and milk products. Semivegetarians eat no red meat but do include small amounts of poultry or fish in their diet.

Vegetarianism based on sound nutrition principles is a healthful choice. Vegetarians tend to weigh less than the average American and to have a lower incidence of atherosclerotic heart disease and high blood pressure. However, similar health status can be achieved with an equally low-calorie diet that includes animal products. The downside of vegetarian eating is that the more restricted the diet, the greater the chance of nutrient deficiency.

Strict vegetarians are at risk for several deficiencies, especially vitamin B_{12}. The other nutrients at risk are riboflavin, calcium, iron, and the essential amino acids lysine and methionine. Vegetarian children not exposed to sunlight are at risk for vitamin D deficiency. Zinc deficiency can occur in vegans because phytic acid in whole grains binds zinc, and there is little zinc in fruits and vegetables. Since B_{12} is naturally present only in animal foods, vegans need to consume B_{12}-fortified foods or take B_{12} supplements.

Strict vegetarianism is not desirable for children under the age of five because it is difficult for vegans to meet children's high requirements for protein and some other nutrients. Growing adolescents may have difficulty getting adequate caloric and nutrient intake from a vegan diet. Nor is strict vegetarianism a good idea for pregnant or lactating women.

Genetic Nutrition

Each of us is born with a genetic blueprint which has, coded within it, tendencies toward most of the chronic diseases we are likely to get. What we eat—and avoid eating—can cause that code to be expressed (i.e., result in disease) or be repressed (not result in disease). Your family history may therefore help guide you toward dietary measures that can prevent or delay various conditions in which heredity is a factor. These facts are symbolized below in the Genetic Pyramid, which adds a "genetic blueprint" base to the U.S. Department of Agriculture's Food Guide Pyramid.

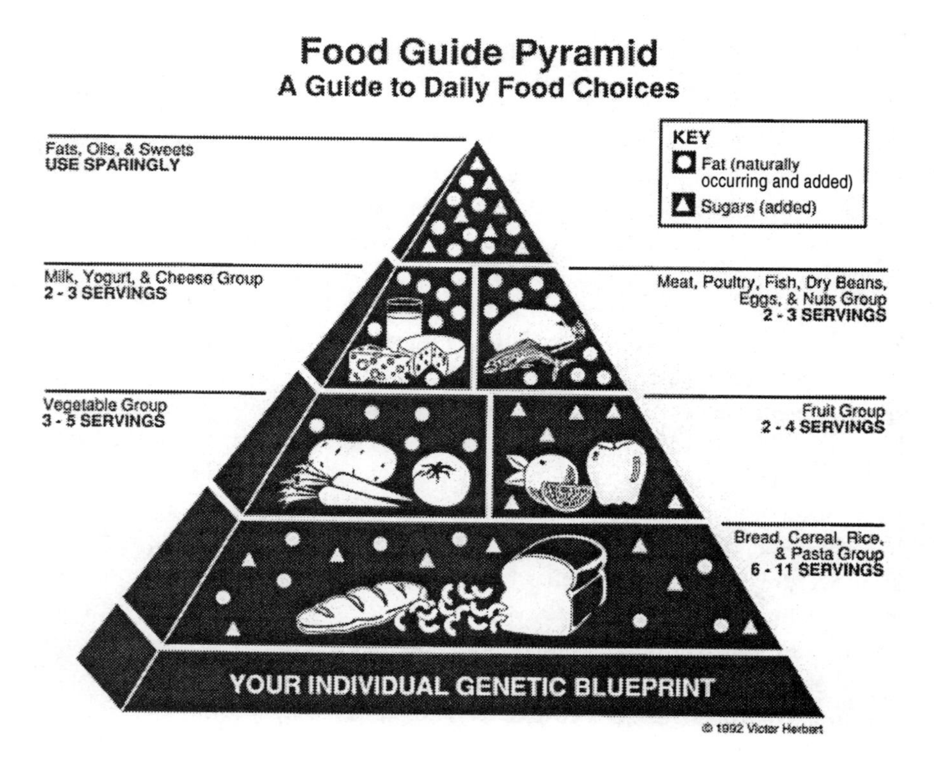

The Genetic Pyramid. The number of servings for each food group are for the "average" American. Serving numbers may need to be increased or decreased according to each individual's genetic blueprint.

Vitamin Facts

A vitamin is an organic (carbon-containing) molecule needed in the diet in tiny amounts. Continued lack of any vitamin in an otherwise complete diet will result in a deficiency disease, the best known of which are beriberi, pellagra, rickets, and scurvy. Vitamins were first discovered by investigators searching for the cause of these diseases.

Thirteen substances are vitamins for humans. Four are fat-soluble (A, D, E, and K) and nine are water-soluble (C and the eight "B-complex" vitamins: thiamine, riboflavin, niacin, B_6, pantothenic acid, B_{12}, biotin, and folic acid). It is unlikely that any new vitamins will be found. The last one was discovered in 1948, and decades of additional research have not uncovered any more. Moreover, patients have lived quite well for years on just intravenous solutions that contain the known nutrients. If there were an undiscovered vitamin, these patients would have shown evidence of a deficiency disease.

Vitamins can function in the body in two ways. In small amounts, they function as *catalysts.* A catalyst is a substance that increases the speed of a chemical reaction without being used up by the reaction. Vitamins help accelerate certain chemical reactions that are essential for health. Without vitamins, these reactions would occur very slowly or not at all. The fact that vitamins are not used up explains why they are needed in only tiny amounts. Unlike foods, they are not a source of energy (calories).

When scientists speak of "excess" vitamins, they mean dosages in excess of the Recommended Dietary Allowances (RDAs) set by the Food and Nutrition Board of the National Research Council. RDAs are not "minimum" values; in fact they are more than most people require. They are set not only to meet body needs, but to allow substantial storage to cover periods of reduced intake or increased need. Amounts of vitamins beyond what the body needs do not function usefully as vitamins but act like *chemicals* or *drugs*. Some excesses of water-soluble vitamins are stored, but most are excreted in the urine. Fat-soluble vitamins, particularly A and D, are more dangerous because excesses accumulate in body fat. Even modest excesses can build up gradually over months or years to toxic levels. The average American eating an average American diet gets so much more than needed of vitamin A that body stores rise with each decade of life. The same is true for vitamin B_{12} until stomach atrophy reduces it absorption.

To clarify in your mind why extra vitamins are not needed, imagine you are hovering in the sky over an intersection (vitamin receptor site) where one police officer (vitamin) at a time is enough to insure that automobile traffic (food) will flow smoothly. Although many cars pass through the intersection (get "used up"), the police officers will need only an occasional replacement when they go off-duty. Bringing more police officers (excess vitamins) to the intersection will not improve the flow of traffic. It will add to taxpayer expense and could cause confusion.

The rapid excretion of excess water-soluble vitamins can be demonstrated by a simple test involving riboflavin, for which the adult RDA is about 1.6 mg. Riboflavin has a bright yellow color. First, urinate. Then swallow two or three vitamin pills that provide a total of 5 mg of riboflavin. Wait two hours and urinate again. The reason why Americans have the most expensive urine and the best-nourished toilets in the world will then be obvious.

To promote supplements, health hustlers misrepresent the concept of "biochemical individuality" (our individual genetic blueprint) to imply that individuals should consume more than the RDAs in case they have greater-than-average nutrient needs. Remember that RDAs are deliberately set considerably higher than virtually all normal people require in order to encompass the range of individual variations and provide for storage of safe amounts. In other words, biochemical individuality has been taken into account. Moreover, if individual variation were as great as the hustlers would have us believe, it would also apply to the inability to tolerate higher doses of nutrients—extra nutrients would be as likely to make people sick as they would be to help them. In fact, because of genetic variability, excess nutrients do more people harm than good.

There are only two situations in which the use of vitamins in excess of the RDAs has proven value. The first is for treatment of medically diagnosed deficiency states—conditions that are rare except among alcoholics, persons with intestinal absorption defects, and the poor, especially those who are pregnant or elderly. The other use is in the treatment of certain conditions for which large doses of vitamins are used as drugs—with full recognition of the risks involved.

The Dangers of Excess Vitamins

Many substances that are harmless in small or moderate doses can be harmful in large amounts or by gradual buildup (body storage) over months or years. Just because a substance (such as a vitamin) is found naturally in food does not mean that it cannot be harmful. In fact, an entire book on this subject, *Toxicants Occurring Naturally in Foods,* was published by a subcommittee of the National Research Council. The book included a chapter on the toxicity of vitamins.

Megadoses of most nutrients have been demonstrated to be harmful. Too much vitamin A can cause lack of appetite, retarded growth in children, drying and cracking of the skin, enlargement of the liver and spleen, increased pressure on the brain, loss of hair, migratory joint pains, menstrual difficulty, bone pain, irritability, and headache.

Prolonged excessive intake of vitamin D can cause loss of appetite, nausea, weakness, weight loss, excess urinary output, constipation, vague aches, stiffness, kidney stones, tissue calcification, high blood pressure, acidosis, and kidney failure which can lead to death.

Large doses of niacin, as recommended by purveyors of megavitamins for mental disorders, can cause severe flushing, itching, liver damage, skin disorders, gout, ulcers, and blood sugar disorders. There is no scientific evidence that megadoses of niacin—or any other nutrient—are effective against mental problems (see Chapter 12). Niacin is a useful drug for improving blood cholesterol values (see Chapter 8), but it should never be used without close medical supervision.

Excess vitamin E can cause headaches, nausea, tiredness, giddiness, inflammation of the mouth, chapped lips, gastrointestinal disturbances, muscle weakness, low blood sugar, increased bleeding tendency, and degenerative changes. By antagonizing the action of vitamin A, large doses of vitamin E can cause blurred vision. Vitamin E can also reduce sexual organ function—just the opposite of the false claim that the vitamin heightens sexual potency. (This claim is based on fertility experiments with rats. Quacks don't tell you that what may be true with rats may be just the opposite with humans!)

Another way to look for health trouble is by taking large doses of ascorbic acid—vitamin C. Here the quacks take great pleasure in linking themselves with one of the truly great men of our age, Linus Pauling, who won Nobel Prizes for chemistry in 1954 and for peace in 1962. Pauling's belief that vitamin C has value against colds and cancer is well intentioned but misguided (see Chapter 17). In some cases, like an antihistamine tablet, vitamin C may reduce the symptoms of a mild cold (thereby creating the impression that no cold occurred). There is no evidence that large doses of vitamin C *prevent* colds, however, so it is not logical to take such doses 365 days a year.

Not a single objective study supports Pauling's claim that megadoses of vitamin C protect against cancer—which he himself has. In fact, among the 10 percent or more Americans born with a gene that leads to increased iron absorption and excessive body iron storage, a high vitamin C intake promotes cancer and heart disease by generating large numbers of harmful free radicals.

Large doses of vitamin C can damage vitamin B_{12} status, converting some

B_{12} to anti-B_{12} molecules. In addition, excess vitamin C may damage growing bone, produce diarrhea, produce "rebound scurvy" in adults and in newborn infants whose mothers took large dosages, cause adverse effects in pregnancy, produce kidney stones, and cause false urine tests for sugar in diabetics. Vitamin C in large doses can also produce false negative tests for blood in the stool and thereby prevent early detection of serious gastrointestinal diseases including cancer.

In 1980, the megavitamin world was rocked by a report of seven cases of unsteady gait and numbness of the feet and hands from taking 2,000 mg or more of vitamin B_6 daily for several months. (The RDA is 2 mg/day.) Although all of them improved greatly within a few months after stopping B_6, their recovery was not complete. Soon afterward, the scientists who made this report heard from at least forty persons with similar symptoms that had improved after stopping their B_6 intake. Some had been misdiagnosed as suffering from multiple sclerosis! In 1987, a survey at a clinic specializing in the treatment of premenstrual syndrome (PMS) discovered that 107 patients had developed neurological symptoms as a result of taking vitamin B_6. Ninety-two had taken less than 200 mg (one hundred times the RDA) daily for more than six months, and twenty had taken less than 50 mg/day. The lowest dosage on which anyone developed symptoms was 20 mg/day for two years; the shortest time was two months of 100 mg/day. Although all of their symptoms resolved when the B_6 was stopped, it is clear that megadoses of B_6 pose considerable risk.

Adverse effects such as those listed above are unlikely to occur with water-soluble vitamins at intake levels below ten times the RDAs, or with fat-soluble vitamins below five times the RDAs. But even if lesser dosages don't harm you physically, if you don't need them, they are a waste of money. The number of reported cases of toxicity is not large, but since there is no evidence that self-prescribed megadoses are helpful, taking them is senseless.

A recent study by the U.S. Centers for Disease Control and Prevention showed that Americans who took supplements had exactly the same mortality rate as those who did not. We interpret this to mean that supplements help some people, harm others, and are a waste of money for most.

Mineral Facts

The important minerals known to be essential to humans are calcium, phosphorus, magnesium, and the trace elements: iron, zinc, copper, manganese, fluoride, chromium, selenium, and molybdenum. Like fat-soluble vitamins, excess amounts of minerals are stored in the body and can gradually build up to toxic levels. An excess of one mineral can also interfere with the functioning of others. There are legitimate reasons for certain people to use mineral supplements, but they should never be used without a competent medical determination that one of these reasons exists.

Iron is needed for blood formation, and new blood is formed rapidly in three groups: children up to age five, boys and girls at the onset of puberty, and women who are pregnant or who must replace blood lost during menstruation. Vegetarians must be particularly careful because vegetable iron is much less absorbable than is iron from animal sources. Iron deficiency is common enough in these groups that they should be evaluated with a blood test for iron deficiency. If it is found, treatment with iron should be administered. Taking iron if you don't have proven iron deficiency is unwise, since it can produce iron overload that can damage the liver, pancreas, and heart. About 6 percent of Americans are in negative iron balance and will profit from supplements of iron and/or vitamin C (which increases iron absorption). However, more than 10 percent are in positive balance and can be harmed by increased iron intake. Thus you should never take an iron or vitamin C supplement unless your blood iron status has been evaluated by a doctor and found to not be elevated.

Fluoride is needed to help form teeth that are strong and resistant to decay. Children whose community water supplies are not fluoridated (either naturally or by addition of fluoride) should take a daily fluoride supplement up to the age of twelve. Except for iron and fluoride, there is little likelihood of mineral deficiency developing in anyone who eats a balanced diet.

Women need to be sure they get adequate amounts of calcium to help prevent osteoporosis. This condition, which involves thinning of the bones, is not simply a deficiency disease but involves hormones and other factors. The best way to get calcium is from milk and milk products. Adults who don't (or can't) consume several portions a day should seek professional advice about possibly taking supplements. Weight-bearing exercise is important because it helps maintain the bones, while cigarette smoking increases the chances of developing osteoporosis. After menopause, estrogen-replacement therapy should also be considered. Men also get osteoporosis, but later than women.

Zinc deficiency may occur in people whose diets are unbalanced with too much fiber (vegetarian diets, for example) because fiber can pull zinc out of the food and into the stool. This can occur even when zinc is eaten in RDA amounts. One portion of meat a day satisfies most mineral requirements.

As with vitamins, the best way to avoid trouble with minerals is to obtain them in the rational packages of natural foods in a balanced diet.

Amino Acid Facts

Proteins, the body's main structural component, are used to make bone, connective tissue, muscle, skin, hair, and cell membranes. Proteins also function as enzymes, hormones, antibodies, and as part of the compounds that transport oxygen to the tissues (hemoglobin and myoglobin).

The proteins in food are too large to be absorbed through the intestines, so they are broken down during digestion into their component amino acids. These smaller components are then absorbed from the intestines and reassembled as needed into the fifty thousand or more proteins needed by the body. Amino acids not used for this purpose are used for energy. There are about twenty amino acids, eight or nine of which are considered essential because they cannot be manufactured by the body and must be included in the diet. The essential amino acids are isoleucine, leucine, lysine, methionine, phenylalanine, threonine, tryptophan, and valine; for infants, histidine also is essential. Protein sources are considered complete or of high quality if they supply all of the essential amino acids in adequate amounts and incomplete or of poor quality if they do not.

Normal people eating a balanced diet will get all the amino acids they need. Vegetarians, particularly those who restrict milk, fish, and eggs as well as meat, have to be more careful. Since animal products are the best source of high-quality proteins, vegetarians who avoid them can get into difficulty if their diet is not varied enough to provide an adequate combination of amino acids. Regardless, it is senseless to consume amino acids as "dietary supplements." A diet that is deficient in one amino acid is likely to be missing more than one—so the problem should be corrected by dietary improvement, not pills or potions. People who use single- or multiple-ingredient amino acid products sold through health-food stores have been misled into thinking they are fat-reducers, pain-relievers, or bodybuilding aids. As noted in Chapters 8 and 11, these products are fakes and have not been shown to be safe.

Richard J. Wurtman, M.D., professor of neuroscience at M.I.T. and Harvard Medical School, is one of the leading researchers on amino acid metabolism. After hundreds of people became seriously ill from taking L-tryptophan supplements (see Chapters 2 and 19), Wurtman described the distribution system of products in health-food stores as "accidents waiting to happen." Like him, we believe that isolated amino acids should not be legal to market unless they can meet regulatory standards for prescription drugs.

Basic Principles of Consumer Protection

The basic premise of this book is the fundamental rule of consumer protection in health matters: *If you can't prove that a product works, you shouldn't sell it.* "Proof" entails two things:

1. Enough testing must be done for the product to become generally recognized by experts as safe, effective, and appropriate for its intended use.
2. New drug products, or new uses for existing products, require FDA approval before marketing them to the public. To gain this approval, there must be substantial scientific agreement that the product is safe and effective for its intended purpose. It is legal and ethical to test an unproven method if there is a logical reason to do so, the test is properly designed, and patients are not charged for the privilege of participating. Large-scale studies require FDA approval of their design.

These principles are codified by federal laws and regulations. Unlike responsible researchers, quacks typically charge high fees and do not keep score of their results.

This book describes how vitamin pushers are violating these principles and selling the American public a bill of antiscientific goods.

2

Thirty Ways to Spot Quacks and Pushers

The doctrines of freedom of speech and freedom of the press give quacks great leeway in deceiving the public. It is perfectly legal to give false or misleading advice as long as the person giving it is not selling the touted product or service at the same time.

Quacks project an aura of sincerity and public interest. They spout (unprovable) "case histories" and glowing tales of personal experience. They cite sloppy and worthless "research" as "the great work of great men." They treat legitimate but *preliminary* research findings as proof that their methods work. Their deceptions dominate the media.

The *Random House Unabridged Dictionary of the English Language* defines "quack" as:

> (1) a fraudulent or ignorant pretender to medical skill; (2) a person who pretends, professionally or publicly, to skill, knowledge, or qualification which he does not possess; a charlatan; (3) being a quack: a quack psychologist who complicates everyone's problems; (4) presented falsely as having curative powers: quack medicine; (5) to advertise or sell with fraudulent claims.

Not all quacks are deliberate frauds, however. Quacks can be classified into three groups based on the nature of their beliefs:

- *Dumb* quacks espouse false ideas out of ignorance. Typically they are well-meaning individuals who have misinterpreted their own experience with a questionable method.

- *Deluded* quacks cling firmly to false ideas despite obvious proof or evidence to the contrary. Their beliefs are based on faulty observations and equally faulty reasoning. Many view themselves as crusaders with a very important mission. Their delusions typically are grandiose ("I can save the world from cancer") and/or persecutory ("The AMA and FDA are out to get us.").
- *Dishonest* quacks lie repeatedly for personal gain. Their primary goal is money. They have no scruples. They have little or no loyalty to others, give plausible rationalizations for their behavior, and lack guilt or remorse when they harm others. Psychiatrists refer to these people as antisocial or psychopathic personalities.

Many people think of quacks as outlandish characters selling snake oil from the back of a covered wagon. But modern quacks tend to wear trappings of science and respectability. Some are physicians, dentists, and nutrition scientists who have gone astray. Some enjoy the support and backing of prominent publishing companies. Many use talented advertising agencies to promote their views and skillful attorneys to protect them. A few have even served in the United States Congress.

How can food quacks and other vitamin pushers be recognized? Here are thirty tips that should make you suspicious.

1. When Talking about Nutrients, They Tell Only Part of the Story.

Quacks tell you all the wonderful things that vitamins and minerals do in your body and/or all the horrible things that can happen if you don't get enough. But they conveniently neglect to tell you that a balanced diet provides the nutrients people need and that the USDA food-group system makes balancing your diet simple. Many supplement manufacturers use subtle approaches. Some simply say: "Buy our product X. It contains nutrients that help promote healthy eyes (or hair, or whatever organ you happen to be concerned about)." Others distribute charts telling what each nutrient does and the signs and symptoms of deficiency diseases. This encourages supplementation with the hope of enhancing body functions and/or avoiding the troubles described. Many of the "vitamin" charts include substances that are not vitamins.

Another type of fraudulent concealment is the promotion of "supplements" and herbal extracts based on incomplete information. Many health-food industry products are marketed with claims based on faulty extrapolations of animal research and/or unconfirmed studies on humans. The most notorious such product was L-tryptophan, an amino acid. For many years it was promoted for insomnia, depression, premenstrual syndrome, and overweight, even though it had not been proven safe or effective for any of these purposes. In 1989, it triggered an outbreak of eosinophilia-myalgia syndrome (EMS), a rare disorder characterized by severe muscle and joint pain, weakness, swelling of the arms and legs, fever, skin rash, and an increase of eosinophils (certain white blood cells) in the blood. Over the next year, more than 1,500 cases of EMS and twenty-eight deaths were reported. The outbreak was traced to a manufacturing problem at the plant of a wholesale supplier. The naked truth is that L-tryptophan should not have been marketed to the public in the first place because—like most single-ingredient amino acids—it did not have FDA approval for medicinal use. In fact, the FDA issued a ban in 1973 but did not enforce it.

2. They Claim That Most Americans Are Poorly Nourished.

This is an appeal to fear that is not only untrue, but ignores the fact that the main forms of bad nourishment in the United States are undernourishment among the poverty-stricken and overweight in the population at large, particularly the poor. Poor people can ill afford to waste money on unnecessary vitamin pills. Their food money should be spent on nourishing food.

With two exceptions, food-group diets contain all the nutrients that people need. One exception involves the mineral iron. The average American diet contains barely enough iron to meet the needs of infants, fertile women, and, especially, pregnant women. This problem can be solved by cooking in a "Dutch oven" or any iron pot or eating iron-rich foods such as soy beans, liver, and veal. Iron supplements should be used only under competent medical supervision. Over 10 percent of Americans are genetically predisposed toward iron-overload disease, which means that supplementation may cause them to accumulate harmful amounts of iron in body tissues. The other common dietary shortfall is fluoride, which should be taken as a supplement by children whose water supply is not fluoridated.

It is falsely alleged that Americans are so addicted to "junk" foods that an adequate diet is exceptional rather than usual. While it is true that some snack foods are mainly "naked calories" (sugars and/or fats without other nutrients), it is not necessary for every morsel of food we eat to be loaded with nutrients. In fact, no normal person following the USDA food-group guidelines is in any danger of vitamin deficiency.

Scientists sometimes use the term "subclinical deficiency" to refer to a person on the road to deficiency from an inadequate diet. But no normal person eating a well-balanced diet is in any danger of vitamin deficiency, subclinical or otherwise. The "subclinical deficiency" quacks talk about does not exist.

3. They Recommend "Nutrition Insurance" for Everyone.

Most vitamin pushers suggest that everyone is in danger of vitamin deficiency and should therefore take supplements as "insurance." Some suggest that it is difficult to get what you need from food, while others claim that it is impossible. Here are two examples, one from the flyer of a prominent supermarket chain, the other from a major department store chain:

> No matter how hard you try, in our fast food society, it's often difficult to make sure you're getting enough essential vitamins and minerals in the food you eat. When you remember that the health of your eyes depends upon a sufficient intake of these vital nutrients, it's not hard to see why neglect of them in your diet can cause needless health problems. Vitamin and mineral supplements, included in your daily diet, can assure you that your body will maintain the level of organic compounds it needs, not only to transform food into energy, but to function properly.
>
> Today's lifestyles, eating habits and processed foods may make it difficult for you to get the vitamins and nutrients your body needs every day to carry on normal cellular functions. . . . Quite possibly deficiencies of many nutrients may be common. Of the approximately 40 nutrients that are considered elemental in meeting daily body requirements, many cannot be manufactured or stored by the body. These nutrients must be ingested daily. Regardless of age, sex, where you live or what you do, proper preventive self care may require the nutritional protection of daily dietary supplements.

Do these sound scary? They are meant to be. Their pitch is like that of the door-to-door huckster who states that your perfectly good furnace is in danger of blowing up unless you replace it with his product. One thing vitamin pushers will never tell you is that few people need their products. Chapter 3 discusses "nutrition insurance" further.

4. They Say That If You Eat Badly, You'll Be OK As Long As You Take Supplements.

The statement is not only untrue but encourages careless eating habits. The remedy for eating badly is a well-balanced diet. If in doubt about the adequacy of your diet, write down what you eat for several days and see whether your daily average is in line with the USDA's guidelines. If you can't do this yourself, your doctor or a registered dietitian can do it for you. In most cases, money spent for a vitamin or mineral supplement would be better spent for a daily portion of fresh fruit, vegetable, milk, grain, or meat product.

5. They Say That Most Diseases Are Due to Faulty Diet and Can Be Treated with "Nutritional" Methods.

This simply isn't so. Consult your doctor or any recognized textbook of medicine. They will tell you that although diet is a factor in some diseases (most notably coronary heart disease), most diseases have little or nothing to do with diet. Common symptoms like malaise (feeling poorly), fatigue, lack of pep, aches (including headaches) or pains, insomnia, and similar complaints are usually the body's reaction to emotional stress. The persistence of such symptoms is a signal to see a doctor to be evaluated for possible physical illness. It is not a reason to take vitamin pills.

Some quacks seem to specialize in the diagnosis and treatment of problems considered rare or even nonexistent by responsible practitioners. Years ago hypothyroidism and adrenal insufficiency were in vogue. Today's "fad" diagnoses—discussed in Chapter 12—are "hypoglycemia," "mercury amalgam toxicity," "candidiasis hypersensitivity," "environmental illness" (also called "multiple chemical sensitivity"), and "Gulf War syndrome." Quacks are also jumping on the allergy bandwagon, falsely claiming that huge numbers of Americans are suffering from undiagnosed allergies, "diagnosing" them with worthless tests, and prescribing worthless "nutritional" treatments. Chronic fatigue syndrome, although not rare, is another diagnosis wrongly applied by some quacks to large numbers of people who consult them. "Parasites" is yet another misdiagnosis percolating through the health-food industry press. Two recent books, for example, claim that 60 percent of Americans are affected, that parasites "thrive on junk food," and that herbal "anti-parasitic formulas," "immune system strengtheners," and "colon cleansings" can eliminate them from the body. These claims are completely unfounded. "Wilson's syndrome," said to be a disorder in which thyroid function goes haywire, is also making its way into the marketplace.

6. They Allege That Modern Processing Methods and Storage Remove all Nutritive Value from Our Food.

It is true that food processing can change the nutrient content of foods. But the changes are not so drastic as the quack, who wants you to buy supplements, would like you to believe. While some processing methods destroy some nutrients, others add them. A balanced variety of foods will provide all the nourishment you need.

Quacks distort and oversimplify. When they say that milling removes B-vitamins, they don't bother to tell you that enrichment puts them back. When they tell you that cooking destroys vitamins, they omit the fact that only a few vitamins are sensitive to heat. Nor do they tell you that these vitamins are easily obtained by consuming a portion of fresh uncooked fruit, vegetable, or fresh or frozen fruit juice each day. Any claims that minerals are destroyed by processing or cooking are pure lies. Heat does not destroy minerals.

7. They Claim That Diet Is a Major Factor in Behavior.

Food quacks relate diet not only to disease but to behavior. Some claim that adverse reactions to additives and/or common foods cause hyperactivity in children and even criminal behavior in adolescents and adults. These claims are based on a combination of delusions, anecdotal evidence, and poorly designed research.

8. They Claim That Fluoridation Is Dangerous.

Curiously, quacks are not always interested in real deficiencies. Fluoride is necessary to build decay-resistant teeth and strong bones. The best way to obtain adequate amounts of this essential nutrient is to augment community water supplies so their fluoride concentration is about one part fluoride for every million parts of water. But quacks are usually opposed to water fluoridation, and some advocate water filters that remove fluoride. It seems that when they cannot profit from something, they may try to make money by opposing it.

9. They Claim That Soil Depletion and the Use of Pesticides and "Chemical" Fertilizers Result in Food That Is Less Safe and Less Nourishing.

These claims are used to promote the sale of so-called "organically grown" foods. If an essential nutrient is missing from the soil, a plant simply doesn't grow. Chemical fertilizers counteract the effects of soil depletion. Quacks also lie when they claim that plants grown with natural fertilizers (such as manure) are nutritionally superior to those grown with synthetic fertilizers. Before they can use them, plants convert natural fertilizers into the same chemicals that synthetic fertilizers supply. The vitamin content of a food is determined by its genetic makeup. Fertilizers can influence the levels of certain minerals in plants, but this is not a significant factor in the American diet. The pesticide residue of our food supply is extremely small and poses no health threat. Moreover, several studies have found that the amounts of pesticide residue in foods labeled organic were similar to those in foods not labeled organic.

The marketplace may become more confusing, however. A federal law passed in 1990 directs the U.S. Secretary of Agriculture to establish "organic" certification standards. Once such standards have been established—which may take several years—violators may face civil penalties of up to $10,000 per offense. Foods certified as "organic" will not be safer or more nutritious than other foods. In fact, except for their high price, they will not be significantly different. Instead of legitimizing nutrition nonsense, our government should do more to attack its spread.

10. They Claim You Are in Danger of Being "Poisoned" by Ordinary Food Additives and Preservatives.

This is another scare tactic designed to undermine your confidence in food scientists and government protection agencies as well as our food supply itself. Quacks want you to think they are out to protect you. They hope that if you trust them, you will buy their "natural" food products. The fact is that the tiny amounts of additives used in food pose no threat to human health. Some actually protect our health by preventing spoilage, rancidity, and mold growth.

Two examples illustrate how ridiculous quacks can get about food additives, especially those found naturally in food. Calcium propionate is used to preserve bread and occurs naturally in Swiss cheese. Quacks who would steer you toward (higher-priced) bread made without preservatives are careful not to tell you that a one-ounce slice of "natural" Swiss cheese contains the same amount of calcium propionate used to retard spoilage in two one-pound loaves of bread. Similarly, those who warn about monosodium glutamate (MSG) don't tell you that the wheat germ they hustle as a "health food" is a major natural source of this substance.

Also curious is their failure to warn that many plant substances marketed as "herbs" are potentially toxic and can cause discomfort, disability, or even death. The April 6, 1979, *Medical Letter* listed more than thirty such products sold in "health food" stores, most used for making herbal teas. Most of these are still sold today.

The value of scare tactics has been acknowledged in *Entrepreneur* magazine's manual for health-food retailers:

> The reason for the market's embrace of health food stores . . . is simple: Negative publicity about chemicals, additives, and sugars in foods has made Americans more aware of what they eat and how they get their

nutrition. Not only that, having made the decision to more or less "go natural," the zealous converted consumer will make few exceptions in his or her new discipline. So the health-food store becomes virtually the only place a devotee shops for foodstuffs.

11. They Charge That the Recommended Dietary Allowances (RDAs) Have Been Set Too Low.

The RDAs have been published by the National Research Council approximately every five years since 1943. They are defined as "the levels of intake of essential nutrients that, on the basis of scientific knowledge, are judged by the Food and Nutrition Board to be adequate to meet the known nutrient needs of practically all healthy persons." The RDAs are determined by the board's Committee on Dietary Allowances (also called the RDA Committee), whose members meet several times a year and engage in extensive correspondence between meetings. Each time the RDAs are updated, they are published in a book that discusses each nutrient and the evidence upon which its RDA is based. The book concludes with a table of RDA values, which winds up—partially or totally—in practically all nutrition textbooks and numerous other publications. The most recent values, published in 1989, were based mainly on the deliberations of the 1980–1985 RDA Committee, of which Dr. Victor Herbert was a member. The committee's work is supported by the National Institutes of Health, but members themselves serve without pay. Most of them are professors at universities and medical schools.

For many years, nutrient contents of vitamin products and many foods have been listed on their labels as "% U.S. RDA." Neither the RDAs nor the U.S. RDAs are "minimums" or "requirements." In fact, because they are deliberately set higher than most people need, they could even be considered "maximum" nutritional levels. The RDA for each vitamin and mineral is usually set by noting the entire range of normal human needs, selecting the number at the high end of that range, and adding a "safety factor" to allow for "reserve" body stores without risking toxicity from overdosage. For example, the range of normal adult need for vitamin C is probably 10–15 mg per day. In setting the RDA at 60 mg, a 45–50 mg "safety factor" is added. (At this intake, the body will store 1,500 mg of vitamin C—enough to last several months if no vitamin C is consumed.) Over the years, some of the RDA values have been lowered as new evidence indicated that the excess over need could be lowered. The RDA for each nutrient varies somewhat with age and sex, and whether a woman is pregnant or lactating.

The U.S. RDAs (U.S. Recommended Daily Allowances), set by the FDA, were based on the largest values for each life-cycle category of the 1968 RDA table. Appendix B discusses the FDA's proposal to update these values.

Some people believe that the RDAs should be redefined and set to achieve "optimal" levels of nutrient intakes to promote health. The prevailing scientific viewpoint, however, is that there are not enough scientific data to do this.

The reason quacks charge that the RDAs are too low is obvious: if you believe you need more than can be obtained from food, you are more likely to buy supplements.

12. They Claim That under Stress, and in Certain Diseases, Your Need for Nutrients Is Increased.

Many vitamin manufacturers have advertised that "stress robs the body of vitamins." One company has asserted that, "if you smoke, diet, or happen to be sick, you may be robbing your body of vitamins." Another has warned that "stress can deplete your body of water-soluble vitamins . . . and daily replacement is necessary." Other products are touted to fill the "special needs of athletes."

While it is true that the need for vitamins may rise slightly under physical stress and in certain diseases, this type of advertising is fraudulent. The average American—stressed or not—is not in danger of vitamin deficiency. The increased needs to which the ads refer are not higher than the amounts obtainable by proper eating. Someone who is really in danger of deficiency due to an illness would be *very* sick and would need medical care, probably in a hospital. But these promotions are aimed at average Americans who certainly don't need vitamin supplements to survive the common cold, a round of golf, or a jog around the neighborhood! Athletes get more than enough vitamins when they eat the food needed to meet their caloric requirements.

Many vitamin pushers suggest that smokers need vitamin C supplements. Although it is true that smokers in North America have somewhat lower blood levels of this vitamin, these levels are still far above deficiency levels. In America, cigarette smoking is the leading cause of death preventable by self-discipline. Rather than seeking false comfort by taking vitamin C, smokers who are concerned about their health should stop smoking. Moreover, since doses of vitamin C high enough to acidify the urine speed up excretion of nicotine, they may even cause some smokers to smoke more to avoid symptoms of nicotine withdrawal. Suggestions that "stress vitamins" are helpful against emotional stress are also fraudulent. Chapter 3 discusses this subject further.

13. They Recommend "Supplements" and "Health Foods" for Everyone.

Food quacks belittle normal foods and ridicule the food-group systems of good nutrition. They may not tell you they earn their living from such pronouncements—via public appearance fees, product endorsements, sale of publications, or financial interests in vitamin companies, health-food stores, or organic farms.

The very term "health food" is a deceptive slogan. Judgments about individual foods should take into account how they contribute to an individual's overall diet. All food is health food in moderation; any food is junk food in excess. Did you ever stop to think that your corner grocery, fruit market, meat market, and supermarket are also health-food stores? They are—and they generally charge less than stores that use the slogan.

By the way, have you ever wondered why people who eat lots of "health foods" still feel they must load themselves up with vitamin supplements? Or why so many "health food" shoppers complain about ill health?

14. They Oppose Pasteurization of Milk.

One of the strangest aspects of nutrition quackery is its embrace of "raw" (unpasteurized) milk. Public health authorities advocate pasteurization to destroy any disease-producing bacteria that may be present. Health faddists and quacks claim that it destroys essential nutrients. Although small percentages of the heat-sensitive vitamins (vitamin C and thiamine) are destroyed during pasteurization, milk would not be a significant source of these nutrients anyway. Raw milk, whether "certified" or not, can be a source of harmful bacteria that cause dysentery and tuberculosis. The FDA has banned the interstate sale of raw milk and raw-milk products packaged for human consumption. In 1989, a California Superior Court judge ordered the nation's largest raw-milk producer to stop advertising that its raw-milk products are safe and healthier than pasteurized milk and to label its products with a conspicuous warning.

15. They Recommend a Wide Variety of Substances Similar to Those Found in Your Body.

The underlying idea—like the wishful thinking or sympathetic magic of primitive tribes—is that taking these substances will strengthen or rejuvenate the corresponding body parts. For example, according to a health-food-store brochure:

> Raw glandular therapy, or "cellular therapy" . . . seems almost too simple to be true. It consists of giving in supplement form (intravenous or oral) those specific tissues from animals that correspond to the "weakened" areas of the human body. In other words, if a person has a weak pancreas, give him raw pancreas substance; if the heart is weak, give raw heart, etc.

Vitamins and other nutrients may be added to the various preparations to make them more marketable. When taken by mouth, such concoctions are no better than placebos. Most won't do direct harm, but their allure may steer people away from competent professional care. Injections of raw animal tissues, however, can cause severe allergic reactions to their proteins. Some preparations have also caused serious infections. Even though "glandulars" are made from glands, most have their hormones removed. A few with their hormones intact have made people seriously ill.

Proponents of "tissue salts" (also called "cell salts") allege that the basic cause of disease is mineral deficiency—correction of which will enable the body to heal itself. Thus, they claim, one or more of twelve salts are useful against a wide variety of diseases, including appendicitis (ruptured or not), baldness, deafness, insomnia, and worms. Development of this method is attributed to a nineteenth-century physician named W.H. Schuessler. Tissue salt products have also been referred to as "homeopathic nutrients." Many are so dilute that they could not correct a mineral deficiency even if one were present.

Enzymes for oral use are another ripoff. They supposedly can aid digestion and "support" many other functions within the body. The fact is, however, that enzymes taken by mouth are digested into their component amino acids by the stomach and intestines and therefore do not function as enzymes within the body. Oral pancreatic enzymes have legitimate use only in diseases involving decreased secretion of one's own pancreatic enzymes. Anyone who actually has a pancreatic enzyme deficiency probably has a serious underlying disease requiring competent medical diagnosis and treatment.

16. They Claim That "Natural" Vitamins are Better than "Synthetic" Ones.

This claim is a flat lie. Each vitamin is a chain of atoms strung together as a molecule. Molecules made in the "factories" of nature are identical to those made in the factories of chemical companies. Does it makes sense to pay extra for vitamins extracted from foods when you can get all you need from the foods themselves?

17. They Suggest That a Questionnaire Can Be Used to indicate Whether You Need Dietary Supplements.

No questionnaire can do this. A few entrepreneurs have devised lengthy computer-scored questionnaires with questions about symptoms that could be present if a vitamin deficiency exists. But such symptoms occur much more frequently in conditions unrelated to nutrition. Even when a deficiency actually exists, the tests don't provide enough information to discover the cause so that suitable treatment can be recommended. That requires a physical examination and appropriate laboratory tests. Many responsible nutritionists use a computer to help evaluate their clients' diet. But this is done to make *dietary* recommendations, such as reducing fat content or increasing fiber content. Supplements are seldom useful unless the person is unable (or unwilling) to consume an adequate diet.

Be wary, too, of questionnaires purported to determine whether supplements are needed to correct "nutrient deficiencies" or "dietary inadequacies." These questionnaires are scored so that everyone who takes the test is judged deficient. Responsible dietary analyses compare the individual's average daily food consumption with the recommended numbers of servings from each food group. The safest and best way to get nutrients is generally from food, not pills. So even if a diet is deficient, the most prudent action is usually diet modification rather than supplementation with pills.

18. They Say It Is Easy to Lose Weight.

Diet quacks would like you to believe that special pills or food combinations can cause "effortless" weight loss. But the only way to lose weight is to burn off more calories than you eat. This requires self-discipline: eating less, exercising more, or preferably doing both. There are about 3,500 calories in a pound of body weight. To lose one pound a week (a safe amount that is not just water), you must eat about five hundred fewer calories per day than you burn up. The most sensible diet for losing weight is one that is nutritionally balanced in carbohydrates, fats, and proteins. Most fad diets "work" by producing temporary weight loss—as a result of calorie restriction. But they are invariably too monotonous and are often too dangerous for long-term use. Unless a dieter develops and maintains better eating and exercise habits, weight lost on a diet will soon return.

The term "cellulite" is sometimes used to describe the dimpled fat found on the hips and thighs of many women. Although no medical evidence supports the claim, cellulite is represented as a special type of fat that is resistant to diet and exercise. Sure-fire cellulite remedies include creams (to "dissolve" it), brushes, rollers, "loofah" sponges, rubberized pants, and vitamin-mineral supplements with or without herbs. The cost of various treatment plans runs from a few dollars for a bottle of vitamins to many hundreds of dollars at a salon that offers heat treatments, massage, enzyme injections, and/or treatment with various gadgets. The simple truth about "cellulite" is that it is ordinary fat that can be lost only as part of an overall reducing program.

19. They Promise Quick, Dramatic, Miraculous Results.

Often the promises are subtle or couched in "weasel words" that create an illusion of a promise, so promoters can deny making them when the "feds" close in. False promises of cure are the quacks' most immoral practice. They don't seem to care how many people they break financially or in spirit—by elation over their expected good fortune followed by deep depression when the "treatment" fails. Nor do quacks keep count—while they fill their bank accounts—of how many people they lure away from effective medical care into disability or death.

Quacks will tell you that "megavitamins" (huge doses of vitamins) can prevent or cure many different ailments, particularly emotional ones. But they won't tell you that the "evidence" supporting such claims is unreliable because it is based on inadequate investigations, anecdotes, or testimonials. Nor do quacks inform you that megadoses may be harmful. Megavitamin therapy is nutritional roulette, and only the house makes the profit.

20. They Routinely Sell Vitamins and Other "Dietary Supplements" as Part of Their Practice.

Although vitamins are useful as therapeutic agents for certain health problems, the number of such conditions is small. Practitioners who sell supplements in their offices invariably recommend them inappropriately. In addition, such products tend to be substantially more expensive than similar ones in drugstores—or even health-food stores. You should also disregard any magazine or newsletter whose editor or publisher sells vitamins.

21. They Use Disclaimers Couched in Pseudomedical Jargon.

Instead of promising to cure your disease, some quacks will promise to "detoxify," "purify," or "revitalize" your body; "balance" its chemistry; bring it in harmony with nature; "stimulate" or "strengthen" your immune system;

"support" or "rejuvenate" various organs in your body; or stimulate your body's power to heal itself. Of course, they never identify or make valid before-and-after measurements of any of these processes. These disclaimers serve two purposes. First, since it is impossible to measure the processes quacks allege, it may be difficult to prove them wrong. Moreover, if a quack is not a physician, the use of nonmedical terminology may help to avoid prosecution for practicing medicine without a license—although it shouldn't.

Some approaches to "detoxification" are based on notions that, as a result of intestinal stasis, intestinal contents putrefy, and toxins are formed and absorbed, which causes chronic poisoning of the body. This "autointoxication" theory was popular around the turn of the century but was abandoned by the scientific community during the 1930s. No such "toxins" have ever been found, and careful observations have shown that individuals in good health can vary greatly in bowel habits. Quacks may also suggest that fecal material collects on the lining of the intestine and causes trouble unless removed by laxatives, colonic irrigation, special diets, and/or various herbs or food supplements that "cleanse" the body. The falsity of this notion is obvious to doctors who perform intestinal surgery or peer within the large intestine with a diagnostic instrument. Fecal material does not adhere to the intestinal lining. Colonic irrigation is done by inserting a tube up to a foot or more into the rectum and pumping up to twenty gallons of warm water in and out. This type of enema is not only therapeutically worthless but can cause fatal electrolyte imbalance. Cases of death due to intestinal perforation and infection (from contaminated equipment) have also been reported.

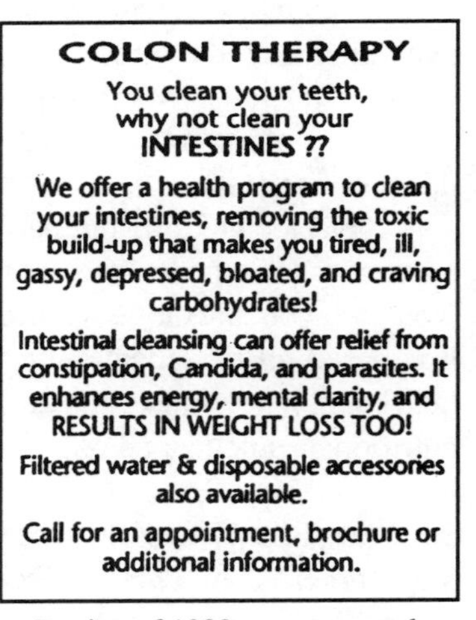

Portion of 1993 newspaper ad

"Balancing body chemistry" typically involves recommendations for supplements based on interpretation of bogus tests or misinterpretation of standard tests. This subject is discussed in detail in Chapter 12.

Many quacks claim that stressful lifestyles and/or environmental toxins weaken the immune system and cause people to become ill. Their solution, of course, is to use whatever they promote to reverse the process. As AIDS focused public attention on the immune system, health-food industry manufacturers began marketing dozens of vitamin concoctions falsely claimed to strengthen the immune system. The FDA has taken action against some of these, but many are still marketed.

Many nonscientific healing systems are claimed to cure disease by stimulating a "vital force" that causes the body to heal itself. This subject is discussed in detail in Chapter 13.

22. They Use Anecdotes and Testimonials to Support Their Claims.

We all tend to believe what others tell us about personal experiences. But separating cause and effect from coincidence can be difficult. If people tell you that product X has cured their cancer, arthritis, or whatever, be skeptical. They may not actually have had the condition. If they did, their recovery most likely would have occurred without the help of product X. Most single episodes of disease end with just the passage of time, and most chronic ailments have symptom-free periods. Establishing medical truths requires careful and repeated investigation—with well-designed experiments, not reports of coincidences misperceived as cause-and-effect. That's why testimonial evidence is forbidden in scientific articles and is usually inadmissible in court.

Never underestimate the extent to which people can be fooled by a worthless remedy. During the early 1940s, many thousands of people became convinced that "glyoxylide" could cure cancer. Yet analysis showed that it was simply distilled water! Many years before that, when arsenic was used as a "tonic," countless numbers of people swore by it even as it slowly poisoned them.

Symptoms that are psychosomatic (bodily reactions to tension) are often relieved by anything taken with a suggestion that it will work. Tiredness and other minor aches and pains may respond to any enthusiastically recommended nostrum. For these problems, even physicians may prescribe a placebo. A placebo is a substance that has no pharmacological effect on the condition for which it is used, but is given to satisfy a patient who supposes it to be a medicine. Vitamins (such as B_{12} shots) are commonly used in this way.

Placebos act by suggestion. Unfortunately, some doctors swallow the advertising hype or become confused by their own observations and "believe in vitamins" beyond those supplied by a good diet. Those who share such false beliefs do so because they confuse coincidence or placebo action with cause and effect. Homeopathic believers make the same error.

Talk-show hosts give quacks a boost when they ask, "What do all the vitamins you take do for you personally?" Then thousands or even millions of viewers are treated to the quack's talk of improved health, vigor, and vitality—with the implicit point: "It did this for me. It will do the same for you." A most revealing testimonial experience was described during a major network show that featured several of the world's most prominent promoters of nutritional faddism. While the host was boasting that his new eating program had cured his "hypoglycemia," he mentioned in passing that he was no longer drinking twenty to thirty cups of coffee a day. Neither the host nor any of his "experts" had the good sense to tell their audience how dangerous it can be to drink so much coffee. Nor did any of them recognize that the host's original symptoms were probably caused by excess caffeine. The average brewed cup of coffee contains 100 mg of caffeine, a significant dose. Excess amounts of caffeine can cause nervousness, irritability, insomnia, heart palpitations, and gastrointestinal symptoms.

Because quackery promoters appear frequently on talk shows, many hosts of these programs have absorbed their ideas and consume supplements by the handful.

23. They Claim That Sugar Is a Deadly Poison.

Many vitamin pushers would have us believe that sugar is "the killer on the breakfast table" and is the underlying cause of everything from heart disease to hypoglycemia. The fact is, however, that when sugar is used in moderation as part of a normal, balanced diet, it is a perfectly safe source of calories and eating pleasure. In fact, if you ate no sugar, your liver would make it from protein and fat because your brain needs it. Sugar is a factor in the tooth decay process, but what counts is not merely the amount of sugar in the diet but how long *any* digestible carbohydrate remains in contact with the teeth. This, in turn, depends on such factors as the stickiness of the food, the type of bacteria on the teeth, and the extent of oral hygiene practiced by the individual.

24. They Offer Phony "Vitamins."

Since vitamins are so popular, why not invent some new ones? Ernst T. Krebs, M.D., and his son Ernst T. Krebs, Jr., invented two of them. In 1949, they patented a substance that they later named pangamate and trade-named "vitamin B-15." The Krebses also developed the quack cancer remedy, laetrile, which was marketed as "vitamin B-17."

To be properly called a vitamin, a substance must be an organic nutrient that is necessary in the diet, and deficiency of the substance must be shown to cause a specific disease. Neither pangamate nor laetrile is a vitamin. Pangamate is not even a single substance; different sellers have put different synthetic ingredients in the bottle. Laetrile contains six percent of cyanide by weight and has actually poisoned people.

Many vitamin pushers refer to bioflavonoids, rutin, inositol, and para-aminobenzoic acid (PABA) as vitamins. These substances are not vitamins for humans and are not needed in the diet. The FDA forbids nutritional claims for them on product labels.

25. They Display Credentials Not Recognized by Responsible Scientists or Educators.

The backbone of educational integrity in America is a system of accreditation by agencies recognized by the U.S. Secretary of Education and/or the Council on Postsecondary Accreditation. "Degrees" from nonaccredited schools are rarely worth the paper they are printed on. In the health field, there is no such thing as a reliable school that is not accredited.

Since quacks operate outside of the scientific community, they also tend to form their own "professional" organizations. In some cases, the only membership requirement is payment of a fee. We and others we know have secured fancy "professional member" certificates for household pets by merely submitting the pet's name, address, and a check for $50. Don't assume that all groups with scientific-sounding names are respectable. Find out whether their views are scientifically based.

Unfortunately, possession of an accredited degree does not guarantee reliability. Some schools that teach unscientific methods (chiropractic, naturopathy, acupuncture, and even quack nutritional methods) have achieved accreditation. Worse yet, a small percentage of individuals trained in reputable institutions (such as medical or dental schools or accredited universities) have strayed from scientific thought.

Some quacks are promoted with superlatives like "the world's foremost nutritionist" or "America's leading nutrition expert." There is no law against this tactic, just as there is none against calling oneself the "World's Foremost Lover." However, the scientific community recognizes no such title.

26. They Offer to Determine Your Body's Nutritional State with a Laboratory Test or a Questionnaire.

Various health-food industry members and unscientific practitioners utilize tests that they claim can determine your body's nutritional state and—of course—what products you should buy from them. One favorite method is hair analysis. For $25 to $50 plus a lock of your hair, you can get an elaborate computer printout of vitamins and minerals you supposedly need. Hair analysis has limited value (mainly in forensic medicine) in the diagnosis of heavy metal poisoning, but it is worthless as a screening device to detect nutritional problems. If a hair analysis laboratory recommends supplements, you can be sure that its computers are programmed to recommend them to everyone. Other tests used to hawk supplements include amino acid analysis of urine, muscle-testing (applied kinesiology), iridology, blood typing, "nutrient-deficiency" questionnaires, and "electrodiagnostic" gadgets. Chapter 7 discusses most of these in detail.

27. They Claim They Are Being Persecuted by Orthodox Medicine and That Their Work Is Being Suppressed Because It's Controversial.

The "conspiracy charge" is an attempt to gain sympathy by portraying the quack as an "underdog." Quacks typically claim that the American Medical Association is against them because their cures would cut into the incomes that doctors make by keeping people sick. Don't fall for such nonsense! Reputable physicians are plenty busy. Moreover, many doctors engaged in prepaid health plans, group practice, full-time teaching, and government service receive the same salary whether or not their patients are sick—so keeping their patients healthy reduces their workload, not their income.

Quacks also claim there is a "controversy" about facts between themselves and "the bureaucrats," organized medicine, or "the establishment." They clamor for medical examination of their claims, but ignore any evidence that refutes them. The gambit "Do you believe in vitamins?" is another tactic used to increase confusion. Everyone knows that vitamins are needed by the human body. The real question is "Do you need additional vitamins beyond those in a well-balanced diet?" For most people, the answer is *no*. Nutrition is a science, not a religion. It is based upon matters of fact, not questions of *belief.*

Any physician who found a vitamin or other preparation that could cure sterility, heart disease, arthritis, cancer, or the like, could make an enormous fortune. Patients would flock to such a doctor (as they now do to those who *falsely* claim to cure such problems), and colleagues would shower the doctor with awards—including the Nobel Prize! And don't forget, doctors get sick, too. Do you believe they would conspire to suppress cures for diseases that also afflict them and their loved ones? When polio was conquered, iron lungs became virtually obsolete, but nobody resisted this advancement because it would force hospitals to change. And neither will scientists mourn the eventual defeat of cancer.

Although most charges of "conspiracy" are too vague to be investigated, some can be directly refuted. In the mid-1980s, the FDA and the Pharmaceutical Advertising Council (PAC) carried out a campaign to call public attention to the problem of health frauds. During the campaign's planning stages, we and a representative from the Council of Better Business Bureaus were asked to evaluate the PAC's application for a $55,000 grant from the FDA to help fund the campaign. All three of us opposed the grant because several members of the PAC (most notably Hoffmann-La Roche and Lederle) had been involved in misleading advertising, but the money was given anyway. Our participation in this process has been cited by critics as evidence that we conspire with drug companies! The charge that drug companies are conspiring against the health-food industry is also ludicrous because the largest vitamin producer is a drug company (Hoffmann-La Roche) that spends millions of dollars each year on ads that stimulate the sale of dietary supplements in health-food stores as well as in pharmacies (see Chapter 16).

28. They Warn You Not to Trust Your Doctor.

Quacks, who want you to trust them, suggest that most doctors are "butchers" and "poisoners." They exaggerate the shortcomings of our healthcare delivery system, but completely disregard their own—and those of other quacks. For the same reason, quacks also claim that doctors are nutrition illiterates. This, too, is untrue. The principles of nutrition are those of human biochemistry and physiology, courses required in every medical school. Some medical schools don't teach a separate required course labeled "Nutrition" because the subject is included in other courses at the points where it is most relevant. For example, nutrition in growth and development is taught in pediatrics, nutrition in wound healing is taught in surgery, and nutrition in pregnancy is covered in obstetrics. In addition, many medical schools do offer separate instruction in nutrition.

A physician's training, of course, does not end on the day of graduation from medical school or completion of specialty training. The medical profession advocates lifelong education, and some states require it for license renewal. Physicians can further their knowledge of nutrition by reading medical journals and textbooks, discussing cases with colleagues, and attending continuing education courses. Most doctors know what nutrients can and cannot do and can tell the difference between a real nutritional discovery and a piece of quack nonsense. Those who are unable to answer questions about dietetics (meal planning) can refer patients to someone who can—usually a registered dietitian.

Like all human beings, doctors sometimes make mistakes. However, quacks deliver mistreatment most of the time.

29. They Sue to Intimidate Their Critics.

The majority of "nutrition experts" who appear on TV talk shows and whose publications frequent the "health" sections in bookstores and health-food stores are quacks and charlatans. Why are they not labeled as such? Many years ago, investigative reporter Ralph Lee Smith answered this question in an exposé of Carlton Fredericks. Smith said it is the "question of libel":

> A reputation for being legally belligerent can sometimes go far to insulate one from critical publicity. And if an attack does appear in print, a threat of legal action will sometimes bring a full retraction.

Smith noted that the threat of legal action can be particularly effective when made against scientific publications, especially those sponsored by universities or publicly supported organizations.

Many people assume that scientists will speak out against nutrition quacks because they have nothing to fear from a libel suit by a quack. Nothing to fear? Defending against an unjustified libel suit can be lengthy and cost tens of thousands of dollars. We need "Good Samaritan" laws to cover the cost of defending libel actions brought by quacks. We also need vigorous use of legal procedures against malicious lawsuits. Any critic sued by a quack should consider a countersuit for malicious harassment, abuse of process, and barratry.

Lawsuits have been used not only against critics, but also against insurance companies who refuse to pay for quack treatments. In some cases, courts have ruled that the company must pay because the language of the insurance policy did not specifically exclude the treatment in question or because the court gave undeserved credibility to claims that the treatment worked. A recent article in the *Journal of the American Medical Association* advised insurance companies to revise their contracts and urged the courts to base their judgments on peer-reviewed scientific literature and opinions from impartial court-appointed experts.

30. They Encourage Patients to Lend Political Support to Their Treatment Methods.

A century ago, before scientific methodology was generally accepted, valid new ideas were hard to evaluate and were sometimes rejected by a majority of the medical community, only to be upheld later. But today, treatments demonstrated as effective are welcomed by scientific practitioners and do not need a group to crusade for them. *Quacks seek political endorsement because they can't prove that their methods work.* Instead, they may seek to legalize their treatment and force insurance companies to pay for it. Judges and legislators who believe in *caveat emptor* (let the buyer beware) and buccaneering free enterprise are natural allies for quacks. One of the surest signs that a treatment doesn't work is a political campaign to legalize its use.

The Bottom Line

Vitamin pushers and food quacks benefit only themselves. Their victims are not only milked financially (for billions of dollars each year), but may also suffer serious harm from vitamin overdosage and from seduction away from proper medical care.

There is nutritional deficiency in this country, but it is found primarily among the poor, particularly among those who are elderly, pregnant, or young children. Their problems will not be solved by the phony panaceas of hucksters but by better dietary practices. The best way to get vitamins and minerals is in the packages provided by nature: foods that are part of a balanced and varied diet. If humans needed to eat pills for nutrition, pills would grow on trees.

The basic rule of good nutrition is moderation in all things. Contrary to the claim that "it may help," the advice of food quacks may harm—both your health and your pocketbook.

We don't mean to imply that everyone who promotes quack ideas is deliberately trying to mislead people. One reason why quackery is so difficult to spot is that most people who spread nutrition misinformation are quite sincere in their beliefs. For them nutrition is not a science but a religion—with quacks as their gurus. Even with this chapter in mind, however, you still may be vulnerable to a sales pitch from someone you would never suspect.

3

"Nutrition Insurance," "Stress Formulas," and Related Gimmicks

The notion behind "nutrition insurance" is that every person on earth needs to take supplements to ensure getting enough vitamins and minerals. It is the central scam of the vitamin industry and has many variations.

Most supplement promoters suggest that it is difficult or impossible to get the nutrients we need from food and that supplements provide a safe, simple way to be sure. For example, General Nutrition Corporation, which operates the nation's largest chain of health-food stores, has distributed a flyer stating:

> It would take a computer and a good deal of conscious effort to devise a diet that each day would give all the nutrients in optimum amounts. . . . From the viewpoint of . . . nutrition, a complete supplement may be the best possible buy in health insurance.

Some promoters of "nutrition insurance" claim that everyone should take supplements because many people eat improperly. Some claim that many population groups have special needs that make it advisable to take supplements. Some claim that diet cannot provide the nutrients we need because our soils are depleted and our food is overprocessed (see Chapter 2). Some claim that large numbers of Americans are suffering from subtle forms of vitamin deficiency (see Chapter 2). Some state that high doses of nutrients should be taken by everyone because they will (or might) protect against the development of heart disease, cancer, and/or other ailments. Some suggest that their products are a form of insurance against "stress."

Every one of the above claims is either false, misleading, or unproven.

The "Busy Lifestyle" Ploy

Many vitamin pushers suggest that being busy, skipping meals, or "eating on the run" places people at risk for dietary deficiency. According to this notion, busy people don't take the time to consume nourishing food. These claims are misleading because preparing or eating a balanced diet takes no more time than preparing or eating an unbalanced diet. During the early 1980s, Hoffmann-La Roche ran a series of ads, pictured below, to encourage "busy" people to take supplements. These ads, which appeared in several prominent magazines, were intended to influence pharmacists (who advise many customers) as well as the general public. The illustrations were also sold as posters.

"I never go out without my vitamins."
"I take my vitamins every day. Just to be on the safe side."
"I've been taking vitamins for years. And they haven't let me down yet."
Don't take chances. Take a supplement.
ROCHE

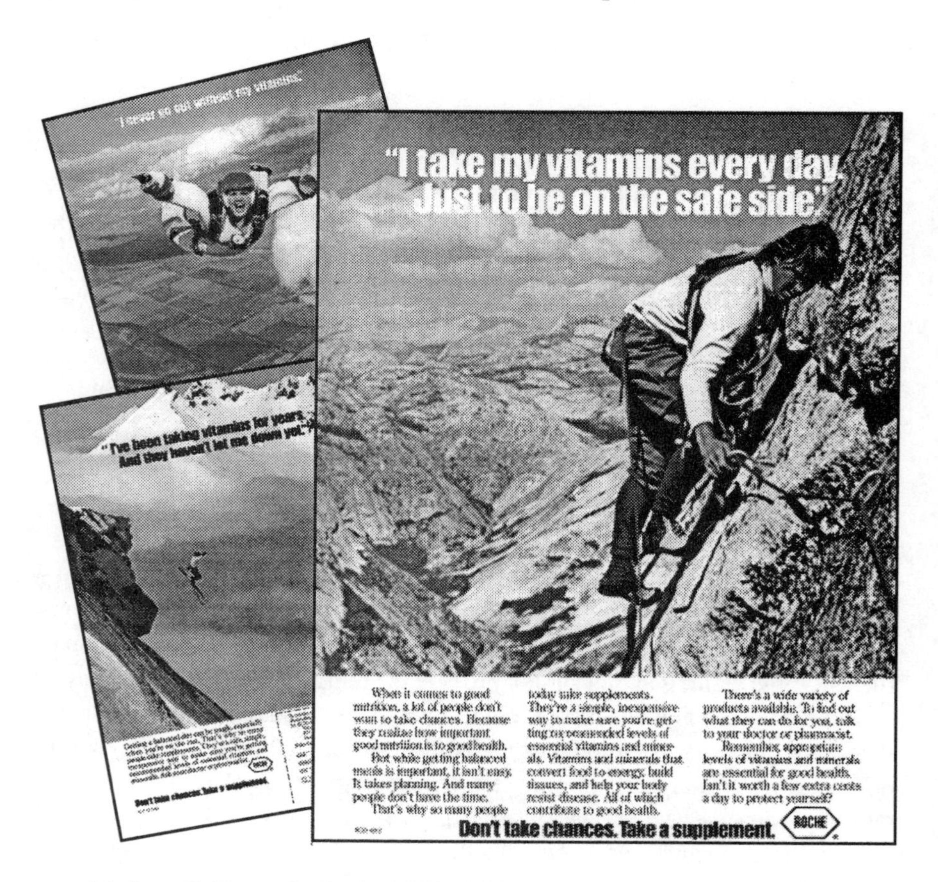

Ads from Hoffmann-La Roche (1983–1984) that promote "nutrition insurance" by falsely representing that it is difficult to get adequate amounts of nutrients from one's diet—especially if one is busy.

Sears Advanced Formula Vitamin Improvement Program, sold during the late 1980s, was pitched as "the easy way to make sure you get the vitamins and minerals you need." To induce sales, the promotional flyer suggested:

> You know how important it is to have proper amounts of vitamins and minerals each day. But, because you're so busy, you may skip a meal or eat on the run. Or you may be on an unsupervised diet, be under stress, or lead an active life. If any of these activities describe you, you may need our Advanced Formula Vitamin Improvement Program. . . . Just one tablet a day will help protect you against possible vitamin and mineral shortages. We think the Advanced Formula Vitamin Improvement Program will help you feel better, help give you more energy, and help you work better.

As an additional selling point, the flyer contained a "potency level chart" showing how *Advanced Formula V.I.P.*® had more active ingredients (25) and a larger total number of milligrams (503) than three other well-known products. Totaling milligrams is a ridiculous way to compare vitamin products. Moreover, *Advanced Formula V.I.P.*® and two of the others contained above-RDA amounts of iron and therefore were irrationally formulated.

"National Vitamin Gap Test"

In 1989, the Council for Responsible Nutrition (CRN), a nutritional supplement industry association, began falsely suggesting that virtually everyone has a "vitamin gap." Through ads in twenty magazines, CRN claimed:

> Even eating three meals a day is no guarantee your body is getting all the vitamins and minerals it needs.
>
> Problems like physical stress and illness rob you of vitamins and minerals. So do smoking and drinking. And birth control pills, pregnancy and lactation also increase nutritional needs. . . .
>
> The fact is, most people reading this ad probably have one or more vitamin and mineral gaps to fill. . . .
>
> So why live at risk? Fill the gap. Take vitamin and mineral supplements every day.

To reinforce this message, CRN invited readers to take the "National Vitamin Gap Test" pictured on the next page. The ads stated that a negative answer to any of the questions may indicate a "gap" that supplements can fill. However, none of the questions was a valid indicator of vitamin shortage.

It is not difficult to construct a questionnaire for determining whether a diet contains adequate amounts of essential nutrients. As we note in Chapter 1 and Appendix A, the U.S. Department of Agriculture's Daily Food Guide

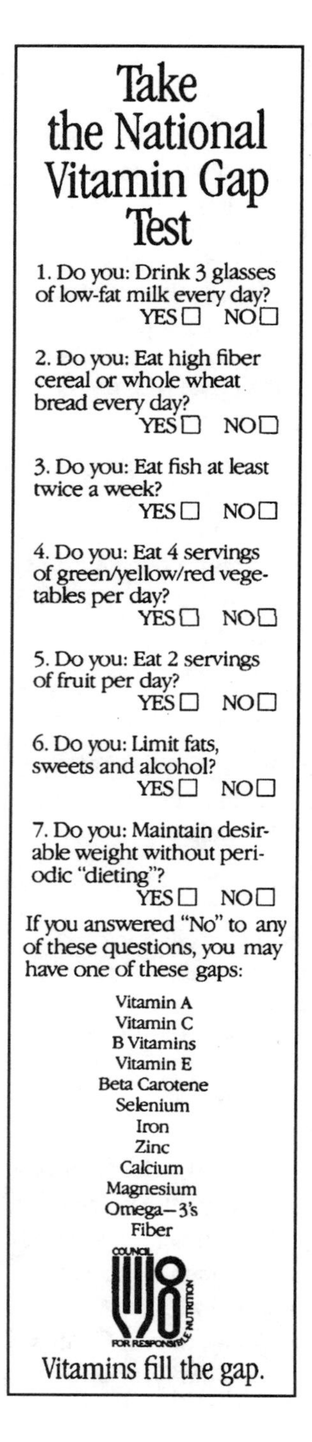
Take the National Vitamin Gap Test

1. Do you: Drink 3 glasses of low-fat milk every day? YES ☐ NO ☐

2. Do you: Eat high fiber cereal or whole wheat bread every day? YES ☐ NO ☐

3. Do you: Eat fish at least twice a week? YES ☐ NO ☐

4. Do you: Eat 4 servings of green/yellow/red vegetables per day? YES ☐ NO ☐

5. Do you: Eat 2 servings of fruit per day? YES ☐ NO ☐

6. Do you: Limit fats, sweets and alcohol? YES ☐ NO ☐

7. Do you: Maintain desirable weight without periodic "dieting"? YES ☐ NO ☐

If you answered "No" to any of these questions, you may have one of these gaps:

Vitamin A
Vitamin C
B Vitamins
Vitamin E
Beta Carotene
Selenium
Iron
Zinc
Calcium
Magnesium
Omega–3's
Fiber

Vitamins fill the gap.

classifies foods into groups according to their major nutrients and indicates how many servings per day from each group are desirable. Valid tests based on this system compare the individual's average daily consumption with the recommended numbers. CRN's test didn't do this and had at least four flaws:

• Some items CRN asked about (such as the amount of fish eaten) are unrelated to nutrient adequacy. Although experts consider it good dietary practice to eat fish once or twice a week, failing to do so will not establish a "vitamin gap."

• Some items didn't conform to the Daily Food Guide. For example, instead of asking whether you consume three servings from the milk *group* (the major nutrient of which is calcium), question #1 asked only about *milk*. Thus people who get adequate calcium from yogurt, cheese, or other dairy products would still have to answer no.

• Instead of asking about average intake, it asked about minimum daily intake. Thus someone who usually eats whole wheat bread or a high-fiber cereal but skips a day would have to answer no to the second question.

• Fruits and vegetables contain similar nutrients. It is not necessary to eat six servings daily to get enough of the nutrients these foods contain.

CRN's "Vitamin Gap" test was intended to frighten people into taking supplements whether they need them or not. However, even well-designed questionnaires may not provide a rational basis for recommending supplements. The safest and best way to get nutrients is generally from food, not pills. So even if a diet is deficient, the most prudent action is usually modification rather than supplementation.

The "Vitamin Gap" campaign was based

> Take a minute to answer these questions—it just may lead to a major change in the way you look at yourself. And the way the world looks at you.
>
> 1. Do you eat balanced meals every day?
>   ❑ yes ❑ no
> 2. Do you often feel fatigued? ❑ yes ❑ no
> 3. Are you under stress? ❑ yes ❑ no
> 4. Do you smoke, diet, or take contraceptives?
>   ❑ yes ❑ no
> 5. Do you drink coffee or tea regularly?
>   ❑ yes ❑ no
> 6. Do you ever miss foods from the recommended daily food groups? ❑ yes ❑ no
>
> If you answered "yes" even once, you may lack key micronutrients essential for good health. Our advice is to strive for a proper balance of correct diet, exercise and rest—and to supplement your meals with the revolutionary system of Clientele Daily Nutrients.

This fraudulent questionnaire is from the Spring/Summer 1985 catalog of I. Magnin, a prominent department store. Questions 1 and 6 are worded so loosely that people with a perfectly adequate overall diet could still answer no. Questions 3 and 5 have nothing to do with nutrient intake or a need to supplement. Question 4 has relevance to long-term, low-calorie dieters but not to smokers or contraceptive users. Question 2 is misleading because dietary imbalance is not a common cause of fatigue.

on market studies conducted during the late 1980s. CRN's "Strategic Plan for a Business Expansion and Nutrition Education Project," developed in 1988, noted "serious concern" among CRN members that the supplement market was not growing and might be starting to decline. "Even more serious is the fact that consumer and health care professional attitudes toward nutritional supplements are not supportive and the consumer base may be eroding," the report said. "Generally, doctors do not recommend vitamins to their patients. The trend is to move the public to eating balanced meals and making them nutritionally aware. . . . People feel they have achieved more balanced diets."

Alarmed by these events, CRN conducted a series of focus groups to determine what motivates consumers to take or stop taking supplements. The

Sure a well-balanced diet is a key to good health, but...
what about the millions of food-faddists, daffy-dieters, junk-food kids and gulp-&-dash execs?
HOW TO LOSE WEIGHT & KEEP YOUR TEETH
22½ DAYS TO LESS YOU
The Cenorsic DIET
Food-faddist
Daffy-dieter
Eat TWADDLES
THE YUMMY FOOD THAT CONTAINS AIR
Gulp-& -dash exec.
Junk-food kid
Maybe they need the additional support of a balanced nutritional supplement.
For information on diet quackery vs. nutritional supplements, call or write:
Public Affairs Department, Lederle Laboratories
Wayne, New Jersey 07470, 201/831-4684
Lederle

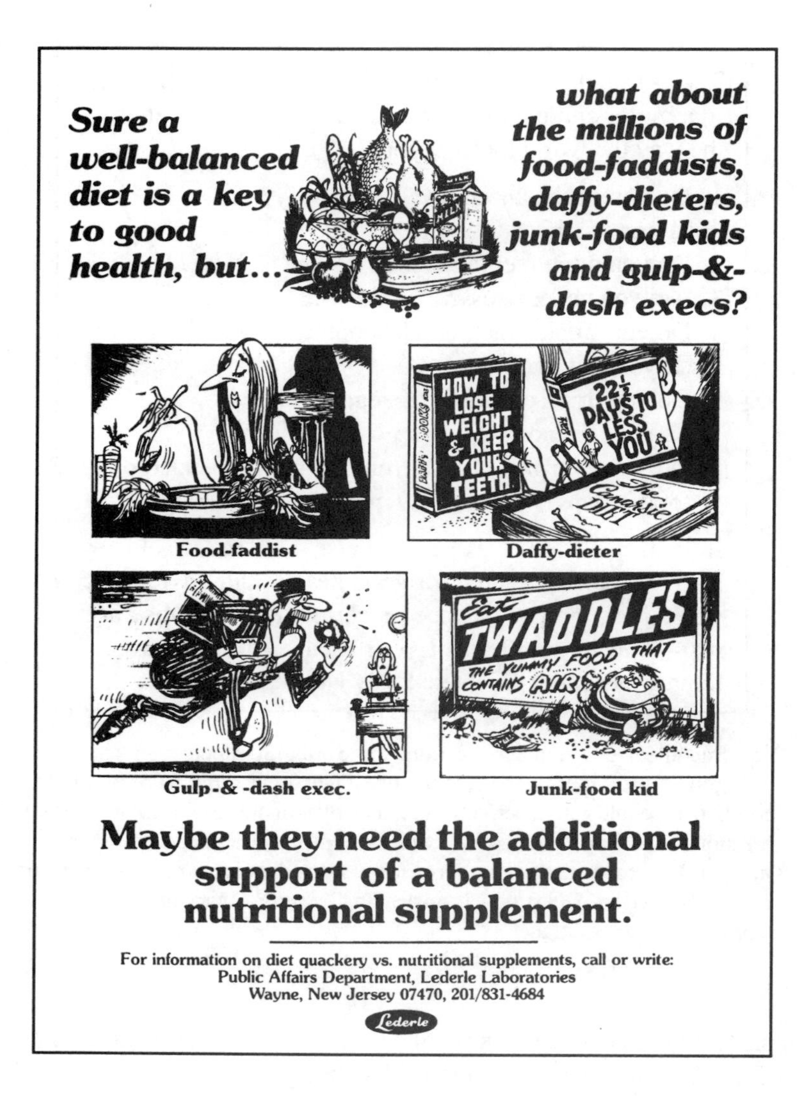

Lederle ad from July 1981 *Columbia Journalism Review* offering an information packet to journalists. The material was largely promotional. One item was a booklet about vitamins and minerals which suggested that many Americans don't get enough of them and that vitamin C megadoses may prevent colds. The booklet also listed "periods of physiologic stress" during which "increased vitamin intake may be needed" and "deficiencies may develop on diets that had previously been adequate." Although an accompanying article said that "nutrition quackery may be today's widespread and most expensive fad," the only vitamin quackery it debunked were claims that vitamin E stimulates the sex drive and that natural vitamins are superior to synthetic ones.

most striking finding was that most users began taking supplements to help cope with stress, fatigue, emotional trauma, or a health problem and that supplements "gave users the feeling they are doing all they can for their physical and psychological health. . . . a means of gaining some kind of control over their traumatic lives." Past users, however, "became vulnerable to negative reports when their stress or problems passed."

CRN's "Vitamin Gap" campaign was designed to convince people that supplements were still needed. First it falsely suggested that vitamins could help against stress. Then it falsely suggested that most Americans were not getting enough nutrients in their diet. A manufacturer using such messages to sell its own products could be prosecuted for fraud. But since CRN sold no products, it was legally free to deceive.

The "Population Studies" Ploy

One of the common arguments used to support "nutrition insurance" is that health and nutrition surveys have found that some segments of the population have intakes of some nutrients below the RDAs. Although such observations have indeed been made, their significance has been greatly exaggerated by vitamin pushers.

The RDAs are not standards for estimating individual vitamin and mineral needs. They were designed to help food-service personnel who prepare food for large groups of people judge whether they were providing large enough amounts of key nutrients. The levels are set high enough to ensure that if the nutrient levels being served meet the RDAs, they will exceed the needs of healthy individuals with the highest requirements. Using the RDA for evaluating individual nutrient intakes is like setting the standard for height at seven feet and concluding that all those under seven feet have suffered growth retardation.

Survey results have additional shortcomings. The vitamins most often identified as "problems" are vitamins C and A. However, findings that vitamin C intakes are below the RDA are misleading because the 60 mg RDA for vitamin C is six times the amount needed to prevent deficiency. Vitamin A presents a different problem. The main food sources of vitamin A (consumed as beta-carotene, which the body converts to vitamin A) include various fruits and vegetables that many people don't eat every day. When dietary surveys measure nutrient intakes for a single day—as they often do—many people score "low" in vitamin A while others have higher-than-necessary intakes. Because vitamin A is stored in the liver for years, a surplus consumed on one day will provide a reserve that is available on subsequent days. Vitamin A intakes should be estimated by averaging daily intake over at least a week. A third pitfall of dietary surveys is that people tend to underestimate the amount of food they eat.

Thus, because of the nature of the RDAs and of dietary surveys, it is not possible to assess nutritional status by comparing estimates of nutrient intakes with the RDA. The only reliable way to determine vitamin status is from clinical observations and/or laboratory measurements. When this is done for research purposes, *very few people are found to be deficient.* Inadequate nutrient intakes occur because of poverty, neglect, illness, alcoholism, and ignorance. In most cases, the nutritional problem should be remedied with appropriate foods rather than dietary supplements.

"Stress Formulas"

Many supplement products are marketed as a form of "insurance" against "stress." While some manufacturers refer only to physical stresses, others include mental stress, overwork, and the like. And some make no health claims at all, but rely on the word "stress" in the product's name to sell it.

"Stress-formulas" typically contain several times the RDA for vitamin C and several B-vitamins. The products manufactured by drug companies do not provide toxic amounts of these ingredients. But some marketed by health-food industry companies contain enough vitamin C to produce diarrhea, and some contain enough B_6 to cause nerve damage over a long period of time. Some formulas contain questionable food substances such as spirulina, bee pollen, and ginseng, to make them appear more "complete." Herbal and homeopathic "stress formulas" are also available. Here are some examples of misleading advertising claims.

• AARP Pharmacy Service has asserted that "A busy lifestyle puts extra demands on your body. That's why you should try . . . *Stress Formula 360*, with biotin and folic acid." The idea that "busy" people need extra vitamins is pure nonsense.

• Abbott Laboratories has advertised that "During illness or stress, the water soluble vitamins are the most quickly depleted. . . . *Surbex-T* restores what the body cannot effectively store."

• Ayerst Laboratories, stating that "just being alive is stressful," has suggested *Beminal Stress Plus* to avoid "stress burnout," a vitamin-deficiency state to which "nobody is immune." Another ad stated that vitamins and minerals were needed to replenish those "lost through . . . the stress you make yourself from dieting, late nights, or even that two-mile jog."

• Barth's *All-Day® Maxi-Stress Tablets* were advised because "stress can affect your health in many ways and can occur at any time." The product was said to contain "all 11 B-vitamins plus calming Tryptophane" to assure "a supply of the right combination of anti-stress nutrients—at the right time—whenever you need it." (There are only eight B-vitamins for humans.)

• General Nutrition Corp. has included "traffic jams, arguments, meeting fast-approaching deadlines, or simply trying to decide what to wear at a party" as sources of emotional stress that "can take their toll on various nutrients in our body, especially vitamin C and B-complex vitamins." A 1988 ad for its *Stress B* stated: "In today's fast-paced world, life's daily routine can rob you of important nutrients. Now you can fight back against this silent 'thief' with the high levels of B vitamins found in our exclusive . . . formula."

• Hoffmann-La Roche, Inc., has advertised that "if you drink, smoke, diet or happen to be sick, you may be robbing your body of vitamins." One of its ads claimed that "the stress of illness" would lower vitamin C plasma levels or that "as part of everyday living you do things that may be lowering the level of vitamins in your body, and robbing you of these vital nutrients." Another ad stated, "Up tight or up in smoke . . . With both acute stress and heavy cigarette smoking, the plasma levels of vitamin C in your blood may be lowered."

• Hudson Vitamins has stated that "the stress of living – whether it's caused by physical or mental or emotional situations in your life – increases your need for certain nutrients. Stress decreases your body's supply of the water-soluble vitamins, B-COMPLEX AND VITAMIN C. Replace them in order to protect your body's nutritional needs." These messages were provided to drugstores on plastic-coated vitamin charts to display near their vitamin sections. The charts also state (falsely) that smoking, alcohol, and oral contraceptives are "vitamin robbers," that PABA, choline, and inositol are vitamins, and that "B-vitamins cannot be stored by your body and therefore must be replaced every day."

• The I. Magnin department store chain has recommended *Clientele Stress Control Nutrients* —in addition to its *Daily Nutrients*, "if you're very active, deal frequently with decision-making or just find yourself drained from everyday events." A 1985 brochure also contained a questionnaire (see below) which suggested that many forms of common behavior provide a reason to take supplements. Neiman-Marcus, another prominent department store that sells through the mail, recommended annual "subscriptions" to the *Stress Control Nutrients* because "a limited supply is produced fresh each month." Subscribing ensures that "a fresh box is reserved for you" and sent automatically for $26.90 per month, with the last two months free. Subscribers also received Clientele's Relaxation Cassette and Biofeedback Band ("valued at $25").

Take a moment to answer
this "Stress Survey" . . .

	YES	NO
1. Do you work under high pressure conditions?	☐	☐
2. Are you under physical or emotional strain?	☐	☐
3. Do you travel frequently?	☐	☐
4. Are you often frustrated, tense, or anxious?	☐	☐
5. Do you become tired, upset, or depressed easily?	☐	☐
6. Do you abuse your health with too much coffee, alcohol, drugs, or cigarettes?	☐	☐
7. Are you physically active or do you exercise often?	☐	☐
8. Have there been major changes in your life recently?	☐	☐

If you answered "yes" to any of the above, your body may be depleting itself of nutrients vital for good health.

Questionnaire from Neiman-Marcus brochure for *Clientele Stress Control Nutrients.* The questions have little or nothing to do with nutrition and provide no basis for concluding that nutrients are being "depleted" or that supplements are needed.

According to Neiman-Marcus's brochure, *Clientele Stress Control Nutrients* can "strengthen the body's natural resistance to disease," "help your body make natural enzymes that may slow the aging process," help to keep skin firm and young looking, "help turn carbohydrates into energy," and "help you cope with stress more easily." The brochure also included a phony "Stress Survey" (see above). In direct-mail ads, Clientele, Inc., stated that if you diet, skip meals, often feel fatigued, are under stress, smoke, drink, or take oral contraceptives, "you are probably lacking nutrients vital to good health. Even if you think that you eat a well-balanced diet."

• Nat-rul Health Products claims: "One of the most important conditions for a person's ability to deal with stress is maintaining proper nutrition levels, especially B-Complex and Vitamin C. Since these vitamins are water soluble, a fresh supply is needed daily, and mega-potencies are preferred when under considerable stress."

• Scandinavian Laboratories, a New Jersey-based firm that markets Royal Harvest supplement products, has advertised that "leading more active and stressful lives, family members often need more nutrients than even a well-balanced diet can supply." It has also advertised that "Stress seems to be a natural part of life today. Unfortunately, many stress formulas . . . aren't natural. *Stress Max* gives you this important advantage in coping with physical and emotional stress." The company describes its *College Stress Formula* as "a wise investment in a student's education."

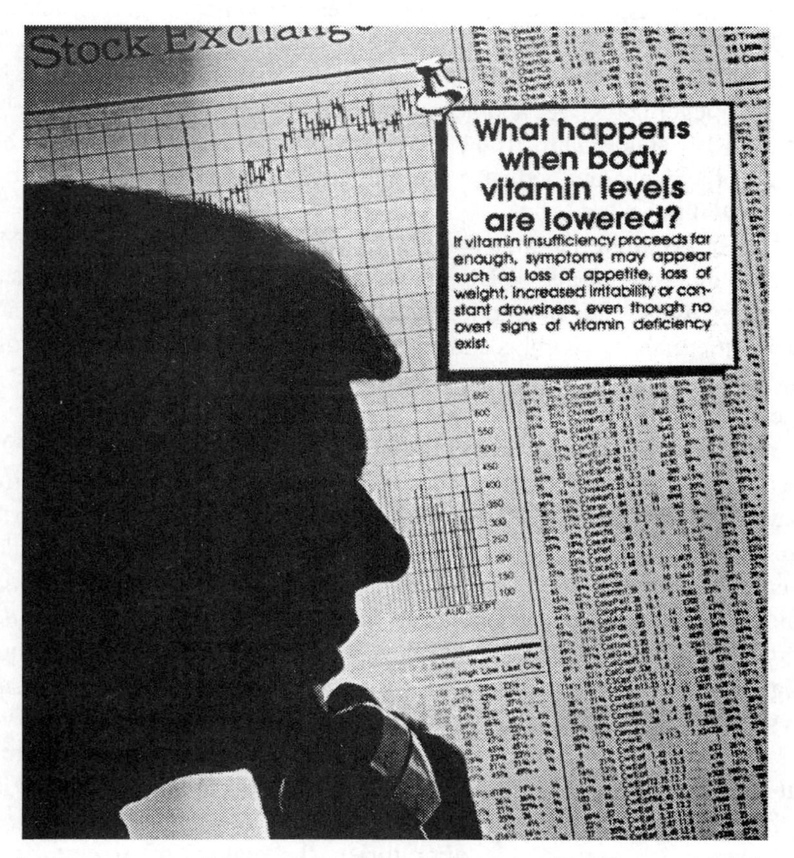

An illustration used to promote the "ultra high potency formulas to combat the effects of stress" listed in the 1984 Sears Shop at Home Service (Puritan's Pride) catalog. Do you think that worrying about the stock market is a reason to take vitamins?

• Sears Shop at Home Service, which in 1985 marketed Puritan's Pride stress formulas, asserted: "Active lives subject us to considerable stress. Working hard and even playing hard creates one type of stress. The weather even affects us. Colds and illness make more demands on our bodies. Of course the everyday pressures of life bring on emotional stress. All these types of stress increase your body's needs for vitamins, especially the water soluble B's and C's. Your body cannot store these vitamins. You need a fresh supply each day and more when stress leaves you depleted."

• The Sharper Image has stated in its mail-order catalogs: "When you get adequate sleep and eat properly, you naturally look and feel better. But in today's world, this isn't always possible. . . . Stress, pollution, caffeine, alcohol, even common aspirin can rob the body of essential health-giving nutrients. . . . Maximum Life Span's Energy/Stress Formula replenishes nutrients. The result is that you not only feel healthier, but look better, too."

• Spiegel added yet another wrinkle in ads for its MDR Fitness Tabs Program. Its catalog claimed that *MDR*'s twice-a-day dosage "helps reduce the chance of leaving your body at a low nutrient level at a time when your body may need it most."

• The Vitamin Shoppe operates several retail outlets in the New York metropolitan area and also sells by mail. Its ads for *Super Stress-Formula* state: "Stress is any physical or emotional strain on the body or mind and it can rob you of important B vitamins and essential nutrients. As daily life gets more hectic, our caps can supply your body with adequate levels of vitamins C and B needed during times of increased physical and emotional demands."

• Vitacrown, Inc., of Hicksville, New York, advertised in the mid-1980s that a fast-paced, stressful lifestyle could be "cheating your body and your mind of the nutrients they need to keep you going strong." The company, described as a subsidiary of Crown Vitamins, Inc., advised readers of the ad to stop taking "weak, standard one-a-day type vitamin brands" and switch to *The Formula.,* which sold for $11.20 per month. The ad also claimed that *"The Formula* 's ingredients will play an important role in relieving or preventing . . . frequent fatigue, headaches, sleep problems, digestive problems, loss of mental or physical vigor, muscular weakness, diminished sex drive, depression, nervous tension, irritability, plus many other deficiency symptoms too numerous to list in this limited space." The ingredients included doses of vitamins A, C, D, and B_6 that were high enough to cause adverse effects.

According to Lederle Laboratories, the makers of *Stresstabs,* the concept of high-dosage stress vitamins is based on a 1952 National Academy of Sciences report called *Therapeutic Nutrition.* The chapter of the report titled "Nutritional Requirements of the Sick, Injured, and Convalescent" recommended extra vitamins for people suffering from stresses such as general surgery, serious burns, and major fractures. However, the report actually stated that "in minor illnesses or injury where the expected duration of the disease is less than 10 days and when the patient is essentially ambulatory and is eating his diet . . . a good diet will supply the recommended dietary allowances of all nutrients."

In other words, when people are so ill that they lose their appetite for a significant period of time, supplementation with water-soluble vitamins may be prudent. Lederle's ads, however, have conveyed a different picture. In 1975, Lederle began advertising that stress "robs the body of vitamins" and can deplete the body's stores of water-soluble vitamins, and that "daily replacement is necessary." The first two of these statements is at best misleading because if stores are depleted, the culprit is lack of food intake, not high body usage. The third statement is a flat lie. Although storage of vitamins is limited, people eating normally will store at least several weeks' supply, and failure to replenish the supply for a few days or even a few weeks is unlikely to cause trouble. A 1978 ad for Lederle's *Stresstabs 600* even claimed that water-soluble vitamins "can't be stockpiled, no matter how much you take in." Other ads have included "chronic overwork" in the list of "stresses" that contribute to "exceptional vitamin needs."

There is absolutely no evidence that emotional stress increases the body's need for vitamins. Leon Ellenbogen, Ph.D., Lederle's chief of nutritional science, readily acknowledged this during an interview noted in the March 1986 issue of *Consumer Reports.* During the interview, which was conducted by Dr. Stephen Barrett, Ellenbogen insisted that "we make it clear in our ads that we're talking about physical stress." Moreover, when asked who *doesn't* need to take a stress vitamin, Ellenbogen (a genuine nutrition scientist) replied: "People who eat a balanced diet do not need stress vitamins—or for that matter, any vitamin supplement at all."

True, ads for Lederle's *Advanced Formula Stresstabs* did not use the words "emotional stress." But they did picture a man working at a paper-strewn desk after dark and touted the product "for people who burn the candle at both ends"—a phrase that most people would interpret as emotional rather than physical stress.

Government Enforcement Actions

In 1986, New York State Attorney General Robert Abrams put an end to Lederle's deception with an agreement under which the company paid $25,000 to the state and promised not to make unsupportable claims that emotional stress causes depletion of water-soluble vitamins, that *Stresstabs* will reduce the effects of psychological stress, or that consumers undergoing ordinary physical stress can't obtain all necessary nutrients by eating a well balanced diet or taking an ordinary-potency (about 100 percent of the U.S. RDA) multiple vitamin

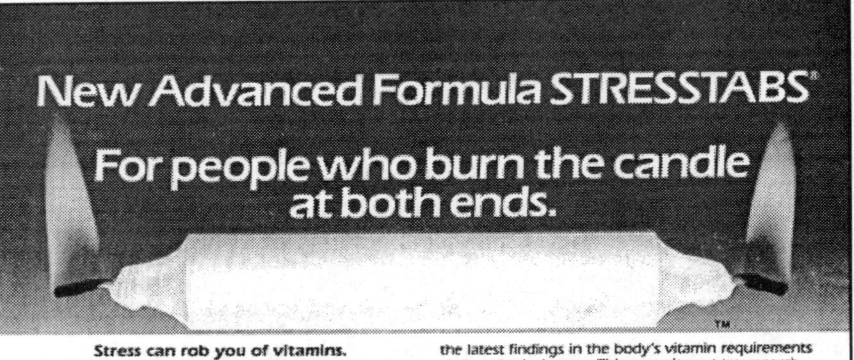

Stress can rob you of vitamins.
It's a fact that during periods of physical stress your body uses up more vitamins than normal. It's also known that unlike such fat soluble vitamins as A and D, which are stored in the body, most of the water soluble vitamins—B-complex and C—should be replaced daily. That's why a good diet is so important. STRESSTABS® high potency stress formula vitamins can help to back up your diet because they concentrate on vitamins your body can't store.

Now biotin makes STRESSTABS even more complete.
New data confirms that biotin is one of many water soluble vitamins that stress can rob. Essential in the conversion of carbohydrates to energy, biotin also plays a large role in the synthesis of fats and in protein metabolism for the building of healthy tissue. Today you'll find the essential biotin extra in all three STRESSTABS high potency formulas.

STRESSTABS. The stress formula vitamin doctors recommend most.
Throughout the years, the Lederle Nutrition Research Group has carefully updated STRESSTABS to reflect the latest findings in the body's vitamin requirements during physical stress. This commitment to research and formula advancement may be part of the reason that physicians continue to recommend STRESSTABS more than any other stress formula vitamin.

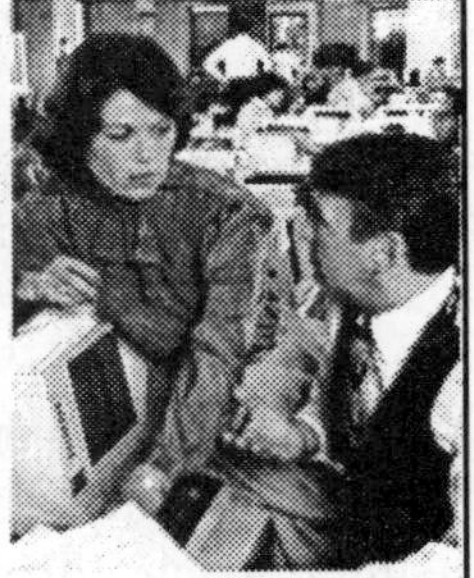

Look for the candle. It's only on Advanced Formula STRESSTABS.
The STRESSTABS candle is your assurance of high quality vitamins from Lederle Laboratories. Look for it on Advanced Formula STRESSTABS, Advanced Formula STRESSTABS plus Iron, and Advanced Formula STRESSTABS plus Zinc. The vitamins for people who burn the candle at both ends.

Advanced Formula STRESSTABS: No other stress formula vitamin can hold a candle to it.

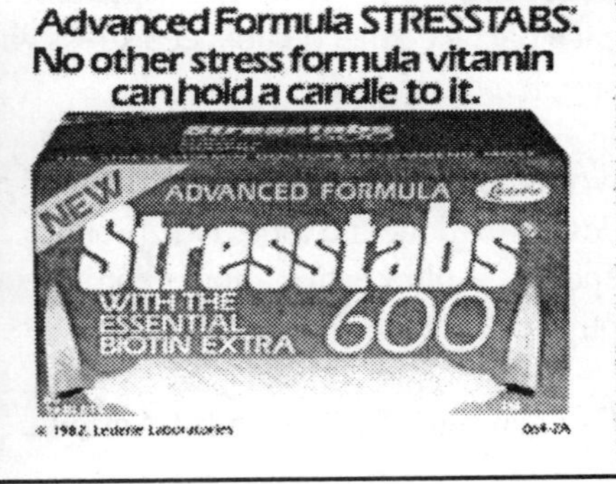

© 1982, Lederle Laboratories

Ad for *Stresstabs 600* used from 1982 to 1985. Although the ad refers to "physical stress," it does not define it. The words and pictures suggest that Stresstabs is a remedy for emotional stress.

supplement. The agreement listed more than a dozen misleading statements from magazine, radio, and television ads.

In 1985, E.R. Squibb & Sons signed a similar consent agreement that included a $15,000 penalty and a pledge to modify the claims made on the package of its *Theragran Stress Formula.* Squibb had been claiming that the product helps relieve stress resulting from "the complications of everyday life" and "that taking the recommended daily allowance would reduce the effects of psychological stress." Its ads had also suggested that biotin is difficult to obtain in an average diet, even though biotin deficiency is virtually nonexistent. (Except in infants, it has been reported only in individuals who ate unbalanced diets containing large amounts of raw eggs, which contain a substance that blocks biotin absorption.)

In 1989, the FTC secured a consent agreement forbidding Miles, Inc., of Elkhart, Indiana, from making unsubstantiated claims for its One-A-Day brand multiple vitamins. According to the FTC complaint, Miles's ads on radio and television had stated:

- Strenuous exercise can actually knock essential minerals right out of your system. But One-A-Day vitamins are uniquely formulated to help put back what your world takes away.
- The stress of daily living can take a lot out of you.... Your B vitamins, for example, are being chipped away by everyday problems and pressures. But One-A-Day puts them back. One-A-Day vitamins are uniquely formulated to put back what your stressful world takes away.
- Defending your lungs against air pollution requires vitamins A, E, and C. Daily stress can chip away at your B vitamins. And rigorous physical training can actually knock essential minerals right out of your system. That's why One-A-Day vitamins are uniquely formulated to help put back what your world takes away. So eat a balanced diet and take One-A-Day, every day.

The consent agreement forbids Miles to represent, directly or by implication, that any vitamin or mineral supplement:

- Affords any protection or benefit to human lungs.
- Is necessary or beneficial in replacing any vitamin and/or mineral lost through physical exercise.
- Is necessary or beneficial in replacing any vitamins and/or minerals lost as a result of, or provides any benefit with regard to, the stress of daily living.

Miles was also barred from making any other unsubstantiated claim for any of its products. This case is highly significant because it involves a large corporation and is the first *federal* case to strike at the heart of fraudulent "stress vitamin" claims.

Miles also signed a three-year "assurance of discontinuance" order with the attorneys general of New York, California, and Texas and agreed to pay $10,000 to each of these three states. The company pledged not to claim that : (1) the average consumer needs a supplement to prevent mineral and vitamin loss; (2) vitamins can prevent or reverse lung damage caused by pollution; (3) routine daily stress depletes vitamins; or (4) routine physical exercise such as the aerobics shown in Miles's television ad depletes essential minerals.

Since these cases were settled, we have seen no ads for "stress supplements" placed by large pharmaceutical companies. (Perhaps they concluded that advertising of stress vitamins doesn't pay unless it is misleading.) Health-food industry manufacturers, however, have continued to use false claims. We note, too, that CRN's "vitamin gap" ad made several misleading claims that would have been illegal in an ad by a manufacturer.

"Special Needs"

Supplement advocates suggest that many population groups have special vitamin needs that may make supplementation advisable. Probably the most elaborate presentation of this concept was contained in "Personal Health Circumstances Benefited by Nutritional Supplementation," a six-page flyer published in 1987 by the Council for Responsible Nutrition (CRN). According to the flyer:

> The analysis of personal nutrition need categories strongly suggests that large groups of people are at risk for a variety of reasons and that their nutritional status, overall quality of health, and consequent mortality and morbidity are affected. Thus it makes good sense to help guide those in these special need categories to take some action that will protect or improve their nutrition status.

In line with these thoughts, the flyer designated eighteen "groups with proven nutrient needs" for which "scientific evidence available today suggests that a nutritional supplement as part of total intake will be beneficial."

CRN was correct that individuals in these groups have "proven nutrient needs." But these needs were taken into account when the RDAs were determined. In 1987, Alfred E. Harper, Ph.D., professor of biochemistry and nutritional sciences at the University of Wisconsin, analyzed each of the eighteen groups in the CRN flyer. Dr. Harper, a prominent nutrition scientist, was chairman of the Food and Nutrition Board of the National Research Council from 1978 to 1982 and has served on other NRC committees involved in determining the RDAs. Here is his analysis, slightly modified by us for this chapter.

• *People taking prescription drug(s): 125 million.* Although certain drugs are known to increase the requirements for specific vitamins, it is improper to assume that drugs automatically increase nutrient requirements. A few drug-nutrient interactions can create clinical problems. Individuals taking such drugs need a recommendation from a physician for the appropriate extra amount of any specific nutrient that is needed. General supplementation is not a rational approach because only the nutrient(s) that will correct the problem will be of any value.

• *Dieters: 95.4 million.* Dieters who consume fewer than 1,200 calories per day should consider whether the food they consume will provide adequate amounts of the essential nutrients. Many dieters do not consume such low levels of calories and, if they do, they usually do so for only a short period of time. If caloric intakes are reduced below 1,000 calories a day for longer than one week, it would make sense to take a vitamin-mineral supplement containing RDA amounts of the essential vitamins and minerals. However, such very-low-calorie dieting should be done under supervision of a physician with the appropriate supplement provided as part of the overall diet plan.

• *Premenopausal women of childbearing age: 55 million.* Premenopausal women of childbearing age are part of the population of normal healthy individuals. The RDAs for healthy adult women are based on their needs. Many of these women need education about appropriate food use, but if they are eating wisely they should not need supplements except during pregnancy, when supplementary folic acid and iron may be appropriate. Premenopausal women whose intake of calcium is inadequate should either consume more dairy products or take a calcium supplement.

• *Smokers: 54 million.* There has been much emphasis on the fact that vitamin C levels in the blood of smokers are lower than those of nonsmokers, even though both groups average several times the level of deficiency. The suggestion that smokers need high doses of vitamin C seems even more incongruous when one considers that most of the subjects used in the major experiments that served as the basis for the present RDA for vitamin C were smokers. Moreover, smoking is so devastating to health that even if vitamin C did offer slight protection against its ravages, it would be senseless to encourage smokers to believe that they can avoid the consequences of smoking through nutritional measures!

• *People with specific gastrointestinal disorders: 40 million.* Most gastrointestinal disorders last only a few days and require no special nutrient supplements. For chronic or prolonged problems, management by a physician is essential, with emphasis on identifying the cause and curing the condition. Supplementation may be desirable while nutrient loss occurs, but it should be done under medical supervision. In malabsorptive diseases—where absorption of specific vitamins is impaired—specific supplementation is advisable until the condition can be brought under control.

• *Postmenopausal women: 39 million.* The major change in nutrient needs of healthy postmenopausal women is reduced energy requirement. From age fifty on, caloric needs decline steadily while the need for essential nutrients remains about the same. The best way to obtain these nutrients while eating less is to choose foods that are rich in essential nutrients. It is also wise for postmenopausal women to maintain and possibly increase their physical activity. This will also help prevent loss of calcium from their bones and will decrease their chances of becoming overweight.

• *The elderly: 28 million.* The active elderly who are healthy have no special needs beyond those covered by the RDA. The elderly who are ill need medical advice and not a general recommendation for a nutrient supplement. The older elderly may have unusually low caloric requirements because of low activity as well as low metabolic rate. Here again, attention should be given to maintaining an adequate intake of foods that are highly nutritious. In some circumstances, food intake may be so low that a supplement is appropriate.

• *Women taking postmenopausal estrogen: 2.3 million.* Women taking postmenopausal estrogens should be no different from the normal healthy elderly. They should maintain calcium intake in the RDA range because the beneficial effect from estrogens on osteoporosis has been shown most clearly when calcium intake is in that range or somewhat higher.

• *People with osteoporosis: 20 million.* There is no evidence that individuals with osteoporosis have any general need for nutrient supplements. Even the evidence of benefits from high intakes of calcium is inconsistent and controversial. For normal bone maintenance, a calcium intake that meets the RDA is needed throughout adult life. This can be obtained from foods, especially dairy products, but dietary surveys show that many elderly women have low total food and calcium intakes. Increased physical activity will enable them to eat more without gaining weight, and tends to reduce bone mineral loss. It is unclear whether calcium supplements alone are helpful in treating osteoporosis. Combined calcium and estrogen therapy is reportedly beneficial, but of course should be done under medical guidance.

• *Poor people: 33.1 million.* The poor need a support system; they need food programs that provide them with adequate quantities of essential nutrients and energy sources. In other words, they need proper food. Supplements of essential nutrients cannot substitute for basic needs for energy sources and protein and are expensive in relation to the income of this group of people.

• *People with chronic or infectious disease(s) or under chronic physical stress: unknown millions.* Chronic and infectious diseases generally cannot be assumed to increase nutrient needs. This is an irrational grouping in relation to nutritional requirements. Infectious diseases are individual problems and should be dealt with by appropriate medical care, not by general recommendations for increased intakes of nutrients. If a chronic or degenerative disease results in severely depressed food intake and weight loss, it may be appropriate to provide a supplement with the food during the period of debilitation.

• *Teenagers: 25.9 million.* Teenagers represent an active part of the total healthy population. Students up to college age are usually physically active and often have caloric intakes that are quite high. They need mainly to learn how to achieve dietary balance by choosing nutritious foods and moderating intake of foods that contain small quantities of essential nutrients. They need nutrition advice, not supplements which tend to distract them from learning about sound food choices.

• *Alcoholics: 25 million.* Supplements are not a solution for alcoholism. Alcoholics need food instead of alcohol and guidance to learn how to control the problem of addiction. If food intake of an alcoholic is extremely low, severe vitamin deficiencies can develop. These need prompt clinical attention and a program of rehabilitation. Inappropriate vitamin supplements may delay the appearance of certain deficiency signs and result in medical treatment being put off until serious deterioration of vital organs has occurred.

• *Women taking estrogen for birth control: 8.8 million.* There have been reports of changes in the metabolism or blood levels of certain essential nutrients in women using birth control pills. However, claims that these provide evidence of nutritional inadequacy have not stood up to rigorous testing.

• *Strict vegetarians: 8.5 million.* Most vegetarians consume eggs and dairy products and obtain adequate quantities of all nutrients including vitamin B_{12}, although some may not. For those who are strict vegetarians, a source of vitamin B_{12} is required. It is also particularly important for vegetarians to select a wide variety of different types of fruits and vegetables and cereal grains because serious malnutrition has been found to occur in individuals who have restricted their intake to a narrow range of foods from plant sources. Supplements are not a substitute for sound diet planning.

• *Pregnant women: 3.6 million.* There are modest increases in needs for essential nutrients during pregnancy. Food consumption usually increases during gestation so the pregnant woman will be eating increased quantities of all nutrients. If food intake declines, a supplement providing about half the RDA for the vitamins most likely to be in short supply, together with iron, would not be inappropriate.

• *Lactating women: 2.16 million.* During lactation, energy needs of women increase substantially. Their increased food intake will normally compensate for the increased quantities of essential nutrients needed for production of milk. For women who are reducing weight during lactation or who have low food intake, a standard vitamin-mineral supplement may be appropriate, but otherwise essential nutrient needs are readily met by diet.

• *Premature infants:* 0.36 million. Premature infants require medical care; their needs should be determined carefully by the physician to ensure that essential nutrient supply is adequate. Essential nutrients are usually provided as part of the formula, not as a special supplement.

The numbers assigned by CRN add up to more than twice the population of the United States because these subgroups overlap. Does CRN think anyone exists who does *not* need supplements? Dr. Barrett explored this issue during a recent phone conversation with CRN president John B. Cordaro:

Q. Would it be correct to say that CRN believes that everyone should take supplements?
A. I believe that almost every person could benefit from using a nutritional supplement at one time or another in their life.
Q. Is there any way to define who would not?
A. Individuals who are healthy, select their foods so they get all of the nutrients they need in the most generous portions to reduce their risk of deficiency and help to prevent chronic disease. . . .
Q. Would someone who meets the RDAs satisfy that?
A. No. Absolutely not . . . because the RDA book talks about [healthy persons]. That's really the issue.
Q. Would a healthy person who meets the RDAs fit your definition?
A. No, because . . . it would not address the issue of optimal intake. The RDA only addresses deficiency.
Q. Is it possible to get the "optimal" amounts of nutrients from food?
A. Certainly not some of the key nutrients. . . . We're talking about . . . trying to select a diet that is as good as possible, and yet supplementing your diet in an appropriate way with responsible dosage levels, so that you fill whatever gaps exist or can add more generous amounts to the diet.

We disagree. The RDAs are designed to provide enough for practically everyone (see Chapter 2). There are not enough scientific data to determine what is "optimal" or to prove that higher amounts will do more good than harm.

"Personalized" Products

Many vitamin companies appeal to the American penchant for custom-made goods. Some products are pitched to meet supposed needs at various ages or stages of life, some are formulated especially for women. Some are purportedly tailored for the individual. Some formulations are based on a modicum of sense, while others are completely irrational. Some are modestly priced, while others are outrageous or beyond. Here are some examples:

• Richardson-Vicks Inc.'s *Lifestage* multivitamins were advertised during the mid-1980s as "a whole new way to look at vitamins." According to the ad, "Lifestage meets your whole family's needs better than any other vitamin brand." The line was composed of *Children's Formula, Teens' Formula, Men's Formula, Women's Formula, Stress Formula for Men,* and *Stress Formula for Women,* each supposedly "customized" for the designated group. Except for the *Children's* Formula, which contained 100 percent of the U.S. RDA for most ingredients, none of the products was a sensible supplement for anyone at any stage of life. The only difference between the men's and women's formulas was that the latter contained 27 mg of iron, which not all women need and is more than women who need an iron supplement should take anyway. Stranger yet, the women's formulas lacked calcium, the nutrient most likely to be appropriate for women to take as a supplement.

• In 1983, A.H. Robins urged consumers to "help protect against vitamin burnout" that occurs when overwork, exercising, dieting, colds, and flu "burn up essential vitamins you need for balanced nutrition every day." To determine the correct *Albee*® formula for each family member (which "depends on eating and working patterns as well as personal lifestyles"), the company advised asking your pharmacist.

• Weider Health & Fitness markets *Actifem Personal R.D.A.*, a women's product whose dosage is adjusted according to daily circumstances. The package insert states: "The Food and Nutrition Board's dietary allowances are *general* recommendations for population *groups*. Individuals vary greatly; therefore, your neighbor, friend or even your sister may not have the same exact nutritional needs as you." To determine your supposed needs, the insert contains a thirty-day chart for checking off which of thirteen items is applicable:

You drank 2 glasses of soda or ate fewer than 3 servings of high-calcium foods
You exercised 1 hour or more
Score an additional point if you exercise 2½ hours or more
You are over 35 years old
You are menstruating or within 1 week of menstruating

You take an oral contraceptive
You are taking medications, or recovering from an injury or illness
You drank more than two glasses of alcohol (includes wine and beer)
You smoke, or spent 4 hours in a highly polluted area
You had a moderate to high intake of processed foods, or ate 1 or more unbalanced meals
You are dieting or skipped 1 meal
Score an additional check if you are following a fad diet or skipped two meals
You have a lot of stress at work, home, or school.

For every item checked, the consumer is advised to take one tablet that day, up to a maximum of eight. Each tablet contains 25 percent of the U.S. RDA for twelve vitamins and six minerals. Eating fewer than three servings of high-calcium foods—if the servings were small—might justify taking extra calcium. But "yes" answers to the rest of the questions are not a rational basis for supplementation. In fact, most of the questions are utterly senseless. Nor is there any reason for routinely taking more than 100 percent of the U.S. RDA.

• Healthbank, a company located in Los Angeles, offered its Matrix "personalized nutritional program" through Jazzercise® and other outlets. Participants fill out a "comprehensive" computer-scored questionnaire composed of fifty items related to health, nutrition, and lifestyle. When Dr. Barrett did so in 1987, he received a "personal health profile" that was mainly general advice about eating a low-fat, high-fiber diet and had little to do with his responses. (For example, he was advised not to take daytime naps even though he had never taken one in his life.) Although his answers indicated that his diet contained adequate amounts of essential nutrients, Healthbank advised him to choose foods daily from the Basic Four food groups and to take its "personalized nutritional formula" containing "vitamins and minerals most appropriate to your personal needs." The formula contained 100 percent of the U.S. RDA of twelve vitamins and four minerals, 50 percent of the U.S. RDA for one mineral, and modest amounts of five other minerals for which no U.S. RDA had been established—the amounts found in many multivitamin/multimineral supplements available for about 5¢ per pill at drugstores. The Matrix program cost $10 for the questionnaire and from $33.45 to $53.45 per month, depending on the amount ordered and whether the purchaser was affiliated with Jazzercise. The monthly supply included two 6-ounce boxes of Fiber Chips, which Barrett characterized as "the most awful-tasting stuff you can imagine."

• Nutrition & Stress Research of Reno, Nevada, has marketed its Energy Quotient Vitamin System (EQV System) primarily through chiropractic offices. Its packaging describes it as "a complete vitamin system" and "a vitamin

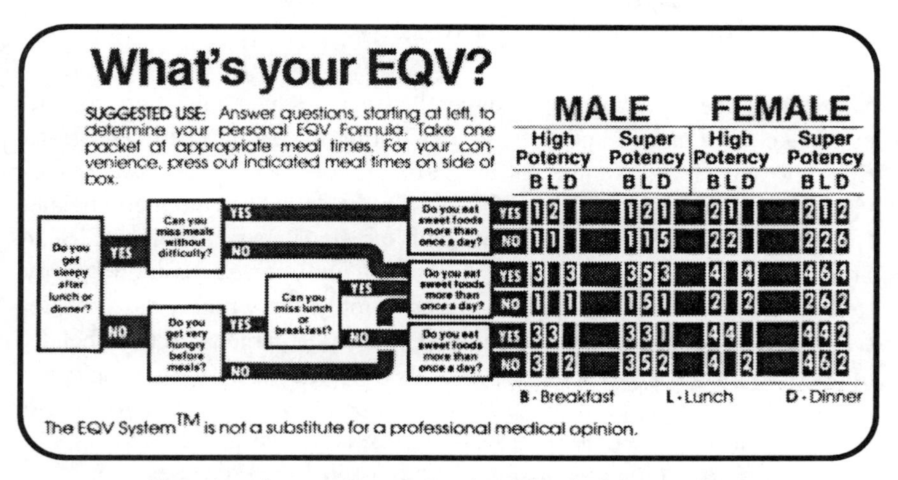

Flow sheet from an *Energy Quotient Vitamin System* package

program unique for you." According to a catalog from a chiropractic distributor:

> In over 5 years of research it was found that most people commonly suffer from energy lows and stress peaks at predictable times of the day resulting from variations in sugar sensitivity (hypoglycemia) and the body's inability to produce energy (cellular oxidation). The EQV system increases energy potential by stimulating cellular efficiency and correcting possible dietary inaccuracies. EQV targets stress to improve energy flow all day long.

The system is based on a flow sheet that asks whether you get sleepy after lunch or dinner, whether you can miss meals without difficulty, whether you get very hungry before meals, whether you can miss lunch or breakfast, and whether you eat sweet foods more than once a day. The flow culminates in a chart with columns for males and female and your choice of "high potency" or "super potency." The chart indicates which of six formulas should be taken with breakfast, lunch, and/or dinner. When Dr. Barrett investigated in 1988, he concluded that following the system would result in an intake of twelve to eighteen pills (two or three packets), which for many users would include unsafe amounts of vitamins A, C, and B_6. The program cost from $1.56 to $2.35/day, twenty to thirty times as much as more sensible multivitamin/mineral pills available through drugstores.

Is there any legitimate reason to seek a "personalized" supplement? In our opinion, the answer is no. For someone determined to take a supplement for "insurance," the best strategy would be to take an inexpensive broad-spectrum product as described below.

Unlimited Hype

Many supplement manufacturers suggest that their products have characteristics that make them unique and/or better than those of their competitors. Nat-rul Health Products, for example, offers "all-day protection" with *timed-release* vitamin-mineral formulas. RichLife offers *OrganiMins,* "the uniquely chelated Organomineral complex that's nutritionally targeted for specific organs." Sears Shop at Home Service's *Vitamin Improvement Program,* assured "purity, freshness, and quality" by shipping a fresh supply every ninety days. Albion Laboratories claims to have discovered "a way to target specific chelated minerals to specific areas of the body." Makers of KAL, in a pitch to people with a busy, active lifestyle, states that its "high-potency" vitamins "dissolve in minutes instead of the hour or more that some lazy vitamins take."

MegaFood "employs nature's unsurpassed Life Processes to actually grow Whole Food Vitamin and Mineral Concentrates" that are "up to 16 times more effective than ordinary 'natural' supplements." JS&A markets a twice-a-day vitamin/mineral product, formulated by "a group of nutritionists, dietitians, dermatologists, biochemists, and physicians," based on the notion that some vitamins are best taken in the morning and others at night. Ortho Molecular Nutrition International states that its vitamins and minerals are "biologically activated with nutrient carriers and absorption factors that make them superior to all other types." (To support this claim, the company states that, in a controlled test, baby rats given *Ortho Molecular* nutrients grew 2206% faster than baby rats given conventional nutrients.") Profitable Nutrition Distributors, Inc., states that its sustained-release, high-potency formula includes "trace minerals which are naturally chelated and are in the exact proportions that exist in ancient sea water from which life arose." Country Life offers "cellular energy activators." NutriLogic promises that its "ultimate blend of highly bioavailable minerals ...transport total nutrition to all parts of your cells. Rainbow Light Nutritional Systems labels its nutrients as "food-grown." IntraCell Nutrition, Inc., describes the nutrients in its *Foodform Manna* as "protein bonded . . . . vitamins and minerals in their original state." American Health's *Total Energy Lift* is a "high-test formula" containing "over 100 'energy-lifting' food source nutrients." *Sun Chlorella* (a type of alga) is "not a substitute for vitamins or minerals, but is an ideal way to get more out of your vitamins and minerals."

Makers of KAL claims that its Multi-*Active* tablets"provide all the Designer Food Activity found in 4 pounds of fresh broccoli, apples, Brussels sprouts, potatoes and alfalfa sprouts combined." (KAL defines Designer Food Actives as "the extraordinary health-giving compounds locked inside fruits and vegetables—that scientists have recently linked with important health benefits.") And so on. (The list is endless.)

Most of these claims are pure hype. "High potency" is a misnomer because above-RDA doses are more likely to cause harm than they are to provide benefit. Nutrients are not "targeted" but are carried throughout the body in the bloodstream and are used as needed. Some nutrients are better absorbed when taken during mealtime, but the time of day is not important. Timed-release supplements are not advantageous because the body does not need a continuous supply of nutrients. Nutrient deficiencies do not develop by the hour—or overnight. Biochemical reactions are driven by nutrients that are stored, as well as by those that are ingested during a given day. People eating a varied and balanced diet will maintain stores that can last for weeks or even years, depending on the nutrient involved. As noted in Chapter 1, the body generally uses what it needs and excretes or stores the rest.

A few situations exist in which absorption characteristics are important. Calcium products vary significantly in their absorbability. And sustained-release niacin, which can be a potent *drug* for treating abnormal blood cholesterol levels, is less likely than ordinary (crystalline) niacin to cause flushing or burning of the skin but is far more likely to cause liver toxicity. It wouldn't surprise us if some of the above products are absorbed more rapidly, more completely, or more steadily than others. But aside from dosage (megadoses are more likely to cause trouble), we doubt that such characteristics make much difference.

Many manufacturers feature supplements that contain no sugar, preservatives, or artificial color or flavor. Others are touted to be "yeast-free." These products are an attempt to capitalize on groundless fears—generated by the health-food industry itself.

Some companies state that their supplement products are patented. The U.S. Patent Office does not require proof that a product actually works; the main requirement is that it be different from previously registered products.

Irrational Dosages

In 1985, two New Haven dietitians surveyed five pharmacies, three groceries, and three health-food stores and concluded that most of their multivitamin products were irrationally formulated. Most people who use these products are seeking "nutrition insurance." For this reason, products were considered appropriate if they contained amounts the dietitians considered suitable for this purpose: 50 to 200 percent of the U.S. RDA for the vitamins and minerals for which U.S. RDAs are available, and no more than 100 percent of others for which Estimated Safe and Adequate Daily Dietary Intakes have been suggested. The authors rated twenty-nine multivitamins (31 percent judged appropriate), 105 multivitamin/mineral preparations (15 percent appropriate), twenty-seven stress formulas (none appropriate), fifty B-complex preparations (none appropriate), fifty children's supplements (half appropriate), and six prenatal supplements (half appropriate). Most products judged inappropriate had too much of some vitamins and not enough of others. These ratings were actually too generous because there is no valid reason to take more than the U.S. RDA of any nutrient for "insurance." But they show how the vast majority of multivitamin products are unsuitable for such a purpose.

Don't Waste Your Money

The best way to get vitamins and minerals is from foods in a balanced diet. If your diet is missing any nutrients, it may also lack components (such as fiber) that will not be supplied by pills. If you think your diet may be deficient, analyze it by recording what you eat for several days and comparing the number of portions of food in the various food groups with those recommended in Appendix A of this book. If you don't feel comfortable doing this yourself, ask a registered dietitian or physician to help you. If you have a shortfall, try to correct it by adjusting your diet. If this is impossible, and you conclude that you need a supplement, purchase one whose label lists nothing above 100 percent of the U.S. RDA or Daily Value—and take one every other day. Since products meeting this description can be obtained for about a nickel per pill, this method would cost no more than a dollar a month. Unless you have been proven anemic with a blood test indicating that the anemia is due to lack of iron, avoid products that contain iron (see Chapter 1).

Remember, too, that vitamins and minerals in foods are biochemically *balanced* because foods contain a large number of other antioxidant, prooxidant, and nonoxidant biochemicals, all of which help balance one another's effects. Supplements are *unbalanced* because they lack the other biochemicals normally found in foods.

Supplementation may be appropriate for children up to two years old, for children who have poor eating habits, for some people on prolonged weight-reduction programs, for pregnant women (who need to have adequate folic acid and iron), for strict vegetarians (those who avoid eggs and milk as well as meat), and for people with certain illnesses, as directed by a physician. Women who eat few or no dairy products should also be concerned about calcium. And supplementary fluoride is vital to help strengthen the teeth of children growing up in nonfluoridated communities—a need that vitamin pushers rarely address.

Don't forget that if you waste money on unnecessary supplements, you are subsidizing an industry that is fundamentally dishonest.

4

More Ploys That Might Fool You

Without a doubt, quacks and vitamin pushers are reaching people emotionally—on a level that counts the most. What sells is not the quality of their products, but the ability to influence their audience. Their basic strategies are to promise the moon and knock the "competition." To one and all, they promise better health and a longer life. They offer solutions for virtually every health problem, including some they have invented. To those in pain, they promise relief. To the incurable, they offer hope. To the nutrition-conscious, they say, "Make sure you have enough." To a public worried about pollution, they say, "Buy natural." For ailments amenable to scientific health care, they offer "safer nontoxic alternatives." And they have an arsenal of ploys for defending themselves against criticism.

Chapter 2 describes how nutrition quackery is promoted. Now let's look further at propaganda techniques. To gain your allegiance it is not necessary to persuade you that all of the statements below are true. Just one may be enough to hook you.

"We really care about you!"

Many quacks are masters at persuading patients that they care about them. Some even post signs to this effect in their office. Although being "cared about" may provide a powerful psychological lift, it will not make a quack remedy effective. It may also encourage over-reliance on an inappropriate therapy.

"We offer alternatives."

Quackery promoters are adept at using slogans and buzzwords. During the 1970s, they popularized the word "natural" as a magic sales word. During the 1980s, the word "holistic" gained similar use. Today's leading buzzword is "alternative." Correctly used, it refers to methods that have equal value for a particular purpose. (An example would be two antibiotics capable of killing a particular organism.) When applied to questionable methods, however, the term is misleading because methods that are unsafe or ineffective are not reasonable alternatives to proven treatment. *For this reason, we place the word "alternative" in quotation marks when it refers to methods not generally accepted by the scientific community and which have no plausible rationale.*

"We treat the whole patient."

There is nothing wrong with giving due attention to a patient's lifestyle and social and emotional concerns in addition to physical problems. In fact, good physicians have always done this. Today, however, most practitioners who label themselves "holistic" are engaged in quackery and embrace the term as a marketing tool. Few actually "treat the whole patient."

"We attack the cause of disease."

Many quacks charge that doctors engage in "crisis medicine" and merely treat symptoms, while they can do much more. This idea is based on the notion that illness occurs because one's "vital force" is impaired and is remedied by strengthening it (see Chapter 13). Quacks claim that whatever they do will not only cure the ailment but will also prevent future trouble. Each of these claims is false. Illness can result from many factors, both internal and external, some of which have been identified and some of which are unknown. Scientific medical care can prevent certain diseases and reduce the odds of getting various others. There is no valid reason to believe that any "vitalistic" method prevents anything except poverty (and perhaps loneliness) among its practitioners.

"No side effects"

"Alternative" methods are often described as safer, gentler, and/or without side effects. If this were true—and often it is not—their "remedy" would be too weak to have *any* effect. Any medication potent enough to help people will be potent enough to cause side effects. FDA approval requires evidence that the likelihood of benefit far exceeds the probable harm.

"We treat medicine's failures."

It is often suggested that people seek "alternatives" because doctors are brusque, and that if doctors were more attentive, their patients would not turn to quacks. It is true that this sometimes happens, but most nutrition-related quackery does not involve medical care. Blaming doctors for quackery's persistence is like blaming astronomers for the popularity of astrology. Some people's needs exceed what ethical, scientific health care can provide. Some harbor deep-seated antagonism toward medical care and the concept of a scientific method. But the main reason for quackery's success is its ability to seduce people who are unsuspecting, gullible, or desperate. Several years ago a survey done in New Zealand found that most cancer patients who used "alternative" therapies were satisfied with their medical care and regarded "alternative" care only as a supplement. With vitamins, particularly with "nutrition insurance," many people feel as though they are making a bet with very little to lose and a great deal to gain.

"Think positive!"

Many quack promoters suggest that use of their method(s) will provide mental benefit that transcends the physical properties of their remedy. This is typically described in terms of "mind/body interaction," "mind over matter," or the power of positive thinking. A positive attitude may make people more apt to comply with an effective treatment regimen. Contrary to "popular wisdom," however, there is little scientific evidence that optimism or faith in a treatment causes people to live longer or to recover faster from an illness. Even if there were, it would not outweigh the dangers of misplaced trust.

"Jump on the bandwagon."

Quacks and vitamin pushers use several strategies to claim that their methods are popular (which may or may not be true), that popularity is a sign of effectiveness (which often is untrue), and that therefore you should try them. The popularity claim may involve endorsements or testimonials (which are inherently misleading) or statistics (which typically are inflated). The statistics can include the number of consumers supposedly using a method, how long the method has been in use, the number of practitioners administering it, and/or the length of time a practitioner or facility has been in business.

Surveys regarding popularity can be difficult to interpret. In 1987, *New Age Journal* reported that almost 100 percent of readers who responded to a questionnaire had used "alternative" health methods and that 97 percent would be willing to choose such methods for treatment of a potentially life-threatening illness. Yet 73 percent said that an "alternative" practice had harmed them and 57 percent felt that closer regulation was needed. The methods most often judged harmful were chiropractic, acupuncture, colonics, fasting, and various "natural" diets.

Have you heard that Americans make more visits to "alternative" practitioners than to medical doctors? This statement, which is false, is based on misinterpretation of figures published in *The New England Journal of Medicine*. Have you heard that "eighty percent of doctors take vitamin E"? This statement, which is false, is based on faulty interpretation of information published in *Medical Tribune*, a newspaper for physicians. As noted in Chapter 18, the media themselves have jumped on the bandwagon by publicizing these statements without examining their lack of validity. Nor do most reporters attempt to examine the true nature of "alternative" practices or what actually happens to people who use them.

"Time-tested"

This ploy suggests that the length of time a remedy has been used is a measure of its effectiveness. Its promoters imply that if the remedy didn't work, it wouldn't remain available. Some promoters claim (sometimes truthfully, sometimes not) that their methods have been handed down from generation to generation, are steeped in folk wisdom, were derived from ancient writings, or the like. The falsity of this ploy is easily seen by noting that astrology has survived for thousands of years with no reliable evidence of any validity. Note, too, that many genuine methods survive briefly because they are replaced by more effective ones.

"Backed by scientific studies"

Since most people regard scientific evidence as a plus, unscientific promoters claim to have it when in fact they do not. Their writings may list dozens or even hundreds of publications that supposedly support what they say. But the references they cite may be untraceable, misinterpreted, outdated, irrelevant, nonexistent, and/or based on poorly designed research. The classic example is Adelle Davis's book *Let's Get Well*, which lists 2,402 references. As we note in Chapter 17, many did not support her viewpoints and some were not even related to the passage in which they were cited. What should count is not the number of references but their quality and relevance—which the average reader will find difficult or impossible to judge.

"Take charge of your health!"

This is probably the most powerful slogan in the quack's bag of tricks. People generally like to feel that they are in control of their life. Quacks take advantage of this fact by giving their clients things to do—such as taking vitamin pills, preparing special foods, meditating, and the like. The activity may provide a psychological lift, but believing in false things tends to carry a high price tag. The price may be financial, psychological (when disillusionment sets in), physical (when the method is harmful or the person abandons effective care), or social (diversion from more constructive activities).

"I can help you."

Self-confidence tends to inspire trust, and quacks tend to exude confidence. Some quacks genuinely believe in themselves, while others are consummate actors. Many can spout one piece of biochemical nonsense after another and appear to believe every word they say. A recent case illustrates how dangerous it can be when vulnerable individuals fall into the clutches of a "healer" who knows no limitations. A few years ago, a Toronto couple, Sonia and Khachadour Atikian, were prosecuted for "failing to provide the necessities of life" for their daughter Lorie, who had died at the age of seventeen months. Courtroom testimony indicated that the child had died of pneumonia and malnutrition after being kept on a meager diet. Mrs. Atikian maintained that she was following the advice of Gerhard Hanswille, a local herbalist who claimed his system could help make Lorie a "superbaby."

Hanswille admitted that on the day before Lorie died, he had treated her with an "electromagnetic machine" and advised wrapping her in cabbage leaves. But he denied influencing Mrs. Atikian against conventional treatment and said he had told her to seek medical advice. Hanswille, who was unlicensed, also told the court that he held a "doctor of naturopathy" degree from Bernadean

University [a nonaccredited correspondence school discussed in Chapter 6]. One witness for the Atikians testified:

> The herbalist was a very impressive man. He just glowed with health and was very charismatic, very jovial, charming, friendly, very nice, very knowledgeable. There was not a question that you could ask that he would not have an answer for. And he told a lot of stories about people who had come to see him and been cured by following his course of treatment.
>
> It's a very difficult thing to communicate just how mesmerizing this man was. He was so good, so positive. He just exuded this powerful aura about him. He told my father that his cancer was completely curable. He had to change his diet because this was the cause of the cancer. He would have to eat strictly fruits and vegetables, raw, or juices of those fruits and vegetables, and by doing this, the tumor would be dissolved. When my father lost weight, the herbalist said this was just the body ridding itself of toxins and poisons. During his final two weeks, my father developed a hole near his rectum and a lesion that grew bigger each day. The herbalist said it was just the radiation coming out, which was a good thing. I now know it was gangrenous tumor. I look back . . . and can't believe that I fell under this man's spell.

The Atikians were actually tried three times. The first trial resulted in a guilty verdict that was overturned on appeal. The second concluded with a hung jury. The third ended when the judge ruled that the prosecutor had wrongfully withheld information from the defense attorneys. As consultants in the case, we thought that it was cruel to prosecute the Atikians and that the real culprit was Hanswille. He disappeared after the third trial when it appeared that the authorities might take action against him.

"Think for yourself."

Quacks urge people to disregard scientific evidence (which they cannot produce) in favor of personal experience (theirs or yours). But personal experience is not the best way to determine whether a method works. When someone feels better after having used a product or procedure, it is natural to give credit to whatever was done. Most ailments are self-limiting, and even incurable conditions can have sufficient day-to-day variation to enable quack methods to gain large followings. In addition, taking action often produces temporary relief of symptoms (a placebo effect). For these reasons, scientific experimentation is almost always necessary to establish whether health methods are really effective. Individual experience rarely provides a basis for separating cause-and-effect from coincidence. Nor can the odds of a treatment working be determined without following participants in a well-designed study and tabulating failures as well as successes—something quacks don't do.

"What have you got to lose?"

Quacks and vitamin pushers would like you to believe that their methods are harmless and therefore there is nothing to lose by trying them. If a method doesn't work, do the odds of it causing physical harm really matter? Moreover, some quack methods are directly harmful; others harm by diverting people from proven methods. All waste people's time and/or money.

"If only you had come earlier."

This phrase is handy when the treatment fails. It encourages patients and their survivors not to face the fact that consulting the quack was a mistake.

"Look who's on our side!"

Endorsements by prominent athletes and movie stars are a standard advertising practice. Vitamin pushers use endorsements (by athletes and vitamin-pushing gurus) in the standard manner, but have added a few wrinkles of their own. Some companies set up "scientific advisory boards" composed of individuals with M.D. or Ph.D. degrees. The few who are respectable scientists usually have nothing to do with the formulation or claims made for the products and may not even know how their names are being used for marketing purposes. Instances have occurred where scientific authorities have been identified as "advisors" without their knowledge or consent.

Some authors of vitamin-pushing books use another name-dropping technique: the acknowledgments section thanks prominent nutrition scientists and/or scientific groups for helping them with the book—even though those named would strongly disagree with the book's contents. The "help" may simply have been a publication that the book cited (and perhaps misinterpreted). Or it may have been a response to a question or two that the author posed in a letter or phone call. In the acknowledgments section of *Dr. Berger's Immune Power Diet,* Dr. Stuart Berger not only thanked twenty-nine "colleagues for their help on this book and in general," but also listed (as the core of his successful practice) more than a hundred "patients who became friends."

"Science doesn't have all the answers."

Quacks use this ploy to suggest looking beyond what scientific medicine has to offer; they also imply that since medical care has limitations, they are entitled to have them too. Medical science doesn't claim to have all the answers, but its effectiveness keeps increasing. The idea that people should turn to quack remedies when frustrated by science's inability to control a disease is irrational. Quackery lacks genuine answers and has no method for finding them.

"Don't be afraid to experiment."

This advice, which appeared in *New Age Journal's 1993–1994 Holistic Health Directory*, was based on the cliché that "what works for one person may not work for someone else with the same problem." Although this statement is literally true, scientific methods enable us to determine which methods are most likely to work and which ones are not worth trying. If a barrel is full of apples that are obviously rotten, does it make sense to sample all of them to see whether one tastes good?

"Let's work together."

This ploy is used to portray quacks as "nice guys" while suggesting that their critics are not. "Since science doesn't have the answers," they may say, "let's put our differences aside and work together for the common good." That would be fine if they had something to offer besides empty promises.

Proponents of "complementary medicine" claim to integrate scientific and "alternative" medicine, using the best of both. Is it helpful to add ineffective methods to effective ones? Does it make sense to go to someone who uses the "best" ineffective methods? Is someone whose reasoning process is faulty enough to believe in such things as homeopathy likely to deliver high-quality medical care? Do "complementary" practitioners use reliable methods as often as they should? From what we have seen, the answer to each of these questions is no.

"Keep an open mind."

Quacks portray themselves as innovators and suggest that their critics are rigid, elitist, biased, and closed to new ideas. Actually, they have things backwards. The real issue is whether a method works. Science provides ways to judge and discard unfounded ideas. Medical science progresses as new methods replace less effective ones. Quack methods persist as long as they remain marketable. Even after they are gone, they still may be glorified.

"Why don't you clean your own house!"

This type of statement comes up most often in debates between scientific and "alternative" practitioners, usually when the latter is not a medical doctor. Its aim is to portray the critic as a meddler or as someone with a grudge. A favorite ploy is, "Why don't you do something about unnecessary surgery?" The simple answer is that the shortcomings of medical care do not justify any form of quackery. Unnecessary surgery is an abuse of something that works and is entirely different from quackery, which is the use of things that do not work. Another big difference is that quackery is organized. There is no national organization of "Surgeons Dedicated to Unnecessary Surgery," but there are national organizations dedicated to quackery. Moreover, unlike members of the scientific community, quacks rarely criticize their own methodology or that of their colleagues.

"Prove me wrong!"

Quacks try to stand science on its head by demanding that their critics prove them wrong. Or they may say, "How do you know it doesn't work if you haven't tried it?" But there are not enough resources to test every idea that is proposed; for this reason, scientists tend to pursue those that seem most promising. Under the rules of science, the burden of proof is on the person who makes the claim. Unproven methods that lack a plausible rationale should be considered worthless until proven otherwise. Personal experience is not a substitute for scientific testing.

"We have no money for research."

When challenged about the lack of scientific evidence supporting what they espouse, promoters of quackery often claim that they lack the money to carry out research. However, preliminary research does not require funding or even much effort. The principal ingredients are careful clinical observations, detailed record-keeping, and long-term follow-up "to keep score." Advocates of "alternative" methods almost never do any of these things. Most who clamor for research do so as a ploy to arouse public sympathy. The last thing they want is a scientific test that could prove them wrong. If a scientific study is performed and comes out negative, proponents invariably claim that it was conducted improperly or that the evaluators were biased.

"I'm too busy getting sick people well."

Quacks use this response when asked why they have not tabulated their supposedly good results and submitted them for publication in a scientific journal. The key question, of course, is how can you know whether a method works without keeping careful score. The correct answer is that you can't. Even simple scorekeeping may provide significant information. In 1983, a naturopath named Steve Austin visited the Gerson Clinic and asked about thirty cancer patients to permit him to follow their progress. He was able to track twenty-one of them through annual letters or phone calls. At the five-year mark, only one was still alive (but not cancer-free); the rest had succumbed to their cancer.

"They persecuted Galileo!"

The history of science is laced with instances where great pioneers and their discoveries were met with resistance. William Harvey (nature of blood circulation), Joseph Lister (antiseptic technique) and Louis Pasteur (germ theory) are notable examples. Today's quacks boldly claim that they, too, are scientists ahead of their time. Close examination, however, will show how unlikely this is. Galileo, Harvey, Lister, and Pasteur overcame their opposition by demonstrating the soundness of their ideas.

"Health freedom"

Quacks use the slogan "health freedom" to divert attention away from themselves and toward victims of disease with whom we are naturally sympathetic. Quacks who insist that "people should have the freedom to choose whatever treatments they want" would like us to overlook two things. First, no one wants to be cheated, especially in matters of life and health. Victims of disease do not demand quack treatments because they want to exercise their "rights," but because they have been persuaded that they offer hope. Second, the laws that outlaw worthless nostrums are not directed against the victims of disease but at the promoters who attempt to exploit them. These laws simply require that products offered in the health marketplace be both safe and effective. If only safety were required, any substance that would not kill you on the spot could be hawked to the gullible.

5

Spreading the Word

Suggestions to take "dietary supplements" seem to be everywhere. Ads on radio and television and in magazines and newspapers warn against deficiencies. Self-appointed "experts," echoed by a chorus of believers, praise the "miracles" of nutrition. Colorful bottles line the shelves—not only in health-food stores but also in pharmacies, supermarkets, discount stores, and department stores. Some doctors even prescribe vitamins as placebos. The great vitamin push now costs consumers more than five billion dollars a year.

Why do people take supplements, and how do they decide which ones to buy?

Most vitamin users believe they are getting "nutritional insurance," but the majority also believe that extra vitamins can give extra energy, improve general health, and prevent disease. Consistent with these beliefs, most supplement users take multivitamin or vitamin-mineral preparations. Smaller numbers of users believe that individual supplements can prevent or relieve specific ailments. The most popular individual supplements are vitamin C, vitamin E, calcium, and the B-vitamins. Surveys suggest that multivitamin users are more likely to shop in pharmacies or supermarkets (where the prices are usually lower), while users of specific supplements are more likely to shop in health-food stores or by mail.

It is clear that many people who use individual supplements believe that these products have medicinal properties. Yet few such products contain health claims on their label. The reason for this is obvious. Unless a claim is backed by proof acceptable to the FDA (which simply means that there is reasonable evidence that it is true), it is illegal for a manufacturer to make that claim on a label or in any other manner related to the sale of a product. This chapter describes how the health-food industry disseminates information that would be illegal on product labels.

How the Law Works

The Federal Food, Drug, and Cosmetic Act defines "drug" as any article (except a device) "intended for use in the diagnosis, cure, mitigation, treatment, or prevention of disease" and "articles (other than food) intended to affect the structure or function of the body." For practical purposes, this means that a manufacturer or distributor who makes a health claim for a product (other than a device) marketed in interstate commerce renders that product subject to regulation as a drug. When dietary supplements are marketed without health claims, they are regulated as "foods," which simply means that their ingredients must be accurately stated on the label and be safe to take as directed. However, if the label contains a health claim—such as "boosts immunity" or "detoxifies the liver"—the law regards the product as a drug. Labeling includes not only the physical label but any written, printed, or graphic material that accompanies a product. Intended use is determined by the facts at hand, such as whether a book or flyer extolling a product's ingredients was shipped together with the product.

It is against the law to market a drug that is not generally recognized by experts as safe and effective for its intended purpose. Marketing such a product in interstate commerce without FDA approval is a federal crime called *marketing an unapproved new drug*. Marketing a drug without adequate directions is a federal crime called *misbranding*. Since adequate directions cannot be written for an unproven product, a manufacturer who makes unproven health claims for a product marketed in interstate commerce would commit at least two federal crimes. Products that are unapproved new drugs or misbranded can be seized and ultimately destroyed by government agencies.

To evade the law's intent, the health-food industry is organized to ensure that the public learns the intended uses of products, even though they rarely appear on product labels. This is done by promoting the *ingredients* of the products through publications, broadcasts, lectures, and person-to-person contacts. In some cases there is collusion between manufacturers and publicists, but in most cases there probably is not. The participants know their roles so well that there is little or no need for collusion.

Manufacturers vary in the extent to which they break the law. Some make no health claims for their products but rely on the print and broadcast media to make the claims for them. Others distribute product literature containing explicit claims, intended as bag-stuffers or for "confidential" use by retailers. Some manufacturers hold seminars, maintain a toll-free information hotline, publish a newsletter, furnish in-store lecturers, and/or advertise in health-food industry trade publications, health-food magazines, other magazines, and/or newspapers. Many manufacturers exhibit at health-food industry trade shows and/or health expos open to the general public, where they may or may not give out violative literature. A few manufacturers use public relations agencies or hold press conferences to boost ingredients in their products. Some manufacturers market through chiropractors, naturopaths, bogus "nutrition consultants," physicians who practice "nutritional medicine," and others who make the claims for them.

Many manufacturers give products names that suggest what they are for. Some names suggest that a product is suitable for a particular group of people. Others suggest that the product can help strengthen some part of the body. Others suggest that the product can enhance metabolism or exert some therapeutic effect. Whether this is illegal depends on the extent to which the name is misleading or creates an "intended use" that would not be legal to place on the product label. In most cases, the message is misleading because the product will not do what the name suggests. The FDA has curbed several products whose name implied that they would boost immunity and therefore might be helpful against AIDS. But most name-claim products have been ignored by government regulators.

The most widely known name-claim product is probably *Stresstabs*, which has no value against ordinary stress and has been marketed deceptively (see Chapter 3). Others include *Brain Power Pack, Candida-Cleanse, Cardio-Maxim, Clear Thinking, Ear-Vites, Fat Metabolizer, Hair-Vites, Immunoplex, Life Extension Mix, Maximum Virility, Nutri-Mem, Paracide Tabs, Prostex, Super Nails, Super-Male Plex,* and *Trymtone 1200.* None of these products can do what its name implies.

Advice from health-food retailers is another major factor in the sale of supplement products. Laypersons (such as health-food store clerks) who diagnose ailments or prescribe products from their stores are *practicing medicine without a license*—which is prohibited by state laws. "Prescribing" can also be construed as the unlawful practice of pharmacy. Although most health-food retailers violate this law routinely, only a few have been prosecuted as criminals.

Now let's examine some of the channels through which information flows.

From Manufacturer to Retailer

The most convenient way for manufacturers to communicate with retailers is through the trade magazines *Health Foods Business, Natural Foods Merchandiser,* and *Whole Foods.* Published monthly, all convey information about industry trends, economic and political developments, marketing techniques, and the alleged uses of various types of products. They also contain reader service cards that can be used to request information from any advertiser simply by circling the numbers corresponding to the ads that interest them. The magazines send computer-generated mailing labels to the manufacturers, who then send information to the stores, either directly or through regional distributors. Manufacturers who wish their ads to appear in issues containing articles promoting the ingredients of their products can easily arrange to do so. Each issue of *Whole Foods* includes a one-page "Consumer Bulletin," which, according to the magazine's publisher, is designed to stimulate sales. These are intended for reproduction and contain space for the store's name and location.

Trade shows (often referred to as "expos") provide opportunities for manufacturers and retailers to network and exchange information. The largest such shows are sponsored by the parent companies of *Natural Foods Merchandiser* and *Whole Foods* and by the National Nutritional Foods Association (NNFA), the largest association of health-food manufacturers, distributors, and retailers. Held annually, they usually feature exhibits by more than five hundred manufacturers and many lectures and seminars on marketing strategies, government regulatory policies, industry developments, "alternative" health practices, and various types of products. The discussions about supplement products focus on their ingredients and include claims that are false or unproven and that would be illegal on product labels. Tape recordings of the sessions can be purchased at the meetings or afterwards. Regional associations also hold annual trade shows.

Some manufacturers publish or sponsor newsletters that describe (or misrepresent) scientific developments related to the ingredients in their products. Some manufacturers and distributors sponsor seminars for retailers and/or "alternative" practitioners in which they recommend specific products or their ingredients for the treatment of diseases. The information conveyed would be illegal on product labels. Chapters 15 and 19 describe seminars that were visited by investigative reporters.

In 1984, investigators for *Consumer Reports* magazine contacted more than seventy companies that sold supplement products. After surveying their catalogs and other product information, the investigators placed orders and asked for additional literature to help explain the products' uses. More than forty of the companies sent literature containing therapeutic claims that were judged illegal by an expert panel assembled by the magazine. The details were published in the May 1985 issue in a cover story called "Foods, Drugs, or Frauds?" The percentage of manufacturers willing to distribute such literature is much lower today than it was ten years ago—thanks to tougher FDA enforcement policies. But the amount of misinformation reaching consumers has not diminished.

From Manufacturer to Consumer

Many manufacturers publish literature to "educate" consumers. Some mention products, others mention only information about ingredients. Some contain no information about the author or publisher, so if the FDA finds such a publication in a store, it may be impossible to hold the manufacturer responsible. Other manufacturers distribute literature from independent sources.

Manufacturers who publish a large amount of promotional material may provide a display rack to hold it. The all-time champion was probably Enzymatic Therapy, of Green Bay, Wisconsin, which provided "some of the best literature in the industry" until stopped from doing so by the FDA (see Chapter 19). Nature's Way, of Springville, Utah, was another prolific supplier.

During the 1980s, Makers of KAL, of Woodland Hills, California, distributed the KAL Self-Education Series, a collection of two-page flyers about various nutrients. Each flyer was loaded with scientific-sounding tidbits about the nutrient under consideration, followed by a list of references "as a service to those who would like to investigate the subject matter through their local college or university library system." The flyers we have collected contain a hodgepodge of research findings, biochemical tidbits, and other information (much of it misleading) that would be difficult or impossible for laypersons (and probably most physicians) to place in perspective. The company has also distributed similar Retailer Information Sheets to help retailers and "other readers" keep up-to-date on the products in their stores.

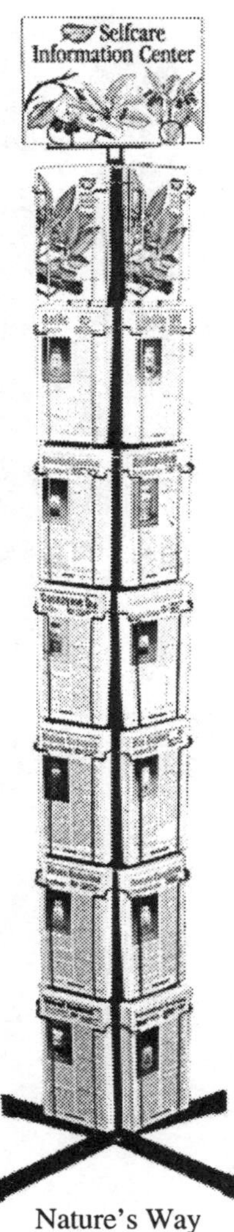

Nature's Way
Display Rack

Similar flyers with no identifiable publisher have been widely distributed through health-food stores. The author of one series was identified as Richard A. Passwater, Ph.D. Passwater, whose "Ph.D." is bogus, is discussed in Chapter 6.

Many manufacturers distribute reprints of magazine or newspaper articles discussing the ingredients in their products. Recently, for example, NuBiologics, Inc., of Downer's Grove, Illinois, sent chiropractors an article titled "Linus Pauling's Prescription for Health," which had appeared in

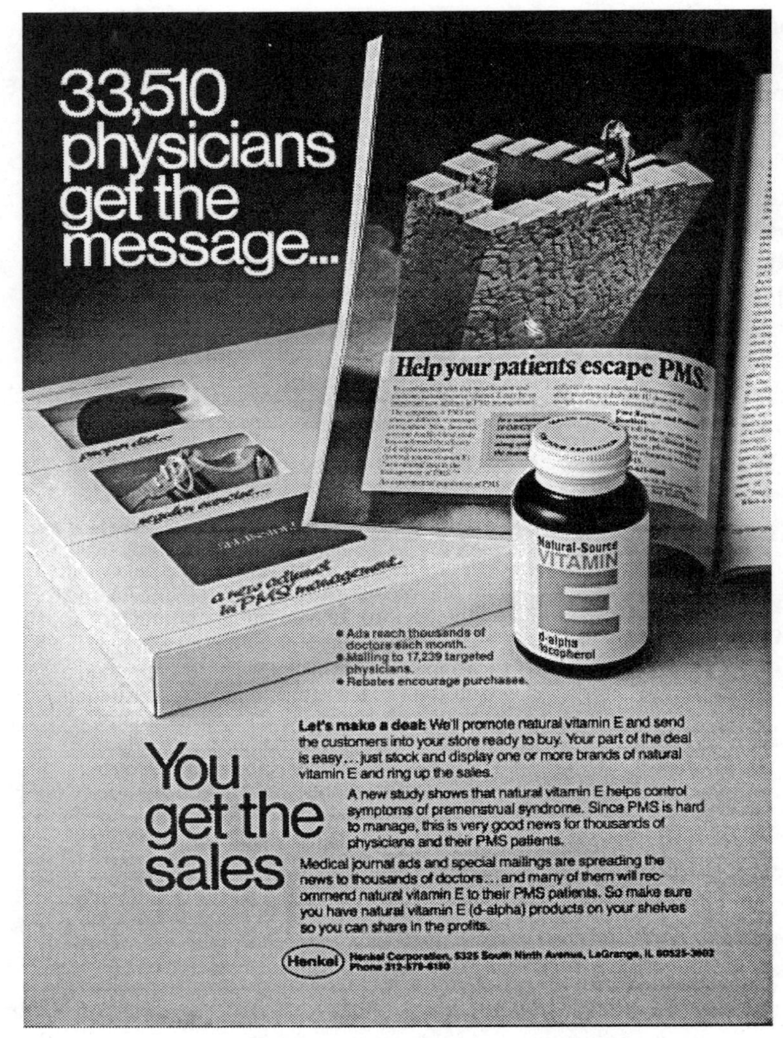

Ad in *Natural Foods Merchandiser*, April 1988

Natural Health magazine. At the bottom of the article the company listed three of its products in a box titled, "Here's a suggestion for following Dr. Pauling's Prescription for Health." Portions of the article pertaining to the ingredients of these products were underlined. The company offered retailers twelve free reprints with each twelve-bottle case of the three products. Its cover letter noted: "The education your patients will get from this article will motivate them to continue taking the nutrients they need for better health. . . . As Dr. Pauling says in the article, nutrients and particularly vitamin C . . . *will cut down the incidence of essentially all diseases.*"

Manufacturers are quick to capitalize on scientific studies that support—or appear to support—their product. 1988, for example, Henkel Corporation gave elaborate publicity to a study of vitamin E and premenstrual syndrome. The company, which is a major bulk wholesaler of vitamin E, advertised in medical journals as well as health-food industry channels. Retailers who responded to Henkel's ad in *Natural Food Merchandiser* received a reprint of the study plus a consumer pamphlet called "Taking Charge of Premenstrual Syndrome (PMS)." The pamphlet mentioned the study and contained a rebate coupon for any brand of "natural source vitamin E." A cover letter stated that more than half a million copies of the pamphlet had been distributed to doctors who requested them. Vitamin E, however, does not "take charge" of PMS.

In 1989, Michael's Health Products, of San Antonio, Texas, advertised in *Natural Foods Merchandiser* that when customers request something for arthritis, "you can offer them . . . everything they need in one tablet." (The fact that this would constitute the illegal practice of medicine was not mentioned in the ad.) Retailers who answered the ad were offered "over 60 different nutritional programs, each providing . . . all the vitamins, minerals, and herbs, plus any other nutrients needed for any specific physical condition." The company's twenty-four best sellers, said one brochure, included *Manpower Caps* (for impotence), *Artho Tabs* (to arrest arthritis), *Diab Tabs* (to provide natural insulin), *Circu Tabs* (to dissolve cholesterol, open arteries, and tone the heart), *Rena-Fit Tabs* (to remove kidney stones), and *Visi Tabs* (for cataracts and glaucoma). The $218.93 "special introductory package"—for products with a retail value of $614.43—included books containing a "scientific explanation of each program for education use," training on how to sell the product, and a lecture in or near the store by the company president, naturopath Michael Schwartz. The promotion was short-lived, however. Within two months, Texas Department of Health officials charged the company with making illegal therapeutic claims for thirty-seven products and issued an embargo to stop their sale. Schwartz agreed to a permanent injunction against advertising alleged curative powers that lack FDA approval. He also agreed to pay $15,000 in fines and costs. Currently, Michael's is offering "*CATA* with Vision factors, *FLX* with joint factors, *NRV* with Nerve factors, *LIPOLECITHIN* with Metabolism factors. . . . and many others."

"Independent" Publications

From the legal viewpoint, of course, it is much safer for manufacturers and retailers if someone else makes the claims for them. That's where independent publishers come in.

In 1993, more than $130 million was spent for books in health-food stores. Nutri-Books, of Denver, Colorado, describes itself as the world's largest supplier of health-related books and magazines. It stocks more than two thousand books, most of which promote questionable ideas and products. Its merchandising manual for retailers states:

> Books and magazines are your "silent sales force." . . .
>
> Books and magazines are designed like billboards. They reach out and "grab" the customer. They call out to your customers' problems—even their most personal and subconscious ones. . . .

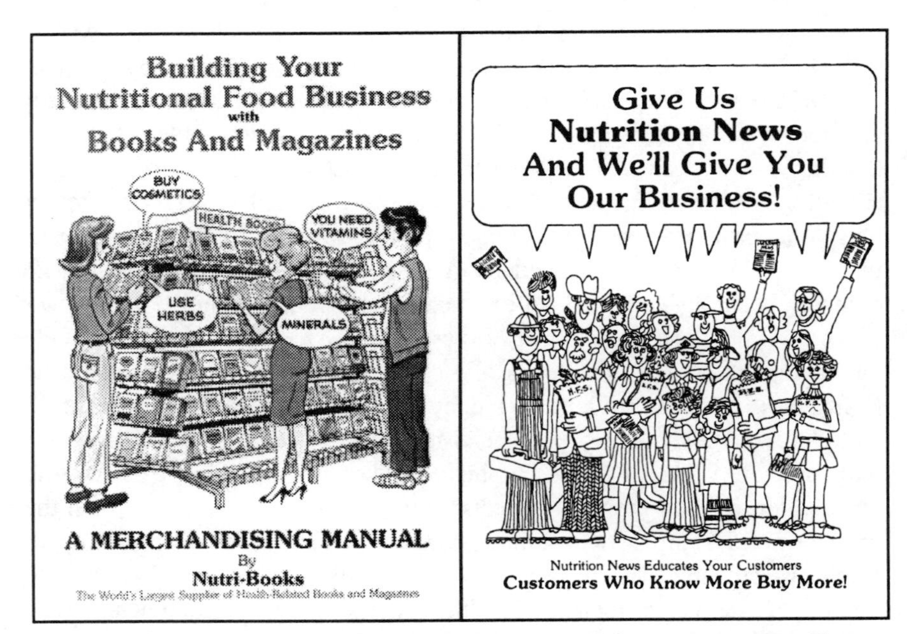

The Nutri-Books brochure depicts how books "call out" to customers. *The Nutrition News* ad promises that "educated" customers will buy more and "well-informed, enthusiastic" employees will sell more.

> They tell your customers what your products will do for them. They explain the ways your products can be used. Very often this is information you may not be able to give—or may not be permitted to discuss. . . .
>
> Sell a pound of wheat germ and it satisfies the customer's need. Sell a book and *it creates* a whole new set of needs in your customers.

The typical "health food" magazine is composed of articles that promote the products sold in health-food stores plus ads by manufacturers of such products. The ads contain no health claims, but the articles invariably contain claims that would not be legal on product labels because they are false or unproven. False claims in the magazine's text, however, are shielded by freedom of the press. Several magazines—most noticeably *Let's Live, Total Health,* and *Health World*—often place ads on the same pages as articles boosting their ingredients. The March 1994 *Let's Live*, for example, has a five-page spread containing an article and three ads for shark cartilage (a fake cancer remedy we discuss in Chapter 18). If there is no actual collusion between the manufacturer and personnel from the magazine, the set-up is legal.

Publications Philosophically Aligned with the Health-Food Industry

Magazines

Better Nutrition for Today's Living; Body, Mind & Spirit; The Choice; Choices; Delicious!; Digest of Alternative Medicine; Energy Times; FACT; Flex; Forefront; Good Medicine; Health Consciousness; Health Counselor; Health Freedom News; Health Science; Health World; Healthier Times; Herbalgram; Holistic Medicine; The Human Ecologist; Innovation; Let's Live; Longevity; Muscle & Fitness; Natural Health (formerly East West); New Age Journal; New Body; Newlife; Nutrition & Fitness; Nutritional Perspectives; Penthouse (Gary Null's articles); Prevention (editorials); Search for Health; Senior Health; Total Health; Townsend Letter for Doctors; Vegetarian Times; Your Health

Newsletters

Alternative Health Issues; Alternatives (published by David Williams, D.C.); Antha; Cancer Chronicles; Dr. Atkins' Health Revelations; Earl Mindell's Joy of Health; Forefront; Fountain; Health & Healing; Health Alert; Health Resource Newsletter; HealthFacts; The International DAMS Newsletter; Malibu Natural Health Letter; Men's Health Newsletter; Nutrition News (edited by Siri Khalsa); The Nutrition Reporter; People's Medical Society Newsletter; Pure Facts; Second Opinion; Vital Communications; Your Good Health

Newspapers

Health News & Review; Health Store News; Nutrition Health Review

Barbara Bassett, who edited and published *Bestways* magazine for more than ten years, addressed this subject at the 1987 NNFA annual meeting. During a panel discussion on "Educating the Consumer" she stated:

> When the need for [a product] is first perceived . . . it comes out in the print media. That's my role. . . .
>
> Manufacturers can't impute or imply the health benefits of their product. We all know that. Linking health benefits to a particular supplement or foods is still the exclusive domain of the press—of the print and broadcast media. . . .
>
> Keep books and magazines up-to-date and well displayed. . . . If possible, be informed of the contents of books and magazines and guide your customer. When they ask for information that you can't give, say, "It's there." . . .
>
> A manufacturer can't say that, "These are the benefits of coenzyme Q_{10}." But in print we can. . . . Display them together. Give your customer the chance to find that material . . . to tell . . . how to use the product. . . . You'll sell both the magazine and the product.

Bassett stressed that her magazine never plugged supplement or herbal products by brand name. However, manufacturers who wish their ads to appear in issues that promote their specific products can ensure this by utilizing the magazine's editorial schedule. Editors know that placing ads near promotional articles will make the ads more effective. All parties involved know that coordinating their efforts will benefit all parties concerned (except the buyers of worthless products). Bassett noted:

> The readers of *Bestways*—as we know from our surveys—93 percent will try new uses from articles. . . . So when you have a product in the store, they see the product in the magazine, and they are presold when they come in to look for it. . . . They spend over three hours reading each issue, and they shop for health-food products more than once a week. But in their shopping they spend less than twenty-five minutes per visit, which tells you that when they come in they already have an idea in their head what they want to buy. They spend over $35 per month.

In 1988, retailers who carried *Bestways* were offered a free monthly newsletter that could be reproduced for distribution to customers. The newsletter, called *Instore,* was imprinted with the store's name and contained summaries of *Bestways* articles.

New Hope Communications, publisher of *Natural Foods Merchandiser,* also publishes *Delicious!* magazine. Each monthly issue is filled with articles and charts that make unsubstantiated claims for foods and supplement ingredients sold in health-food stores. From 1987 to 1991, *Delicious!* contained a

"Shopping Guide" that listed manufacturers of products whose ingredients were mentioned in the articles. Some issues listed brand names as well. *Better Nutrition for Today's Living*, another magazine that promotes the gamut of supplement and health-food products, claims that its recent readership profile found that 79.3 percent of readers had purchased a product based on an ad or article they had read in the magazine. Many stores distribute free copies of one or both of these magazines to their customers.

Nutrition News, produced by Gurumantra and Siri Khalsa, is an independent newsletter that was launched in 1976. Each issue contains four pages and "presents a different health-related topic featuring products you carry in your store"—most often the supposed relationships between one or more "health-promoting nutrients" and various health problems. The newsletter is available by individual subscription and is sold in bulk to health-food stores for free distribution to customers. Mastheads can be customized, and back issues are available so that storekeepers have about seventy-five topics to choose from. "Your customers want to know what your products can do for them," said a recent solicitation. "Each month we publish an attractive, topical newsletter geared specifically to inform them and motivate them to buy those products. . . . Put *Nutrition News* in your store and you put the finest sales builder money can buy right into your customers' hands." Another solicitation stated: "Since retailers know topics in advance they can plan in-store promotions with sales support from us. More important, retailers report making back nearly $3 for every $1 they spend on *Nutrition News*."

Keats Publishing, of New Canaan, Connecticut, is by far the most prolific publisher of unscientific health and nutrition information. Established in 1971, it has issued more than four hundred books, of which over two hundred are still in print. It has also published more than ninety "Good Health Guides," booklets that focus on products or product categories.

Health Foods Business has published many articles describing how books can enhance the sales process. A 1977 issue, for example, describes how a proprietor "keeps a couple of nutrition textbooks handy under the sales counter and when a question arises about the function or use of a product, he looks it up. He's very careful to stress that he is not a physician and that what he says should be taken as informative rather than authoritative." In another issue, a storekeeper stated:

> *We can avoid prescribing through the use of books. . . .*
>
> In our stores we provide an area near the book display where people can sit and look at the books. . . . Sometimes they will then purchase one or more of the books, but even if they don't, they have

> usually found a suggestion of at least one product they will buy before leaving. . . .
>
> Any time we sell a book, we know that it will help to generate sales of other items within our stores.

The book most widely used as a sales tool is Avery Publishing Group's *Prescription for Nutritional Healing* (1990), by James F. Balch, Jr., M.D., and Phyllis A. Balch, "C.N.C." Its back cover describes Dr. Balch as a urologist who "has helped patients to assume a portion of responsibility for their own well-being" and has a newspaper column and a radio show. Mrs. Balch is described as a "certified nutrition consultant" who works in her husband's practice and has established a health-food store. The dubious nature of the "C.N.C." credential is described in Chapter 6.

About 250 of the book's 378 pages are devoted to an A-to-Z compendium of health problems and the authors' lists of nutrients that are "essential," "very important," or "helpful." Some lists contain more than thirty items. The authors recommend daily dosages of 3,000 mg or more of vitamin C for everybody ("for maintaining good health") and higher doses (up to 30,000 mg/day "under a doctor's supervision") for dozens of problems. They also recommend daily dosages of vitamin A ranging from 50,000 to 100,000 IU for many conditions and 75,000 IU for "maintaining healthy eyes." The vitamin C dosages are high enough to produce severe diarrhea; the vitamin A dosages are high enough to cause liver injury.

From a scientific viewpoint, the book's advice is loony from beginning to end. But from the supplement industry's standpoint, it is a gold mine. According to a 1992 flyer from the publisher:

> With over 175,000 sold during its first nine months, *Prescription for Nutritional Healing* has become the health-food industry's best-selling reference on supplementation available. . . . This complete and authoritative guide to dealing with health disorders through nutritional, herbal and supplemental therapies contains a complete listing of vitamins, herbs, and supplements—each with information on use, dosages, and benefits.
>
> Let *Prescription for Nutritional Healing* provide your customers with all the information they need to know to make informed purchasing decisions.

From Retailer to Customer

NNFA's handbook on giving information to customers lists five things that "You May Not Do Or Say!" These guidelines—which reflect NNFA's "Code

Increase your sales—
Sell our natural resources.

Prescription For Nutritional Healing

A Practical A-Z Reference to Drug-Free Remedies Using Vitamins, Minerals, Herbs, & Food Supplements
By James Balch, M.D. & Phyllis Balch, C.N.C.

The authors of health food store best seller *Nutritional Outline for the Professional*, now bring you the most up-to-date, comprehensive guide to good health-through-supplementation available to the general public in book form. Dr. Balch is an M.D. and health columnist, and his wife, Phyllis, is a certified nutritional consultant and owner of Good Things Naturally, a health food store in Indiana. They have combined over 35 years of professional experience in the fields of medicine, nutrition, and health food retailing, to provide a practical A-Z reference for both consumers and professionals. Not only does *Prescription for Nutritional Healing* provide your customers with nutritional treatments for over 250 common ailments and disorders, but IT also suggests a complete wellness program using the products you sell.

This complete and authoritative A-Z guide to dealing with health disorders through nutritional, herbal, and supplemental therapies contains a complete listing of vitamins, minerals, herbs, amino acids, enzymes, and food supplements—each with information on use, sources and proper dosages, explaining which nutrients will combat the condition, and then listing traditional remedies and therapies which can be used in conjunction with the suggested [illegible]. Insets throughout

A COMPREHENSIVE AND UP-TO-DATE SELF-HELP GUIDE

Prescription for
NUTRITIONAL HEALING

A PRACTICAL A-Z REFERENCE TO DRUG-FREE REMEDIES USING VITAMINS, MINERALS, HERBS & FOOD SUPPLEMENTS

JAMES F. BALCH, M.D. • PHYLLIS A. BALCH, C.N.C.

- Based on revolutionary ODA (Optimum Daily Allowance) requirements
- Includes recent breakthroughs on the healing value of nutrients including omega–3, coenzyme Q_{10} and SOD
- Information on chelation, juicing, and [illegible] surgical remedies/therapies [illegible] to yeast infection, ascorbic [illegible]ca, boron to zinc—a com[illegible]tional resource that will [illegible] customers select products [illegible]ctively
- Authors on extensive 24-city U.S. tour, including Dallas, Miami, New York, and San Diego. Scheduled appearances on national television and radio shows
- Planned space ads in *Prevention, Health World, Let's Live*
- Not just another book to sell: a book that *sells* your products!

THE GLOBAL BEST SELLING
VITAMIN & HERB GUIDE
The Ultimate Sales Tool
*Guaranteed to increase your sales in 6 major departments
ORDER TODAY FOR TOMORROW'S PROFITS
The Vitamin Herb Guide
NATURAL TREATMENTS
The best selling "VITAMIN & HERB GUIDE" holds the proven track record in sales of Vitamins, Minerals, Herbs, Tissue Salts, Amino Acids & Related Health Guides.
This invaluable selling tool has increased supplement sales by over 40% in the Canadian Health Food Stores in only three months.
Global Health has now revised & updated this best selling guide for the U.S. market so your stores can now take advantage of the overwhelming increase in sales that this guide creates.
This highly acclaimed and comprehensive guide is designed to give your customers more information in less reading time, at such an affordable price. That's precisely why busy people around the world rely on the "VITAMIN & HERB GUIDE".
AN INFORMED CUSTOMER IS YOUR BEST CUSTOMER!
*Global Health Guarantees Results — In the event that you do not see a significant increase in retail store sales, simply return the unsold guides within 120 days of purchase with your proof of purchase to, GLOBAL HEALTH, Box 18, Site 1, RR 2, Tofield, Alberta, Canada T0B 4J0 for a full and complete refund.

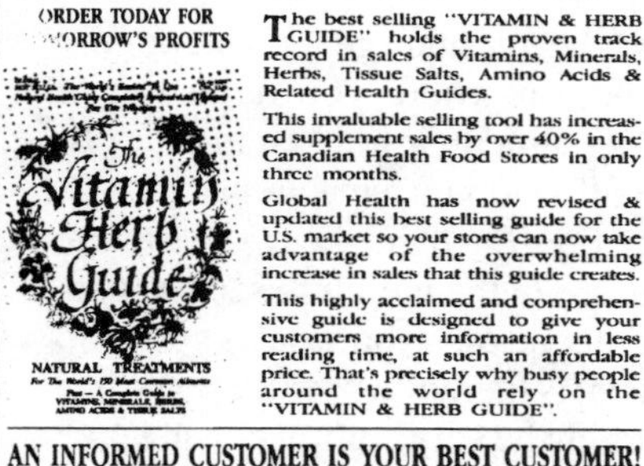

In ads to retailers, Avery Publishing's *Prescription for Nutritional Healing* is promised to "provide your customers with nutritional treatments for over 250 common ailments and conditions." Global Health's *Vitamin & Herb Guide* is said to have increased supplement sales in Canadian health-food Stores by over 40 percent in only three months.

of Ethics" as well as its legal advice—are meant to apply to telephone inquiries and public lectures as well as to situations within the store:

1. Do not diagnose! . . . This is the practice of medicine.
2. Do not prescribe! . . . This again involves the practice of medicine and should be scrupulously avoided.
3. Do not make claims that your products (or any specific product) is good for the treatment or cure of any disease condition! . . . Such statements could be construed not only as the dispensing of medical advice, but may also be construed as drug claims converting the food products which you sell into drugs. This then could entail the unlicensed practice of medicine and/or pharmacy.
4. Do not recommend any particular books or literature as being descriptive of the value of your products! . . . Avoid the temptation to recommend any particular book which you know to contain a discussion of the product or nutrient involved because such a recommendation would, as a matter of law, convert that book into labeling and claims for the product. . . . If you are confronted with a question asking you to recommend nutritional literature, you should refer your customer to the book section of your store and advise him that there he may find many interesting books and writings on a variety of subjects in the field of nutrition.
5. Do not display a particular book with a particular product! . . . It is likely that the book will be construed as labeling for the product if there is even the remotest connection between the two. This may be avoided by leaving the book in the book section of your store.

NNFA attorney Scott Bass informs retailers that the key to providing information without legal risk is to have a "real literature section" in their store. At the 1988 NNFA convention he advised:

> Make it separated from the products. Make it contain general literature. Don't make it an advertisement section where you have every company's specifically named product with their brand name. . . . If you have newspaper articles to reprint, fine. If you have books, fine. If you have articles people have sent you, fine. Put them there. Give them to your customer. But make sure they are in the literature section and you are not handing them out when someone asks you what is good for curing cancer or arthritis. . . . Say: "There is literature over there on that topic and I think it's very good and it might be very helpful to you." Let the customer make the decision.

Although industry leaders have devised ways to convey advice "indirectly," retailers actually risk little by making direct oral claims in the relative privacy of a store. Government enforcement efforts, which are limited, are directed primarily against manufacturers. Retailers are generally quite willing to give advice about supplements to their customers.

• In 1976, Eric Faucher, a *National Enquirer* reporter, visited sixteen health-food stores in major American cities and complained of afternoon fever, weight loss, insomnia, and fatigue—symptoms that could indicate a serious disease such as cancer. Only one salesperson told him to see a doctor. The rest prescribed various supplements for such diagnoses as "high blood pressure," "imbalance of energy," and "hypoglycemia." "One salesgirl was stumped by my symptoms," Faucher reported, "so she called up her mother (the store owner) who prescribed vitamin E without ever seeing me!"

• In 1980, Sheldon S. Stoffer, M.D., and three associates from the Northland Thyroid Laboratory in Southfield, Michigan, described what happened when several of their employees consulted a supervisor or "nutritionist" at ten health-food stores. The investigators stated that their goiter was being treated with thyroid hormone and asked whether any of the store's products would help. All ten retailers said yes. Two advised stopping the hormone treatment, six advised kelp, two advised iodine tablets, two advised a raw-gland preparation containing thyroid, parathyroid, pituitary and adrenal gland extracts, and one advised a raw thyroid preparation. (Health-food-store products made from animal glandular tissues are not legally permitted to contain potent amounts of hormones. Some do, however, as noted in Appendix C, but they are not reliable because the dosage is variable.) Other phony remedies included turnip tops, parsnips, parsley, malt tablets, and vitamin and mineral supplements.

• In 1981, Julian DeVries, seventy-six-year-old medical editor of the *Arizona Star*, visited a health-food store complaining of weight loss, loss of appetite, insomnia, leg cramps at night and psoriasis (a skin disorder). "Two young clerks sold me an assortment of vitamins for $124.34 that, according to a doctor, easily could have worsened the conditions I told them I had," DeVries reported. Instead of being referred to a physician for diagnosis of his possibly serious symptoms, he was sold megadoses of several vitamins; a product containing ginseng and an adrenal substance; digestive enzyme tablets; an iron-and-molasses compound; tryptophan tablets; skin cream containing vitamin E and PABA; and a book that suggested a nutritional cure for almost every ailment known to humans. The clerks said that their recommendations were authoritative because they had taken a three-week course in vitamin nutrition in which the book was used.

• In 1983, researchers from the *Columbus Monthly* contacted nine health-food stores in central Ohio, by phone or in person, posing as women suffering from an undiagnosed eye condition, a mother-to-be seeking nutrition information for her pregnancy, a recent heart attack victim, and a would-be weightlifter seeking to build muscles. They concluded that although the store clerks appeared to be sincere, their advice was "like flipping a coin."

• In 1983, three investigators from the American Council on Science and Health made 105 inquiries by phone or in person at stores in New York, New Jersey, and Connecticut. Asked about eye symptoms characteristic of glaucoma, twelve retailers attempted to diagnose the problem (all incorrectly) and seventeen out of twenty-four suggested a wide variety of products for the investigator's "mother." None recognized that urgent medical care was needed. Asked over the telephone about sudden, unexplained fifteen-pound weight loss in one month's time, nine out of seventeen recommended products sold in their store; only seven suggested medical evaluation. Seven out of ten stores carried "starch blockers" (bogus diet pills) despite an FDA ban. Nine out of ten recommended bone meal and dolomite, products considered hazardous because of contamination with lead. Nine retailers made false claims of effectiveness for bee pollen, and ten did so for RNA. The investigators concluded that most health-food store clerks give advice that is irrational, unsafe, and illegal.

• In 1986, Claire Aigner, R.D. posed five similar questions to ten health-food store proprietors in eastern Pennsylvania and concluded that fewer than half the answers were correct.

• In 1991, Julia M. Haidet, a student at Kent State University, made thirty phone calls to ten stores in Central Ohio for advice about headaches, kidney stones, or abnormal thirst, dizziness, and fatigue. She received no appropriate advice.

• In 1993, armed with a hidden camera, "Inside Edition" visited four health-food stores in New York City to ask whether they carried anything for fatigue and headaches; blurred vision; arthritis; shortness of breath of a "grandmother who just had bypass surgery"; strengthening the immune system; improving memory; and/or "cleansing the blood." Products were recommended in response to every question. When asked for a product that could help people with AIDS, one GNC store manager recommended an amino acid product that he said was one of the store's top sellers. He also said the product was supposed to "help block the chemical inhibiting the growth of the virus" and did not have the toxic side effects of AZT. When confronted later, however, he denied recommending the product for AIDS.

• In 1993, "CBS Evening News" showed: (1) a GNC clerk recommending a vitamin product to prevent hair loss, (2) a Nature Food Centres clerk endorsing a fish-oil product as an arthritis cure, and (3) another retailer recommending "E, C, A, shark-oil capsules, all of these things help" for cancer. The program reported that CBS News had sent fifty vitamin and mineral product to independent laboratories for analysis to see whether they contained the amounts claimed on their labels. Many were found to contain too little or too much. Michael Jacobson, Ph.D., executive director of the Center for Science in the Public Interest, commented that going into a health-food store "is like being the victim of one hundred different snake oil salesmen."

• In 1993, FDA agents visited local health-food stores throughout the United States, posing as prospective customers. The investigators asked, "What do you sell to help high blood pressure?" "Do you have anything to help fight infection or help my immune system?" and/or "Do you have anything that works on cancer?" Of 129 requests for information, 120 resulted in recommendations of specific dietary supplements. In twenty-three cases, the retailer looked up the answer in *Prescription for Nutritional Healing* or advised the agent to refer to or purchase the book.

• John Renner, M.D., president of the Consumer Health Information and Research Institute and a board member of the National Council Against Health Fraud, has sought advice for health problems at more than a hundred health-food stores in twenty states and the District of Columbia. In all but two stores, he was advised to buy products. Renner also observed hundreds of customers shopping at these stores. More than half asked for advice about a health problem, and almost all questions led to inappropriate advice.

The prevalence of bad advice is not surprising. Retailers absorb much of their misinformation from the very same sources as their customers. In fact, many retail clerks are former customers. The American Entrepreneurs Association's health food/vitamin store business manual states:

> One of the best sources of informed employees is your customer base; the type of people who trade with you will consist of people who are enthusiastic about nutrition and health matters. . . . Some operators . . . get 90 percent of their new employees from the ranks of current customers and have found this more effective than hiring a totally untrained or uncommitted individual. You can easily see that a person who is "presold" on health consciousness is more likely to do the kind of salesmanship that you need for building volume.

From Store to "Star"

Many retailers appear on local radio or TV shows where it is legally safe to give advice as long as specific products are not recommended. "Getting on a talk show is not difficult," says an article in *Health Foods Business,* entitled "From Store to Star":

> Nutrition is a popular and controversial subject these days, and you, a health food store owner, are—by definition—an expert on the subject. . . . Chances are good that a station in your area would like to do a talk show on the subject, particularly if the guest is an area businessperson.

Some retailers host their own radio programs. Many others are hosted by dedicated promoters of quackery and food faddism. In the New York City metropolitan area alone, there are a dozen shows that specialize in dispensing unsound nutrition and health advice. Some radio stations permit advertisers to either suggest guests or come on the program themselves to discuss their products and related health issues. Manufacturers commonly subsidize such programs either directly or through dollars spent advertising their products. For example, former NNFA president Stan Jacobson has organized a program called "Natural Grocer" which is aired in several states. Sponsored by seventy-five stores and twenty manufacturers, the program has store owners and "nutritionists" as local hosts. Its guests include authors, "nutritionally oriented doctors," and store representatives.

NNFA itself sponsored a talk show that began in 1970 and aired for about ten years. Called "Viewpoint on Nutrition," it was broadcast by more than forty radio and TV stations. Most of the program's guests were food faddists, and its conversations invariably recommended "natural" foods and food supplements. Its host was Arnold Pike, D.C., who was NNFA's public information director. On the programs we saw, Pike was introduced as "Dr. Arnold Pike" and not identified as a chiropractor. Nor was his affiliation with NNFA revealed.

"Here's to Your Health" is broadcast by Independent Broadcasters Network to more than 140 affiliates coast to coast. In an interview in *Natural Foods Merchandiser*, hostess Deborah Ray said that the show receives more responses than any other on the network, more than 130 calls per day, and three hundred letters a week. The program promotes the gamut of health-food industry ideas as well as information on new products. Listeners who ask for further information are referred to local stores who help sponsor the program.

Catalog Sales

Dietary supplement products also are sold through mail-order catalogs. Some companies market their own lines of products in this manner. Others include a few pages of supplement products in general merchandise catalogs. A few compete with health-food stores by carrying the products of many manufacturers at discounts of 20 percent or more. The three largest discounters appear to be Swanson's Health Products, of Fargo, North Dakota; L&H Vitamins, of Long Island City, New York; and The Vitamin Shoppe, of West Bergen, New Jersey. All three issue newspaper-style catalogs filled with articles that promote specific products or product ingredients and are accompanied by display ads for the products. Until recently, most of these products were promoted with claims that would be illegal on product labels. These companies also sell promotional books.

The largest company selling its own product line by mail is probably Nature's Bounty, of Bohemia, New York, doing business as Puritan's Pride. During the past ten years, its catalogs have contained false and misleading claims for scores of products. In November 1990, postal officials filed a false representation complaint charging that at least nineteen Puritan's Pride products were falsely advertised. The products included *Cholesto-Flush, Fatbuster Diet Tea, Kidney Flush, Memory Booster, Prostex, and Stress B with 500 mg Vitamin C.* In May 1991, the case was settled with a consent agreement under which Nature's Bounty admitted no wrongdoing but agreed to stop making the

NNFA Code of Ethics

As a member of the National Nutritional Foods Association I will strive to adhere to the following Code of Ethics:

- I will sell or supply only those foods, food supplements and accessories that may be helpful to consumers who seek to maintain or improve physical fitness and good nutrition, or seek to correct nutritional deficiencies.
- I will not engage in the treatment, diagnosis, or prescribing for any pathology.
- I will not knowingly sell or supply those foods that contain harmful chemical food additives or artificial ingredients that are alien to the recognized concept of natural foods, nor will I knowingly deal in products that are untruthfully advertised.
- I will not engage in false or misleading advertising.
- I will support public measures that protect the environment, safeguard our natural resources, and improve the quality of life.
- I will cooperate with all professional, educational, civic, and consumer organizations that support greater nutritional information and consumer rights.
- To help implement this Code, NNFA designated the month of April as NATURAL FOOD MONTH in which special efforts will be made to enlighten the public about the importance of improving health and nutrition through natural farming methods, protecting the environment and conserving our natural resources.
- In pursuit of these goals, I will vigorously defend our first amendment right to freedom of speech and press to impart truthful information concerning diet and nutrition and will defend the health freedom right of consumers to obtain such data from the sources that they may choose.

How many of these guidelines do you think health-food manufacturers and retailers follow?

challenged claims. Subsequent catalogs contain no blatant therapeutic claims but promote "nutrition insurance" with misleading statements.

Another active marketer is Home Health Products, Inc., of Virginia Beach, Virginia, which specializes in "natural products for a holistic approach to health care" and bills itself as an "official supplier of Edgar Cayce products for health, beauty, and wellness." (Cayce was an alleged clairvoyant who combined "psychic readings" with spiritual and dietary advice.) Home Health's own products include skin conditioners, laxatives, and a few supplements, but its catalog also offers supplements made by other companies. Its offerings have included: (1) *ANF-22*, touted as "powerful relief from the pain, swelling and stiffness of arthritis"; (2) *Aphro* "Herbal Love Tonic"; (3) *Bio Ear*, said to provide "all-natural relief for ringing, buzzing, and noise in the ear"; (4) *Brain Waves*, described as a mental stimulant; (5) *Cata-Vite* (formerly *Cata-Rx*), said to be "a safe non-prescription formula which counteracts nutritional deficiencies associated with age-related cataracts"; (6) *His Ease*, alleged to "increase seminal fluid and sexual virility"; (7) *Kidney Flush*, claimed to "help flush away urinary infections"; (8) *Liva-Life*, for "toxic overload"; (9) *Liver Tonic Detoxifier*, "an all-natural mixture that detoxifies and cleanses the liver"; (10) *Prostate Plus*, proposed as an alternative to surgery; (11) *Ribo Flex*, "muscle/joint nourishment that reduces painful muscle spasms and enhances natural flexing action"; (12) *Sugar Block*, said to "prevent absorption of unwanted sugar"; (13) *Thyro-Vital*, claimed to "improve thyroid function"; and (14) *Jerusalem Artichoke Capsules*, an Edgar Cayce product described as "a natural equivalent to insulin injections."

Consumer Beware!

The health-food industry espouses a huge number of "treatment" methods. Thousands of supplement products are produced by hundreds of manufacturers, and a wide variety of foods are promoted for their supposedly special health-giving properties. The overall industry philosophy seems to be that virtually anything is worth trying and that "more is better" when it comes to dosage. Its salespeople may not understand biochemistry, but they do know how to sell.

The degree of danger in following advice from a popular publication, a talk show, a health-food store clerk, or a mail-order catalog varies with the degree of customer belief and the presence or absence of significant illness. Reliance upon a questionable method can endanger your health or your life in addition to your pocketbook. Federal regulation has driven most false claims from product labels. But it is clear that the health-food industry has little difficulty in reaching consumers through other means.

6

Dubious Credentials

In 1983, Jacob W. Kulp, D.C., of Cheektowaga, New York, pled guilty to a charge of violating federal drug law by claiming that wheat bran tablets would improve a patient's nutrient absorption by eliminating "black intestinal plaque"—a condition unknown to medical science. The "patient" was an undercover agent for the U.S. Postal Inspection Service who paid $25 for the advice. Kulp was sentenced to six months' probation with special conditions that he not pose as a nutritionist or give nutritional advice through broadcast media unless he acquires a graduate degree in nutrition from an accredited college or university.

In 1985, New York State Attorney General Robert Abrams filed a civil suit accusing Gary Pace, of Garden City, N.Y., of practicing medicine without a license, false advertising, and illegal use of educational credentials. Pace's schemes, said Abrams, induced hundreds of consumers to pay him for improper physical examinations, worthless laboratory tests (including hair analysis and herbal crystallization analysis), bogus nutritional advice, and unnecessary vitamin, mineral, and herbal supplements. The case against Pace was supported by affidavits from thirteen aggrieved clients and two undercover investigators, all of whom had been advised to take supplements. Some of the female clients reported that Pace had examined their breasts or genitals. Several clients underwent significant expense to obtain medical reassurance that they did not have various diseases that Pace said they had. One was advised by her medical doctor to stop taking vitamin A because her palms had become yellow as a result of overdosage. Abrams said that at least 251 clients had paid Pace an average of $307 during the previous four years. Many had been attracted by his ad

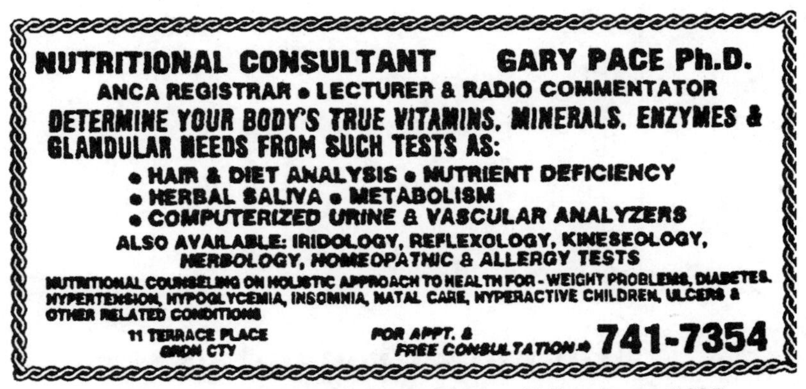

Ad by Gary Pace, "Ph.D.," in Nassau County Yellow Pages (1985)

(pictured above), which was the largest of eleven listings in the "Nutritionists" section of the Nassau County Yellow Pages. Pace also taught in the extension division of a local community college and hosted a radio program. The investigators discovered that the "free consultation" promised in Pace's Yellow Page ad was merely the brief telephone conversation in which he advised prospective clients to make an appointment. The case was settled with an injunction forbidding Pace from engaging in the unlawful practice of medicine or using "Ph.D." or "Dr." in dealings with the public unless he obtains a degree from an institution recognized by New York State. Pace agreed to pay $2,000 to the state and to make restitution to dissatisfied clients. He also agreed not to do further "nutritional counseling" unless he obtains proper credentials or posts a $150,000 bond.

Kulp and Pace had two things in common: (1) they were not qualified to practice medicine or give nutrition advice; and (2) each sported a "Ph.D. degree" in nutrition from Donsbach University, a nonaccredited correspondence school.

Why Reliable Credentials Are Important

During the past century or so, educational authorities have established a system of accreditation whose goal is to ensure that schools meet appropriate standards of quality. At the same time, state governments have established licensing systems for many professions to ensure that practitioners meet appropriate standards of competence. In many fields, professional groups have established certification procedures that recognize additional levels of expertise. In the field of health and nutrition, accreditation, licensure, and certification are important because laypersons rarely can evaluate professional competence.

Accreditation means that a school's credits can be transferred to other schools and be used as a basis for entering various professions. In the United States, educational standards are set by a network of accrediting agencies approved by the U.S. Secretary of Education or the Council on Postsecondary Accreditation. Attendance at an accredited school does not guarantee that a health or nutrition practitioner is competent, but the vast majority are.

In most health-related fields, licensure requires a degree from an accredited school plus passage of an examination. Licensure indicates that the state government has recognized the achievement of a basic level of competence. Certification conveys an additional endorsement of expertise. There are many subjects in which self-taught individuals can acquire expertise with little or no formal education. However, the fields of health and nutrition are sufficiently complex that home study cannot produce an expert. In fact, *lack of accredited training virtually guarantees incompetence.*

The accreditation system is not perfect. Accreditation is not based on soundness of academic content, but on such factors as record-keeping, physical assets, financial status, makeup of the governing body, catalog characteristics, nondiscrimination policy, and self-evaluation system. In recent years, accrediting agencies have been recognized for schools of chiropractic (see Chapter 15), naturopathy (see Chapter 13), and acupuncture (see Chapter 12), all of which teach unscientific concepts. A few other accredited schools grant health-related "Ph.D." degrees based on "research" that would be unacceptable in a standard university-based program. All states license chiropractors; and some states license practitioners of naturopathy, acupuncture, homeopathy, and Chinese medicine. Licensing of these professions was based on their ability to garner legislative support and not on soundness of their practices.

During the past fifteen years, nonaccredited correspondence schools and other organizations have issued thousands of "degrees" and certificates which suggest that the recipient is a qualified expert in nutrition. These documents have been promoted as though they are equivalent in meaning to established credentials—which they are not. Some were obtained by licensed professionals such as chiropractors, but most were acquired by health-food retailers and others who, like Pace, set up shop as a "nutrition consultant."

Now let's look at how credentials like these have been generated.

The Mercurial Kurt Donsbach

Kurt W. Donsbach, D.C., has played an important role in keeping the health-food industry several steps ahead of the law. From 1975 through 1989 he was chairman of the board of governors of the National Health Federation (NHF), the health-food industry's militant lobbying arm (see Chapter 20). Throughout most of this period, he directed nonaccredited programs that issued "degrees" and other "credentials" in nutrition. His other activities have been so numerous and complex that no one—including Donsbach himself—seems able to document all of them with certainty.

Donsbach (pronounced Dons'-bah) graduated in 1957 from Western States Chiropractic College, in Portland, Oregon, and practiced as a chiropractor in Montana, "specializing in treatment of arthritic and rheumatoid disorders." Later he acquired a license to practice naturopathy in Oregon, based on a degree from the Hollywood College School of Naturopathy. From 1961 to 1965 he worked in "research development and marketing" for Standard Process Laboratories (a division of Royal Lee's Vitamin Products Company) and the Lee Foundation for Nutritional Research, headquartered in Milwaukee, Wisconsin (see Chapter 20).While working for Lee, Donsbach lived in California, did literature research, and gave nutrition seminars (primarily to chiropractors) on how to determine nutritional deficiencies. After Lee became ill, Donsbach left his employ and opened Nature's Way Health Food Store, in Westminster, California, and Westpro Laboratories, in Garden Grove, California, which repackaged dietary supplements and a few drugs.

In 1970, undercover agents of the Fraud Division of the California Bureau of Food and Drug observed Donsbach telling customers in his store that vitamins, minerals, and/or herbal tea were effective against cancer, heart disease, emphysema (a chronic lung disease), and many other ailments. Most of the products Donsbach "prescribed" were packaged by Westpro Labs. Charged with nine counts of illegal activity, Donsbach pleaded guilty in 1971 to one count of practicing medicine without a license and agreed to cease "nutritional consultation." He was assessed $2,750 and served two years' summary probation.

In 1973, Donsbach was charged with nine more counts of illegal activity, including misbranding of drugs; selling, holding for sale, or offering for sale, new drugs without having the proper applications on file; and manufacturing drugs without a license. After pleading "no contest" to one of the "new drug" charges, he was ordered to pay a small fine and was placed on two years' summary probation with the provision that he rid himself of all proprietary interest in Westpro Labs. In 1974, he was found guilty of violating his probation and was fined again.

Donsbach sold the company to RichLife, Inc., of Anaheim, California, for $250,000. He was also promised $20,000 a year for occasionally conducting seminars and operating the company's booth at trade shows. The agreement gave RichLife sole right to market Dr. Donsbach Pak Vitamins, which RichLife later described as "specialized formulas" to "help make your life less complicated, more healthy." Among the products were *Arth Pak, Athletic Pak, Dynamite Pak, Health and Beauty Pak,* and *Stress Formula Pak.*

In 1975, after briefly operating another vitamin company, Donsbach began producing a large series of "Dr. Donsbach tells you everything you always wanted to know about . . ." booklets on such topics as acne, arthritis, cataracts, ginseng, glandular extracts, heart disease, and metabolic cancer therapies. The booklets were published by the International Institute of Natural Health Sciences—operated by Donsbach—which sold distribution rights to RichLife. Donsbach says that his books and booklets have sold more than fourteen million copies. Donsbach also produced *Dr. Donsbach's Nutritional Tape Cassettes,* which were sold through health-food stores. Nutri-Books, which distributed twelve such tapes, said they were "like having Dr. Donsbach as your personal physician right in your own home. Each . . . gives pertinent information and direction to aid in diagnosis and remedial action."

In 1980, the District Attorney of Orange County charged RichLife with making false and illegal claims for various products, including some originally formulated by Donsbach. In a court-approved settlement, RichLife paid $50,000 and agreed to stop making the claims. In 1986, RichLife was charged with violating this agreement and was assessed $48,000 more in another court-approved settlement.

In 1984, Donsbach was sued by Jacob Stake, of Urbana, Illinois, who became ill and was hospitalized as a result of ingesting large amounts of vitamin A over a two-and-a-half-year period. The suit papers state that Stake began taking the vitamin at age sixteen because it was recommended in Donsbach's booklet on acne. The case was settled out of court for about $35,000.

During the mid-1970s, Donsbach affiliated with Union University, a nonaccredited school in Los Angeles, where he says he acquired a master's degree in molecular biology and a Ph.D. in nutrition. In a deposition in the Stake case, he testified that he also was awarded an honorary doctor of science degree from Christian University, a nonaccredited school which had operated in Los Angeles. However, two reporters have said he told them that his "D.Sc." was obtained from a Midwest Bible college. In 1977, Union University formed a Department of Nutrition—"with Kurt Donsbach, Ph.D., Sc.D., as Dean of the Department." RichLife, which still was selling "Dr. Donsbach" supplements, offered scholarships to retailers who carried its products and wished to work toward a degree at Union. Soon afterward, Donsbach launched and became president of his own school, Donsbach University, which in 1979 was "authorized" by California to grant degrees. This status had nothing to do with accreditation or other academic recognition, but merely required the filing of an affidavit describing the school's program and asserting that it had at least $50,000 in assets.

Donsbach University, which operated mainly by mail, initially offered courses leading to B.S., M.S., and Ph.D. "degrees" in nutrition at fees ranging from $1,495 to $3,795, with a 20 percent discount for advance payment. Most of the "textbooks" required for the "basic curriculum" were books written for the general public by promoters of questionable nutrition practices, including Donsbach, Carlton Fredericks, Lendon Smith, and Robert Atkins. The original "faculty" had seven members, including Donsbach and Alan Nittler, M.D., a physician whose California medical license had been revoked for using "nutritional therapies." But ads for the school promised "the finest quality nutrition education available anywhere." Donsbach University also offered courses in iridology, homeopathy, herbal therapy, and chiropractic business administration, as well as a $495 "mini-course" for health-food retailers who wanted a "Dietary Consultant" certificate.

The fact that Donsbach University was not accredited did not deter Donsbach from claiming that it was—by the National Accreditation Association (N.A.A.) of Riverdale, Maryland. But this "agency" had no official standing. It was formed in 1980 by a California chiropractor and granted "accreditation" to Donsbach University a few months later. In 1981, Dr. William Jarvis, President of the National Council Against Health Fraud, visited N.A.A. in Maryland. He reported that its "office" was a telephone in the living room of the executive director, who said he received $100-a-month salary. Although N.A.A. correspondence had designated the man as holding a "Ph.D." from the Sussex College of Technology in England, the British Embassy informed Jarvis that it did not consider the "school" or its diplomas valid. N.A.A. quietly disappeared after the California Department of Education warned Donsbach to stop misrepresenting the significance of N.A.A. "accreditation."

In 1979, Donsbach launched the International Academy of Nutritional Consultants, which offered general memberships (to anyone) for $10 per year and "professional memberships" for $50 per year. The $50 fee included a directory listing plus a "beautiful certificate for your office." During 1983, the International Academy of Nutritional Consultants merged with a similar group to become the American Association of Nutritional Consultants. The only requirement for "professional membership" in either of these groups was submission of a name, an address, and a check for $50. Several investigators, including both of us, had no difficulty in obtaining such membership in the name of a household pet.

In 1985, New York Attorney General Robert Abrams brought actions against Donsbach, his university, and the International Institute of Natural Health Sciences, charging that they lacked legal authorization to conduct business within New York State and that it was illegal to advertise a nonaccredited degree to state residents. Abrams also charged that the institute's Nutrient Deficiency Test was "a scheme to defraud consumers" by inducing them to buy dietary supplements to correct supposed deficiencies reported with the test.

This test was composed of 245 yes/no questions about symptoms. When the answers were fed into a computer, a report of supposed nutrient deficiencies and medical conditions was printed out. The questions did not provide a basis for evaluating nutritional status. Moreover, a scientist with the FDA's Buffalo district office who analyzed the test's computer program as part of the Kulp investigation found that no matter how the questions were answered, the test reported several "nutrient deficiencies" and almost always recommended an identical list of vitamins, minerals, and digestive enzymes. The questionnaire also contained a section with questions about the subject's food intake during the past week. However, the answers given did not affect the printout of supposed deficiencies.

In 1986, Donsbach and the institute agreed to: (1) stop marketing in New York State all current versions of its nutrient deficiency questionnaire and associated computer analysis services, (2) place conspicuous disclaimers on future versions of the questionnaire to indicate that the test should not be used for the diagnosis or treatment of any disease by either consumers or professionals, and (3) pay $1,000 in costs. Donsbach and the University agreed to disclose in any direct mailings to New York residents or in any nationally distributed publication that the school's degree programs are not registered with the New York Department of Education and are not accredited by any accrediting commission recognized by the U.S. Department of Education. The university also agreed to pay $500 to New York State. In 1989, a New Jersey judge who issued an injunction against another Donsbach University alumnus, Raymond J. Salani, Jr., referred to Salani's"Ph.D." as "a Mickey Mouse degree."

In 1987, Donsbach abandoned his school, which was renamed International University for Nutrition Education but soon went defunct. He also began operating the newly-built Hospital Santa Monica, in Baja, Mexico, "a full care facility specializing in the treatment of chronic degenerative diseases including cancer and multiple sclerosis." This appears to be his principal activity today. He also launched the Donsbach/Whiting International Institute of Nutritional

Science, another nonaccredited correspondence school whose "Ph.D." students were required to spend two weeks of "residency" at Donsbach's Mexican clinic "to obtain practical experience in laboratory technique and diet kitchens" before getting their degree. The school's catalog listed Kurt Donsbach, "D.Sc., D.C., N.D., Ph.D." as professor of nutrition and Steven E. Whiting, a Donsbach University "Ph.D.," as professor of nutrition and director of education. Prospective students were assured that the degree would be recognized by the Confederation of Health Organizations (whose founder and board chairman was Donsbach). The confederation's magazine identified Whiting as "an orthomolecular nutritionist" whose background includes "extensive research with cardiovascular disease and chelation therapy."

Having seen no publicity for either the institute or the confederation for several years, we assume they are no longer active. However, Rockland Corporation, which markets Dr. Donsbach's "Professional" product line, noted recently that Donsbach plans to resume his "educator" role with a new facility, the University of the Healing Arts, which will be housed in Chula Vista, California. At least two of Rockland's current products, *Cardio-Eze* and *Prost-Aid*, are unapproved new drugs and misbranded because their names imply therapeutic usage that lacks FDA approval and because they lack adequate directions for their intended use.

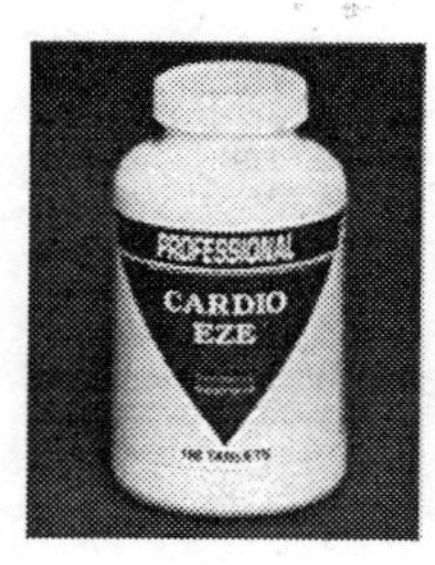

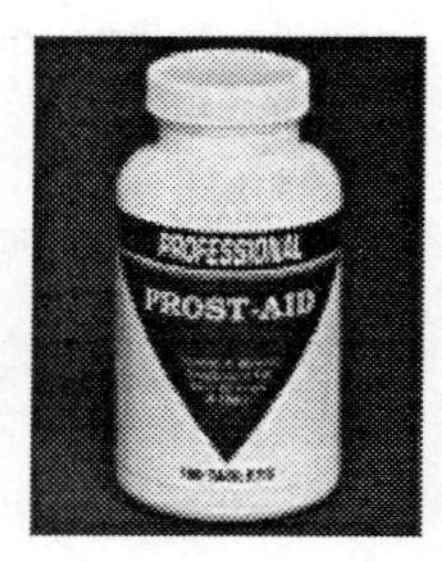

Donsbach himself was involved in a scandal involving credentials. In 1988, the Arizona Naturopathic Physicians Board of Examiners revoked the naturopathic license of Jess Franklin Lee after determining that he had used a counterfeit credential to obtain it— a diploma dated "17st June 1961" from the "Hollywood College School of Naturopathy" in Los Angeles. The authorities concluded that no such school had existed and that the "diploma" was created by making a photocopy of an altered 1961 diploma from the Hollywood College School of Chiropractic. Authorities in Oregon then determined that Donsbach and four others had done the same thing to become licensed as naturopaths in Oregon.

Donsbach has claimed that thousands of people enrolled in Donsbach University and that more than a thousand have graduated. As his graduates began representing themselves to the public as nutrition professionals, the American Dietetic Association began a drive for passage of state laws to restrict use of the word "nutritionist" to qualified professionals with accredited training.

The health-food industry, which does not want the government to help consumers tell the difference between qualified professionals and supplement pushers, has worked hard to thwart passage of such laws. At the same time, the industry has developed various "credentials" of its own.

American College of Nutripathy

For more than ten years, ads in many magazines invited readers to "come help transform the world" by becoming a "Doctor of Nutripathy." According to its creator, Gary Martin, of Scottsdale, Arizona: "Nutripathy is the condensation of most all natural healing and counseling techniques available today. . . . It is the basics 'boiled' from literally hundreds of different therapies and techniques." The "degrees" offered by correspondence were Associate Degree in Nutripathy ("N.A."), Bachelor of Science in Nutrition ("B.S."), Master of Science in Nutrition ("M.S."), Doctor of Nutripathy ("D.N.), Doctor of Philosophy in Nutrition ("Ph.D."), Doctor of Theology ("Th.D."), and Doctor of Nutripathic Philosophy ("Ph.D."). The school was advertised as "accredited" and touted approval by the International Accrediting Commission for Schools, Colleges and Theological Seminaries. However, a reporter discovered that this "commission" operated from the home of a couple in Holden, Missouri, and was not recognized by the U.S. Department of Education or any other government body.

A school brochure claimed that "in mastering nutripathy, you will be in possession of the true art of healing. You will know more about the Science of Health and Nutrition than the medical profession, chiropractic profession, osteopathic profession, homeopathic school and the so-called wholistic health school. . . . You will have accomplished in a few months what the medically oriented school of nutrition has not achieved in all of its existence." The brochure also says, "We do not cater to the complicated and extensive body of trivia and irrelevance that today goes under the name of nutritional science." Another brochure stated that most nutripathy graduates entered private practice and some made $100,000 per year.

During the mid-1980s, degrees from the American College of Nutripathy's "Department of Nutrition" cost $1,995 each with advance payment or $2,495 in installments. People who generated referrals by placing brochures in health-food stores were promised a recruiting bonus of $200 for each person who signed up for one of these courses. Participating stores were also promised $200. Students were required to get the bachelor's and master's degrees in nutripathy before pursuing a doctorate.

For fees ranging from $30 to $400, the nutrition department also offered twenty-five "mini-courses," including "Nutripathic Arthritis Studies," "To Cleanse or to Surgery," "Nutripathic Emotional Recovery Studies," "Nutripathic Master Herbalist Course," and "Sin, Fear and Guilt Removal." Upon request, "a beautiful Certificate of Completion" was available for all mini-courses. Students who wished to use nutripathy "on a professional basis" and desired "proper internship certification" were urged to take a $100 two-day internship, which Martin described as "the highlight of nutripathic education" and provided them with a "certification plaque." In 1989, a brochure stated that the school's curricula were "accepted for full credit" toward "earned, accredited" bachelor's, master's, and Ph.D. degrees in "holistic science" by the International Institute of Holistic Sciences in Glendale, Arizona, at an additional cost of about $100 per degree.

Martin also operated Nutripathic Formulas (which sold more than five hundred nutrition products, educational materials, and other items by mail) and Natural Health Outreach, a clinic where he practiced for "suggested donations" of up to $700. According to a clinic brochure, "Dr. Martin and Staff counsel and teach nutritional counseling, bio-chemical analysis, symptomatology, reflexology, iridology, sclerology, nutripathic therapy, mineral (hair) analysis, kinesiology, color therapy, radiesthesia techniques, stress counseling, colonic therapy, massage therapy and awareness techniques." In the Yellow Pages—under "Nutritionists"—the clinic advertised that its doctors could handle weight loss, fatigue, and other physical and mental matters. Martin also offered counseling by mail for a suggested donation of $25.

Martin claimed that nutripathic tests can detect "imbalances which, if left to mature, must ultimately manifest as some form of disease process." He claims "to discover the root cause of the disease while it is still in the PREDIAGNOSABLE stage." The most notable test was a urine/saliva test developed about fifty years ago by Cary Reams, a self-proclaimed biophysicist who was prosecuted during the 1970s for practicing medicine without a license. Reams, who also claimed to be guided by God, devised "a mathematical formula for perfect health, based on the biophysical frequencies of living matter." The formula, which Martin called "your Nutripathic Portrait," looks like this:

1.5   6.4 / 6.4   7   1   3 / 3

According to Martin's book, *Nutripathy: The Final Solution to Your Health Dilemma,* the first three numbers represent sugars excreted in the urine and the acidity (pH) of the urine and saliva, and indicate how much "energy input" you have. The other numbers, said to represent your "mineral salts index, urine debris index and nitrate nitrogens over the ammoniacal nitrogens index," indicate how much energy your metabolism is using. "A low energy input and high energy drain," says the book, "means degeneration, rot, decay and death."

Martin's book claims that "a properly combined diet of natural foods will allow a person to live in a state of perfect health." But students were still urged to buy the products they'd be selling to patients, including "flower formulas" to overcome depression, a solution that supposedly killed the urge to smoke, oral drops to relieve arthritis and inhibit aging, aphrodisiac herbs, and a water filter. The school also sold a laboratory kit for $750, a urine/saliva manual ($1,000), and a manual called *How to Prosper as a Natural Health Practitioner* ($100).

Martin denied that his graduates diagnosed or treated illness; they merely "guide patients to the elimination of disease." A school brochure warned that a special Nutripathic Disclaimer and Contract should be used "with every client, no matter how well you know the person or how you are related." Applicants to the school had to sign a statement acknowledging that "Nutripathy is a religious science of health" and that "Nutripathic methods are not for the purpose of diagnosing, alleviating, mitigating, curing, preventing or caring for 'disease' in any manner whatsoever." They must also agree not to use the knowledge they obtain for any such purpose and to "release the College, authors, publishers and/or any instructors from any damages, claims or liability whatsoever, as a result of the information presented."

The American College of Nutripathy appears to have granted hundreds of "degrees" to people throughout the United States. In 1987, one of its graduates pled guilty to practicing medicine without a license in New York City and was placed on a year's probation. Another graduate we know of practiced in an East Coast city and wrote local newspaper columns, some of which identified her as "Dr." without indicating the source of her credential. The harm caused by Martin's other graduates cannot be measured, but it is difficult to imagine their rendering any worthwhile service as "health professionals."

Bernadean University

Another school that issued mail-order diplomas is Bernadean University, which opened in Las Vegas, Nevada, and later moved to Van Nuys, California. Bernadean was founded and operated by Joseph M. Kadans, "Ph.D., J.D., N.D., Th.D.," whose *Encyclopedia of Medicinal Herbs* (1970) is filled with unfounded advice. Kadans's credentials appear to be just as dubious as the ones he distributed. He claimed to have obtained a law degree in 1943 from Eastern College of Commerce and Law (a nonaccredited law school), and to have earned Ph.D. and N.D. degrees from the International University in New Delhi, India. However, an investigation by the Nevada State Board of Bar Examiners could not confirm that Kadans had enrolled in the New Delhi School. The investigation was ordered by the Nevada Supreme Court after Kadans petitioned to take the state bar examination, even though he lacked an accredited law degree. The board concluded that he had received a doctor of theology degree from Berean Christian College in Kansas in exchange for a degree from Bernadean to the President of Berean Christian College!

Bernadean University was never authorized by the State of Nevada to operate or grant degrees. State investigators reported that it operated out of a small office with no classrooms and had four "faculty" members (who merely helped grade student papers), only one of whom even possessed a high school diploma. The investigators also found that law books Kadans claimed to have written were merely "an incomplete compilation of texts written by other authors" which Kadans had copied on Xerox machines. In 1977, the Nevada Supreme Court turned down Kadans' petition, stating, "We agree with the Board's conclusion that Kadans' operation of the dubious Bernadean University and his misrepresentations concerning the nature of the University cast serious doubt upon Kadans' moral suitability to practice law in this state." During the same year, the Nevada courts ordered Bernadean to stop issuing degrees.

Undaunted, Kadans moved his "university" to Van Nuys, California, where it continues to operate without state authorization. Besides guiding his new operation as "Dean of Students," Kadans was also executive director of the "International Naturopathic Association," which claimed a membership of two thousand and had the same Nevada address as Bernadean University. In 1981, the group's name was changed to "International Association of Holistic Health Practitioners (Naturopathic)," but its executive director and address remained the same.

In 1978, Benjamin Wilson, M.D., a surgical resident concerned about quackery, examined Bernadean's offerings and made a series of inquiries. One course that was offered was "Child. 101," which cost $90 and was described as: "Comprehensive course in home delivery, with section on natural birth control. Certificate as Mid-Wife." "Can. 401," offered for $120, was described as "a special research course in cancer theories and therapies. Degree as Master of Cancer Theories (Ct.M.)." Other offerings included a three-credit course in basic nutrition, resulting in a certificate as a "Nutritionist," for $120. A "Cancer Researcher" certificate could be obtained after a two-credit-hour course costing $80. Holders of a bachelor's degree could obtain a master's degree if they wrote a "thesis" or took "some short course with the school." A doctoral degree ("Ph.D." or "Sc.D.") could then be obtained by taking thirty-six credit hours (@ $40 per credit) or writing an "equivalent" thesis. "Doctoral" degrees in acupuncture, reflexology, iridology, naturopathy, and homeopathy were also available. The naturopathy course cost $800 or $2,400. Both were said to have the same contents, but the more expensive version included unlimited toll-free telephone calls with Kadans plus "free consultations," a tape recorder, and a tape of a health talk with each lesson. Any student who satisfactorily completed a course could apply for designation as a "school mentor" who then could tutor new students. Mentors were also referred to as "Adjunct Professors."

Kadans was assisted in his California operation by Howard Long, "Th.D., D.Sc.," a former health-food store operator who also was executive director of the Adelle Davis Foundation. From 1962 through 1972, Long had been vice president in charge of membership, promotion, education, public relations, and conventions for the National Health Federation. In 1978, Wilson asked whether Bernadean would award him an honorary M.D. or Ph.D. degree in return for a contribution of several hundred dollars. Wilson stressed that he needed one in a hurry because he was about to publish a book. Long replied that the M.D. degree "will not be offered by the University under any circumstances," but a Ph.D. was possible—"with the necessary credentials" plus payment of $1,000.

In, 1981, Virginia Aronson, R.D., obtained a "Nutritionist" certificate from Bernadean, even though she deliberately attempted to fail the course. On the first "test," she answered the thirty-five true/false questions in accordance with nutrition facts. Since nearly one third of her answers contradicted information given in the school's lessons, she expected to get a grade of 70 or below. However, the test was returned with a grade of 90, with a letter from the "office administrator" stating: "You may use the book for answers as it is an open book course. I just seem to feel that you put the answers in the wrong column." On the second test, Aronson answered all the questions accurately so that her grade—based on information given in the course—should have been a zero. Yet she received a grade of 100 percent and an accompanying note congratulating her on the "excellent manner in which you have completed the Nutrition course." The above "Nutritionist"

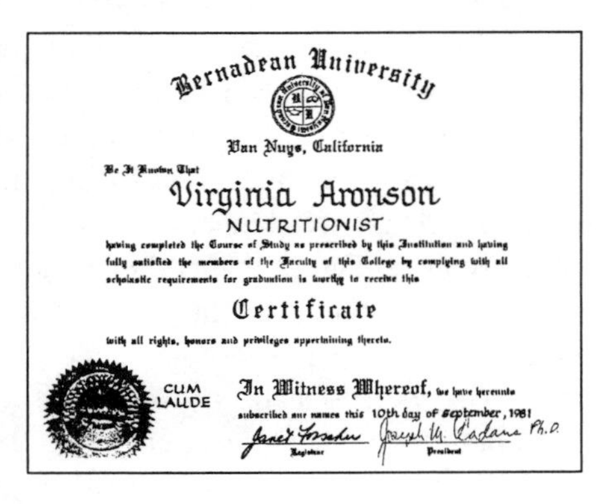
Bernadean University
Van Nuys, California
Be It Known That
Virginia Aronson
NUTRITIONIST
having completed the Course of Study as prescribed by this Institution and having fully satisfied the members of the Faculty of this College by complying with all scholastic requirements for graduation is worthy to receive this
Certificate
with all rights, honors and privileges appertaining thereto.
CUM LAUDE
In Witness Whereof, we have hereunto subscribed our names this 10th day of September, 1981
Registrar
President

certificate, obtained for an additional $10, contains an attractive gold seal and indicates that she graduated "cum laude"!

In 1990, the Nevada Commission on Postsecondary Education refused to process an application from Kadans to operate a correspondence school to grant law degrees. An official wrote:

> Your past history and practices make it evident that you are unqualified to be licensed as a postsecondary school in the state of Nevada. I am aware of your history as Bernadean University and its predecessor. . . .
>
> Pursuant to [Nevada laws], you are required to be of good reputation and character. . . . In . . . 1977 . . . our Supreme Court found that you indulged in misrepresentations in . . . the operation of Bernadean University in Las Vegas and found that you were morally unfit to practice law in Nevada. In addition, we have evidence that Bernadean University issued a diploma in 1986 to an inmate at Leavenworth for the degree of Juris Doctor and Master of Theology without the academic achievement consistent with such diplomas.

Bernadean's best-known alumnus is probably Richard A. Passwater, "Ph.D.," whose books include *Cancer and Its Nutritional Therapies*, *Supernutrition,* and *Selenium As Food and Medicine.* Passwater is director of research for Solgar Company, Inc. (a supplement manufacturer) and writes regularly for *Whole Foods*, a health-food-industry trade magazine. Another purported "graduate" was "herbalist/naturopath" Gerhard Hanswille, whose advice led to the death of a seventeen-month-old girl (see Chapter 4).

Another Bernadean "graduate" is Chester P. Yozwick, "C.N.A., N.D., P.M.D.," author of *How to Practice Nutritional Counseling Legally Without Being Guilty of Practicing Medicine Without A License,* a forty-two-page manual for "natural health" practitioners. The booklet's foreword, written by Kadans, calls Yozwick "a highly regarded graduate of Bernadean University."

The key to avoiding legal trouble, says Yozwick, is not to "diagnose, treat or sell anything or collect fees for anything under the promise that it will cure disease." He advises readers to watch their language, to avoid naming organs of the body, and to say what they would do if they had their client's problem. He advises screening clients with a questionnaire, verifying their identity, and taking other steps to keep out "undesirables" (such as government investigators). He advises using a disclaimer stating that the advice given is not a substitute for medical treatment but is "for the sole purpose of teaching people how to build their own health." He also advises joining a professional nutritional association that can provide sound legal advice, nutrition news, group malpractice insurance, increased prestige, and news of "detrimental" legislative developments.

Accredited, But Still Questionable

The American Academy of Nutrition, a correspondence school located in Corona del Mar, California, offers its "Comprehensive Nutrition" course for $1,185. The school's catalog states that the course will help graduates prepare nutrition plans for personal use and enhance their ability to perform as a private nutrition counselor; writer for health and nutrition magazines; vitamin sales representative; owner, manager, or employee of a health-food store; nutrition counselor in a doctor's office; and nutrition advisor to a health club, weight-loss clinic, or athletic team. "Comprehensive Nutrition" includes "Essentials of Nutrition Counseling"—available separately for $290—"only for health professionals who possess a very high level of nutrition knowledge." Graduates can "proudly display the Academy diploma on the wall and enjoy new respect and credibility with their clients, as well as an increased level of confidence."

In 1989, according to its catalog, the American Academy of Nutrition "became the first and only home study school devoted to nutrition education to be accredited by the National Home Study Council [now called the Distance Education and Training Council], which is the only United States Department of Education listed agency solely accrediting home study schools." The school's major text, *Understanding Nutrition*, is a highly respected textbook used in hundreds of colleges and universities throughout the United States. Nevertheless, there is good reason to be suspicious.

The academy was founded in 1985 by Sandy Berwick, who "began to study nutrition in the late 1970s and . . . has been involved in the nutrition field since 1980." The school's catalog describes her as nutrition advisor to many prominent athletes, a frequent television and radio talk show host and guest, and a frequent "spokesperson for the National Home Study Council to encourage people to continue their education through home study." Berwick's biographical-sketch flyer does not indicate that she holds any type of academic degree. The other six individuals listed under "Administration and Faculty" in the school's catalog include Ann Louise Gittleman, M.S., and Bruce B. Miller, D.D.S., both of whom promote many unscientific nutrition concepts. The others include Peter Berwick, an attorney "with many years of independent study of nutrition in sports nutrition and fitness," a woman with a master's degree in public health, and a medical doctor described as "a writer and lecturer in preventive nutrition."

Gittleman is author of *Guess What Came to Dinner: Parasites and Your Health*, a book that misrepresents the prevalence of parasitic infections among Americans. For those who have them—or think they do—she recommends using laxatives and other "intestinal cleansers," colonic irrigation, plant enzymes, dietary measures, and homeopathic remedies—none of which would actually provide effective treatment for any type of parasite. She also states that "folklore instructions suggest that any course of treatment for worms should begin around the full moon when the parasites become more active in the system." Although she correctly indicates that "many effective drugs are used against parasite infections," she incorrectly suggests that they are more likely to cause harm than good. One way to obtain Gittleman's book is by calling the toll-free number of Uni-Key Health Systems, of Bozeman, Montana, which Gittleman publicizes. The book is then shipped with a brochure and a form for ordering herbal "non-drug parasite eliminators" and other dubious products touted by the book.

Miller has produced a large number of audiotapes, videotapes, and booklets, some of which have been used by Shaklee distributors to promote products. The booklets were published as "A Better Health Series" by Bruce Miller Enterprises or its subsidiary, The Institute for Preventive Health Care. They include about a dozen by Miller and several by James Scala, Ph.D., former director of research for the Shaklee Corporation. The biographical sketch in Miller's booklets states that he practiced "nutritionally oriented dentistry" in Dallas, Texas, until 1983, when he decided to concentrate on researching, writing, and consulting. His booklet "Do I Need Food Supplements?" lists twenty-three questions to help readers decide "if supplements are for you." A single "yes" answer to any of these questions indicates that "safe use of supplements may give your health a boost your body will appreciate." However, only two of the questions provide a legitimate basis for considering supplements. The illegitimate questions include "Are you one of 17 million adolescents?" "Are you depressed?" and "Would you like to feel better?"

Even if all of the American Academy of Nutrition's academic material is scientifically sound, can such a school qualify people to do nutrition counseling? The answer is no. *The professional skills needed to counsel people cannot be acquired by mail.* Proper training requires several years of full-time scientifically-based schooling that includes counseling many clients under responsible expert supervision.

"Professional" Groups

> Whatever your specialty, one thing is certain. If you offer nutrition or dietary counseling as part of your service, you should proclaim your professional status by joining the American Association of Nutritional Consultants. When you display the prestigious A.A.N.C. Membership Certificate on your wall, you make your clients, patients, and profes-

> sional colleagues aware of your commitment to high standards and professional competence in Nutrition Counseling. And you demonstrate your dedication to the cause of good health through nutrition by supporting your Professional Association.

So stated "An Open Letter To All Health Professionals" in several issues of *The Nutrition & Dietary Consultant,* the monthly publication of the American Association of Nutritional Consultants, of Las Vegas, Nevada. The certificate—printed on imitation parchment paper and complete with gold seal and red ribbon—does indeed look attractive and professional. But those who encounter it would be wise to look closely at what it signifies.

AANC began operations in 1981 as the American Association of Nutrition & Dietary Consultants (AANDC). During 1983, AANDC assumed its current name and absorbed Kurt Donsbach's International Academy of Nutritional Consultants (IANC). AANC's membership structure was similar to that of IANC: associate membership cost $30, professional membership cost $50, sustaining membership cost $100, and lifetime membership cost $250. In 1989, AANC listed about 240 lifetime members, the most noteworthy of whom was Barbara Reed, "Ph.D.," author of *Food, Teens & Behavior.*

Reed, whose "Ph.D." came from Donsbach University, is a former probation officer who claims that a five-year study she conducted during the 1970s proved that dietary changes plus supplementation with vitamins and minerals could prevent teens on probation from getting into trouble. She also claims that half the people in American suffer from hypoglycemia and that virtually all addictions are caused by "altered biochemistry." Although her study lacked a control group and had other flaws in its design, it apparently impressed several judges and received favorable publicity in a front-page story in 1977 in the *Wall Street Journal.* Her book states that the article led to "media appearances and speaking engagements all over the country" and "encouraged other probation departments, correctional institutions and programs for the behaviorally impaired to experiment with the orthomolecular [megavitamin] approach."

AANC's "journal" has been published under various names and in several formats. It began in 1983 as a tabloid newspaper called *The Nutrition & Dietary Consultant* and was renamed *The Nutritional Consultant* later that year. When IANC and AANC merged, their publications merged to become *The Nutritional Consultant & Health Express* ("The Magazine People Read For Nutritional Advice"). Toward the end of 1984, it was called *Your Nutritional Consultant* ("The Magazine America Reads for Nutritional Advice"). In 1985, it again became *The Nutrition & Dietary Consultant* ("America's Only Journal

For The Practicing Professional"). In 1986, it reverted to tabloid newspaper format in order to save money.

For the first few issues after the merger that formed AANC, its national board of counselors was listed on the journal's masthead with Donsbach as chairman. But a few months later, this listing was dropped and Donsbach's name appeared as contributing editor. At various times, AANC's letterhead had listed seven, eight, or nine members on its national board of counselors, one of whom—until his trouble arose—was Gary Pace.

Shortly after the attorney general sued Pace, AANC notified its members in northeastern states that Pace had temporarily obtained permission to solicit funds to set up New York and northeastern chapters of AANC. The notice stated that Pace had announced his election as president of the New York chapter without actually holding elections, that he had refused to render a financial accounting to AANC headquarters, and that he was "illegally circulating a letter on AANC stationery soliciting funds in the name of AANC." Pace was then removed from the AANC board, and Donsbach's name disappeared from the masthead of *The Nutrition & Dietary Consultant.*

AANC said its journal is "edited specifically for you who do now, or plan in the future, to earn all or part of your income through counseling on good health or proper nutrition, and for those of you who offer nutritional advice as part of your overall professional services." During the 1980s, each issue contained articles promoting unscientific practices as well as ads for questionable products, some of which were subjected to government enforcement action for misbranding.

AANC's 1986 *National Profile Directory of Nutritional Consultants* listed 686 practicing "professional nutritionists," but stated that since listing requires a written request, the list "in no way represents the total membership of AANC which at press time stood at 5,618." (This number was probably inaccurate because it was identical with the number listed in the 1985 directory.) The directory was intended to facilitate member-to-member referrals and to be distributed free at health shows, seminars, conventions, and other distribution points where it can reach potential clients. Listings included the consultant's name, address, telephone number, tests utilized, modalities offered, and areas of specialization. Nineteen percent of those cited were chiropractors. Nine percent had no listed degree, 12 percent a B.A. or B.S., 10 percent an M.A. or M.S., 23 percent a Ph.D., and 3 percent a medical degree. The rest displayed one or more of some forty sets of initials, many of which we could not recognize.

"Tests utilized" included complete workup by a medical doctor, hair analysis, herbal crystallization, urine analysis, blood analysis, a test to determine metabolic type, a saliva test, iridology, kinesiology, computerized questionnaires, diet analysis, and cytotoxic testing. "Modalities offered" included acupressure, acupuncture, intravenous chelation therapy, oral chelation therapy, general medicine, detoxification, herbology, homeopathy, hypnosis, naturopathy, nursing, optometry, osteopathy, reflexology, colonic irrigation, chiropractic, dentistry, biofeedback, hydrotherapy, massage, yoga, and megavitamin and mineral therapy. The "nutritional support specialties" were allergies, cancer, diabetic nutrition, drug rehabilitation, endocrine disturbances, general nutrition, geriatric nutrition, hypoglycemia, pediatric nutrition, skin conditions, smoking cessation, sports nutrition, stress management, temporomandibular joint dysfunction, weight control, premenstrual syndrome, prenatal nutrition, heart and blood conditions, digestive problems, and spines, bones, joints.

It is clear that membership in AANC and its predecessors has been open to anyone. In 1983, Sassafras Herbert (a poodle) became a professional member of AANDC and Charlie Herbert (a cat) secured professional membership in IANC. Both were household pets of Dr. Victor Herbert, who merely submitted their name and address plus $50.

Soon after a front-page story in the *Washington Post* exposed the bogus nature of AANC's application process, AANC began asking applicants to complete an application form that requested their name, address, phone number, school attended, major, degree and year earned, how long the applicant had been involved professionally in the field of nutrition, names of other health associations to which the applicant belonged, and the names of two nutrition-oriented health care professionals who could provide references. After this process began, one of us submitted the form under an assumed name, listing a degree from a nutrition diploma mill and providing appropriate references. Membership was granted as soon as the application was received. AANC did write to the persons listed as references—not for information about the applicant, but to ask them to join AANC! Another person bypassed the formidable "credential check" and simply submitted $50 plus the name and address of her daughter's pet hamster. She too was notified of acceptance within a few days and received the certificate shown here. A few months later, AANC reduced its application process to submission of a coupon that asked only for the applicant's name, address, and "degree initials, if any." Currently, the longer form is used.

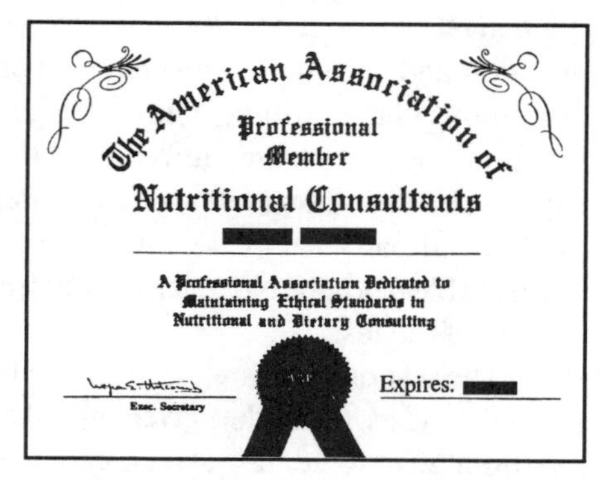

AANC's professional members are also invited to become "Certified Nutrition Consultants." According to AANC, "The trademark designation CNC after a Nutritional Consultant's name testifies to the world that the practitioner's qualifications have been certified by his or her Professional Association—that he or she has met professional requirements in addition to, and beyond, normal academic studies and/or professional experience." Some AANC literature refers to an "RNC" designation for "Registered Nutritional Consultant." In 1989, AANC listed about two hundred "Certified Nutritional Consultants," including James F. Balch, Jr., M.D., and his wife Phyllis, coauthors of *Prescription for Nutritional Healing*, an irresponsible book that many health-food retailers use to prescribe products for their customers (see Chapter 5).

According to AANC's executive director, CNC applicants must be professional members in good standing in AANC "and have met the high eligibility requirements for membership." However, the CNC application form asks nothing about training, experience, or qualifications, but merely requests the names of three professional references (which are not contacted). Applicants must pay a $150 fee, demonstrate knowledge of practice management and the laws pertaining to nutritional consulting, and pass a self-administered 2,000-question test on general and applied nutrition. They must acknowledge in writing that information presented in the certification program "is not intended as a substitute for licensed medical care, and is offered for educational purposes only." And they must release AANC "from any damages, claims, or liabilities whatsoever resulting from the information presented." "Successful" applicants receive an attractive certificate.

In 1986, when one of us obtained a copy, the CNC nutrition exam was divided into sections on basic anatomy, principles of nutrition, vitamin therapy, nutrition and common ailments, biochemical individuality, higher nutrition, orthomolecular nutrition, nutrition against disease, diet and disease, child nutrition, geriatrics, acquired body toxins and their elimination, and psychodietetics. Candidates were required to submit a notarized statement that no "second party" helped with the test, but they were given a list of books, purchasable from AANC, each of which could help answer the questions in one section of the test.

The test questions were divided about equally into multiple-choice and true/false types. Candidates were asked to choose "the most accurate" answer, even though in some cases, "if the candidate is real sharp and wants to get tricky, he or she might be able to point to special cases or circumstances where none of the choices is correct." Many questions had no correct answer, and the test contained many misspelled words. The clinical significance of some questions—like one about whether whole wheat flour can support the life of weevils—was rather obscure.

Another organization, the American Nutrition Consultants Association (ANCA) is open to "anyone interested in the fields of nutritional science and nutritional consultation, and in developing, perfecting and updating one's scope of nutritional knowledge." The only requirements for membership appear to be payment of $25 and completion of an application form that asks for one's name, address, telephone number, gender, age (optional), and professional activities (also optional). Members receive a certificate suitable for framing and *Lifelines*, the monthly ANCA newsletter. The ANCA catalog defines a "nutrition consultant" as:

> one who is trained in the science of dietetics and nutrition for the purpose of providing information to the public as a consultant in the matters of achieving proper dietary regimens for maintaining a state of optimal health. The profession is often practiced in conjunction with the distribution of health foods and food supplements.

ANCA's president, James D. Flaherty, Ph.D., is also administrator and sole faculty member for a course in nutrition consultation sponsored by his organization. Flaherty's doctoral degree in nutrition is from nonaccredited Union University. According to him, "The world is waiting for people knowledgeable in nutrition for the purpose of maintaining a state of optimal health. . . . These people have the opportunity of becoming a part of the biggest boon to humanity since time began." His sixty-lesson course, which costs $675 and must be completed within six months, is based on manuals and an audiotaped lecture series that he prepared. Students who finish the course with a "C" average or better receive a "Diploma in the Science of Nutritional Consultation," while those who complete it with lower grades are given a "certificate of completion." Graduates are invited to register as a "Registered Nutrition Consultant (RNC)" and be listed in the *International Registry of Consulting Nutritionists,* which ANCA publishes.

An ANCA brochure states that "every normal, healthy man, woman and child should seek the advice of a nutritionist for evaluation of his/her nutritional needs." So should people involved in active sports, children, teenagers, pregnant women, persons suffering from chronic diseases, individuals on medication, people with weight problems, people over sixty and people in job- or life-related stress situations. (Do you know anyone not covered by this list?)

The American Holistic Health Sciences Association, of St. Charles, Illinois, formed in 1979 but became defunct during the mid-1980s. It charged $70 for first-year membership and $40 per year thereafter. Members received

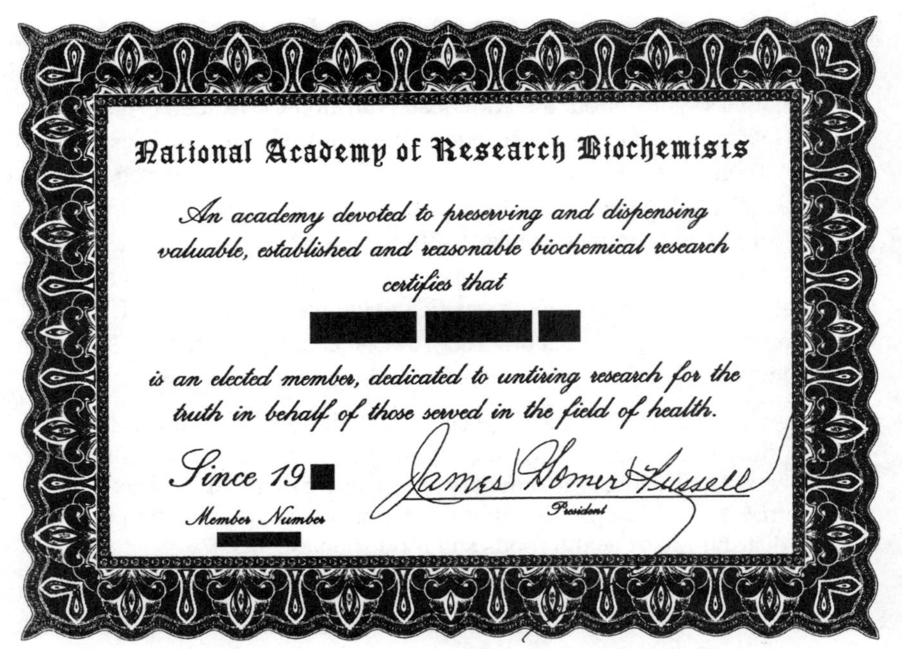

National Academy of Research Biochemists

An academy devoted to preserving and dispensing valuable, established and reasonable biochemical research certifies that

is an elected member, dedicated to untiring research for the truth in behalf of those served in the field of health.

Since 19

Member Number

President

This certificate was issued to a chiropractor who was not a biochemist, did no research, and was not elected to membership.

a hand-calligraphed certificate stating that they had "been elected by the A.H.H.S.A. board of examiners as a Fellow of the Society of Nutrition and Preventive Medicine in recognition of the contributions made towards the promotion and advancement of scientific nutrition and preventive healthcare." Each also received a certificate from AHHSA's National Board of Registration and Examination stating that he has "completed all required prerequisites . . . and is hereby recorded as a Registered Holistic Practitioner." Members also received a free copy of Chester Yozwick's *How To Practice Nutritional Counseling Legally Without Being Guilty Of Practicing Medicine Without A License*.

The National Association of Research Biochemists (NARB) confines its activities to publishing a "journal," selling a small line of taped seminars, and issuing a certificate (pictured above) to new members. As with the other groups, NARB's only membership requirements are a name, an address, and payment of a modest membership fee.

The most elaborate "paper conglomerate" we've seen was launched in Indiana in 1983 as the American Nutritional Medical Association (ANMA). Its stated purpose was to promote increased public understanding and legal recognition of "nutritional medicine and alternative holistic health care." Its manifesto stated:

> NUTRITIONAL MEDICINE . . . refers to that branch of alternative health care which deals with the treatment or prevention of disease through the use of vitamins, minerals, herbs, amino acids, homeopathy, and natural health care education and counseling. This is NOT a branch of allopathic medicine, and practitioners of NUTRIMEDICAL ARTS and SCIENCES should never let their patients think so!

ANMA members were offered "registration and/or certification" in various "alternative health care specialties." Its members could become Fellows of such august bodies as the American Board of Family Nutrimedicists, the American College of Naturopathy, the American College of Otology, the American Board of Homeopathy, and the American Board of Nutrimedical Obstetricians and Gynecologists. Certification was also available as a chiropathic therapist, massage therapy technician, nutritional medical counselor, nutrimedicist, and naturodermacist. (None of these "credentials" is recognized by the scientific community.)

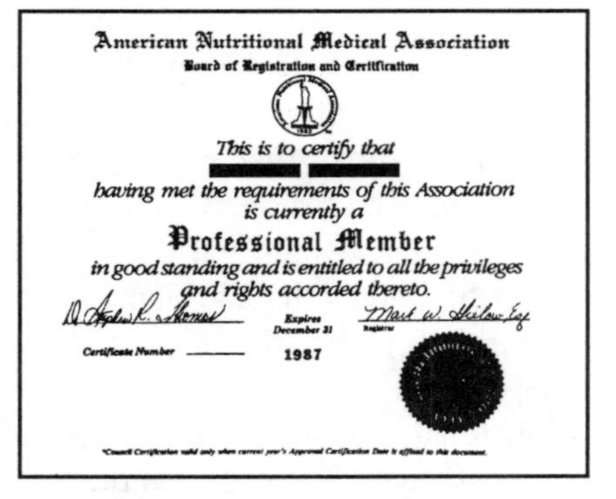

American Nutritional Medical Association
Board of Registration and Certification

This is to certify that

having met the requirements of this Association is currently a

Professional Member

in good standing and is entitled to all the privileges and rights accorded thereto.

Expires December 31 — Registrar

Certificate Number ______ 1987

*Council Certification valid only when current year's Approved Certification Date is affixed to this document.

The original cost of "professional membership" in ANMA was $100 for the first year and $50 per year thereafter, but discounts were sometimes offered. Associate membership cost $60 for the first year and $40 thereafter. Although the application asked for education and professional affiliations, these were not verified. A $5 commission was offered for each new member recruited. For an additional $25, ANMA members could join the United Natural Health Association, from which they would receive a Certificate of Fellowship.

ANMA also operated John F. Kennedy College of Nutrimedical Arts & Sciences (American Nutrimedical University), which offered correspondence courses leading to a "degree," "diploma," or certificates in "nutritional medicine," "chiropathic medicine," "naturodermatology," homeopathy, hypnotherapy, "neuroreflex therapy," and "nutrimedical" counseling. Its one-year Doctor of Nutritional Medicine (N.M.D.) course cost $1,895, but ANMA publications indicate that "nonacademic N.M.D. degrees" were awarded to members holding a doctoral degree or qualified through other experience. The one-and-a-half-year Doctor of Chiropathy (D.C.M.) course cost $2,400. The Nutritional Medical Counselor (N.M.C.) course cost $800. ANMA members received a 10 percent discount. Passage with lower than a C average would yield a certificate of completion rather than a diploma. We assume that the "N.M.D." was its most popular "degree" because the public might think it was a type of medical (M.D.) credential.

In 1987, ANMA moved to Colorado and evolved into the American Nutrimedical Association and International Alliance of Nutrimedical Associations. Around the time of the move, holders of an N.M.D. diploma were invited to exchange it for one from Lafayette University. But not long afterward the degree's name was changed to "Doctor of Nutrimedicine" and designated "the official degree of the Nutrimedical Arts and Sciences offered by the Colorado College of Nutrimedicine." Other "professional" activities and their corresponding "organizations" were renamed, probably bringing the total of possible ANMA-related credentials to over a hundred. By 1991, however, ANMA's directory listed only eighty-three "professional members" in the United States, fewer than half the number listed in 1986.

A Step toward Professionalization?

Health-food-store salespeople typically acquire their "knowledge" of nutrition by reading popular "nutrition" books and magazines, attending seminars sponsored by supplement manufacturers and distributors, and possibly self-experimentation. About fifteen years ago, an article in *Health Foods Business* suggested that health-food stores should work toward achieving professional status. "It's likely that the health food store of the future will have a certified nutritionist on its staff—the equivalent of a pharmacist in a drug store," the article stated. "Health food store owners—and the whole industry—should begin thinking about how such a system of accreditation from a recognized and respected institution might work."

Since that time, two industry-affiliated programs have been developed. One is the National Institute of Nutritional Education (NINE), which is now located in Aurora, Colorado. The other is an outreach of Bastyr University, a naturopathy school in Seattle, Washington.

NINE became incorporated in 1982, began enrollment in its "Certified Nutritionist" ("CN") program in 1983, and held its first "graduation" in 1985. The CN course outline was produced by Jeffrey Bland, Ph.D., whose views and activities are described in Chapter 17 of this book. The course is a mixture of sense and nonsense. The eleven "textbooks" used initially included some standard nutrition textbooks. But they also included *Nutrition Against Disease,* by Roger Williams, M.D.; *Diet and Disease* by Emanuel Cheraskin, M.D., D.M.D., W.M. Ringsdorf, D.M.D., and J.W. Clark, D.D.S.; *Guide to Healing with Nutrition,* by Jonathan V. Wright, M.D.; and Bland's *Medical Applications of Clinical Nutrition*—all of which promote unproven and irrational uses of dietary supplements. Books added later included *Nutritional Guidelines for Correcting Behavior,* by Barbara Reed, and *Nutrition and Behavior*, by Alexander G. Schauss, who, like Reed, has promoted the false notion that diet is a major factor in criminal behavior. During the mid-1980s, NINE was rejected for accreditation by the National Home Study Council. NINE's board of advisors includes Richard Passwater (holder of a Bernadean University "Ph.D.") and Joseph Montante, M.D., whose "Nutrabalance" system is detailed in Chapter 7 of this book.

In 1987, a CN study guide stated that the Williams and Cheraskin books were "not the typical text" but were selected because "they are considered 'industry textbooks,' books that most of us would have in our stores or personal library." Later these books were dropped. Another study guide promised that students would learn teach "a new vision of reality: the systems view and the holistic ecologic health care model." The topics associated with this approach included Chinese medicine, homeopathy, herbal medicine, and visualization to treat cancer.

The "CN" credential was developed to provide training and credentials for health-food retailers, but "progressive health professionals" have also been solicited:

> Just think what having a Certified Nutritionist, CN, on your staff could do for your practice:
>
> • Increase your credibility and prestige in the new Health Centered Age of the 1990's.
>
> • Make your practice stand out . . . up and above others still functioning in the outdated Disease Model.
>
> • Substantially increase your patient/client load.
>
> • Target more specifically the "health-minded" patients you most enjoy working with.

An article in the January 1993 issue of *Health Foods Business* states that NINE had awarded the CN designation to about 735 people (at least half of whom were affiliated with health-food stores, and many others who are health professionals) and had "educated" an additional seven thousand. The courses were all given by correspondence until 1992, when NINE added a small classroom teaching program. CNs can join the Society of Clinical Nutritionists, which was founded in 1985.

In 1987, NINE began offering a Retailer Training Course (RTC), which covers business aspects, foods, and nutrition. The business aspects appear sound, and so does the "textbook" on foods. However, the "nutrition text"

(*Nutrition Almanac*) is filled with advice that is questionable, inaccurate, and/or potentially dangerous. The book's worst part—Section IV—specifies large dosages of vitamins, minerals and other supplements which the author (incorrectly) claims may be beneficial for more than a hundred ailments, including cancer, leukemia, multiple sclerosis, and venereal disease. NINE originally intended to award a "Certified Health Food Store" designation to stores whose employees complete the program. This was not done, however, "so as not to compete and to avoid confusion" with chains that have their own system for "certifying" stores. NINE also offers a "Nutritionist" program.

NINE's purpose was described by its founder and President James R. Johnston, Ph.D., in the February 1987 issue of *Health Foods Retailing*. In an article called "Professionalism or Bust," Johnston outlined five steps toward "professionalization." He stated:

> Step Four is the stage marked by a determined and arduous fight for public and legal recognition. Few would argue that individuals and businesses that comprise the natural food industry at all levels are fighting more and more for public recognition, for the right to provide the information and sell the products traditional to the industry. Hassles with the FDA, the Victor Herberts, the dietitians, and others are all examples.

In another article, Johnston suggested that retailers should do "nutrient deficiency testing" and should position their business "as a concept somewhere between a retail store and a doctor's office."

Johnston's "Ph.D." degree, said to be in educational psychology, does not appear to be accredited. In 1989, he telephoned Herbert to complain about criticism on a radio program. When asked where his degree was from, he replied "Occidental University . . . in St. Louis," which he said was not accredited. The school was not listed in 1988-89 *Accredited Institutions of Postsecondary Accreditation* or even in *Bear's Guide to Non-Traditional College Degrees*, the most comprehensive guide to nonaccredited schools. Herbert's criticism had included unkind remarks about a "Health Appraisal Questionnaire" for "Low Blood Sugar Condition" which contained thirty-six "yes/no" questions about symptoms that have no diagnostic significance in diagnosing hypoglycemia. The questionnaire, with NINE's name and address at the top, had been deployed by Johnston at a "NINE" booth at a mall in Denver that Herbert had visited in 1988.

NINE's 1992 catalog states that the CN designation is "far more than a title; it is a precise definition of a person's competence, experience and intelligence in the complex profession of nutrition counseling." The catalog claims that students will be prepared to support the premise that "diet and diet supplementation can help many problems usually treated with drugs and surgery." The "Philosophy" section states: "While we in the United States may be one of the best fed people in history, we are also one of the most malnourished."

Naturopathic Connections

In 1991, Bastyr University, a naturopathic college, began marketing "The Natural Foods Education Program" to NNFA members. This two-part program was sponsored by NNFA and supported by grants from many health-food-industry manufacturers. Its $99 Level I "New Employee Orientation" includes two videos and a workbook. Its $450 Level II "Basic Training Program" includes five videotapes, ten audiotapes, thirty lessons in booklet form, a store owner's manual and employee workbooks with lesson-by-lesson self-tests. The Level II topics include vitamin and mineral supplementation, accessory food factors (other supplements), herbs, oriental medicine, homeopathy, and sports nutrition. Most of the booklets were written by Bastyr faculty members, but a few were written by the ever-present Jeffrey Bland. Not surprisingly, most make inappropriate recommendations. Although the programs state plainly that retailers should not diagnose or prescribe, the course contains information that encourages them to do so. Course materials also encourage retailers to refer customers who need "professional care" to naturopaths.

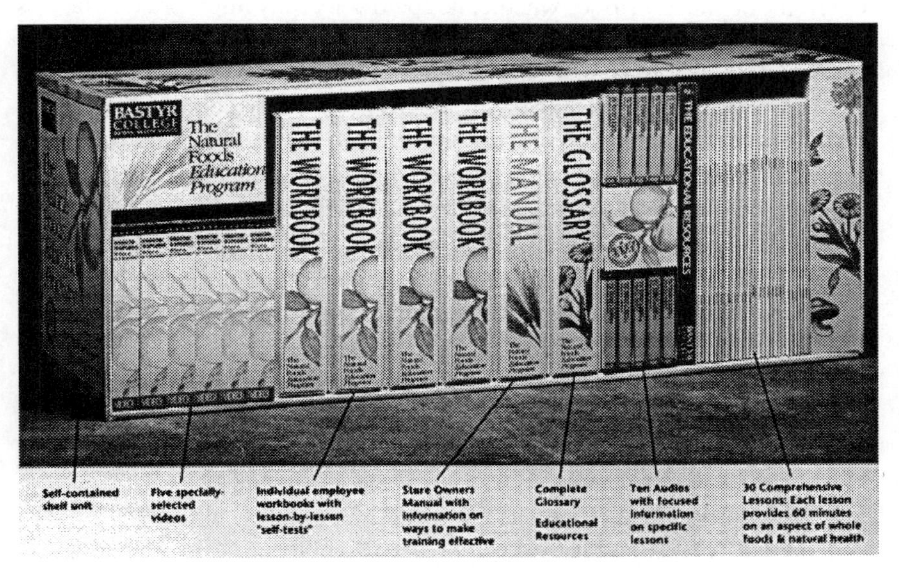

Natural Foods Education Program

Each salesperson at an NNFA-member store who completes Levels I and II (or has long-term industry experience or other background nutrition education) and passes a hundred-question exam will be designated as a Nutrition Product Specialist (NPS), receive an official "Certificate of Registration," and be able to operate as a "registered nutrition advisor." In an interview reported in *Natural Foods Merchandiser,* NNFA's executive director said that the knowledge imparted to store managers and employees through the NPS program "can only lead to greater public confidence and a more professional industry." She likened the registration program (which entails all of forty hours of instruction) to the program for registered nurses (who typically spend three or four years full-time) and registered dietitians (who spend at least five years full-time)! The education program's manual suggests having a party and issuing a press release each time an employee gets registered.

Recently, the American Dietetic Association (ADA) approved a didactic program in dietetics at Bastyr, whose nutrition department is chaired by a registered dietitian with a Ph.D. in nutrition. The approval involved review of a detailed application but did not require an on-site visit to determine precisely what would be taught. Dr. Barrett telephoned an ADA official to ask why ADA had approved a program at a school whose teachings include health nonsense and whose graduates have opposed ADA's campaign to license nutritionists. He was told that the application had met ADA's criteria for approval and that a lawsuit could result if ADA does not follow its own rules. When he asked to review the application to see whether he could detect any improprieties, he was told that the approval process is confidential.

Students who complete Bastyr's new course will be eligible to compete for entry-level jobs in dietetics. Any who subsequently complete an ADA-approved clinical internship will become eligible to take the examination for Registered Dietitian examination. Do you think a naturopathy school is likely to attract students motivated to learn scientific nutrition? Or prepare students for a scientifically based practice? More important, how much will naturopaths gain by being able to (mis)represent ADA's approval as evidence that "naturopathy is gaining acceptance by the scientific community"? Bastyr's dietetics course appears based on standard nutrition textbooks, and its contents may be 100 percent scientific. Even so, we do not think ADA should have approved it.

The Yellow Page Minefield

In 1993, a thirty-two-state survey sponsored by the National Council Against Health Fraud found that 286 (46 percent) of 618 Yellow-Page listings under the heading "Nutritionists" were spurious and seventy-two (12 percent) were suspicious. The volunteer surveyors were asked to contact every business they did not recognize as reliable and to request information about credentials, methods and, if possible, advice to clients. Listings were considered "spurious" if the advertiser used an invalid method of diagnosis, treatment, or nutritional assessment (applied kinesiology, hair analysis, iridology, or chelation therapy) or publicized a degree from a nonaccredited school. Listings were rated "suspicious" if the practitioner did not comply with a request for information on credentials or methods used.

Dubious nutrition practitioners were also found under the headings "Acupuncture," "Health & Diet Products," "Health, Fitness & Nutrition Consultants," "Herbs," "Holistic Practitioners," "Weight Control Services," and "Wellness Programs." Many listings under these headings were for chiropractors, homeopaths, naturopaths, "holistic" physicians, health-food stores, and multilevel distributors for such companies as Herbalife International, Nu Skin International, Shaklee Corporation, and Sunrider International. The credentials sported by these practitioners included CCN (certified clinical nutritionist), CN (certified nutritionist), CCT (certified colon therapist), CMT (certified massage therapist), CNC (certified nutrition consultant), DC (doctor of chiropractic), HMD (homeopathic medical doctor), L.Ac. (licensed acupuncturist), MLD (manual lymph drainage), NC (nutrition counselor), ND (doctor of naturopathy), NMD (doctor of nutrimedicine), and OMD (oriental medical doctor).

Among twenty-four individuals identified as "Ph.D." in their ad, three were Donsbach graduates and fourteen others had equally spurious credentials. Among 231 listings under the heading "Dietitians," twenty-one (9 percent) were spurious, including several from GNC stores. When a GNC employee was asked why her store was advertised this way, she replied, "Because we have literature in our store to help people." The study was headed by Ira Milner, R.D., coordinator of NCAHF's Task Force on Diploma Mills.

"Nutritionist" Licensing Is Needed

During the past fifty years, perhaps fifty individuals without valid credentials have pretended to be medical doctors and actually managed for a time to practice. So far as we know, no one has ever been exposed as a fake dentist, podiatrist, optometrist, or even chiropractor. But in nutrition, nonaccredited correspondence schools and other organizations have issued thousands of "degrees" and certificates that falsely suggest that the recipient is a qualified expert in nutrition.

In most states, it is legal for anyone to set up shop as a "nutritionist." In response to this problem, dietitians have been seeking laws that define "nutrition practice," restrict it to licensed practitioners, and restrict use of the word "nutritionist" to individuals with recognized credentials. The health-food industry—whose "credentials" are no better than its products—is adamantly opposed to this effort. Although many states now license dietitians, few have passed laws to curb quack "nutritionists."

We believe it is unfair to expect consumers to check the credentials of every health practitioner they encounter. Rather, state governments should set licensing standards and prevent individuals who don't meet the standards from representing themselves as equivalent to those who do. Nutritionist licensing can't protect against every form of nutrition practice conducted in private between consenting adults. Nor can it halt the activities of licensed health professionals who practice unscientifically. But it can make it difficult for unlicensed vitamin pushers to proclaim to the world that they are nutrition experts.

7

Phony Tests

Vitamin pushers have developed their own methods of "diagnosis" based on misinterpretations of physical findings, laboratory tests, and/or questionnaires. They use the results of these tests as a basis for suggesting dietary changes and recommending supplements, and/or herbs that they typically sell. This chapter discusses hair analysis, amino acid analysis, iridology, live-cell analysis, herbal crystallization analysis, bogus questionnaires, Essential Metabolic Analysis, computerized blood chemistry analysis, and the lingual vitamin C test. Information on other invalid tests can be located by looking in the index of this book under "Diagnostic tests, dubious."

Hair analysis

Hair analysis is a test in which a sample of a person's hair, usually from the back of the neck, is sent to a laboratory for measurement of its mineral content. The customer and/or the referring source usually get back a computerized printout that indicates "deficiencies" or "excesses" of minerals. Some also report supposed deficiencies of vitamins. The test usually costs from $25 to $60. This type of analysis is used by chiropractors, "nutrition consultants," physicians who do chelation therapy, and other dubious practitioners who claim that hair analysis can help them diagnose a wide variety of diseases and can be used as the basis for prescribing supplements. Proponents also claim that hair analysis can help to determine whether heavy metal pollutants are the cause of a patient's symptoms.

These claims are false. Although hair analysis has limited value as a screening device for exposure to lead and other heavy metals, it is *not* reliable for evaluating the nutritional status of individuals. Hair analysis cannot detect vitamin deficiency because there are normally no vitamins in hair except at the root (below the skin surface). Nor can it identify mineral deficiencies because the lower limits of "normal" have not been scientifically established. Moreover, the mineral composition of hair can be affected by a person's age, natural hair color, and rate of hair growth, as well as the use of hair dyes, bleaches, and shampoos.

In 1983 and 1984, Dr. Stephen Barrett sent hair samples from two healthy teenage girls to thirteen commercial laboratories performing multimineral hair analysis. Each lab received two identical samples from each girl, three weeks apart, under different assumed names. In 1985, Barrett sent paired samples from one of the girls to five more labs. The reported levels of most minerals varied considerably from sample to sample and from laboratory to laboratory. The laboratories also disagreed about what was "normal" or "usual" for many of the minerals, so that a given mineral value might be considered low by some laboratories, normal by others, and high by others. These results demonstrated that even if hair analysis were a valuable diagnostic tool, most of the laboratories were not performing it accurately.

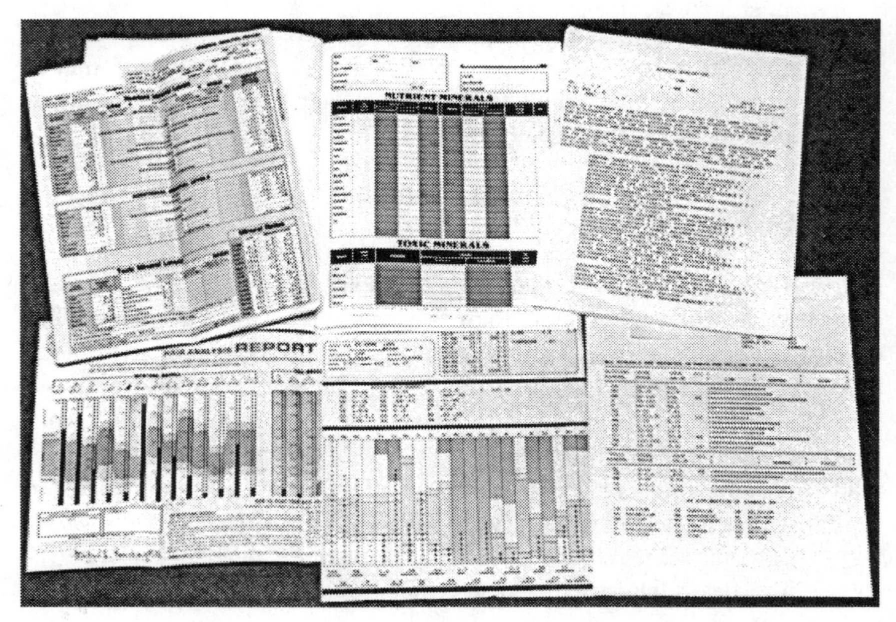

Portions of reports from five hair analysis labs (1983–1984)

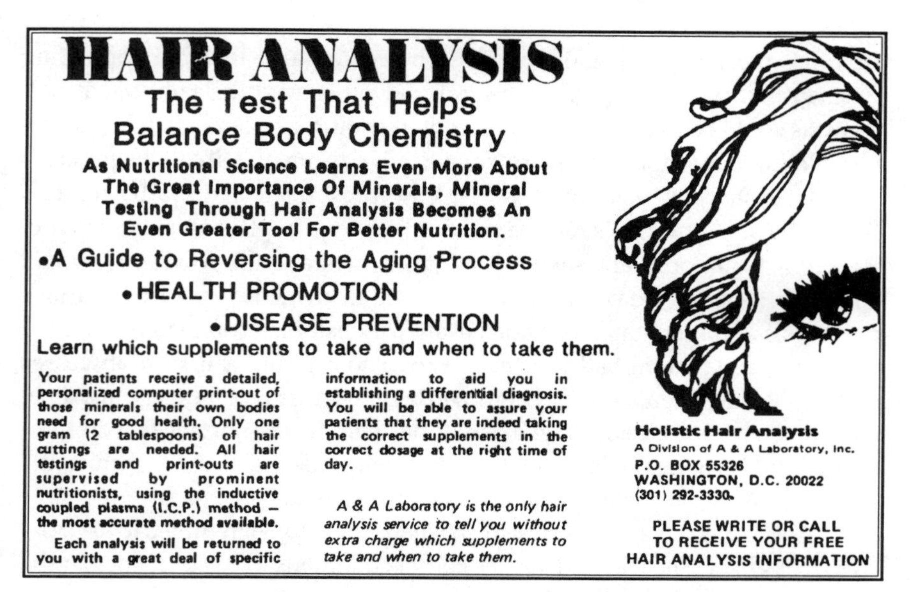

Ad in the September 1981 *ACA Journal of Chiropractic.* This laboratory, operated by the Furman family, also advertised directly to the public in health-food magazines and through posters in health-food stores. The lab ceased operations in 1984 after the Federal Trade Commission filed a complaint. Although the lab grossed 1.5 million between 1979 and 1983, no fine or restitution was ordered.

Most reports contained computerized interpretations that were voluminous and potentially frightening to patients. The nine labs that included supplement advice in their reports suggested them every time, but the types and amounts varied widely from report to report and from lab to lab. Many of the items recommended were bizarre mixtures of vitamins, minerals, nonessential food substances, enzymes, and extracts of animal organs. One report diagnosed twenty-three "possible or probable conditions," including atherosclerosis and kidney failure, and recommended fifty-six supplement doses per day. Literature from most of the laboratories suggested that their reports were useful in managing a wide variety of diseases and supposed nutrient imbalances.

One of the laboratories was owned by Arthur Furman, a dentist who had lost his license for insurance fraud. In an interview in *Health Foods Business*, he had stated:

> Hair analysis is a super good marketing tool. It's a neat, clean way of telling a customer what he specifically needs. It's the only way, with any specificity, that the health food store owner can tell scientifically what nutrients and minerals a customer needs.

In 1985, the Federal Trade Commission secured a court order forbidding Furman and two family members from advertising to the public that hair analysis could be used as a basis for recommending supplements. The laboratory closed as a result, and others stopped advertising directly to the public.

Hair analysis was involved in a case prosecuted in 1980 by the Los Angeles City Attorney's Office. According to the official press release, Benjamin Colimore and his wife, Sarah, owners of a health-food store, would take hair samples from customers in order to diagnose and treat various conditions. Prosecution was initiated after a customer complained that the Colimores had said she had a bad heart valve and was suffering from abscesses of the pancreas, arsenic in her system, and benign growths of the liver, intestine, and stomach—all based on analysis of her hair. Two substances were prescribed, an "herbal tea" which turned out to be only milk sugar, and "Arsenicum," another milk-sugar product that contained traces of arsenic.

Another sample of hair was taken when the customer returned to the store five weeks later. She was told that the earlier conditions were gone, but that she now had lead in her stomach. A government investigator received similar diagnosis and treatment. After pleading "no contest" to one count of practicing medicine without a license, the Colimores were fined $2,000, given a sixty-day suspended jail sentence, and placed on probation for two years.

Amino Acid Analysis

Proponents claim that amino acid analysis of blood and/or urine is useful in uncovering a wide range of nutrition and metabolic disorders. As with hair analysis, the test report may be accompanied by a lengthy computer printout containing speculations about the patient's state of health. According to one laboratory, the test "not only measures important metabolic factors that affect many bodily systems but also directly reveals a wide variety of *functional vitamin and mineral deficiencies.* This makes Amino Acid Analysis *one of the most cost effective tools* for the clinician practicing medicine." A flyer from the lab claims the test has proven useful for managing chronic fatigue, food and chemical sensitivity, *Candida albicans* infections, headaches, trauma, depression/anxiety, learning disorders, cancer (prevention), hypoglycemia/diabetes, cardiovascular disease, seizures, behavioral disorders, immune system disorders, arthritis, eating disorders, and athletic performance.

These claims are false. Like hair analysis, amino acid analysis is not valid for determining the body's nutritional or metabolic state.

Iridology

Iridology, also called iris analysis, is a system of diagnosis devised by Ignatz von Peczely (1822–1911), a Hungarian physician who was also drawn toward homeopathy. It is based on the premise that each area of the body is represented by a corresponding area in the iris of the eye (the colored area surrounding the pupil). Iridologists claim that states of health and disease can thus be diagnosed according to the color, texture, and location of various pigment flecks in the eye. Iridology practitioners purport to diagnose "imbalances" and treat them with vitamins, minerals, herbs, and similar products. They may also claim that the eye markings can reveal a complete history of past illnesses as well as previous treatment. One textbook, for example, states that a white triangle in the appropriate area indicates appendicitis but a black speck indicates that the appendix had been removed by surgery.

Advocates of the "Rayid Method" of iridology claim that iris analysis can determine learning and communication modes, latent behavioral traits, parent-child relationships, introversion-extroversion tendencies, and right or left brain dominance, and that "all this and more can be assessed prior to the age of three."

To "insure the highest standards of iridology practice," the Iridology Research Association, of Santa Fe, New Mexico, sponsors seminars and

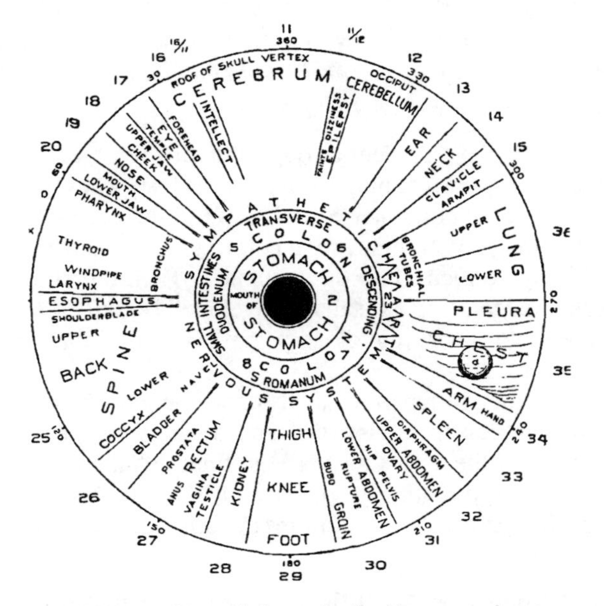

Iridology chart of left eye devised by a prominent naturopath more than seventy years ago.

awards certification to those who complete twenty-four hours of instruction, twenty-four hours of supervised externship, and "an original thesis which contributes to the field."

Bernard Jensen, D.C., the leading American iridologist, states that "Nature has provided us with a miniature television screen showing the most remote portions of the body by way of nerve reflex responses." He also claims that iridology analyses are more reliable and "offer much more information about the state of the body than do the examinations of Western medicine." But in 1979, he and two other proponents failed a scientific test in which they examined photographs of the eyes of 143 persons in an attempt to determine which ones had kidney impairments. (Forty-eight had been so diagnosed on the basis of creatinine clearance tests, and the rest had normal kidney function.) The three iridologists showed no statistically significant ability to detect which patients had kidney disease and which did not. One iridologist, for example, diagnosed 88 percent of normal patients as having kidney disease, while another judged that 74 percent of patients sick enough to need artificial kidney treatment were normal.

More recently, five leading Dutch iridologists flunked a similar test in which they were shown stereo color slides of the right iris of seventy-eight people, half of whom had gall bladder disease. None of the five could distinguish between the patients with gall bladder disease and the people who were healthy. Nor did they agree with each other about which was which.

But don't despair. In *Visions of Health: Understanding Iridology* (1992), Jensen promised greater accuracy was on the way:

> Currently under development through Bernard Jensen International, Inc., is the Neuroptic Scanning Computer. Iridology has been waiting a long time for the computer to arrive. With the computer, we can digitize the image of an iris from a color video camera and feed the digitized image directly into the computer. Then the computer can analyze the image using a database developed by skilled iridologists who have been working closely with professional computer programmers. . . .
>
> The computerization of iris analysis will assure objectivity in the examination process from iris to iris and from person to person. . . . The special ability of the computer to see in finer detail and with greater accuracy than is possible by the naked eye will bring out many heretofore undreamed-of possibilities in both the scope and accuracy of iris analysis.

The AMA Council on Scientific Affairs has noted that iridology charts are similar in concept to those used years ago in phrenology, the pseudoscience that related protuberances of the skull to the mental faculties and character of the individual. Another critic of iridology has collected twenty iridology charts that show differences in the location and interpretation of their iris signs.

Live Cell Analysis

Live cell analysis is carried out by placing a drop of blood from the patient's fingertip on a microscope slide under a glass coverslip to keep it from drying out. The slide is then viewed with a dark-field microscope to which a television monitor has been attached. Both practitioner and patient can then see the blood cells, which appear as dark bodies outlined in white. The practitioner may take polaroid photographs of the television picture for himself and the patient, and the results are used as a basis for prescribing supplements. The procedure is also called live blood analysis, dark-field video analysis, and several other names. According to a flyer from a Los Angeles chiropractor:

> NutriScreen Live Blood Analysis is a simple procedure for obtaining a quick and accurate assessment of your blood. With only a sample, taken virtually without pain from your finger, NutriScreen is able to provide a composite of over 25 aspects from your live blood. Darkfield microscopy now allows us to observe multiple vitamin and mineral deficiencies, toxicity, tendencies toward allergic reaction, excess fat circulation, liver weakness and arteriosclerosis.

These claims are sheer bunkum. Dark-field microscopy is a valid scientific tool in which special lighting is used to examine specimens of cells and tissues. The objects being viewed stand out against a dark background—the opposite of what occurs during regular microscopy. This allows the observer to see things that might not be visible with standard lighting. Connecting a television monitor to a microscope for diagnostic purposes is also a legitimate practice. However, live cell analysis is not. It merely misinterprets the significance of various blood cell characteristics, the amount of clumping of red blood cells, and several artifacts that occur as the blood sample dries.

During the mid-1980s, one company marketing live cell equipment projected that a practitioner who persuades one patient per day to embrace a supplement program based on the test would net over $60,000 per year for testing and supplement sales. Another company estimated that with five new patients a day (twenty-two days a month) paying $30 for the test and $50 for supplements, practitioners would gross over $100,000 per year just on initial visits. James Lowell, Ph.D., vice president of the National Council Against Health Fraud, watched three practitioners demonstrate live cell analysis at health expositions. Lowell noted that none took precautions during the preparation of the slides to prevent the blood from drying out or clotting. He also noted that "some of the patterns one practitioner saw resulted from his microscope being out of focus and disappeared when I adjusted it properly."

Herbal Crystallization Analysis

This test is performed by adding a solution of copper chloride to a dried specimen of the patient's saliva on a slide. The resultant crystal patterns are then matched to those of about eight hundred dried herbs to determine which "body systems" supposedly have problems and which herbs should be used to treat them. Herbal crystallization analysis is said to be based on the work of Rudolf

Sample Herbal Crystallization Test Report

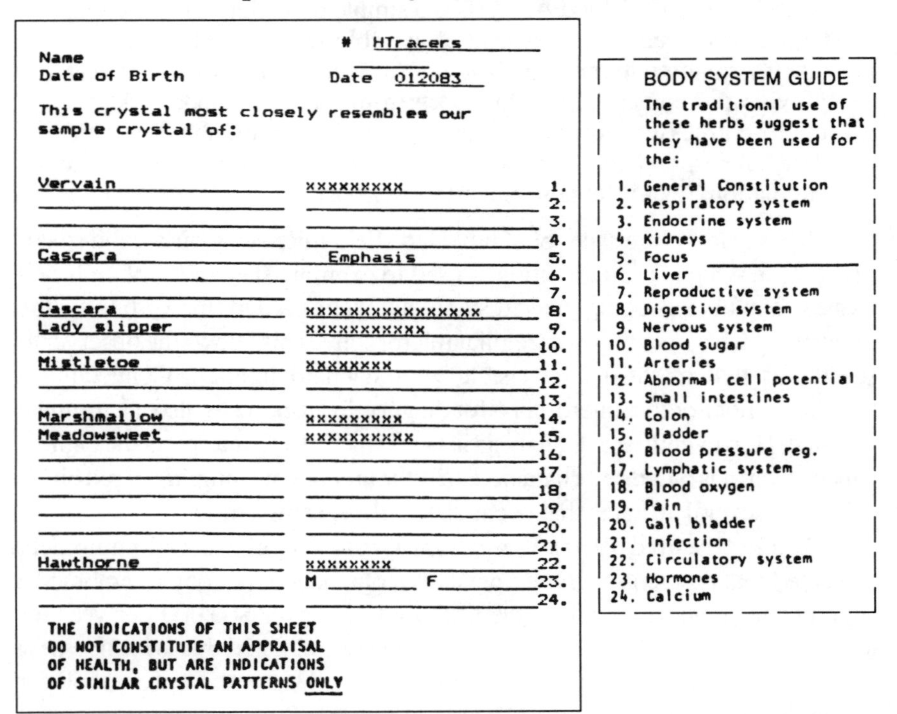

Name — # HTracers

Date of Birth — Date 012083

This crystal most closely resembles our sample crystal of:

Herb		No.
Vervain	xxxxxxxxx	1.
		2.
		3.
		4.
Cascara	Emphasis	5.
		6.
		7.
Cascara	xxxxxxxxxxxxxxxx	8.
Lady slipper	xxxxxxxxxxx	9.
		10.
Mistletoe	xxxxxxxx	11.
		12.
		13.
Marshmallow	xxxxxxxxx	14.
Meadowsweet	xxxxxxxxxx	15.
		16.
		17.
		18.
		19.
		20.
		21.
Hawthorne	xxxxxxxx	22.
	M ______ F ______	23.
		24.

THE INDICATIONS OF THIS SHEET DO NOT CONSTITUTE AN APPRAISAL OF HEALTH, BUT ARE INDICATIONS OF SIMILAR CRYSTAL PATTERNS ONLY

BODY SYSTEM GUIDE

The traditional use of these herbs suggest that they have been used for the:

1. General Constitution
2. Respiratory system
3. Endocrine system
4. Kidneys
5. Focus ______
6. Liver
7. Reproductive system
8. Digestive system
9. Nervous system
10. Blood sugar
11. Arteries
12. Abnormal cell potential
13. Small intestines
14. Colon
15. Bladder
16. Blood pressure reg.
17. Lymphatic system
18. Blood oxygen
19. Pain
20. Gall bladder
21. Infection
22. Circulatory system
23. Hormones
24. Calcium

The box on the left shows the format of the report, which the practitioner deciphers by lining up the body system guide on the right. The number of x's supposedly indicates how much help the corresponding organs need.

Steiner, an occultist who, in the 1920s, developed a system of identifying botanical specimens by crystallizing the sap with a copper sulfate solution. Neither the procedure nor the theory behind it has the slightest validity.

During the mid-1980s, Herbal Tracers, Ltd., of Hewlett, N.Y. promoted the test to retailers, chiropractors, and the general public. Its mailing to retailers promised that "the average test will pick up 6 to 8 herbs of varying importance to the client. . . . We feel that any retailer who fully participates in a healthcare professional/retailer referral program with a fully participating health professional will, at a minimum, double their herbal clients and sales, and potentially herbal sales records will be broken." In 1984, Dr. Barrett prepared specimens by licking one slide with the left side of his tongue and the other slide with the right side of his tongue, and submitted them under different names to Herbal Tracers. One report found crystal patterns "closely resembling" those of nine herbs; the other listed only one of these but identified six others. Most of the "body systems" did not match either. In 1985, New York Attorney General Robert Abrams filed suit against the company. Its owners agreed to pay $5,000 for court costs and penalties and to stop representing that the test is valid for use in the diagnosis, prevention, or treatment of disease.

Bogus Questionnaires

Many questionnaires have been devised to help persuade people they need supplements. Some are related to ideas that extra nutrients are needed to cope with factors in people's lifestyle or environment. Others falsely assert that a wide variety of symptoms are related to nutrient deficiency.

A few years ago, Great Earth Vitamin Stores, then the nation's second largest health-food-store chain, advertised a twenty-nine-question "Nutritional Fitness Profile." The ads stated that "Great Earth's highly trained Vitamiticians" were prepared to analyze the results and "tailor a nutritional support program" that's "just right for each individual's physical makeup and lifestyle." However, the questions provided no rational basis for recommending supplements or even analyzing anyone's diet.

James J. Kenney, Ph.D., R.D., a nutritionist at the Pritikin Longevity Center in Santa Monica, California, visited two Great Earth stores to see how the Nutritionist Fitness Profile is used. Each question has three possible answers, with #1 indicating no problem, #2 indicating a slight problem, and #3 indicating a significant problem. Kenney found that for each question where he checked #3, the "vitamitician" recommended one or more products. The recommended products included digestive enzymes to combat flatulence

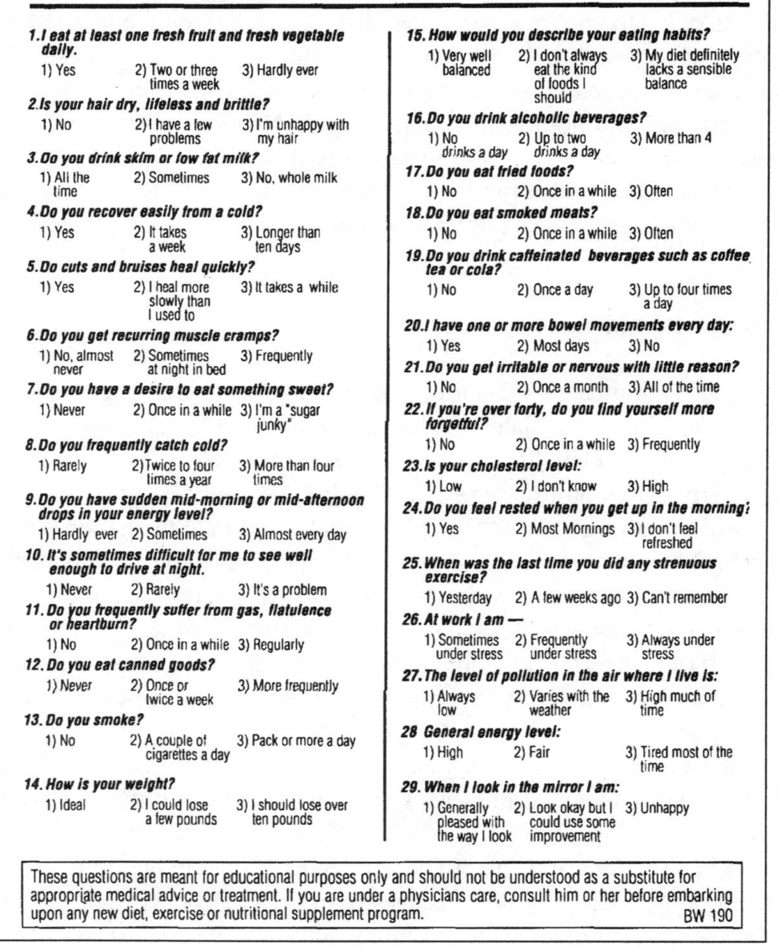

NUTRITIONAL FITNESS PROFILE

DEVELOPED BY DR. IRA A. MORRIS M.D.

Although no two people have the exact same nutritional needs, research has shown that lifestyle "patterns", when supported by a controlled diet, exercise and nutritional supplements, lead to better health and longer life. For example: a person who ignores fruits and vegetables and who smokes heavily may need as much as twenty times the amount of Vitamin C daily as a non-smoker who has orange juice or grapefruit regularly. A woman taking birth control pills may require ten times the RDA of vitamins B-12, B-6 and Folic Acid.

The following profile takes into account lifestyle factors. It can help indicate the nutritional fitness of your lifestyle patterns.

DIRECTIONS: Complete the questionnaire and bring it to a Vitamitician at any Great Earth Vitamin Store

1. I eat at least one fresh fruit and fresh vegetable daily.
1) Yes 2) Two or three times a week 3) Hardly ever

2. Is your hair dry, lifeless and brittle?
1) No 2) I have a few problems 3) I'm unhappy with my hair

3. Do you drink skim or low fat milk?
1) All the time 2) Sometimes 3) No, whole milk

4. Do you recover easily from a cold?
1) Yes 2) It takes a week 3) Longer than ten days

5. Do cuts and bruises heal quickly?
1) Yes 2) I heal more slowly than I used to 3) It takes a while

6. Do you get recurring muscle cramps?
1) No, almost never 2) Sometimes at night in bed 3) Frequently

7. Do you have a desire to eat something sweet?
1) Never 2) Once in a while 3) I'm a "sugar junky"

8. Do you frequently catch cold?
1) Rarely 2) Twice to four times a year 3) More than four times

9. Do you have sudden mid-morning or mid-afternoon drops in your energy level?
1) Hardly ever 2) Sometimes 3) Almost every day

10. It's sometimes difficult for me to see well enough to drive at night.
1) Never 2) Rarely 3) It's a problem

11. Do you frequently suffer from gas, flatulence or heartburn?
1) No 2) Once in a while 3) Regularly

12. Do you eat canned goods?
1) Never 2) Once or twice a week 3) More frequently

13. Do you smoke?
1) No 2) A couple of cigarettes a day 3) Pack or more a day

14. How is your weight?
1) Ideal 2) I could lose a few pounds 3) I should lose over ten pounds

15. How would you describe your eating habits?
1) Very well balanced 2) I don't always eat the kind of foods I should 3) My diet definitely lacks a sensible balance

16. Do you drink alcoholic beverages?
1) No drinks a day 2) Up to two drinks a day 3) More than 4

17. Do you eat fried foods?
1) No 2) Once in a while 3) Often

18. Do you eat smoked meats?
1) No 2) Once in a while 3) Often

19. Do you drink caffeinated beverages such as coffee tea or cola?
1) No 2) Once a day 3) Up to four times a day

20. I have one or more bowel movements every day:
1) Yes 2) Most days 3) No

21. Do you get irritable or nervous with little reason?
1) No 2) Once a month 3) All of the time

22. If you're over forty, do you find yourself more forgetful?
1) No 2) Once in a while 3) Frequently

23. Is your cholesterol level:
1) Low 2) I don't know 3) High

24. Do you feel rested when you get up in the morning?
1) Yes 2) Most Mornings 3) I don't feel refreshed

25. When was the last time you did any strenuous exercise?
1) Yesterday 2) A few weeks ago 3) Can't remember

26. At work I am —
1) Sometimes under stress 2) Frequently under stress 3) Always under stress

27. The level of pollution in the air where I live is:
1) Always low 2) Varies with the weather 3) High much of time

28 General energy level:
1) High 2) Fair 3) Tired most of the time

29. When I look in the mirror I am:
1) Generally pleased with the way I look 2) Look okay but I could use some improvement 3) Unhappy

These questions are meant for educational purposes only and should not be understood as a substitute for appropriate medical advice or treatment. If you are under a physicians care, consult him or her before embarking upon any new diet, exercise or nutritional supplement program. BW 190

Portion of two-page ad in March 1990 *Bestways.*

(question 11), high doses of niacin to lower cholesterol (question 23), and vitamin E to combat air pollution (question 27). He was also advised to take a high-dose multivitamin/mineral product, even though he described a more-than-adequate diet and said he was already taking a product that contained 100 percent of the RDAs.

The advice Kenney received was not merely useless. Although niacin can be valuable for controlling blood cholesterol levels, it should never be used outside of a comprehensive, medically supervised program that begins with attention to diet, exercise and other factors related to heart disease risk. When niacin use is appropriate, the dosage should be built up gradually to minimize the incidence of side effects, and blood tests should be performed regularly to detect liver problems or other adverse effects. But neither "vitamitician" mentioned the potential dangers.

Later, Kenney telephoned and asked a third "vitamitician" about her training. She replied, "There really wasn't any . . . All you really have to know is how to sell supplements."

Several years ago, Dee Cee Laboratories, a food supplement company that markets to chiropractors, offered to provide "nutritional questionnaires" for their patients to complete. The forms were analyzed by a computer that supposedly could "evaluate the nutrients you are presently low in." The form stated that it "is not designed for the purpose of diagnosing, prescribing or treatment of disease. Its purpose is to evaluate your nutritional status and to determine if you are consuming the right nutrients in the proper proportions." The computer was programmed to recommend various Dee Cee formulas which could be purchased from the chiropractor (at two to three times his cost) or shipped directly from Dee Cee to the patient. The report cost the doctor $10, and its suggested cost to the patient was $20 or $25.

Although ads for the questionnaire suggested that it was "a complete nutritional evaluation," only four of its 132 questions even asked about the patient's eating habits. The rest referred to nonspecific symptoms. Some of the symptoms might occur in vitamin deficiency disease or glandular dysfunction, but many of them had nothing whatsoever to do with nutritional status. Nor was there any reason to believe that any of Dee Cee's products were useful for glandular disorders. Kurt Donsbach's "Nutrient Deficiency Test" (see Chapter 6) and William H. Lee's "Personal Computerized Nutrition Profile Questionnaire" (see Chapter 16) contain about twice as many questions and are invalid for the same reason. NutriPro's "Personalized Optimal Nutrient Analysis Program," which supposedly compares the individual's dietary and "optimal" nutrient intakes, is also invalid (see Chapter 20.

Nutrition professionals may use a questionnaire as part of an evaluation for dietary counseling. But no questionnaire can provide a legitimate basis for prescribing dietary supplements. Questionnaires covering symptoms, illnesses, health habits, and other lifestyle factors can be a valuable part of a comprehensive medical evaluation. However, symptom-based questionnaires used for the purpose of providing supplement recommendations are invariably bogus. Thus, to protect yourself from being misled, reject any questionnaire connected with the promotion or sale of supplement products.

Essential Metabolic Analysis

SpectraCell Laboratories, Inc., of Houston, Texas, claims that the majority of Americans have nutrient deficiencies and that "intracellular nutrient deficiencies" even occur in over 40 percent of the more than one hundred million Americans taking multivitamins as "insurance." Furthermore, according to a company flyer:

> If you are one of the many people who have nutrient deficiencies, a treatment program to correct these deficiencies could greatly contribute to better health. Until recently, however, it was difficult to measure a person's nutrient status. As a result, many cases of nutrient deficiency have gone undetected.
>
> Today, there is a scientific way to precisely measure your nutrient status. It's a personal nutrient analysis called Essential Metabolics Analysis (EMA) and it's available only from SpectraCell Laboratories. The EMA is like a window on your cells, allowing your physician to look inside and identify individual nutrient needs. A targeted, tailored plan of dietary changes or supplements can then be prescribed with confidence.
>
> Everyone can benefit from SpectraCell's EMA, since so many illnesses can be directly or indirectly linked to diet. . . .
>
> But the EMA is not just for sick people. It's for anyone who wants to feel their best, perform their best and lay the groundwork for future good health.

SpectraCell's information packet for doctors states that the test is performed by placing lymphocytes (a type of white blood cell) from the patient's blood into ninety-six petri dishes that contain various concentrations of nineteen nutrients. Three days later, technicians add nutrients to the cultures and identify the dishes in which "greatest cell growth—or feeding frenzy" takes place, which supposedly points to a deficiency. The patient's doctor then gets a report that "this otherwise normal patient has a serious deficiency." Based on these findings the doctor may recommend a change of diet or a dietary supplement and have the patient retested in six months "to confirm they've corrected the deficiency." Company literature states that 90 percent of patients tested are "functionally deficient," with an average of three deficiencies per patient, and that patients experiencing arthritis, cancer, cardiovascular disease, chronic fatigue, diabetes, immune disorders, multiple sclerosis, obesity, and several other health problems "can benefit from the SpectraCell's EMA, since these conditions are directly or indirectly linked to nutrient deficiencies."

SpectraCell's EMA costs $250 to practitioners and $325 if billed directly to the patient. If its promoters are correct that "everyone can benefit," the cost of screening the American population and retesting those who are "seriously deficient" would exceed one hundred *billion* dollars.

Properly performed lymphocyte cultures have a legitimate role in testing for certain nutrient deficiencies. But they are not appropriate for general screening or for diagnosing "nutrient deficiencies" in the manner used by EMA. The average lymphocyte is three months old, so if the test could show anything, it would be the patient's nutritional status three months before the test. More important, SpectraCell's methodology is not valid. The correct way to use lymphocyte cultures to diagnose nutrient deficiency was developed years ago by Dr. Victor Herbert and several other scientists to detect deficiencies of vitamin B_{12} and folic acid.

The test actually measures the rate of DNA production as the lymphocytes reproduce. In Herbert's test, the patient's lymphocytes are given a reproductive stimulus and cultured with and without extra B_{12} or folic acid in the media. If the patient has been deficient during the previous few months, the cells exposed to extra vitamins will grow more rapidly. The SpectraCell procedure is done by culturing the patient's lymphocytes for seventy-two hours, during which time they use up their internal supplies of various nutrients. When they are stimulated and given the "missing" nutrients, they reproduce rapidly. This merely demonstrates that if lymphocytes are "starved" for three days they will become nutrient-deficient. It has nothing to do with nutrient deficiency in the patient!

SpectraCell Laboratories is not only using an invalid test, but also appears to be encouraging those who use it to defraud insurance companies. It is against the law to bill an insurance company for individual procedures that are actually components of a single procedure. Thus, when a single blood chemistry test measures twenty components of the blood, it would be illegal to bill for it as twenty separate tests. This practice is called "unbundling" and is considered a form of fraud. SpectraCell Laboratories has supplied its clients with a list of diagnostic codes for twelve separate lab tests to use for billing purposes.

Computerized Blood Chemistry Analysis

In 1984, Joseph Montante, M.D., and Mark Shusterman, M.D., of Boulder, Colorado, doing business as Total Health Enterprises, Inc., launched a computerized program called Nutrabalance. The program was promoted through seminars and ads and was targeted to physicians, dentists, "nutritionists," and chiropractors. One ad in a chiropractic journal stated:

> Would you believe us if we told you we had a comprehensive nutritional program that would improve your patient care and your profitability? Well, we do. . . .
>
> Nutrabalance is a scientifically and clinically based nutritional analysis program that uses high-tech computerized accuracy to create a balanced, individualized nutritional regimen specifically tailored to match the unique health care needs of your patients. . . .
>
> Because Nutrabalance is comprehensive your recommendations can be efficiently targeted to the underlying source of your patients' problems and not just their symptoms.

A Nutrabalance flyer added:

> Using blood and urine test results, which are processed through our Computer Center, Nutrabalance develops a complete nutritional profile for your patients.
>
> Each profile includes an in-depth evaluation and discussion of any physiologic imbalances your patient may have and comprehensive nutritional recommendations geared towards correcting these imbalances. The Nutrabalance system uses a unique classification system based on glandular organ functions.

The evaluation is based on the results of a blood chemistry profile and a urinalysis performed at a legitimate laboratory and submitted to Nutrabalance for interpretation. Nutrabalance then issues a lengthy computerized report which classifies the patient according to fourteen "metabolic types," lists supposed health problem areas, and recommends dietary changes and food supplements from a manufacturer chosen by the patient's doctor. The process is similar to hair analysis schemes except that, unlike the hair tests, the blood and urine tests are legitimate. (In fact, Nutrabalance arranged for three of the nation's largest medical laboratories to identify the combination of tests as a "Nutrabalance Profile" so that they could be ordered efficiently.) The metabolic types—most of which are named after a gland or other body organ, do not correspond to anything known to medical science, and the supplement recommendations are nutritionally senseless. The interpretation of the tests is also improper. Laboratories list a normal "clinical range" for each laboratory value.

Nutrabalance uses a narrower "physiologic range," which means that some normal lab values will be classified as abnormal.

To clarify the intent of the Nutrabalance program, doctors who wished to use the company's services were required to sign the following statement:

> I understand that the Nutrabalance recommendations made by Total Health Enterprises, Inc., are meant to be solely educational to the patient, informational to me as the health care practitioner, and are not meant to diagnose or treat disease. I also understand that these recommendations are not designed to take the place of traditional methods of medical treatment. As the health care practitioner using these recommendations, I further consent that no guarantee has been offered in terms of a cure or the outcome from their use in the treatment of any patient.

In 1985, an undercover investigator sent two sets of blood and urine test results to Nutrabalance for interpretation. The blood test values were almost identical, but the investigator drank two glasses of water between urine specimens, which made their pH (acidity) and specific gravity differ. The first report classified the "patient" as: "Primary Type: Adrenal, Secondary Type: Posterior Pituitary, Acid/Alkaline Condition: Acid" and recommended an "acid food plan" plus thirteen supplement pills per day. The second report classified the patient as: "Primary Type: Adrenal, Secondary Type: Liver Spleen, Acid/Alkaline Condition: Balanced" and recommended a "balanced food plan" plus ten supplement pills per day. Both reports identified a large number of glandular "imbalances." The treatment program includes two weeks of daily "cleansing enemas," using coffee or licorice powder administered through a tube inserted "8 to 12 inches into the rectum." A Nutrabalance spokesperson said the company had about four hundred clients and was processing about a thousand reports per month.

Recently, an official of the American Chiropractic Association Council on Nutrition recommended a simpler "computerized blood chemistry analysis" for use in chiropractic offices. About forty blood test results are entered into a computer, which compares each laboratory value with the average for that value and reports on the significance of each "deviated lab result . . . based on body physiology at the molecular tissue and organ level." The five-page report also suggests which supplement products will correct the alleged "deviations." The company marketing the computer program also sells supplements and promises that approximately thirty tests will pay for its cost ($695). According to the official, "This is a concise learning and adjunctive assessment tool that will enhance any doctor's practice." However, "computerized blood chemistry analysis" does not provide a legitimate basis for recommending supplements.

Lingual Vitamin C Test.

This test is performed by placing a drop of 2,6-dichloro-indophenol on the tongue and noting the time required for the color to change from blue to pink. Proponents claim that this indicates whether there is enough vitamin C in the body. However, two published studies have demonstrated that the test is not valid. In one study, no correlation was found between lingual test results and serum vitamin C concentration in fifty male dental students. In the other, seventeen volunteers were tested with the Vitamin C Self Test Kit, after which a sample of their blood was analyzed using high-pressure liquid chromatography. The test subjects also kept a food diary for the day preceding the tests. No significant correlation was found between the lingual test result and the serum concentration or dietary intake of vitamin C.

The Bottom Line

The tests described in this chapter have two things in common: (1) they are not appropriate, and (2) the people administering them usually want to sell you something. No test is valid for screening whole populations for nutrient status. Nor should any test be used as the sole basis for recommending supplements. If you encounter anyone who utilizes such a test, seek your health care elsewhere.

8

Promises Everywhere

Since ancient times, people have sought at least four types of magic potions: the love potion, the fountain of youth, the cure-all, and the athletic superpill. Quackery has always been willing to cater to these desires. It used to offer "unicorn horn," special elixirs, amulets, and magical brews. Today's scams are "antioxidants," aromatic oils, bee pollen, herbs, Gerovital, "glandular extracts," "energy-enhancers," "sports vitamins," and many more.

Products of this type are sold by health-food stores, drugstores, supermarkets, unscientific practitioners, multilevel distributors, and mail-order vendors. The Vitamin Shoppe, a large mail-order discounter, lists about fourteen thousand items in its catalog. The total number of supplement, herbal, and homeopathic products in the marketplace has never been tabulated, but probably exceeds twenty-five thousand. The vast majority have no useful purpose. Among those for which no therapeutic benefit is claimed, only a small percentage are rationally formulated. Among those for whom therapeutic benefit is claimed, most don't work and the few that do are not suitable for self-medication.

The health-food industry almost seems to operate a "supplement-of-the month" club. Manufacturers never miss an opportunity to exaggerate the significance of preliminary research or to exploit reports in tabloid newspapers, "television magazines," and talk shows. The most recent example is the boom in shark cartilage sales triggered by a "60 Minutes" broadcast (see Chapter 18). Government regulatory actions or reports of toxic effects can dampen sales or even drive an occasional substance from the marketplace, but the number of products has been expanding.

In 1992, according to *Health Foods Business,* the "top ten supplements" sold through health-food stores were multivitamins, vitamin C, vitamin E, calcium, B-complex, beta-carotene, zinc, calcium-magnesium, multiminerals, potassium, and iron. The magazine also identified "up and coming" products alleged to improve brain function, lower cholesterol, enhance immunity, and contribute to muscle growth. Joe Bresse, vice-president of sales and marketing for General Nutrition Inc., predicted that "herbs are the wave of the future."

"Antioxidants" (and Other Phytochemicals)

Today's hottest supplement product category is antioxidants. The health-food industry promotes antioxidants as though they have proven benefit and zero risk—neither of which is true. The typical pitch for them—as stated in a recent catalog from The Vitamin Shoppe—goes like this:

> Our bodies are constantly bombarded by free radicals—atoms or groups of atoms that cause damage to our cells. Free radicals are present in tobacco smoke, air pollution, radiation, herbicides and other toxic chemicals. . . .
>
> Premature aging, impaired immune function, cancer, heart disease and numerous other major health complications have been linked to tissue damage from free radicals. The introduction of free radicals into the body can set off a chain reaction as thousands of free radical reactions can occur within seconds.
>
> Antioxidants, also known as free radical scavengers, are a family of nutrients that protect our body.

The most publicized dietary antioxidants are vitamin C, vitamin E, and beta-carotene (which the body converts into vitamin A). They are among dozens of chemicals involved in the production and control of free radicals within the body. Free radicals promote beneficial oxidation that produces energy and kills bacterial invaders. In excess, however, they produce harmful oxidation that can damage cell walls and cell contents. Vitamins C and E and beta-carotene are mischaracterized by describing them as "antioxidants." They are in fact redox agents—antioxidant in some circumstances (often so in the physiologic quantities found in foods), but prooxidant in others, producing billions of harmful free radicals (often so in the pharmacologic quantities found in supplements). Supplement pushers mention only the potential benefits.

Two large studies published in 1993 in *The New England Journal of Medicine* found that people who took vitamin E supplements had fewer deaths from heart disease. No similar association was found with vitamin C or beta-carotene. These studies did not prove that taking vitamin E was useful because they did not rule out the effects of other unmeasured lifestyle factors or consider death rates from other diseases. In addition, other studies have had conflicting results. The only way to settle the question scientifically is to conduct long-term double-blind clinical studies comparing vitamin users to nonusers and checking death rates from all causes. Meanwhile, caution is in order.

Medical Poll Reveals 8 Out of 10 Doctors Take an Antioxidant for Good Health

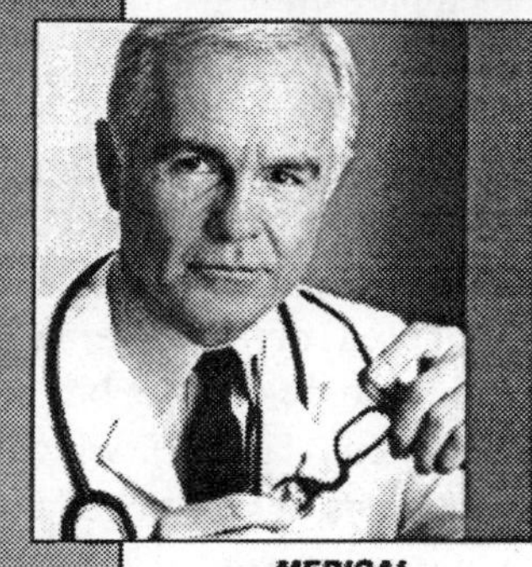

MEDICAL BREAKTHROUGH OF THE 90S!

Medical news from around the world now reveals the increasing need for antioxidants in our diet. As study after study continues to emerge, we now find 8 out of 10 doctors taking an antioxidant to promote longterm health.*

The most compelling new studies come from such prestigious research centers as the National Cancer Institute (NCI), the National Institute on Aging, Johns Hopkins University, Harvard University and the American Heart Association. With each new study, we find exciting breakthroughs on antioxidants isolated from fruits and vegetables and how they function within our body's cellular and tissue systems.

We now know that specific fruits, vegetables and other plant foods carry hundreds of protective compounds, called *phytonutrients*.

These newly discovered compounds protect our bodies against the devastating effects of free radicals. Similar to out-of-control "pac-men", these molecules seek out, attack and can virtually destroy our cells and tissues. Today, we find the very elements we need to sustain life: air, water, food and even sunlight – can now pose a serious threat to our health. Pollution, food preservatives, heavy metals, UV radiation and stress are among the biggest culprits of free radical production.

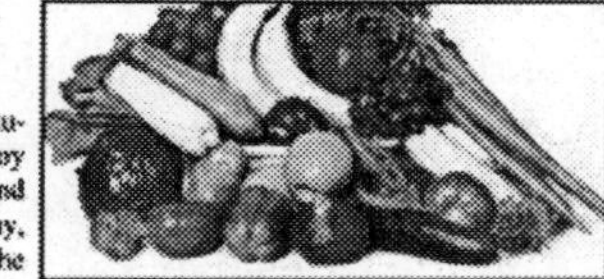

NATURE'S HEALTH CARE PLAN!

Although current research consistently reveals the need for antioxidant rich fruits and vegetables, an astounding 80% of us do **not** eat the recommended 5-9 daily servings. As a result, we are severely lacking in these powerful health protectors!

Now you can get the same health coverage as many of our leading doctors and scientists...with KAL's **Body Defense**. Unlike other products which contain only Beta Carotene, C and E, this breakthrough in nutritional research provides a *dual-system* approach to maximize health defense!

First, **Body Defense Multiple** provides mega potencies of essential vitamins, minerals, *Fruit & Veg Actives* antioxidants and other defenders to safeguard your daily nutrient intake!

As a complement to your Multiple, the **Body Defense Antioxidant** is packed with an exclusive complex of *Fruit & Veg Actives* to boost health defense even more! These remarkable phytonutrients are isolated from a wide array of fruits, vegetables and other plant foods. Each active is designed to target their actions to specific areas in the body most prone to free radical damage. As **Body Defense** supplies a full spectrum of phytonutrients, not just a few, our formulas help provide **Total Body Coverage!**

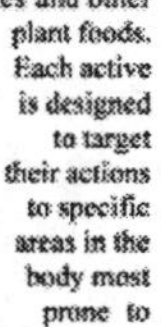

The Body Defense Antioxidant System

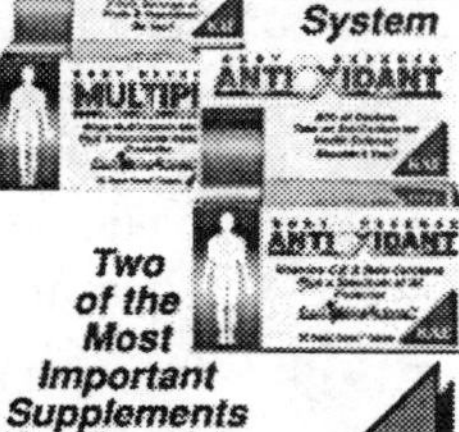

Two of the Most Important Supplements You Can Take Today!

KAL

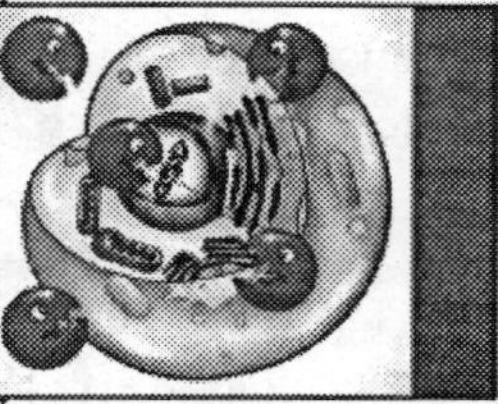

Free Radicals Attacking a Human Cell

*1992 Medical Tribune

Ad from May 1994 issue of Whole Foods. The "poll" it mentions did not show that eight out of ten doctors take antioxidants.

In 1994, *The New England Journal of Medicine* reported on the first two large clinical trials done to test whether supplementation with "antioxidants" would lower the incidence of cancer. The first trial compared the effects of vitamin E, beta-carotene, and a placebo. Much to the dismay of vitamin pushers, the researchers found no benefit from vitamin E and 18 percent more lung cancer among those who received beta-carotene! Not only that, but the overall death rate of beta-carotene recipients was 8 percent higher. There is evidence that vitamin E can help prevent atherosclerosis by interfering with the oxidation of low-density lipoproteins (LDL). However, vitamin E also has an anticoagulant effect, which, like that of aspirin, may promote excessive bleeding. Sure enough, those who took vitamin E had a higher frequency of hemorrhagic stroke. The second study found no evidence that supplementing with vitamin C, vitamin E, or beta-carotene prevented colorectal cancer.

It is known that people who eat adequate amounts of fruits and vegetables have a lower incidence of cardiovascular disease, certain cancers, and cataracts. But it is not known which factors are responsible. Vitamins A and C and beta-carotene constitute a tiny part of a large group of compounds called phytochemicals (plant chemicals). Plants contain hundreds of these chemicals, including isothiocyanates, which may protect against some cancers but promote others, and cyanogenic glycosides like amygdalin (laetrile), which is poisonous. Each individual plant food contains hundreds of phytochemicals whose presence is dictated by hereditary factors. Only well designed long-term research can determine whether any of these chemicals, taken in a pill, would be useful for preventing any disease.

The key question for today is whether supplementation with antioxidants (or other phytochemicals) has been *proven* to do more good than harm. The answer is no, which is why the FDA will not permit any of these substances to be labeled or marketed with claims that they can prevent disease.

In 1994, Makers of KAL began claiming that a survey conducted in 1992 by *Medical Tribune* (a newspaper for physicians) found that eight out of ten doctors take an antioxidant. Similar claims have been made by other manufacturers and health-food-industry publicists. However, *Medical Tribune* did not conduct a survey. Its editor merely asked doctors to share their experiences with vitamin E. Eighty percent of responders wrote positive statements. The percentage of doctors who do or don't take vitamin E cannot be determined this way. In addition, some doctors are just as gullible as other college graduates to incessant promotions.

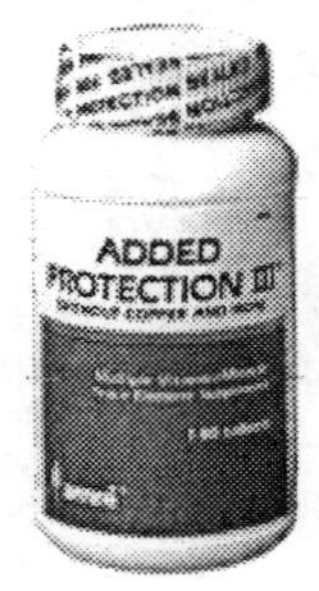

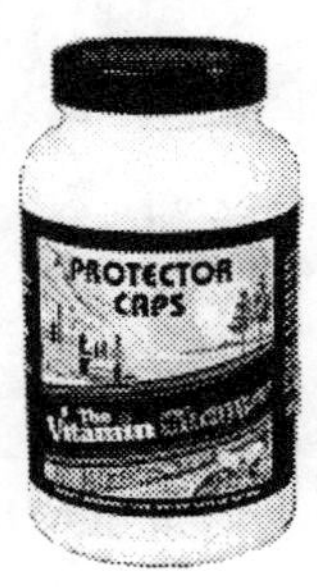

Many other manufacturers are marketing products that "protect against free radical damage" or are characterized as "protector vitamins"—a deceptive term introduced by Hoffmann-La Roche during the 1980s to describe vitamins C and E and beta-carotene. These claims are misleading but have not yet triggered federal regulatory action. Dr. Victor Herbert has petitioned the FDA to do something to rectify this situation.

Making Dollars out of Scents

Aromatherapy (sometimes called aroma therapy) is described by its proponents as "the therapeutic use of the essential oils of plants." These oils are said to be highly concentrated substances extracted from flowers, leaves, stalks, fruits, and roots, and also distilled from resins. They are alleged to contain hormones, vitamins, antibiotics, and antiseptics and to represent the "life force," "spirit," or "soul" of the plant. The oils are administered in small quantities through inhalation, massage, or other applications to the skin. Occasionally, a product is taken internally. The products include diffusers, lamps, pottery, candles, pendants, earrings, shampoos, skin creams, lotions, bath salts, and shower gels. *Health Foods Business* estimated that the total of aromatherapy products sold through health-food stores during 1992 was $26.5 million.

The leading American manufacturer, Aroma Vera, Inc., of Los Angeles,

Claims Made for Aromatherapy Products

Product Name	Features/Benefits
Calming	Lends a slight sense of euphoria - perfect for unwinding after a stressful day
Clear Mind	Freshens and sharpens the mind, making it more alert
Drainer/ Detoxification	Promotes elimination of toxins, helps tone and firm the body
Meditation	Facilitates deep relaxation
Mental Power	Designed for sustained intellectual power and focus
Purifier	Ideal to rid the atmosphere of smoke and heavy odors
Respiration	Helps open the lungs and clear respiration
Sacred	Helps open higher energy centers
Slimming/ Circulation	Promotes circulation and encourages elimination of excess fluids

claims that "essential oils have the power to purify the air we breathe while they relax, stimulate, soothe or sharpen our senses . . . a wonderful antidote to the air pollution and 'scentsory' imbalance of modern life." It also claims that inhaling the scents "balances the biological background," "revitalizes the cells," and produces a "strong energizing effect on the sympathetic nervous system." Charts in Aroma Vera's brochures explain how its products can be used (see previous page). Another company touts aromatherapy's promise as "a mood alternative, as biofeedback tied in to relaxation, stress release, concentration and meditation." Yet another describes the oils as "an alternative to synthetic drugs to feel good." A practitioner has claimed that the technique "addresses the nervous system and the energy fields of the body. It soothes the body, cleans the body, clears the body, and tones the body."

The Complete Book of Essential Oils and Aromatherapy, by Valerie Ann Worwood, states that there are about three hundred essential oils and that they constitute "an extremely effective medical system." It claims:

> Natural plant oils can be used to treat your child's flu, or called upon when you want to create a delicious and exciting new dish when the boss is invited to dinner. They will get rid of the fleas on your dog's coat as easily as the aphids from your garden plants. . . . With essential oils you can take control of your life and environment, secure in the knowledge that your well-being will be improved.

Aromatherapy for Common Ailments, by Shirley Price, tabulates which oils are to be used for more than forty problems, including depression, sex-drive problems, bronchitis, athlete's foot, high blood pressure, cystitis, and head lice. Her table identifies from three to nine oils "likely to help" each problem. She reassures:

> With self-help aromatherapy, you will be using oils recommended for a particular ailment or preventative treatment, but it should not take you long to discover which of them work best for you as an individual, particularly since simply liking the aroma of an oil may indicate that it will help you.

The Aromatherapy Workbook charts more than one hundred therapeutic applications. Author Marcel Lavabre maintains:

> Even though it can relieve symptoms, aromatherapy primarily aims at curing the causes of disease. The main therapeutic action of essential oils consists in strengthening the organs and their functions, and acting on the defense mechanisms of the body. They do not do the job for the body; they help the body do its own job and thus do not weaken the organism. Their action is enhanced by all natural therapies that aim to restore the vitality of the individual.

The American Alliance of Aromatherapy, a trade association, publishes a quarterly *Journal of Aromatherapy* to inform its readers about pertinent research, books, and news. The American Aromatherapy Association offers "certification" based on attendance at two three-day weekends plus submission of a thesis that includes case studies. The course includes such topics as internal methods of treatment, essential oils in healing, addressing common health problems, and how to market yourself. The International Association of Aromatherapists has "accredited" an eleven-month correspondence course with six seminars and two final exams. Completion of the program leads to "certification" as an "Aromatherapist Practitioner." Aromatherapy Seminars, the educational division of Aroma Vera, offers "five-day certification" and other courses and claims to have over 3,500 graduates.

The FDA regulates perfumes as cosmetics, which it defines as "articles to be introduced into or otherwise applied to the body to cleanse, beautify, promote attractiveness or alter appearance." A general claim that a perfume's aroma is good or beneficial is a cosmetic claim that does not require FDA approval. In 1986, the agency warned that marketing a scent with a preventive or therapeutic claim would make the product a drug subject to regulatory action. Although several manufacturers have done so, the FDA has not made them stop.

Arthritis Quackery

"Arthritis" is a group of more than a hundred conditions. Although the term literally means "inflammation of a joint," some types of arthritis involve pain without inflammation. People tend to lump them all together when applying folk remedies, and quacks rarely differentiate between the various types when making claims for "cures." Except for gout, no clear relationship exists between nutrition and arthritis. It is unlikely that a dietary change will be effective for most types of arthritis or even for most people with the same type. Even with gout, the primary treatment is medication, not diet.

Most types of arthritis can have a variable course, with periods of improvement and worsening. If improvement occurs following use of a questionable remedy, the patient may become convinced that the remedy caused the improvement. Although medical researchers continue to explore the role that diet may play in certain types of arthritis, so far it seems that only a tiny percentage of individuals with arthritis have idiosyncratic reactions to food. Only carefully controlled experiments can determine whether dietary manipulation actually works for a given person. So far, no compelling evidence exists that any diet is consistently helpful for arthritic conditions. Yet myths persist that dietary factors can cause or cure them. A 1986 FDA survey found that about one out of three people with arthritis said they had tried at least one method considered questionable by the survey's designers. The most frequently tried methods included vitamins (17 percent), special diets (12 percent), alfalfa tablets (9 percent), honey/vinegar (8 percent), and cod liver or fish oil (8 percent). L-canavanine, a toxic amino acid in alfalfa, can promote some types of arthritis (see Appendix C).

Diets based on raw foods, foods without chemical additives, and other supposedly "natural" nutrition items are being hustled by the health-food industry. So are misleading books, several of which have been best sellers. Many of these approaches are based on the notion that arthritis and other "degenerative diseases" are caused by a buildup of (unspecified) toxins that can be corrected by whatever method they happen to advocate.

Green-lipped mussel has been promoted by the book *Relief from Arthritis* by John Croft, as well as through articles in health-food magazines and tabloid newspapers. The mussel is harvested in New Zealand, made into supplement capsules, and marketed by various American companies. In 1976, the FDA banned importation of green-lipped mussel preparations. In 1983, the agency seized a large quantity of products and raw materials from the Aquaculture Corporation of Redwood City, California, manufacturer of *Neptone*. The company contested the seizure on the grounds that their product was a food rather than a drug. However, FDA documents proved that the company had distributed literature and suggested in advertisements that green-lipped mussel preparations were effective against arthritis. Similar products are still marketed—as "mucopolysaccharides." Their labels contain no claims, but the ingredients are promoted by health-food-industry publications. Other supplements, such as shark cartilage, are falsely claimed to increase joint flexibility.

Capsules of omega-3 fatty acids—commonly referred to as "fish oils"—have been marketed with claims that they are effective against several types of arthritis. A few experiments in both animals and humans have had positive results, but it is not known whether there is a dose that is both practical and safe. Fish oil supplements can interfere with blood clotting and increase the risk of stroke, especially when taken with aspirin or other nonsteroidal antiinflammatory drugs. Fish oils can also cause diarrhea and upset stomach. Responsible medical authorities believe that including oily fish (mackerel, salmon, sardines, or lake trout) in the diet is far preferable to taking fish oil supplements.

Cod liver oil was popularized by *Arthritis and Common Sense*, whose author, the late Dale Alexander, was endearingly referred to as "the Codfather." The book states that he was inspired by treating his mother's crippling arthritis. He concluded that the basic cause of arthritis is "poorly lubricated joints" and that dietary oils (particularly cod liver oil) relieve arthritis by lubricating the joints. This theory is ludicrous. The lubricating fluid within the joints is not oil but a fluid that resembles blood plasma and is secreted by the tissue lining the joints. Moreover, dietary oils can't reach the joints intact because they are broken down into simple substances by the digestive process. Alexander also stated that arthritics should allow at least six months to assess the results of taking cod liver oil because "it could take that long for the whole body to lubricate itself." That, of course, would be sufficient time for many arthritics to undergo spontaneous improvement.

Authors and book publishers are not the only ones who profiteer in print at the expense of arthritis victims; media that accept ads for misleading books are equally to blame. And so are the health-food industry's publications, which abound with claims that food supplements can help virtually every health problem. In 1990, the year Alexander died, his theories appeared in a two-page interview in Swanson's *Health Shopper* together with an ad for Twin Laboratories' *Emulsified Norwegian Cod Liver Oil*, the label of which bore Alexander's signature. Other supplement manufacturers market products that contain no claims on their labels but the names of which (e.g., *Ar Pak, Artho-Plex, Arthritis Relief Tablets*) falsely suggests effectiveness against arthritis.

Homeopathic products, discussed in Chapter 9, are also promoted for arthritis. In a recent issue of *Let's Live,* a leading homeopath stated that there may be 150 remedies available for different types of arthritis and that they work by stimulating the body to heal itself. He claimed, "Mild or relatively recent cases can be cured completely. Cases of many years' duration can usually be greatly relieved, sometimes cured, and, at the very least, the degenerative process can be halted." There is no reliable evidence to support these claims.

Most bogus arthritis remedies are nontoxic, but some are dangerous. Since the late 1970s, Oriental arthritis remedies said to be "all-natural" herbal products have been illegally marketed in the United States under the names *Chuifong Toukuwan, Black Pearls,* and *Miracle Herb.* Government agencies have found that in addition to herbs, these products contain various potent drugs not listed on their labels. The FDA has banned importation of these products and helped Texas authorities obtain criminal convictions against several marketers. However, they may still be marketed through clandestine channels.

Multiple Sclerosis "Cures"

Multiple sclerosis (MS) is a degenerative disease of the brain, spinal cord, and optic (eye) nerves, in which patches of inflammation and scarring interfere with the function of the brain, spinal cord, and/or the nerves to the eyes. Its symptoms include muscular weakness, loss of coordination, and difficulty with speech and vision. It occurs chiefly in young adults and, like arthritis, can have a very variable course. Some people have only a few attacks in a lifetime, recover from these, and experience no disability except during attacks. Others have frequent attacks from which they don't recover completely, but which cause only partial disability. Still others have a slow progression of disability over a period of ten to twenty-five years, which eventually leaves them helpless. When attacks occur, symptoms may come and go suddenly and may even vary from hour to hour.

MS's extreme variability makes it a perfect disease for quacks. The only way to know whether a treatment is effective is to follow a large number of patients for *years* to see whether those who receive the treatment do better than those who do not. Quacks don't bother with this kind of testing, however. They simply claim credit whenever anyone who consults them improves. And since the majority of attacks are followed by complete or partial recovery, a persuasive quack can acquire patients who swear by whatever he recommends.

The Therapeutic Claims Committee of the International Federation of Multiple Sclerosis Societies has analyzed more than fifty alleged treatments and published the results in a book called *Therapeutic Claims in Multiple Sclerosis*. Each analysis includes a description of the method, the proponents' rationale, a scientific evaluation, estimate of risks and/or costs, and the authors' conclusion. With respect to nutrition, the committee concluded: (1) supplementation with polyunsaturated fatty acids and fish oils should be regarded as "investigational" because the evidence for it is conflicting; (2) low-fat diets, allergen-free diets, the Kousmine Diet, gluten-free, raw food (Evers), MacDougall Diet, pectin- and fructose-restricted diet, liquid VLC diets, and the sucrose- and tobacco-free diet should be considered unproven because there is no generally accepted rationale for their use and they have not been tested by properly controlled studies; (3) supplementation with cerebrosides, aloe vera, or enzymes should be considered unproven, and (4) megavitamin and megamineral therapies are unproven and potentially hazardous.

Bee Pollen and Royal Jelly

"Bee pollen" is actually pollen from flowers that is collected from bees as they enter the hive or is harvested by other means. Promoters call it "the perfect food" and stress that it contains all of the essential amino acids and many vitamins and minerals. However, none of these nutrients offers any magic, and we obtain all of them easily and less expensively from conventional foods. Bee pollen has also been claimed to improve athletic and sexual performance; prolong life; promote both weight loss *and* weight gain; prevent infection, allergy, and cancer; and alleviate more than sixty other health problems. There is no scientific support for any claim that bee pollen is effective against any human disease. The few studies that have been done to test its effect on athletic performance have shown no benefit. Royal jelly, which is used to make and feed queen bees, comes from the salivary glands of bees. It too has been falsely claimed to be especially nutritious, to provide buoyant energy, and to have therapeutic properties.

Bee pollen and royal jelly should be regarded as potentially dangerous because they cause allergic reactions. People allergic to specific pollens have developed asthma, hives, and life-threatening anaphylactic shock after ingesting pollen. Recently, an eleven-year-old Australian girl suffered a fatal asthma attack after receiving 500 mg of royal jelly.

Both bee pollen and royal jelly have been involved in recent federal enforcement actions. In 1992, a federal court ordered destruction of quantities of *Bee Alive*, a royal jelly and herb combination in honey seized from Bee-Alive Inc., of Valley Cottage, N.Y. In 1989, the FDA had warned the company that promotional material distributed with a similar product had made illegal statements that the product was useful in treating or preventing chronic Epstein-Barr virus syndrome, gastrointestinal ulcers, colitis, low blood pressure, arteriosclerosis, nervous breakdowns, infertility, impotence, depression, rheumatoid arthritis, Alzheimer's disease, anemia, asthma, hemorrhoids, migraine headaches, and other problems. Despite a promise to stop distributing literature making these claims, the company continued to advertise that Regina Royal Jelly could help children resist childhood ailments, "offers daytime vitality and nighttime tranquillity," increases mental and physical stamina, and "seems to improve the immune system."

In 1992, the CC Pollen Company, of Phoenix, Arizona, and its owners (Bruce R. Brown, Carol M. Brown, and Royden Brown) agreed to pay $200,000 to settle charges that they falsely represented that bee-pollen products could produce weight loss, permanently alleviate allergies, reverse the aging process, and cure, prevent, or alleviate impotence or sexual dysfunction. The company and its owners were also charged with falsely stating that bee-pollen products are an effective antibiotic for human use and cannot result in an allergic reaction. Under the agreement, the company and its owners are prohibited from making all of these claims and are required to have scientific evidence to support any other health-related claims about any other product for human consumption. Some of the false claims were made in "infomercials" that were misrepresented as news or documentary programs, even though they were paid ads. During one infomercial, entitled "TV Insiders," host Vince Inneo falsely implied that the program was part of a series of independent investigations. The products offered during the infomercial were *Bee-Young, Pollenergy* (to "restore missing energy'), *Royal Jelly* ("to keep sexually active at any age"), *President's Lunch,* and *First Lady's Lunch Bar.*

Although violation of an FTC consent agreement can trigger a penalty of up to $10,000 per day, Brown continued to promote bee pollen illegally. In May 1994, a few weeks before Brown had a fatal accident, S&S Public Relations Inc., of Chicago, issued a letter stating: "It's allergy season, but many sufferers aren't suffering anymore. They're using *Aller-Bee-Gone,* bee pollen tablets that are credited with relieving the symptoms of allergies, asthma, and other respiratory ailments." The accompanying news release added:

> Bee pollen is used to enhance athletic performance. Called the 'edible fountain of youth,' been pollen is a regular part of the diet for 94-year-old New York marathon runner Noel Johnson, as well as for former President Ronald Reagan.
>
> Royden Brown's lifetime goal now is to eliminate degenerative disease worldwide through the use of bee pollen.

"Energy Enhancers"

Hundreds of products have been marketed with false or misleading claims that they will reduce fatigue and/or make people more energetic. Sometimes the claim is implied by the product's name or by an ad that depicts an energetic person. In a recent report in *Health Foods Business,* one retailer advised placing photographs of people engaged in vigorous activities near the "energy boosters" section.

Most such products contain various combinations of vitamins, minerals, and/or herbs. Although vitamins and minerals are necessary to help release energy (calories) from food, the amount released is not increased by taking extra vitamins or minerals. Herbal products that contain stimulant drugs (such as guarana, which contains caffeine) can increase alertness and may prevent fatigue—as would a cup of coffee—but whether it is wise to use them habitually is another matter.

Nature's Plus, of Farmingdale, New York, refers to its products as "the Energy Supplements." A recent flyer touts its *Source of Life* formulas "for a guaranteed burst of energy." Its "multivitamin and mineral with whole food concentrates" is claimed to provide a unique "broad spectrum of ingredients ...

combined to create the powerful, synergistic effects that result in an incredible 'Burst of Energy.'" This claim is pure hype. The product contains more than forty ingredients, most of which have no caloric or energy value. The few that do—such as bee pollen, spirulina, and octacosanol, provide insignificant amounts of calories.

One widely advertised "energizer" was *Essential Factors,* marketed by Sharper Image Corporation, an upscale company that sells through retail outlets and a widely distributed mail-order catalog. The product was said to contain vitamins, minerals, antioxidant and immune factors, plus a patented form of potassium-magnesium aspartate. According to Sharper Image's 1989 and 1990 catalogs:

> Oxy-Energizer is the first nutritional supplement ever to be granted a US patent. Supported by over 300 independent clinical trials, this anti-fatigue formula consistently demonstrated increases in stamina, endurance, recovery time, and cardiovascular function, results that simply can't be duplicated by any other nutritional supplement. . . . Oxy-Energizer contains a trade secret blend of potassium, magnesium and aspartic acid. Double-blind swimming, running, and aerobics studies consistently show improvements in stamina and endurance for subjects who regularly take these active ingredients. It can help you accomplish more at the office because you're not fighting tiredness. After work, you have more energy to enjoy sports or a late evening out.

The ad also stated that fitness authority Kathy Smith got extra energy from the product and had used it daily for five years to help maintain her busy pace. A two-month supply cost about $1.25 per day.

Since government enforcement efforts give priority to false claims involving the treatment of disease, "energy-enhancing" claims are seldom regulated. In 1993, however, Sharper Image Corporation and its president, Richard Thalheimer, signed an FTC consent agreement not to make unsubstantiated claims that any U.S. Government agency has recognized the product as effective for relieving fatigue or producing energy. The FTC order did not address other false claims in the ad. Do you believe that *Oxy-Energizer* underwent three hundred scientific trials? We don't.

Tonics for the Heart

Many companies market "cholesterol-lowering" nostrums and other supplement products said to be effective in preventing or treating heart disease. These products include niacin, oat bran tablets, fish oil, lecithin, vitamins, minerals, herbs, and various other substances, either alone or in multiple-ingredient products. A few of these substances may play a useful role in a *medically supervised* program for cholesterol control, but no product of this type is suitable for self-medication.

High doses of niacin can be very effective in improving blood cholesterol levels. They can also damage the liver and elevate blood sugar and uric acid levels. For this reason, people who take niacin should have periodic blood tests to detect trouble before it becomes serious. Drugs should rarely be considered unless dietary modification and exercise are unable to modify cholesterol levels sufficiently. If a drug is appropriate, the choice and dosage of the drug and the target levels of the treatment program should depend on various factors that are best analyzed by a physician.

Oat bran is potentially useful but should not be taken in pill form. Although increasing the amount of soluble fiber in the diet can lower cholesterol levels, pills containing fiber usually contain too little to be significant. Moreover, it is better to get fiber from foods, as part of a low-fat diet, because foods contain a greater variety of fibers.

Fish oil capsules present a different problem. Epidemiological research has found that populations whose diet is rich in certain fatty acids tend to have less heart disease. Other research has found that supplements of omega-3 fatty acids (found in fish oils) can help lower blood cholesterol levels and inhibit clotting, which means they may be useful in preventing heart attacks. However, it is not known what dosage is appropriate or whether long-range use is safe or effective for any purpose. Eating fish once or twice a week is advantageous, but fish oil capsules are not suitable for use by the general public. They can increase the tendency toward strokes and—since they are high in fat—may even increase blood cholesterol levels.

A few studies have found that people given daily garlic or garlic extract had lowered their blood cholesterol levels. However, this evidence is preliminary and does not indicate which people might benefit, whether high doses of garlic are safe, effective, or practical for long-term use, or how garlic products compare to other drugs whose effects have been thoroughly studied. Garlic can produce bad breath, heartburn, and flatulence and can inhibit blood clotting.

Lecithin is also claimed to help prevent and/or treat coronary heart disease. But there is no scientific evidence that it is effective for this purpose.

Vitamin E is being studied to see whether high doses can prevent atherosclerosis by preventing oxidation of low-density lipoproteins (LDL) in the blood. Experiments now under way may settle this question, but they will take several years to complete (see discussion above under "Antioxidants").

Many multiple-ingredient products sold as "dietary supplements" are

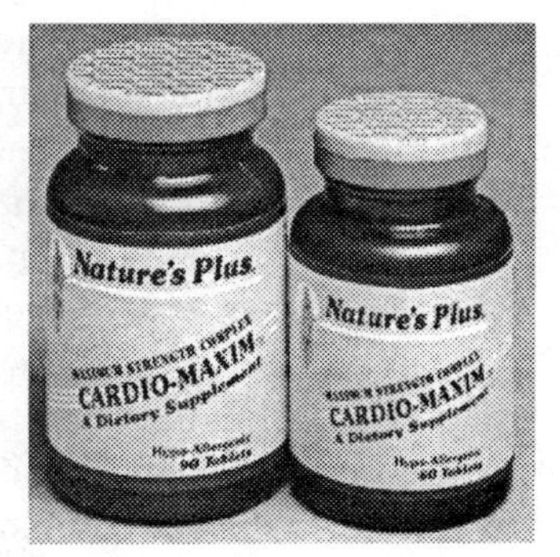

claimed to help "protect," "strengthen," "nourish," or "support" the heart or prevent or correct heart disease. All such products are worthless. *Cardio-Maxim*, sold by Nature's Plus, is an example. This product contains 25 mg of niacin, a dose too small to have any beneficial effect. Its other six ingredients have nothing whatsoever to do with preventing heart disease. Yet its promotional literature claims:

> Cardio-vascular disease is the number one killer in America. Therefore, strengthening the body's vital organs is an essential part of preventative health. . . .
>
> Cardio-Maxim [is] a sophisticated foundation of nutrients for those who are interested in this very special supplementation.

Cardio-Maxim is noteworthy because the president of Nature's Plus is leading the health-food industry's campaign to cripple FDA regulation of dietary supplements (see Chapter 20).

Many entrepreneurs have marketed "oral chelation" products with claims that they can clean out atherosclerotic coronary arteries. These concoctions, all of which are bogus, contain various amounts of vitamins, minerals, amino acids, and/or other substances. The FDA has banned them, but a few are still sold.

A maximal program to protect against heart disease should be based on an analysis of risk factors: cigarette smoking, obesity, high blood pressure, elevated blood cholesterol levels, diabetes, and lack of exercise. If you have any of these risk factors, you should become well informed and make significant changes in the way you live. Quackery may appear to offer easy solutions, but it can't deliver them.

"Immune-System Boosters"

Public focus on AIDS has spawned a host of products and procedures claimed to work by influencing the immune system. In recent years, many "alternative" practitioners have adopted the "immune system" as a focus of their treatment. Cancer quacks allege that cancer occurs because the immune defenses fail to destroy cancer cells before they multiply out of hand. Acupuncturists, naturopaths, chiropractors, homeopaths, natural hygienists, and other types of so-called vitalistic healers equate their various forms of "life force" with immune mechanisms. "Clinical ecologists" insist that millions of people have become ill because their immune system was overloaded. And the health-food industry has promoted countless nutrient concoctions purported to "strengthen" the immune system.

In 1986, the trade magazine *Health Foods Retailing* reported that vitamin sales had increased sharply in response to *Dr. Berger's Immune Power Diet,* by Stuart M. Berger, M.D., which claimed that weight control can be achieved by "rebuilding" one's immune system with dietary change and food supplements (see Chapter 17). According to the magazine's editor, the problem of AIDS had stimulated public concern about the immune system. During the same year, *Health News & Review,* a bimonthly "health food" newspaper for the general public, reported "growing public recognition that AIDS, cancer, arthritis, even colds—very nearly the whole spectrum of infections and degenerative diseases—become manifest dangers only when the immune system is depressed. Strengthening the immune system . . . is clearly emerging as a health priority." The report then described how promoters of a wide variety of unproven nutrition practices related them to supposed immunological factors. Sugar, food allergies, and mercury fillings, for example, were said to weaken the immune system, while vitamin C, zinc, beta-carotene, and certain herbs were said to strengthen it. Although no scientific evidence supported any of these claims, "health food" marketers began marketing new products and recasting old ones as "immune boosters."

One manufacturer whose ads were particularly blatant was Futurebiotics, of Brattleboro, Vermont. One ad stated:

> To provide as broad a spectrum of immune defenders as possible, Futurebiotics has created MAXIMUM IMMUNE SUPPORT. . . .
>
> You can't read a magazine or newspaper, listen to the radio or watch TV today without some mention of clear and present dangers such as cancer and AIDS and all the lifestyle and environmental agents implicated in this health crisis. Everyone is exposed to billions of viruses, bacteria, pollutants and toxins all the time. This constant bombardment . . . can be held off and destroyed only by our healthy immune system. As in any battle, ammunition is vital. The ammunition required to supply our immune systems is a vast array of varied life-promoting nutrients.

In 1989, volunteers of the Houston-based Consumer Health Education Council telephoned forty-one health-food stores and asked to speak with the person who provided nutritional advice. The callers explained that they had a brother with AIDS who was seeking an effective alternative to standard drugs. The callers also explained that the brother's wife was still having sex with her husband and was seeking products that would reduce her risk of being infected, or make it impossible. All forty-one retailers offered products they said could benefit the brother's immune system, improve the woman's immunity, and protect her against harm from the virus. The recommended products included vitamins (forty-one stores), vitamin C (thirty-eight stores), immune boosters (thirty-eight stores), coenzyme Q_{10} (twenty-six stores), germanium (twenty-six stores), lecithin (nineteen stores), ornithine and/or arginine (nine stores), gamma-linolenic acid (seven stores), raw glandulars (seven stores), hydrogen peroxide (five stores), blue-green algae (five stores), homeopathic salts (five stores), Bach Flower Remedies (four stores), cysteine (three stores), and herbal baths (two stores). Thirty retailers said they carried products that would cure AIDS. None recommended abstinence or use of a condom.

In June 1993, the New York City Department of Consumer Affairs charged four supplement companies with deceptively promoting products characterized as "immune boosters." The action was taken under a city consumer protection law, passed in 1990, which regulates advertising of products and services claimed or implied to "boost, enhance, stimulate, assist, cure, strengthen or improve the body's immune system." Under this law, no such effect can be claimed without an accurate statement about whether or not the product or service is effective in preventing HIV infection or improving the health of an infected individual. The cited products were *Immune Protectors* (Twin Laboratories, Inc.), *Immunizer Pak Program* and *Immune Nectar* (Nature's Plus), *Pro-Immune Anti-Oxidant* (Nutritional Life Support Systems), and *Ecomer* (a shark liver oil capsule marketed by Scandinavian Natural Health & Beauty Products, Inc.).

The FDA has acted against several companies that marketed bogus products with "immune" or "immu-" in their name. The most noteworthy involved a seizure in 1988 of nine Futurebiotics products, one of which was *Maximum Immune Support*. The case was settled by a consent decree ordering destruction of the products and prohibiting the company from making false or unsubstantiated claims in the future.

Despite government actions, however, many such products are still sold. In fact, since the potential market for "immune boosters" is everyone, supplement concoctions of this type will continue to be promoted even after a cure for AIDS is found.

"Life Extension" Products

Since the early 1980s, several books have suggested to the public that life can be extended by using various dietary methods, nutritional supplements, and/or drugs. The claims are based mainly on misinterpretations or inappropriate extrapolations of animal experiments. The leading book has been *Life Extension: A Practical Scientific Approach*, which was published in 1982. Despite its many inaccuracies (or perhaps because of them), it topped best seller lists for many weeks. Its authors, Durk Pearson and Sandy Shaw, have also licensed several lines of supplement products sold by others.

Life Extension outlined an extensive program of supplements and drugs, combined with laboratory testing to look for signs of improvement or toxicity. They claimed that their program might extend an average individual's life span by several decades and improve quality of life as well. The book's success inspired many manufacturers to market "life extension," "life expander," and "antiaging" products, which included substances characterized as antioxidants, antioxidant cofactors, cellular rejuvenators, immune-system stimulants, growth-hormone releasers, anti-crosslinking factors, and membrane stabilizers. In 1983, *Health Foods Business* listed thirty-nine "age-fighting agents" that "when used alone or in compounds, are said to slow down the aging process and/or reduce its degenerative aspects."

Another leading promoter of life-extension mythology is Saul Kent, author of *The Life Extension Revolution*, who founded the Life Extension Foundation in Hollywood, Florida. The foundation's stated purpose is to "mobilize support for life extension, provide the public with products and services, and raise money for life extension research." Regular membership costs $50 a year and entitles members to product discounts, a directory of "life extension" doctors, a directory of "innovative medical clinics," a copy of *The Physician's Guide to Life Extension Drugs*, and two monthly newsletters. The Foundation also sells supplement products, many of them based on the theories of Pearson and Shaw. One of them, *Life Extension Mix*, resembles the formula Pearson and Shaw said they had used for themselves. In 1986, the foundation marketed Mother's and Father's Day gift packages containing the book, the mix, and either *Rejuvenex* (an "antiaging" face cream for women) or *Mineral Orotate Complex for Men* (said to help prevent heart disease).

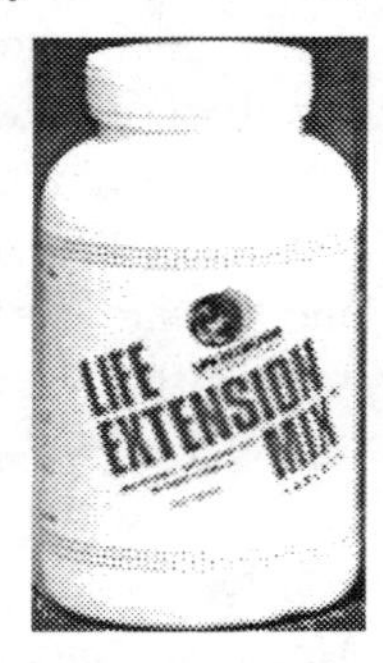

In 1987, FDA officials and U.S. marshals raided the foundation and seized large quantities of *BHT* (promoted for herpes and AIDS), *DMSO* (for arthritis and bursitis), *Coenzyme Q10* (for cardiovascular disorders and increased longevity), and *Cognitex* (to enhance mental function). In November 1991, a twenty-eight-count indictment was filed in the Southern District Court of Florida charging Kent and the company's vice president with importing and selling unapproved new drugs and misbranded prescription drugs. According to an FDA report, the products were imported from Europe, labeled as nutritional supplements, and promoted for cancer, AIDS, herpes, senility, heart and lung disease, and other illnesses.

Gerovital H3 (GH3) was developed by Dr. Anna Aslan, a Rumanian physician. It has been promoted by the Rumanian National Tourist Office and a few American manufacturers as an antiaging substance—"the secret of eternal vigor and youth." Claims have been made that GH3 can prevent or relieve a wide variety of disorders, including arthritis, arteriosclerosis, angina pectoris and other heart conditions, neuritis, deafness, Parkinson's disease, depression, senile psychosis, and impotence. It is also claimed to stimulate hair growth, restore pigments to gray hair, and tighten and smooth skin. The main ingredient in GH3 is procaine, a substance used for local anesthesia. Although many uncontrolled studies describe benefits from the use of GH3, controlled trials using procaine have failed to demonstrate any. Noting that para-aminobenzoic acid (PABA) appears in the urine of people receiving procaine injections, a few American manufacturers have sold "procaine" tablets containing PABA with false claims similar to those made for GH3. The FDA has taken regulatory action against several companies marketing "GH3" products, but other brands still are marketed.

Dubious Weight-Control Products

Nonprescription diet aids sold in health-food stores, in pharmacies, and by mail enjoy popularity despite their questionable effectiveness. Ads for some of them make dieting sound like more fun than eating. Some products are accompanied by a printed diet that, if followed, will produce weight loss. But the pills themselves have little or no value.

Pills claimed to block food components from being absorbed into the body are hardy perennials in the diet-fraud marketplace. In the early 1980s, "starch blockers" led the field. These products were claimed to contain an enzyme extracted from beans that could block the digestion of significant amounts of starch. The enzyme works in the test tube, but the human body produces more starch-digesting enzymes than these products could possibly block. Moreover, if large amounts of undigested starch did reach the large intestine, they would be fermented by the bacteria normally present, producing gas and digestive disturbances. In 1982, the FDA received more than a hundred reports of abdominal pain, diarrhea, vomiting, and other adverse reactions among users of "starch-blockers." As the reports poured in, the agency took regulatory action and drove most of these products from the marketplace.

"Bulk producers," containing glucomannan or other dietary fiber, have been claimed to suppress appetite by swelling within the stomach. Even if this method actually could reduce food intake, the amount of fiber in "diet pills" is too small to accomplish this. One double-blind study found no evidence that glucomannan supplements affect hunger ratings or weight loss, but some of the individuals taking them developed bloating and gas.

The most notorious fiber product in recent years was *Cal-Ban 3000*, a guar gum product claimed to cause "automatic" weight loss by decreasing appetite and blocking the absorption of fat. When taken by mouth, guar gum forms a gel within the stomach that may contribute to a feeling of fullness and may block some nutrients so they are not absorbed. However, it has not been shown that either of these things is enough to produce weight loss consistently. Many overweight people keep eating even when their stomach signals that it is full.

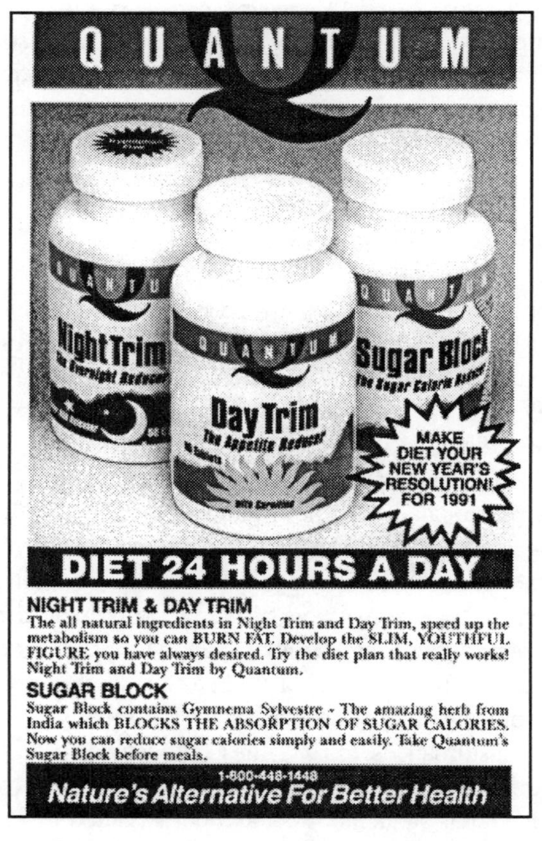

Misleading ad for three weight-control products.

Moreover, if food absorption is decreased, the individual may eat more often to compensate.

Another supposed bulk-producer was Schering Corporation's *Fibre Trim*, which was hyped as effective for weight loss, weight control, and weight maintenance. The product was made of fiber from citrus and grain compressed into tablets. Ads said it could provide a feeling of fullness and could "take the edge off hunger." In 1991, an FTC administrative law judge ruled that there was no scientific evidence to substantiate such claims. A company document suggested that most of *Fibre Trim*'s sales were to consumers "looking for the magic pill" and who "want a product that will do the work." The judge ordered Schering to refrain from making unsubstantiated claims that *Fibre Trim* (a) is a rich source of fiber, (b) could provide any health benefit associated with the intake of fiber, or (c) could provide any appetite-suppressant, weight-loss, or weight-control benefit.

Extracts of *Gymnema sylvestre*, a plant grown in India, are being heavily promoted through health-food stores. These products are claimed to cause weight loss by preventing dietary sugar from being absorbed into the body. According to Purdue University's Varro E. Tyler, Ph.D., a leading authority on plant medicine, chewing the plant's leaves can prevent the taste sensation of sweetness. But there is no reliable evidence that the chemicals they contain can block the absorption of sugar into the body or produce weight loss.

Many companies have marketed programs and products claimed to remove "stubborn fat," which they refer to as "cellulite." Widespread promotion of the "cellulite" concept in the United States followed the 1973 publication of *Cellulite: Those Lumps, Bumps and Bulges You Couldn't Lose Before,* by Nicole Ronsard, owner of a New York City beauty salon that specialized in skin and body care. Cellulite is alleged to be a special type of "fat gone wrong," a combination of fat, water, and "toxic wastes" that the body has failed to eliminate. Anticellulite products include "loofah" sponges, cactus fibers, special washcloths, horsehair mitts, creams to "dissolve" cellulite, vitamin-mineral supplements with herbs, bath liquids, massagers, rubberized pants, exercise books, brushes, rollers, and toning lotions. Many salons offer treatment with electrical muscle stimulation, vibrating machines, inflatable hip-high pressurized boots, "hormone" or "enzyme" injections, heating pads, and massage. Some operators claim that five to fifteen inches can be lost in one hour. However, cellulite is not a medical term or even a legitimate one; the areas so named are ordinary fatty tissue. Strands of fibrous tissue connect the skin to deeper tissue layers and also separate compartments that contain fat cells. When fat cells increase in size, these compartments bulge and produce a waffled appearance of the skin. No equipment, exercise, or nonsurgical treatment can produce "spot-reduction." The amount of body fat is determined by the individual's eating and exercise habits, but the distribution of fat is determined by heredity. Reduction of a particular part can be accomplished only as part of an overall weight-reduction program or, in some cases, by liposuction.

"Growth hormone releasers" have been claimed to cause overnight weight loss by stepping up the body's production of growth hormone. These products typically contain one or more amino acids. Their promoters claim that ingesting them on an empty stomach triggers the pituitary gland to produce growth hormone, which burns fat and results in weight loss. This concept is invalid. Although blood levels of growth hormone can be raised temporarily by injecting large amounts of arginine, the commercially marketed pills don't accomplish this. Even if they could, it wouldn't help because increased blood levels of growth hormone don't cause weight loss. If elevated blood levels could be maintained, the result would be acromegaly, a disease in which the hands, feet and face become abnormally large and deformed. Federal and state enforcement actions have driven some so-called "growth hormone releasers" from the marketplace, but many are still available.

Many types of herbs are touted as effective for controlling weight. No herbal product has been approved by the FDA as safe and effective for weight control. In fact, many contain laxatives that cause adverse effects. Another dangerous ingredient is ma huang, which contains ephedrine.

Homeopathic products, such as drops placed on the tongue or adhesive dots applied to "acupuncture points" on the wrist, are said to suppress appetite. Such products are total frauds.

Spirulina, a type of alga sold in tablet or powder form, is claimed to "bolster willpower" and to suppress hunger by making biochemical changes in the brain. Although these claims are false, spirulina gained a market toehold in 1981 after the *National Enquirer* published an article with a front-page headline touting it as an appetite suppressant. Although the FDA has stated that spirulina may not be legally sold as an appetite suppressant, many health-food entrepreneurs still do so.

Kelp, lecithin, cider vinegar, and B_6—accompanied by a 1,000-or-so-calorie diet will cause weight loss—as a result of the diet alone. The kelp and other supplements have no useful purpose in a weight-reduction program.

"Slimming teas," Oriental or otherwise, have no proven value for appetite suppression or any type of "automatic" weight loss. Some teas are said to be "thermogenic," which is a scientific term for "heat-producing." However, they are not. They neither raise body temperature nor speed metabolism.

Mail-order products are typically marketed with claims that they can cause weight loss of several pounds a week without exercise or calorie restriction. Some of these products are claimed to suppress appetite through hormonal manipulation ("growth-hormone releasers"). Others are supposed to block the absorption of fat, carbohydrate, sugar, or calories in general. We have never seen a product advertised in this manner that was not a complete fake. Not only that, but countless people have complained to government agencies and Better Business Bureaus that money-back "guarantees" for such products were not honored.

Juicing

According to the cover of his book *The Juiceman: the Power of Juicing*, Jay "the Juiceman" Kordich offers a "revolutionary program for staying healthy, looking young, staying trim, and feeling great—all by taking advantage of the natural healing power of fresh fruit and vegetable juices." Kordich claims that at age twenty, he became gravely ill with a cancer and was told he might not live. Inspired by literature about the Gerson diet, he began drinking thirteen glasses of carrot-apple juice every day. "Two and a half years later," he says in the book, "I was a well man." After more than twenty years of hawking juice extractors from town to town, Kordich gradually harnessed the power of television to boost "juicing" into a nationwide fad with sales in the tens of millions annually. Health-food stores are profiting from the fad by selling more juice extractors and "organic" foods.

Kordich's book is filled with fanciful physiologic tidbits and farfetched claims that juices boost energy and are effective against scores of ailments. His recipes include "Pancreas Rejuvenator" (carrot-apple-lettuce-string bean-Brussels sprout juice), "Body Cleanser" (carrot-cucumber-beet juice), "Graying Hair Remedy" (cabbage-spinach-carrot juice), and other concoctions for anemia, anxiety, arthritis, gallstones, impotence, and heart disease. He claims that for the more serious diseases, "the right nutrients may retard or reverse the manifestations of some of these diseases by feeding the immune system and making the body healthier and stronger overall."

According to Kordich, "live foods" are superior to cooked or processed foods because they contain "active enzymes." These, he claims, help break down foods in the digestive tract, "thus sparing the body's valuable digestive enzymes. . . . This allows vital energy in the body to be shifted from digestion to other body functions such as repair and rejuvenation." Of course, "organic foods" are preferable because "the corporate giants use deadly chemicals." Further:

> The abundance of live, uncooked foods flushes your body of toxins,

> leaving you refreshed, energized, and relaxed all at the same time. The pure foods make your skin glow, your hair shine, your breath fresh, and your entire system so regulated you will never have to give it another thought. Colds and flu become fewer and farther between; many people report that arthritic joints loosen with renewed flexibility; and gums and teeth become less prone to bleeding and cavities.

All of the above notions are utter nonsense.

Juice extractors cut food into tiny pieces that are then spun to separate the juice from the fiber-containing pulp. Ordinary juicer machines leave the pulp in the juice. Since the fiber in fruits and vegetables is an important part of a balanced diet, there is no reason to remove it while making juice. In December 1992, *Consumer Reports* tested Kordich's "Juiceman II" extractor and concluded that several competitive products worked better, were easier to clean, and cost far less.

Safer Cigarettes?

Perhaps the strangest products sold through health-food stores are those of the Santa Fe Natural Tobacco Company—all prepared without the use of chemical additives and preservatives. The products are said to be "for smokers who use tobacco the way Native Americans intended," who "have wanted to stop smoking but could not," or who "smoke out of choice rather than out of habit." A 1991 mailing to retailers stated that Santa Fe's cigarettes taste better and are less addictive than most mass-market brands and that its pouch tobacco was grown organically. The mailing also said: "We all know that it would be better for us health-wise if we did not smoke. However, if you cannot stop smoking (or choose not to stop), then we believe it makes sense to smoke the purest cigarettes available." Some health-food retailers think it is unethical for them to sell tobacco products. Other retailers are willing to do so.

The Herbal Minefield

In 1993, health-food-store patrons spent an estimated $679 million for capsules, tablets, bulk herbs, and herbal teas. Although many of these items are consumed for their flavor, most are probably used for supposed medicinal qualities. Sales by multilevel distributors amount to hundreds of millions more for products that are obviously intended for self-medication (see Chapter 10). Herbs are also marketed through the mail and in the offices of naturopaths, acupuncturists, iridologists, chiropractors, and unlicensed "herbalists," many of whom prescribe them for the entire gamut of health problems.

Herbal advocates like to point out that about half of today's medicines were derived from plants. (Digitalis, for example, was originally derived from leaves of the foxglove plant.) This statement is true but misleading. When potent natural substances are discovered, drug companies try to isolate and synthesize the active chemical in order to provide a reliable supply. They also attempt to make derivatives that are more potent, more predictable, and have fewer side effects. In the case of digitalis, derivatives provide a spectrum of speed and duration of action. Digitalis leaf is almost never used today because its effects are less predictable.

In the United States, herbs intended to be used for preventive or therapeutic purposes would be regulated as drugs under federal laws. To evade the law, these products are marketed as "foods" or "nutritional supplements," without health claims on their labels. However, information on their alleged use is readily available through other channels. Since herbs are not regulated as drugs, no legal standards exist for their processing, harvesting or packaging. In many cases, particularly for products with expensive raw ingredients, contents and potency are not accurately disclosed on the label. Purdue University's Varro E. Tyler, Ph.D., a leading authority on plant medicines, has observed:

> The literature promoting herbs includes pamphlets, magazine articles, and books. Practically all of these writings recommend large numbers of herbs for treatment based on hearsay, folklore, and tradition. The only criterion that seems to be avoided in these publications is scientific evidence. Some writings are so comprehensive and indiscriminate that they seem to recommend everything for anything. Even deadly poisonous herbs are sometimes touted as remedies, based on some outdated report or a misunderstanding of the facts. Particularly insidious is the myth that there is something almost magical about herbal drugs that prevents them, in their natural state, from harming people.
>
> Many herbs contain hundreds or even thousands of chemicals that have not been completely cataloged. Some of these chemicals may turn out to be useful as therapeutic agents, but others could well prove toxic. With safe and effective medicines available, treatment with herbs rarely makes sense. Moreover, many of the conditions for which herbs are recommended are not suitable for self-treatment. Consumers are less likely to receive good value for money spent on herbal "remedies" than for almost any other health-related product.

Most publications related to herbs appear to be published independently, but some are published by trade associations and manufacturers. Twin Laboratories, which markets a product line called *Nature's Herbs*, publishes a newsletter called The *Herbal Healthline,* whose editor, Michael Weiner, Ph.D., also hosts a radio show sponsored by the company.

Herbs are not only marketed for disease but for "purifying," "cleansing," "detoxifying," "energizing," and "revitalizing" the body. Nature's Secret, of Santa Barbara, California, offers *A.M./P.M. Ultimate Cleanse*, "a complete internal body cleansing program" said to contain twenty-six herbs and five types of fiber. The company was founded in 1991 by R. Lindsey Duncan, a "nutritionist" in Santa Monica who "studied for 7 years" with iridologist/chiropractor Bernard Jensen (see Chapter 7) and was "asked by Dr. Jensen to carry on his work." Duncan's patients are said to include Ringo Starr, Demi Moore, Mariel Hemingway, Englebert Humperdink, and other prominent entertainers. An *A.M./P.M.* brochure states:

> We clean our home, our office, our car, our kitchen, our bedroom, our shower, our clothes, our mouth. . . . When our drain clogs, we clean it out. If our toilet backs up, the problem demands our immediate attention. . . .
>
> When was the last time you cleaned your liver, your heart, your lungs, or your body's sewage system?

The brochure claims that "when we don't have 2 to 3 GOOD bowel movements per day, toxins ferment and decay in the colon." Although this idea has no scientific support, Duncan says he has "consulted with over 7,000 clients [and has] yet to meet an individual with a toxin-free body." How he determined this is not stated in the brochure.

Set-N-Me-Free, of Portland, Oregon, is marketing an "inch-loss program" claimed to slenderize by "cleansing your body of the toxins that hold cellulite in place." The program consists of an herbal body wrap plus *Reducing Herb Capsules* "to help in curbing the appetite as well as nourishing the parts of the body to reduce fat percentage." The "telephone presentation" instructions given to prospective retailers and salon-keepers suggests stating "We have an average of 7 to 10 inches lost with each wrap . . . . using cotton cloth strips that have been soaking in our all-natural aloe vera and herb solution." A brochure advises consumers who have weight to lose to be wrapped once or twice a week. It was not clear from the promotional material which "7 to 10 inches" would be lost or what would happen to a client over a month's time. Would some people disappear altogether? (We're kidding, of course. Body wrapping does not produce shrinkage of anything but the customer's wallet.)

Eden's Secrets, of Portland, Maine, sells *The Purifying Program,*™ "a unique combination of twenty-eight herbs," which costs a mere $79.45 for a four- to six-week supply. A mailing from the company claims that headaches,

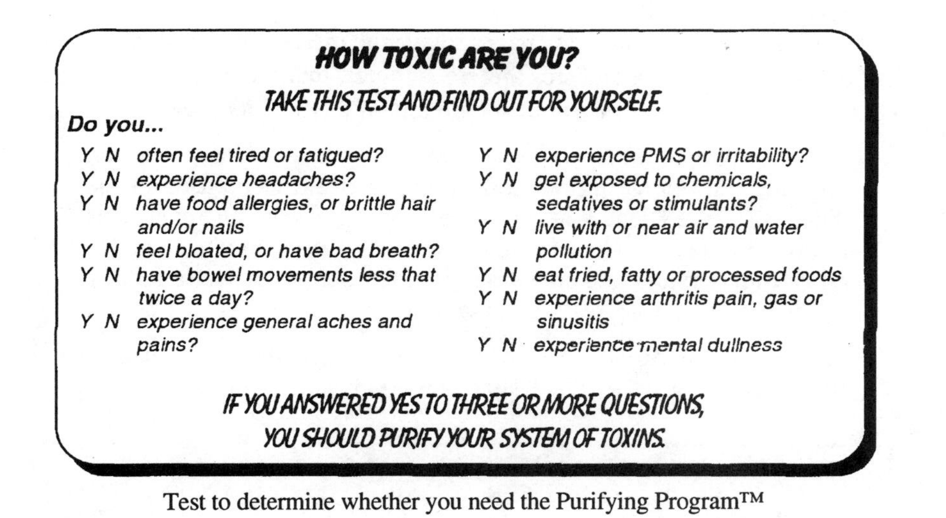

Test to determine whether you need the Purifying Program™

fatigue, poor digestion, and general aches and pains are due to toxins, additives, and other impurities that accumulate in the body. But when *The Purifying Program*™ is taken regularly, "you feel more alert, you have more energy, and you'll tend to lose weight more easily, without changing your eating habits!" The mailing included a phony self-test to determine whether the program is needed.

The most aggressive mail-order marketer of herbs is the Health Center for Better Living (HCBL), of Naples, Florida. Individuals on its mailing list receive multiple copies of its catalog, which currently is a seventy-two-page booklet called "A Useful Guide to Herbal Health Care." The booklet lists "five main benefits of herbs":

1. CLEANSING (Herbs help cleanse and purify the body without side effects)
2. NORMALIZES BODY FUNCTION (Herbs regulate and tone the glands to function normally)
3. EXTREMELY NUTRITIONAL (Herbs are high in vitamins, minerals, and other nutrients that nourish and build the body)
4. RAISES THE ENERGY LEVEL OF THE BODY (Herbs allow the body to have extra energy to maintain good health)
5. STIMULATES THE BODY'S IMMUNE SYSTEM (Herbs help to promote the body's naturally occurring beneficial bacteria)

HCBL's catalog has many pages filled with medicinal claims, including an "easy-to-use herb/ailment cross-reference chart" that occupies twelve pages (illustrated below). A note near the beginning of the booklet states:

> The information contained on the following pages . . . has been written only for educational purposes. It is not intended to be used in the diagnosis, cure, treatment, or prevention of disease in man. This information is not to be used to promote the sale of products, nor to replace the services of a physician. By all means, see a doctor for any condition which may require his services.

Disclaimers like this provide no legal protection to those who make them. The FDA is aware of HCBL's activities and listed many its products in a report

Easy to Use Herb/Ailment Cross Reference Chart

A=Excellent Remedy
B=Very Good Remedy
C=Good Remedy

AILMENT → / ↓ HERB ↓	EYES	GALL BLADDER	GAS	GOUT	HAIR	HEADACHE	HEART	HEMORRHOID	IMMUNE	INSOMNIA	KIDNEY/BLADDER	LIVER	LUNGS	MENOPAUSE	MENSTRUAL	NERVES	PAIN	PROSTATE	SEXUAL	SINUS	SKIN	ULCER	VARICOSE VEIN	WATER RETENTION	WEIGHT LOSS
Dill Weed																									
Dong Quai Rt															A	A									
Echinacea Rt									A									A		A					
Elder Leaf																									
Elecampane Rt																									
Eucalyptus Lf																									
Eyebright	A																								
Fennel Seed	A		A	A								B													A
Fenugreek Sd						A							B									B			
Feverfew Herb						A						B													
Garlic Bulb							A		A																
Gentian Root												A			B										
Ginger Root											A														
Ginkgo Lf	A												A			A									
Ginseng Rt																			A			A			
Golden Seal Rt								A			A									A		A	A		
Gota Kola																A									
Gravel Root											A														
Green Barley									A																
Hawthorne							A			B															

Portion of the "herb/ailment" chart from *A Useful Guide to Herbal Health Care.* The full chart rates 162 herbs for forty-seven types of problems on unsubstantiated claims presented at a Congressional hearing in 1993. The report describes serious adverse effects associated with the use of chaparral, comfrey, yohimbe, lobelia, germander, willow bark, jin bu huan, ma huang, and Chinese herbal preparations containing *Stephania* and *Magnolia.* Other FDA reports have listed more. The FDA has sent warning letters to HCBL and several other manufacturers. However, it lacks the resources to clean up the herbal marketplace.

The American Herbal Products Association (AHPA), which has 150 current members, is making efforts toward industry self-regulation. In 1993, its board of trustees adopted a forty-eight page code of ethics that became mandatory for 1994 membership renewal. The code states that all products must be labeled completely and accurately, that claims must be verifiable, and that products must be safe for their intended use. AHPA is developing a "restricted use list," which now includes comfrey (which contains liver toxins) and ma huang (which poses risks for individuals with high blood pressure, glaucoma, and several other conditions). However, Mark Blumenthal, executive director of the American Botanical Council, recently warned:

> There are really two herb industries. One is comprised of businesses which are attempting to increase . . . the quality of information to consumers, as well as increase the overall quality and confidence in herb products themselves. On the other hand, there are numerous companies that . . . do not appear interested in increasing herb standards and quality on an industry-wide basis. Many of the latter appear to be "only in it for the money."

What should consumers do? The most prudent course of action is to forget about using herbs for medicinal purposes. In fact, it is wise not to use *any* product sold in a health-food store for self-medication.

9

The Ultimate Fake

Homeopathic "remedies" enjoy a unique status in the health marketplace: they are the only quack products legally marketable as drugs. This situation is the result of two circumstances. First, the 1938 Federal Food, Drug, and Cosmetic Act, which was shepherded through Congress by a homeopathic physician who was a senator, recognizes as drugs all substances included in the *Homeopathic Pharmacopeia of the United States.* Second, the FDA has not held homeopathic remedies to the same standards as other drugs. Although they are not nutritional products, they are discussed here because most of their marketing is done through health-food stores and because manufacturers are capitalizing on the apparent freedom to make unsubstantiated claims for them.

Basic Misbeliefs

Homeopathy originated in Europe in the late 1700s when Samuel Hahnemann (1755–1843), a German physician, began formulating its basic principles. Hahnemann was justifiably distressed about bloodletting, leeching, purging, and other medical procedures of his day that did far more harm than good. He was also critical of medications like calomel (mercurous chloride), which was given in doses that caused mercury poisoning. Thinking that these treatments were intended to "balance the body's 'humors' by opposite effects," he developed his "law of similars"—a notion that symptoms of disease can be cured by substances that produce similar symptoms in healthy people. The word "homeopathy" is derived from the Greek words *homoios* (similar) and *pathos* (suffering or disease).

Although ideas like this had been espoused by Hippocrates in the fourth century B.C.E., and by Paracelsus, a fifteenth-century physician, Hahnemann was the first to use them in a systematic way. He and his early followers conducted "provings" in which they administered herbs, minerals, and other substances to healthy people, including themselves, and kept detailed records of what they observed. Later these records were compiled into lengthy reference books called *materia medica,* which are used to match a patient's symptoms with a "corresponding" drug. The basis for inclusion in the *Homeopathic Pharmacopeia* is not scientific testing in patients, but homeopathic "provings" conducted during the 1800s and early 1900s.

Hahnemann declared that diseases represent an impairment in the body's ability to heal itself and that only a small stimulus is needed to begin the healing process. He either failed to recognize or rejected the fact that illnesses produce changes in the body that are now studied as part of the science of pathology—to him, disease was chiefly a matter of disturbing the body's "spirit." At first he prescribed small doses of accepted medications. But later he used enormous dilutions and theorized that the smaller the dose, the more powerful the effect—a principle he called the "law of infinitesimals." That, of course, is just the opposite of what pharmacologists have demonstrated in dose-response studies.

Many homeopaths maintain that certain people have a special affinity to a particular remedy (their "constitutional remedy") and will respond to it for a variety of ailments. Such remedies can be prescribed according to the person's "constitutional type" (also called "bodymind type")—named after the corresponding remedy in a manner resembling astrologic typing. The "Ignatia Type," for example, is said to be nervous and often tearful, and to dislike tobacco smoke. The typical "Pulsatilla" is a young woman, with blond or light-brown hair, blue eyes, and a delicate complexion, who is gentle, fearful, friendly but shy, romantic, and emotional. The "Nux Vomica Type" is said to be aggressive, bellicose, ambitious, and hyperactive. The "Sulfur Type" likes to be independent. And so on. Does this sound to you like a rational basis for diagnosis and treatment?

The "Remedies" Are Placebos

Homeopathic products are made from minerals, botanical substances, and several other sources. If the original substance is soluble, one part is diluted with either nine or ninety-nine parts of distilled water and/or alcohol and shaken vigorously; if insoluble, it is finely ground and pulverized in similar proportions with powdered lactose (milk sugar). One part of the diluted medicine is diluted, and the process is repeated until the desired concentration is reached. Dilutions of 1 to 10 are designated by the Roman numeral X (1X = 1/10, 3X = 1/1,000, 6X = 1/1,000,000). Similarly, dilutions of 1 to 100 are designated by the Roman numeral C (1C = 1/100, 3C = 1/1,000,000, and so on). Most remedies today range from 6X to 30X, but products of 30C or more are marketed.

A 30X dilution means that the original substance has been diluted 10^{30} times. Assuming that a cubic centimeter of water contains fifteen drops, 10^{30} is greater than the number of drops of water that would fill a container more than fifty times the size of the Earth. Imagine placing a drop of red dye into such a container so that it disperses evenly. Homeopathy's "law of infinitesimals" is the equivalent of saying that any drop of water subsequently removed from that container will possess an essence of redness. Robert L. Park, Ph.D., a prominent physicist who is executive director of The American Physical Society, has noted that since the least amount of a substance in a solution is one molecule, a 30C solution would have to have at least one molecule of the original substance dissolved in a minimum of 10^{60} molecules of water. This would require a container more than thirty billion times the size of the Earth!

Actually, the laws of chemistry state that there is a limit to the dilution that can be made without losing the original substance altogether. This limit, called Avogadro's number (6.023×10^{23}), corresponds to homeopathic potencies of 12C or 24X (1 part in 10^{24}). Hahnemann himself realized that there is virtually no chance that even one molecule of original substance would remain after extreme dilutions. But he believed that the vigorous shaking or pulverizing with each step of dilution leaves behind a "spirit-like" essence—"no longer perceptible to the senses"—which cures by reviving the body's "vital force." This notion is utter nonsense. Moreover, if it were true, every substance encountered by a molecule of water might imprint an "essence" that could exert powerful (and unpredictable) medicinal effects when ingested by a person.

Because homeopathic remedies were actually less dangerous than those of nineteenth-century medical orthodoxy, many medical practitioners began using them. But as medical science and medical education advanced, homeopathy declined sharply, particularly in America, where its schools either closed or converted to responsible methods.

Since many homeopathic remedies contain no detectable amount of active ingredient, it is impossible to test whether they contain what their label says. They have been presumed safe, but unlike most potent drugs, few have actually been tested and none has been proven effective.

In 1988, a French scientist working at a prestigious laboratory claimed to have found that high dilutions of substances in water left a "memory" that would provide a rationale for homeopathy's "law of similars." However, a subsequent investigation by experts revealed that the research had been improperly carried out. In 1990, an article in *Review of Epidemiology* analyzed forty randomized trials that had compared homeopathic treatment with standard treatment, a placebo, or no treatment. The authors concluded that all but three of the trials had major flaws in their design, that only one of those three had reported a positive result, and that there is no evidence that homeopathic treatment has any more value than a placebo.

Proponents trumpet the few "positive" studies as proof that "homeopathy works." Even if their results could be consistently reproduced (which hasn't happened), the most that the study of a single remedy for a single disease could prove is that the remedy is effective against *that* disease. It would not validate homeopathy's basic theories or prove that homeopathic treatment is useful for other diseases.

In 1986, Dr. Stephen Barrett sent a questionnaire to the deans of all seventy-two U.S. pharmacy schools. Faculty members from forty-nine schools responded. Most said their school either didn't mention homeopathy at all or considered it of historical interest only. Hahnemann's "law of similars" did not find a single supporter, and all but one respondent said his "law of infinitesimals" was wrong also. Almost all said that homeopathic remedies were neither potent nor effective, except possibly as placebos for mild, self-limited ailments. About half felt that homeopathic products should be completely removed from the marketplace.

Students at Purdue University are taught about homeopathy in a single lecture that is part of a history of pharmacy course given by Varro E. Tyler, Ph.D., professor of pharmacognosy and former dean of Purdue's pharmacy school. In it, Tyler shares some interesting speculations about homeopathy's popularity here and abroad:

- Homeopathy may be popular in Britain because of its use by the royal family—Queen Elizabeth, Prince Charles, and other relatives. The editors of various British journals are well aware of this implied endorsement and seem amenable to publishing papers on this subject that would not be accepted elsewhere.

- Homeopathy retains its popularity in Germany because it was devised there. The Germans, like many other peoples of the world, are not about to give up a medical system that was devised by one of their own, even though most medical and pharmacy professionals in that country recognize that it simply does not work.

- Homeopathy has enjoyed a resurgence in the United States because practically no one here understands it. It is no longer taught in medical or pharmacy schools, so most professionals know little or nothing about it. Not understanding it themselves, they cannot explain it to patients and consumers; and since the FDA permits homeopathic products to be sold, people think they must be good.

Sources of Remedies

Homeopathic products are available from practitioners, health-food stores, drugstores, discount chains, and other retail outlets, as well as from manufacturers who sell directly to the public. Products are also sold person-to-person through multilevel marketing companies. Several companies sell home remedy kits. The size of the homeopathic marketplace is unknown because many manufacturers keep their sales figures private. However, *Health Foods Business,* which conducts an annual survey of health-food retailers, has estimated that their 1992 sales totaled about $160 million. New Hope Communications, publisher of *Natural Foods Merchandiser*, pegged the total 1992 United States market at over $200 million, with $99 million through health-food stores, $40 million through medical professionals, $30 million through multilevel companies, and $34 million through supermarkets, supercenters, and drugstores.

In most states, homeopathy can be practiced by any practitioner whose license includes the ability to prescribe drugs. Arizona, Nevada, and Connecticut have separate licensing boards for homeopathic physicians—a situation that the National Council Against Health Fraud calls "a haven for untrustworthy practitioners." In 1988, the *Las Vegas Review-Journal* reported that at least ten of the thirty-two people licensed by the Nevada board had been in hot water with medical boards in other states for questionable or unlawful practices—and that four licenses had been obtained by submitting "phony credentials from imaginary schools or licensing boards."

Even though chiropractors are not legally permitted to prescribe drugs, a 1991 survey by the National Board of Chiropractic Examiners found that 36.9 percent of 4,835 full-time chiropractic practitioners who responded said that they had prescribed homeopathic remedies within the previous two years. The 1994 directory of the National Center for Homeopathy (NCH), in Alexandria, Virginia, lists about four hundred licensed practitioners, about half of them physicians and the rest mostly naturopaths, chiropractors, acupuncturists, veterinarians, nurses, dentists, or physician's assistants. Although several hundred physicians and naturopaths not listed in the NCH directory practice homeopathy to some extent, they appear to be greatly outnumbered by chiropractors.

Laypersons are also practicing homeopathy in ways that violate medical practice laws—with some getting referrals through health-food stores.

The practice of Classical Homeopathy is a safe, natural, wholistic science which considers all aspects of the patient's symptomatology. Your specific symptoms, no matter what the disease or disorder, are most significant in determining the cure for you as an individual. Conditions of the most difficult diseases can be cured: CFS to HIV. The immune system is always improved. Homeopathic remedies are non-toxic and have no side-affects.

█████ █████ is a renowned homeopath, highly respected for her thoroughness, personal care, and expertise in constitutional prescribing for chronic diseases and disorders. She is a graduate in Advanced Homeopathy with honors from the British Institute of Homeopathy. **For more information, to schedule an appointment or telephone consultation.**

Recent ad in *Newlife* magazine by a New York City homeopath who appears to be practicing without a license to do so.

Consumers interested in homeopathic self-treatment can obtain guidance through lay study groups, books, and courses sponsored by NCH. Membership in the center, open to anyone, costs $35 per year and includes a subscription to its monthly newsletter *Homeopathy Today.* The center now has about seven thousand members. A similar organization, the International Foundation for Homeopathy, is located in Seattle, Washington. Both groups train health professionals as well as laypersons. Courses leading to certificates or "degrees" have been offered by other nonaccredited schools, some of which operated only by mail.

Two "experienced homeopathic nurses" are advertising a $75 home-study course that teaches how homeopathy "fits into [holistic] nursing practice, both legally and philosophically." The ad promises "practical information about homeopathic remedies for first aid and acute conditions, such as fevers, upper respiratory tract infections, influenza, pharyngitis, coughs, digestive problems, abdominal cramps, colic, minor skin problems and more," plus an introduction to "the specific skills needed for effective prescribing for these conditions."

Homeopathic physicians who follow Hahnemann's methods closely take an elaborate history to "fit the remedy to the individual." The history typically includes standard medical questions plus many more about such things as emotions, moods, food preferences, and reactions to the weather. The remedy for symptoms on one side of the body may differ from that for identical symptoms on the other side of the body. The remedy is then selected with the help of a *materia medica* or computer program.

Other practitioners, whose approaches have not been systematically tabulated, may spend little time with patients. In the 1992 *Digest of Chiropractic Economics*, for example, Frank J. King, Jr., D.C., N.D., a chiropractor who markets homeopathic products, described how he had treated someone with a history of hay fever, allergies, sinusitis, postnasal drip, frequent cough, cold hands and feet, skipped heart beats, unhealthy skin, insomnia, abdominal bloating, and slowness in healing skin sores. The bill—for eleven visits totaling 107 minutes —came to $1,007.24. King's *Physician's Reference Manual*, given free to prospective customers, states:

> **WHAT KIND OF DIS-EASES CAN HOMEOPATHY TREAT?** Homeopathy does not treat dis-eases per se. Homeopathy ACTIVATES THE BODY'S OWN HEALING PROCESSES in both the PHYSICAL AND MENTAL/EMOTIONAL LEVELS. THE RANGE OF PROBLEMS IN WHICH

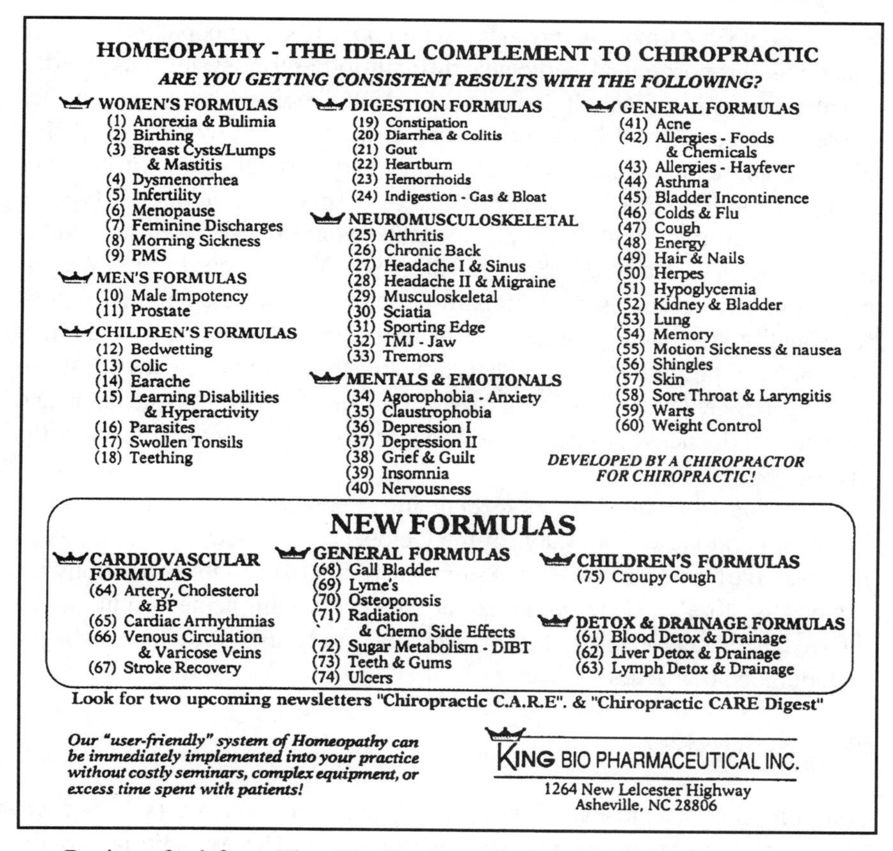

Portion of ad from King Bio Pharmaceutical Inc., which offers "practice enhancement and management materials" and "complimentary consultations" concerning the conditions listed (two of which are misspelled). The company's reference manual suggests which products should be used for more than two hundred problems, including epilepsy, Hodgkin's disease (a form of cancer), hookworm, jaundice, kidney stones, manic depression, and multiple sclerosis. Do you think these problems are amenable to homeopathic treatment or suitable for management by chiropractors?

HOMEOPATHY CAN BE EFFECTIVELY UTILIZED IS EXTENSIVE AND INCLUDES FIRST AID, ACUTE ILLNESSES, and ALL MANNERS OF CHRONIC CONDITIONS.

HOW SOON CAN RESULTS BE EXPECTED? In ACUTE ILLNESSES, the appropriate remedy CAN ACT WITHIN MINUTES. It is commonplace to see a child who is screaming out in pain with an earache, drop off to sleep in one or two minutes after a dose of THE APPROPRIATE REMEDY. In CHRONIC CONDITIONS, results can be slower. Roughly, for every year of ILLNESS, it may take a month to achieve maximum results.

About fifty American physicians who prescribe homeopathic remedies practice anthroposophical medicine, a difficult-to-describe system based on the occult philosophy of Rudolf Steiner (1861–1925). Steiner's teachings encompassed: (1) a system of body movements termed "eurythmy"; (2) a peculiar educational method that stresses art, drama, and spiritual development; (3) a bizarre theory of medicine; and (4) "biodynamic" agriculture, a type of "organic" farming. Anthroposophical remedies are marketed in the United States through Weleda Inc. of Spring Valley, New York. According to a Weleda brochure, each plant used to prepare remedies is "selected for its unique 'personality,' revealed in form, color, pattern of growth, with consideration of its beneficial properties" and is "harvested when its growth forces are strongest." Proponents also state that "seasonal changes" and "solar, lunar and planetary influences" are taken into account in deciding when to harvest the plants.

During 1993, retail stores specializing in homeopathic products opened in Boston and New York City. In the October 1993 issue of *Health Foods Business,* the founder of the Boston store said he hopes to establish a nationwide chain. His store's policy requires that customers with acute conditions be referred to a doctor. The store's reference guide lists local practitioners, including ten homeopathic doctors.

"Electrodiagnosis"

Some physicians, dentists, and chiropractors use "electrodiagnostic" devices to help select the homeopathic remedies they prescribe. These practitioners claim they can determine the cause of any disease by detecting the "energy imbalance" causing the problem. Some also claim that the devices can detect whether someone is allergic or sensitive to foods, vitamins, and/or other substances. The procedure, called Electroacupuncture according to Voll (EAV) or electrodiagnosis, was initiated during the 1970s by Reinhold Voll, M.D., a West German physician who developed the first model of the device. Subsequent models include the *Vega, Dermatron, Accupath 1000,* and *Interro.*

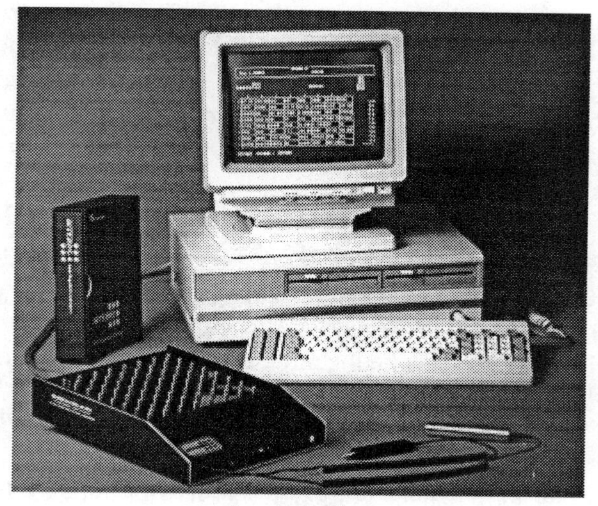

Interro device

Proponents claim these devices measure disturbances in the body's flow of "electro-magnetic energy" along "acupuncture meridians." Actually, they are little more than fancy galvanometers that measure electrical resistance of the patient's skin when touched by a probe. One wire from the device goes to a brass cylinder covered by moist gauze, which the patient holds in one hand. A second wire is connected to a probe, which the operator touches to "acupuncture points" on the patient's other hand or foot. This completes a low-voltage circuit and the device registers the flow of current. The information is then relayed to a gauge that provides a numerical readout. (The size of the number actually depends on how hard the probe is pressed against the patient's skin.) Recent versions, such as the *Interro* pictured above, make sounds and provide the readout on a computer screen. The treatment selected depends on the scope of the practitioner's practice and may include acupuncture, dietary change, and/or vitamin supplements as well as homeopathic remedies. Regulatory agencies have seized several types of electroacupuncture devices but no systematic effort has been made to drive them from the marketplace.

The Expanding Marketplace

FDA officials have noted that homeopathic remedies used to be marketed on a small scale by a few long-established companies, mainly to serve the needs of licensed practitioners. The products bore little or no labeling for consumers because they were intended for use by homeopathic physicians who would make a diagnosis and either compound a prescription, dispense the product, or write a prescription to be filled at a homeopathic pharmacy. During the past fifteen years, however, the homeopathic marketplace has changed drastically. New firms have entered the field and sold all sorts of products through health-food stores and directly to consumers. Today, more than a hundred manufacturers are involved.

In 1986, Jay P. Borneman, whose family has marketed homeopathic remedies since 1910, readily admitted to Dr. Barrett:

> There is a lot of insanity operating under the name of homeopathy in today's marketplace. Companies not committed to homeopathy's principles have been marketing products that are unproven, untested, not included in the *Homeopathic Pharmacopeia,* and combination products that have no rational or legal basis. Some are simply quack products called homeopathic for marketing purposes.

Perhaps the most blatant promotion was that of Biological Homeopathic Industries (BHI) of Albuquerque, New Mexico, which, in 1983, sent a 123-page catalog to almost two hundred thousand physicians nationwide. Its products included *BHI Anticancer Stimulating, BHI Antivirus, BHI Stroke*, and fifty other types of tablets claimed to be effective against serious diseases. In 1984, the FDA forced BHI to stop distributing several of the products and to tone down its claims for others. However, BHI has continued to make illegal claims. Its 1991 *Physicians' Reference* ("for use only by health care professionals") inappropriately recommends products for heart failure, syphilis, kidney failure, blurred vision, and many other serious conditions. The company's publishing arm issues the quarterly *Biological Therapy: Journal of Natural Medicine*, which regularly contains articles whose authors make questionable claims. An article in the April 1993 issue, for example, listed "indications" for using BHI and Heel products (distributed by BHI) for more than fifty conditions—including cancer, angina pectoris, and paralysis. And the October 1993 issue, devoted to the homeopathic treatment of children, includes an article recommending products for acute bacterial infections of the ear and tonsils. The article is described as selections from Heel seminars given in several cities by a Nevada homeopath who also serves as medical editor of *Biological Therapy.*

In 1988, the FDA took action against companies marketing "diet patches" with false claims that they could suppress appetite. The largest such company, Meditrend International, of San Diego, instructed users to place one or two drops of a "homeopathic appetite control solution" on a patch and wear it all day affixed to an "acupuncture point" on the wrist to "bioelectrically" suppress the appetite control center of the brain.

In 1991, the U.S. Postal Service took action against the marketers of a homeopathic product called *Oncor,* which had been claimed to alleviate impotence and increase sexual desire in men. An Administrative Law Judge concluded that the product was neither safe nor effective and that the television infomercial used to promote it had been falsely represented as an independent talk show.

During the past few years, many other companies have offered dubious homeopathic products for over-the-counter sale. Some examples are: *Arthritis Formula, Bleeding, Kidney Disorders, Flu, Herpes, Exhaustion, Whooping Cough, Gonorrhea, Heart Tonic, Gall-Stones, Prostate Pain, Candida Yeast Infection, Candida-Away, Cardio Forte, Thyro Forte,* and *Worms.*

Natra-Bio of Bellington, Washington, states that its homeopathic

Natra-Bio Home Pharmacy™ Remedy Guide

Natra-Bio products can be used individually, or for maximum relief, used in combination. To use this chart, locate ailment in left column. Principal remedy to be used is located in next column to right. Appropriate tissue salts and glandular tinctures follow. The numbers listed are for your convenience in locating the correct product(s). Every Natra-Bio product has its own number.

		Remedy	Tissue Salts	Glandular Tinctures
Colds & Flu	Cough	502	304, 308	403, 414
	Fever	505	304	403
	Sore Throat	509	304, 305	403
	Chest Cold	512	304, 311, 305, 307	403, 414
	Head Cold	513	307, 309	403
	Flu	527	304, 307, 311	403
Pain	Injuries	504	302, 301	401
	Neuralgic Pain	506	308	401
	Arthritis Pain	508	310	401
	Earache Pain	514	308	403
	Headache & Pain	515	308, 304, 306	
Stress & Nerves	Nervousness	503	306	401, 406
	Insomnia	523	306	
	Exhaustion	528	306	
	Emotional	529	309	
Allergies	Sinus	507	305, 312, 309	401, 403
	Hayfever	519	307, 309	401
	Eye Irritation	530	309	
Children	Bedwetting	518	306	
	Colic	524	311	
	Teething	532	302	
Gastro-intestinal	Indigestion	501	302, 306, 310, 311	406, 412
	Nausea	511	302, 310, 309	412
	Hemorrhoids	520	307, 301, 312	
	Laxative	521	301, 309, 312	
	Bladder Irritation	522	304	
Male & Female	Menstrual	510	308, 304, 309	405, 407
	Prostate	516	301	404, 407
	Menopause	517	313	405, 407
	Varicose Veins	533	301	
Skin	Injuries	504	302, 301	401
	Cold Sores	525	309, 312, 303	403
	Acne	526	303, 309, 312	
	Teeth & Gums	531	312, 302	
	Hair & Scalp	534	309, 312	
	Insect Bites	535	313	401
	Poison Oak & Ivy	536	313	401

Natra-Bio's Home Pharmacy™ Remedy Guide states which of the company's remedies are intended for various problems.

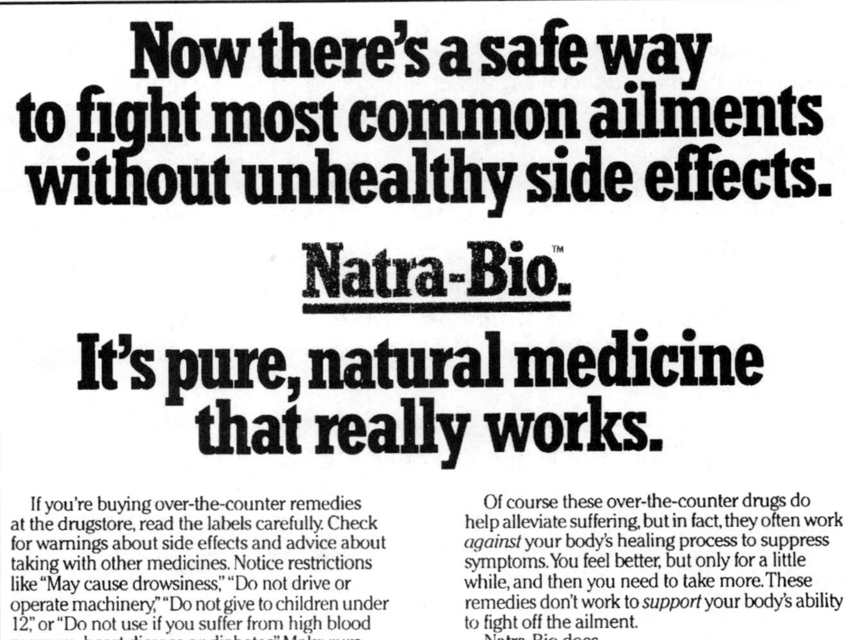

Natra-Bio's flyer "Getting Well Without Chemicals" falsely suggests that standard over-the-counter drugs are inferior to homeopathic products. Products that never produce side effects are too weak to exert therapeutic effects.

products offer a "safe way to fight most common ailments without unhealthy side effects." Its "glandular tinctures" (*Adrenal Gland, Kidney, Liver, Lungs, Ovaries, Pancreas, Pituitary, Testes, Thymus,* and *Thyroid*) are said to "stimulate and support" the function of the organ or gland whose name they bear. Its "tissue salts" are for "improving" more than forty ailments, including bronchial phlegm, stomach cramps, muscular weakness, and pimples. Its other fanciful products have included *Bedwetting, Chest Cold, Hemorrhoids, Nervousness, Smoking Withdrawal Tablets,* and *Detoxification* ("for the relief of constipation, lack of energy, and headaches due to overindulgence in food and alcohol"). The company's *Homeopathic Reference Manual* for retailers states:

> Unlike any other form of medicine, the patient can confidently listen to their own body and determine for themselves what they need to do. In homeopathy, there is no harm in taking the wrong medicine or too much medicine.

Retailers who submit nine or more correct answers to the eleven-question

Natra-Bio Test for Certification can receive a "Certificate of Completion of Homeopathic Knowledge" to display in their store.

According to a recent ad by Nova Homeopathic Therapeutics of Albuquerque, New Mexico:

> Developed in a doctor's office for patients with similar conditions, Nova's clinically tested homeopathic remedies are proven performers. Just ask any of the thousands of satisfied customers that already use Nova's products.
>
> With more than 44 different remedies to choose from, it's like having a doctor's office in your store.
>
> Nova's homeopathic remedies sell themselves! Symptoms associated with the remedy are clearly listed on the front of the box.

For many years, Ellon USA, Inc., of Lynbrook, New York, marketed the Bach Flower Remedies, a line of thirty-eight products said to alleviate "negative" emotions. These remedies—considered a homeopathic offshoot—were developed about sixty years ago by Edward Bach, a British bacteriologist and homeopath, who reportedly observed ailing animals licking the dew from flowers and intuited how each flower influences different emotional states. According to the company's literature, Bach believed that "the only way to cure illness was to address the underlying emotional causes of disease." Remedies could be selected according to responses to a 116-item questionnaire published by Ellon USA. Someone who feels overwhelmed with work, for example, is advised to take the product called *Elm,* while someone who has strong opinions and is easily incensed by injustices is advised to use *Vervain.* In 1993, after another company purchased the distribution rights for the Bach brand, Ellon USA launched its own line of "Traditional Flower Remedies . . . made in strict accordance with Dr. Bach's methodologies."

The National Center for Homeopathy keeps close track of homeopathy's portrayal by the media. Its newsletters from July 1993 through January 1994 rated 161 articles and broadcasts and concluded that 125 (78 percent) were favorable, twenty (12 percent) were unfavorable, and sixteen (10 percent)) were neutral. Most reports simply parrot the claims of homeopathy's promoters. To help ensure that homeopathy's viewpoint is represented by its ablest spokespeople, NCH members have been urged to inform the group's headquarters if they become aware that a story is being prepared. When a critical report appears, homeopathic believers may respond with hundreds or even thousands of protest messages.

In the United States, homeopathy's most prolific publicist is probably Dana Ullman, M.P.H., an NCH board member who is president of the Foundation for Homeopathic Education and Research. Nature's Way, of

Springville, Utah, is marketing a "Medicine from Nature" line formulated by Ullman, which includes: *Insomnia, Sinusitis, Migraine Headache, Vaginitis, Menopause* (for women), and *Earache* (for children). The company has promised an "aggressive marketing strategy"—with ads in healthcare, women's, and parenting magazines—intended to "make homeopathy a household word." Its ads claim that "homeopathic medicine offers a significant advantage over its orthodox counterparts" and that "medicines from Nature works in harmony with the body's own natural defenses and gets to the cause of your illness or discomfort."

Ullman also directs Homeopathic Educational Services, a mail-order service for homeopathic books, cassette tapes, remedies, toothpaste, and computer software. At a recent meeting, he told Dr. Barrett that his foundation, despite its name, does not fund research because he does not have sufficient time for fundraising. Ullman's book *Everybody's Guide to Homeopathic Medicines* states:

> Homeopathy . . . . offers a way to gently stimulate our inner healing resources through recognizing and reinforcing the adaptive reactions of our natural defense processes. By choosing the correct, individually suited homeopathic medicine . . . you can successfully stimulate the body's own defenses.

Dangerous Promotions

According to press reports, some parents feel that homeopathic remedies enable them to take care of their children's minor accidents and self-limiting illnesses without becoming overly dependent on a physician. These parents also report having less concern about accidental poisoning because a child could consume an entire bottle of a homeopathic remedy and not have any side effects. Do you think these are logical reasons to use placebos?

In 1993, Video Remedies Inc. of Davie, Florida, began marketing a videotape called "Homeopathic Care of Infants and Children," which features Lendon Smith, M.D., advising members of a local homeopathic study group. Even though Smith relinquished his medical license several years ago (see Chapter 17), he is portrayed as a practicing physician. The video is intended to guide the use of a homeopathic home remedy kit that has Smith's picture on its case. During the tape Smith explains what homeopathy is about, suggests that vaccinations do more harm than good, and advises how to use the remedies in the kit for bedwetting, chicken pox, colds, colic, constipation, coughs (including purulent and bloody coughs), diarrhea, earache and otitis media, flu, headaches, measles, mumps, sore throats, and teething. A "remedy chart" booklet enclosed with the video advises: "Take the remedies 3 times a day for 3 days or *until you see a change.* If there has been no change, either check the chart and try another remedy, or call your doctor." However, when Smith discusses ear infections during the video, he states that if an acute earache does not respond within a day or so to a homeopathic remedy, another should be selected. The fact that prompt antibiotic therapy may prevent needless suffering or complications due to bacterial infections such as otitis media, strep throat, croup, or pneumonia does not seem to have occurred to the video's participants. The videotape is being marketed through health-food stores and through ads in health-food publications. Some ads describe the video and kit as "a complete program of gentle, non-toxic health care for infants and children."

Another dangerous message was aired in February 1994 on "Rolonda," a syndicated television talk show hosted by Rolonda Watts. One of the guests was a man who maintained that homeopathy had cured him of cancer. The homeopath, who also appeared, said she was not a medical doctor but had been "educated as a homeopath and naturopath and is doing something actually between the zones of legality." (Actually, it was quite illegal because she was not licensed as a health professional.) The man said that four years ago he had undergone surgery and radiation for a cancer but had become alarmed when a "suspicious" spot later appeared on an x-ray film. His doctor suggested watchful waiting to see whether the spot required further investigation. The man, however, felt he needed something more and wound up in the office of the homeopath—who prescribed a remedy and assured him he would be cured. When the spot did not appear on a follow-up x-ray, the man became convinced that the homeopath had cured a recurrence of his cancer. The fact that harmless x-ray changes often occur after radiation therapy had no effect on his beliefs.

Minimal Federal Regulation

Federal laws and regulations require that drugs be safe, effective, and properly labeled for their intended use. However, the FDA has not demanded that homeopathic remedies be proven *effective* in order to remain on the market. Its current guidelines, issued in 1988, state:

> Homeopathic drugs cannot be offered without prescription for such serious conditions as cancer, AIDS, or any other requiring diagnosis and treatment by a licensed practitioner. Nonprescription homeopathics may be sold only for self-limiting conditions recognizable by consumers. . . . [Their] labeling must adequately instruct consumers in the product's safe use.

Of course, if products don't work, there is no such thing as safe use.

The Federal Trade Commission could take effective action against homeopathic manufacturers that make false claims in their ads. Since no homeopathic product now advertised has been proven effective, and since few if any have even been reliably tested, it is hard to imagine how therapeutic claims for them could stand up in court. However, the FTC has shown no inclination to regulate homeopathic advertising.

The health-food industry is well aware of the unique regulatory status of homeopathic remedies. (While it is illegal to make unproven therapeutic claims for dietary supplements, the FDA tolerates most such claims for homeopathic remedies.) A recent article in a trade publication said that "there is more freedom in selling homeopathy than most other categories." Another article even

The Cold, Flu, and Cough Medicines Designed with You in Mind

One cold & flu medicine relieves all your symptoms. Another has a sleep-aid added. The third is specially formulated for kids. Our cough & bronchial syrup soothes your throat relieves coughs, and helps clear your lungs. The special kids formula is 100% sugar free. All-natural, homeopathic. No synthetic medicines. No known side effects.

Alpha CF for Colds & Flu
The first and only all-natural cold & flu medicine clinically proven to relieve all major cold & flu symptoms: fever, chills, sneezing, runny nose, stuffed-up nose, coughing, headache, and body aches and pains. Tablets or liquid.

New! Alpha CF Nighttime *(Liquid)*
The first and only all-natural cold & flu medicine to contain a sleep-aid. Relieves all major cold & flu symptoms plus the sleeplessness that sometimes accompanies colds & flu. No sleeping pill hangover. No known side effects.

Children's Alpha CF for Colds & Flu
The first and only all-natural medicine, specially formulated for children, that relieves all major cold & flu symptoms. (It's part of our best-selling line of children's remedies.)

B&T Cough & Bronchial Syrup
Relieves coughs due to viruses and air pollution. Soothes irritated throat membranes and helps remove the phlegm that causes irritation. Relieves bronchial congestion and wheezing by helping bronchial tubes to drain. No habit-forming drugs. No synthetic cough suppressants.

B&T Cough & Bronchial Syrup for Children
The first and only all-natural children's cough syrup that is sugar-free! Helps soothe the throat, relieve the cough, and clear the lungs. Special children's formula created by homeopathic physicians. Soothing honey base, natural cherry flavor. No artificial color. No artificial flavoring. No habit forming drugs. No synthetic cough suppressants.

... the better alternative!

B&T **Boericke & Tafel, Inc.**
2381 Circadian Way, Santa Rosa, CA 95407

Portion of ad for homeopathic remedies available in health-food stores. Do you believe these products can fulfill the claims made in the ad? Do you believe that *Alpha CF* can relieve all major flu symptoms? Or that directions for safe use can be written for a homeopathic remedy for bronchial congestion and wheezing in children?

suggested that "when a customer comes into your store complaining of an earache, fever, flu, sore throat, diarrhea, or some other common health problem . . . one word that should immediately come out of your mouth is 'homeopathy.'" A third article said that, because of an FDA crackdown on several nutritional supplements, "more and more companies were turning to herbs and homeopathy to regain sales." Another article stated: "Homeopathy is natural medicine's favorite son in the 1990s. Suddenly the category is appearing everywhere—in newspapers, on radio talk shows, on special television programs. . . . For natural products retailers, it can be a dream come true." In the latter article, a marketing manager for a homeopathic manufacturer stated: "Retailers can say exactly what's on the package—if it's to alleviate sinusitis or influenza, they can say that too. It doesn't matter if they are selling directly to an FDA agent." Yet another article called homeopathy "a sure sales cure." Other articles have suggested that homeopathic products offer an opportunity for "add-on sales"—whereby supplement customers can be persuaded that a homeopathic product offers additional benefit. (And, of course, homeopathic users are prospects for "add-on" supplements.)

Bastyr University (a naturopathic school), with support from the National Nutritional Foods Association, has produced an "educational" program for health-food retailers (see Chapter 6). Its booklet, "Introduction to Homeopathy," states:

> Do not recommend homeopathic remedies for your customers unless you have been specifically trained and licensed to do so. . . . Without training, however, you can learn to recommend homeopathic remedies for first-aid and minor illnesses if it is legal in your state to do so.
>
> Encourage your customers to see a well-trained naturopathic or homeopathic physician for proper diagnosis of any chronic illnesses or very severe acute conditions. . . . Referrals can also be made to physicians and lay people who, after attending a two to five week course, received a Certificate of Completion from the International Foundation for Homeopathy . . . or the National Center for Homeopathy.

As its final absurdity, the booklet advises that conventional medications can "interfere with or stop the action of a homeopathic remedy."

Political Shenanigans

Homeopathy proponents form what amounts to a cult that is prepared to do battle for its beliefs. In 1985, for example, when Arizona's homeopathic licensing board was in danger of being abolished, the state's homeopaths joined forces with health-food retailers to lobby vigorously to preserve it. According to the National Health Federation, a health-food-industry group that helped with the campaign, close to two thousand supporters attended hearings and state legislators got hundreds of handwritten letters supporting homeopathic licensing. The reauthorization bill passed unanimously.

In 1986, the North Carolina Board of Medical Examiners conditionally revoked the license of George A. Guess, M.D., the state's only licensed homeopathic physician, after concluding that he was "failing to conform to the standards of acceptable and prevailing medical practice." In 1992, after an appeal to the courts had failed, Guess relocated his practice to Virginia. But in 1993, following intense lobbying triggered largely by Guess's case, the North Carolina legislature passed a law barring the medical board from revoking a license solely because a practitioner departs from accepted medical practices, unless "the board can establish that the treatment is not generally effective." Medical science and consumer protection laws place the burden of proof on the person who makes a claim. Proving that health claims are false may be difficult, if not impossible, and might be prohibitively costly. Guess now appears free to resume practice in North Carolina.

Homeopaths are working hard to have their services covered under national health insurance. They claim to provide care that is "safer," "gentler," "natural," and less expensive than conventional care—and more concerned with prevention. The "prevention" claim is particularly odious because homeopathic treatments prevent nothing and many homeopathic leaders preach against immunization.

If the FDA required homeopathic remedies to be proven effective in order to remain on the market—the standard it applies to other remedies—homeopathy would face extinction in the United States. However, there is no indication that the agency is considering this. FDA officials regard homeopathy as relatively benign and believe that other problems should get enforcement priority. If the FDA attacks homeopathy too vigorously, its proponents might even persuade Congress to rescue them. Regardless of this risk, the FDA should not permit worthless products to be marketed with claims that they are effective. Nor should it continue to tolerate the presence of quack "electrodiagnostic" devices in the marketplace.

10

The Multilevel Mirage

Many companies that sell health-related products are systematically turning customers into salespeople. Multilevel marketing ("MLM")—also called network marketing—is a form of direct sales in which independent distributors sell products, usually in their customers' home or by telephone. In theory, distributors can make money not only from their own sales but also from those of the people they recruit. National Council Against Health Fraud president William T. Jarvis, Ph.D., calls MLM "the most effective system ever devised to turn ordinary people into quacks." We agree with him.

The recruitment process includes humanitarian pitches as well as financial ones. "When you share our products," says the sales manual of one company, "you're not just selling. You're passing on news about products you believe in to people you care about. Make a list of people you know; you'll be surprised how long it will be. This list is your first source of potential customers."

"Recruiting is the lifeblood of your business," says another sales manual. "If you believe that our company is the greatest in the world, if you believe that your products are the finest products you have ever discovered or used, and if you believe the opportunity is the greatest financial opportunity in the world—then your conviction, belief and excitement will make you a good recruiter, providing you share your conviction with everyone you meet."

The goal is not merely to sell products but to encourage your more enthusiastic customers to become salespeople themselves. The more you sell, the more "distributors" you recruit and supervise, the higher your potential profit percentages and bonuses. Topflight sales leaders can earn a car allowance, free vacation trips, and more than $1 million a year while "working to benefit humanity." Those who work out of their home can also deduct a portion of their household expenses as business deductions.

Becoming an MLM distributor is simple and requires no real knowledge of health or nutrition. Many people do so initially in order to buy their own products at a discount. For a small sum of money —usually between $35 and $100—these companies sell a distributor kit that includes product literature, sales aids (such as a videotape or audiotape), price lists, order forms, and a detailed instructional manual. Most MLM companies publish a magazine or newsletter containing company news, philosophical essays, product information, success stories, and photographs of top salespeople. The application form is usually a single page that asks only for identifying information. Millions of Americans have signed up.

The American Entrepreneurs Association's business manual for multilevel marketing offers the following advice about recruiting:

> Every time you look at a person you should view him as a potential recruit. *Every person.* Try to determine whether that person is interested in making more money. . . . Look for people who are frustrated or dissatisfied in their present occupations. People who are already successful and satisfied will be poor choices. . . .
>
> Mention the reasons that people want or need more money, such as a new home, a vacation, a new car, college for their children, etc. Tell them that if they join your organization these needs can be met. Discuss security, luxury items, increased income potential—all the things your organization offers them the chance to achieve. Talk about the tangible and intangible benefits, naming items that are beyond the average income (yachts, second homes). Discuss the freedom of being in business for themselves. Stress the independence they will realize in terms of both money and time. . . .
>
> Once you have their mouths watering, then, and only then, should you tell them about your company. Describe the nature of the business. . . . Then hit them with the real income potential of multilevel selling. Draw a picture of a "pyramid" type organization on the blackboard. Explain how few people they'll need to build a successful sales organization of their own.

Financial Opportunity?

MLM distributors can buy products "wholesale," sell them "retail," and recruit other distributors who can do the same. When enough distributors have been enrolled "downline," the recruiter is eligible to collect a percentage of their sales. Companies suggest that this process provides a great opportunity to make money and "fulfill the American dream." However, people who don't join during the first few months of operation or become one of the early distributors in their community are unlikely to build enough of a sales pyramid to do well. And many who stock up on products to meet sales goals get stuck with unsold products that cost thousands of dollars.

In the June 1987 issue of *Money* magazine, Ginnie Gemmel, of Emmaus, Pennsylvania, described how that had happened to her. In 1983, she answered a local newspaper ad looking for someone to start a small business. She purchased a Shaklee distributor kit for $18 and was warmly welcomed by other distributors at her first sales meeting. She decided to go all-out and stockpiled enough vitamins to meet the minimum monthly quotas needed for a substantial commission on the sales of distributors in her downline. She worked sixty hours a week and spent thousands of dollars on products, telephone calls, and demonstrations. She told *Money*'s reporter:

> At one point, I had signed up eighty distributors. They ranged from a teenager to widows and my friends and relatives. We all thought we would get rich. But I had to bug people to get orders, and my downline shrank to three people. I might get ten people for customers but soon lose eight or nine of them. It was a road to empty dreams.

Two former Nu Skin distributors related a similar story in the November 1991 issue of *Kiplinger's Personal Finance Magazine.* After many months of hard work, Tammy and Charlie Kuhn of Fort Lauderdale, Florida, built a downline of 1,500 distributors and received a monthly check as high as $8,300. In order to maintain high commissions ("overrides"), they had to recruit constantly. When they realized that Fort Lauderdale had become saturated with distributors, they moved to Jacksonville, only to find that it too was saturated. After twenty months in the business, they gave up. As the article explained:

> All along, the Kuhns had resorted to buying products themselves, placing phantom orders in the names of inactive distributors, to keep sales volume at the level needed to qualify for override checks. As their business came apart, they had to put in more and more. . . .
>
> In 1990, they grossed $50,000 from Nu Skin, but their expenses for the year totaled about $47,000. . . . They are deeply in debt and are declaring bankruptcy.
>
> The Kuhns were so bitter about their experience that they joined a $75 million class-action lawsuit against the company.

A pyramid scheme is an illegal scam in which many people at the bottom

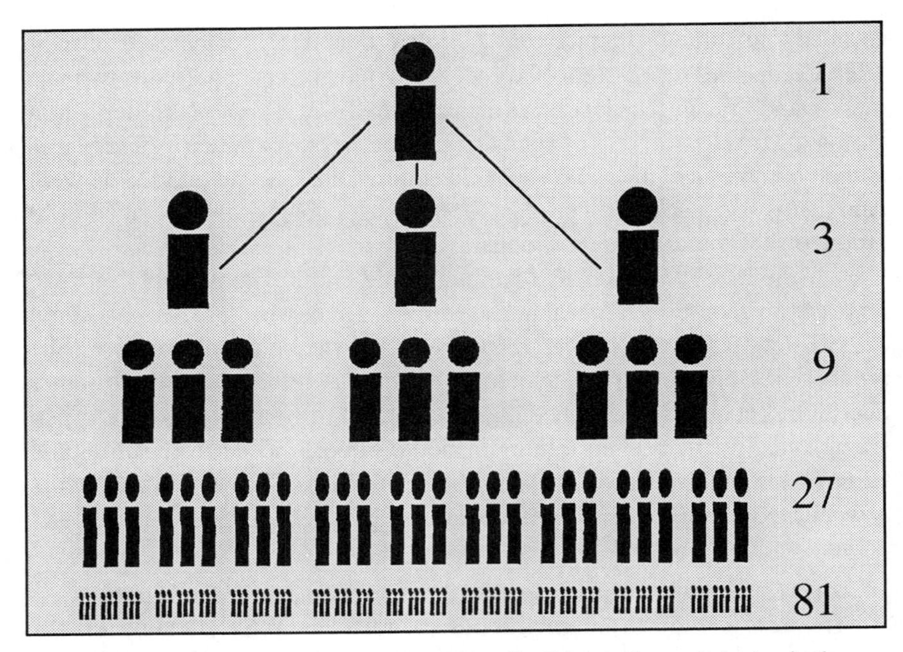

If every distributor manages to recruit three distributors, the total number in the first distributor's downline will be 120. Diagrams like these do not take into account the high dropout rate or the odds against latecomers achieving large downlines. In order for all distributors in the lowest row to reach a downline that big, 29,523 would have to sign up. Big money can be made only by continuously recruiting and/or finding large numbers of retail customers.

of the pyramid pay money to a few at the top. Each new participant pays for the chance to move toward the top and profit from payments from others who might join later. It may appear that recruits will quickly recover their investment from others and that the operation can go on forever with everyone making money and no one being hurt. To maintain the process, however, the number of new participants must keep multiplying—which is impossible. When the supply of recruits dries up, the pyramid will collapse, leaving almost everyone but the earliest participants as losers.

A multilevel company that makes most of its money by selling distributorships and makes little or no effort to market products would be an illegal pyramid scheme. To avoid that pitfall, a company's distributors must engage in genuine retail selling and not just in recruiting other distributors. However, profiting from retail sales is difficult to do—particularly with health products—because even if steady customers can be found, most will become distributors in order to purchase their products "wholesale."

MLM industry folklore holds that 20 percent of American millionaires made their fortunes in multilevel marketing. However, despite thorough investigation, *Money* magazine staff members were unable to find anyone able to document that figure.

Illegal Health Claims

Most multilevel companies that market health products claim that their products can prevent or cure disease. When clear-cut therapeutic claims are made in product literature, the company is an easy target for government enforcement action. Some companies run this risk, hoping that the government won't act until their customer base is well established. Other companies make no claims in their literature but rely on distributors to supply anecdotes, testimonials, and independently published literature. MLM distributors typically encourage people to try their products and credit them for any improvement that occurs.

Most multilevel companies tell distributors to make no claims for the products except those found in company literature. (That way the company can deny responsibility for what distributors do.) However, many companies hold sales meetings at which people are encouraged to tell their stories to the others in attendance. Some companies sponsor telephone conference calls during which leading distributors describe their financial success, give sales tips, and describe their personal experiences with the products. Testimonials may also be published in company magazines, audiotapes, and videotapes. Testimonial claims can trigger enforcement action, but since it is time-consuming to collect evidence of their use, government agencies seldom bother to do so.

Some multilevel companies merely suggest that people will feel better, look better, or have more energy if they supplement their diet with extra nutrients. These suggestions are usually accompanied by warnings about faulty diet, food additives, soil depletion, "overprocessed" foods, air and water pollution, rising cancer rates, and other statements of the type we have described in Chapters 2 and 3—all calculated to alarm the recipient. The proposed solution, of course, is to correct these alleged problems by consuming the company's "natural and scientifically formulated" products.

Multilevel companies that market health products typically begin with the most blatant therapeutic claims they think they can get away with. Each time a government enforcement agency protests, the company will withdraw or tone down just enough claims to avoid a courtroom confrontation. Government enforcement action against multilevel companies has not been vigorous. These companies are usually left alone unless their promotions become so conspicuous and their sales volume so great that an agency feels compelled to intervene. Even then, few interventions have substantial impact once a company is well established. If the original sales push has been effective, the company will have established a base of distributors who believe in the products and don't need official company literature to sell them. Many will use their own testimonials and print their own "unofficial" flyers.

Now lets look at the activities and products of various companies.

In the Beginning . . .

MLM's roots are intertwined with those of the Amway Corporation and its Nutrilite product line. The "Nutrilite concept" is said to have originated about sixty years ago in the mind of Carl Rehnborg, an American businessman who lived in China from 1917 to 1927. According to Amway publications, this gave Rehnborg "ample opportunity to observe at close range the effects of inadequate diet." He also "became familiar with the nutritional literature of his day." Concluding that a balanced diet was needed for proper bodily function, he began to envision a dietary supplement which could provide people with important nutrients regardless of their eating habits.

After seven years of "experimentation," Rehnborg produced food supplements which he gave to his friends to try. According to his son, Sam, who is now Nutrilite's president and chief operating officer:

> After a certain length of time, Dad would visit his friends to see what results had been obtained. More often than not, he would find the products sitting on the back shelves, unused and forgotten. It had cost them nothing and was therefore, to them, worth nothing. . . . It was at this point that he rediscovered a basic principle—that the answer was merely to charge something for the product. When he did, the friends, having paid for the product, ate it, liked it, and further, wanted their friends to have it also. When they asked my dad to sell the product to their friends, he said, "You sell it to them and I'll pay you a commission."

Carl Rehnborg's food supplement business, which began as the California Vitamin Corporation, was renamed Nutrilite Products in 1939 when it moved to larger quarters. According to Federal District Court records, significant out-of-state distribution of Nutrilite supplements began in 1945 when a company operated by Lee S. Mytinger and William S. Casselberry became exclusive national distributor. The pair had sold these products since 1934, but in 1941 they had established the first MLM plan. Rehnborg acted as "scientific advisor" in the distributional scheme and would explain to sales groups that his supplements contained a secret base of unusual therapeutic value and were the answer to man's search for health.

Gross sales soared to $500,000 a month, but the promoters also ran afoul of the law. In 1947, the FDA began a four-year struggle to force Mytinger, Casselberry, Rehnborg, their respective companies, and some fifteen thousand door-to-door agents to stop making wild claims about their products. Potential customers were being given a booklet, "How to Get Well and Stay Well," which represented Nutrilite as effective against "almost every case" of allergies, asthma, mental depression, irregular heartbeat, tonsillitis, and some twenty other common ailments. The booklet, which contained testimonial letters, also implied that cancer, heart trouble, tuberculosis, arthritis, and many other serious illnesses would respond to *Nutrilite* treatment.

After Mytinger and Casselberry, Inc., was asked by the government to show cause why a criminal proceeding for misbranding should not be started, the booklet was revised. A "new language" was devised which referred to all diseases as "a state of non-health" brought about by a "chemical imbalance." Nutrilite would cure nothing—the patient merely gets well through its use. Most direct curative claims were removed from the booklet, but illustrative case histories were added. Although continued governmental pressure led to removal of the case histories, the booklet remained grossly misleading. In 1951, the Court issued a permanent injunction forbidding anyone who sold Nutrilite products from referring to any edition of "How to Get Well and Stay Well" and more than thirty other publications that misrepresented the significance of food supplements. The court decree also contained a long list of forbidden and permissible claims about nutrition and Nutrilite products.

Amway's founders, Rich DeVos and Jay Van Andel, were friends who became *Nutrilite* distributors after high school graduation. They were extremely successful and built a sales organization with over two thousand distributors. Fearing that Nutrilite might collapse, they formed a new company, the American Way Association, later renamed Amway. They began marketing biodegradable detergent products and other household cleaning products and later diversified the product line to include beauty aids, toiletry, jewelry, furniture, electronic products, and many other items. Gross sales have risen steadily from half a million dollars in 1959 to over a billion dollars in the early 1980s and over four billion dollars today. DeVos and Van Andel are now billionaires and are closely connected to the Republican party. DeVos has served as the party's finance chairman, and Ronald Reagan has spoken several times before Amway audiences.

Nutrilite Double X, the company's leading food supplement, contains twelve vitamins and eleven minerals, most in amounts approximating their U.S.

RDAs or a little bit more. A one-month supply, which cost about $20 in 1950, now retails for $48. During the early 1980s, the official sales pitch was simple and low-keyed, based on the misleading concepts of "subclinical deficiency" and "nutrition insurance" described in Chapters 2 and 3 of this book. Prospective customers were given a sixty-page booklet, "Food and Your Family," which explained the importance of nutrients, listed reasons why people's diets may be inadequate, and asked whether they thought there was room for improvement in their own diet. The booklet stated that hundreds of thousands of Americans had used *Nutrilite* " morning, noon and night for more than forty years." If this claim was accurate (which is questionable), most of these lucky customers would have wasted close to $10,000 for their pills.

Nutrilite's current official sales pitch is more subtle but still misleading. Amway's 1994 video, "Nutrilite... Now You Know," is filled with scenes of people who look healthy, happy, and energetic. After stating that good nutrition is available through diet alone, the narrator warns that some people make unwise food choices, that "normal cooking actually destroys some of the essential nutrients in the food we *do* eat," and that "regular exposure to physical stress, tobacco smoke, alcohol, and air pollution can rob our bodies of certain nutrients." The video also contains a segment in which Sam Rehnborg pitches a "three-step plan": (1) *Nutrilite Double X* as "basic nutritional insurance" for the entire family, (2) *Nutrilite Double Edge* (an "antioxidant" product) "to guard against the increased risks that many people believe accompany a high-stress, high-energy lifestyle," and (3) other products that "best complement your lifestyle"—as determined by an Amway distributor.

Steve Butterfield, a professor of English at Castleton State College in Vermont, became an Amway distributor in 1978 and went all-out for two years until he quit in disgust. In *Amway: The Cult of Free Enterprise* (1985), he states: (1) distributors were expected to completely convert to Amway products within a few months of getting into the business, even though these products were more costly than similar products they were accustomed to using; (2) distributors were expected to maintain product inventories and purchase audiotapes and tickets to special meetings; (3) during the early 1980s, over 97 percent of active distributors made no money; (4) although believers advertise Amway as "people helping people," the reality is that the higher-up distributors exploit the cheap labor of the rest; and (5) the whole MLM edifice depends upon sustaining the faith of people on the bottom who have just bought their distributor kit.

The Shaklee Way of Life

Shaklee Corporation was founded in 1956 by Forrest C. Shaklee (1894–1985), a retired chiropractor said to have a lifelong interest in "improving health by working with Nature." According to company literature, he was sickly at birth, but eventually "learned to overcome his deficiency with a program of exercise and nutrition."

During his teens, Shaklee became interested in the ideas of Bernarr Macfadden. In 1912, at the age of eighteen, he helped Macfadden tour midwestern cities to spark interest in "physical culture." According to a biography sold by the Shaklee Corporation:

> Parades were held on the main street of each town, and consisted of a pride of muscular youths (including Shaklee), some musicians, and a flatbed wagon. . . . When enough of a crowd had been gathered around the flatbed, each of the youths was to exercise with a given piece of equipment. This was preceded by a discourse by Macfadden, extolling health through nature, diet and especially non-diet (he tended to look upon fasting as a blanket cure-all) and, of course, strenuous exercise. . . .
>
> The pièce-de-resistance of these outdoor displays was the lifting of an iron ball which appeared to weigh easily 500 pounds. Secured to the ball was a massive link chain, which one of the youths would grasp and which, with much concentration and apparent straining, he would raise gradually over his head. The crowds, watching in awed silence at the beginning of the feat, would break into cheers and applause when the ball was finally lifted. When it was his turn at the ball, Forrest discovered that lifting it was easily accomplished; the ball was hollow!

Within the next few years, Shaklee graduated from chiropractic school and began to treat patients with a substance he developed and called "vitalized minerals." He then headed several chiropractic clinics where he "concentrated on treating patients who had nutritional disorders." In the early 1940s, he stopped clinical practice but continued to lecture on "nutrition." In 1956, he and two sons began marketing a few products he had used during his practice. These included *Pro-Lecin*, (a combination of protein and lecithin), *Herb-Lax* (an herbal laxative) and *Vita-Lea* (a multiple vitamin-mineral supplement). Later a wide variety of other supplements, food products, cleaning products, and cosmetics were added to the company line.

"Basic to the Shaklee Way of Life," said the 1980 version of *The Shaklee Sales Manual*, "is the belief that you have the right to prosper through your own personal efforts." The manual advised new distributors to sell to their friends "as a natural extension of your friendship." Other prospects could be contacted with a letter that begins: "Dear Mrs. Jones: Would you be interested in learning how you can simplify your shopping and at the same time provide total care for your family?" ("Total care," however, was not defined.) In 1980, Shaklee's sales approach was similar to that of Amway, but some of its authorized practices were a bit more misleading. A section of the manual called "Appearances Can Deceive" suggested a variety of ways to make people worry that they are not getting enough nutrients in their food. The importance of each nutrient was described in detail, "individuality" of needs was stressed, and various situations were described wherein nutrients supposedly might be lacking. The fact that vitamin deficiency is rare, of course, was not mentioned.

Many Shaklee distributors have made claims that went far beyond those officially authorized by the company. In 1981, Susan Fitzgerald and Pete Mekeel of the *Lancaster (Pa.) New Era* found that distributors in their county tended to follow the example of their local leadership. At local sales meetings, the reporters observed a wide variety of testimonials:

> People stand up at meetings and in the best spirit of an old-fashioned revival tell how Shaklee products have rid them of arthritis, saved their marriage, enabled them to have two bowel movements a day, and kept them from breaking a leg when they fell off a ladder. If there are any doubters, they keep quiet.

When the reporters consulted Shaklee distributors as potential clients, they were advised to buy a "Basic Five Plan" of supplements and *Herb-Lax* that would cost close to $600 per year per person. Similar observations were made at sales meetings in 1982 by Kristan Dale, a research assistant for the American Council on Science and Health. Our recent investigation did not uncover any company-produced sales aids indicating why people should buy Shaklee vitamins. However, the distributor with whom we dealt gave us a handout in which he offered "nutritional programs for arthritis, diabetes, asthma, nervousness, children's nutrition, heart disease, brain and memory, skin problems, weight control, cholesterol, anemia, alcoholism."

Shaklee became a publicly owned corporation in 1973 and was listed on the New York Stock Exchange from 1977 through 1989, when it was purchased by Yamanouchi Pharmaceuticals Co., a Japanese manufacturer. Shaklee's annual reports indicate that its gross worldwide sales rose steadily from $75 million in 1973 to $539 million in 1983 but dropped to about $400 million by 1986. Nutritional products accounted for about 75 percent of these figures. In 1990, Shaklee was reported to have more than five thousand full-time sales leaders and more than 400,000 part-time distributors.

Neo-Life's Scare Tactics

Neo-Life Company of America was co-founded in 1958 by Donald E. Pickett, who served for many years as chairman of its board of directors. In the late 1970s and early 1980s, Neo-Life publications described him as a man who was "deeply concerned about human survival in this over-chemicalized world," and was "nationally recognized as a nutritional expert." Although the publications did not describe Mr. Pickett's background or provide any basis for considering him a nutrition expert, Neo-Life's *Counselor* magazine did spell out how to sell vitamins:

> Do you meet people who complain about being tired, sluggish or listless? Would they like to feel better, look better and have more energy? Maybe their nutritional fuel level is low, their diet is lacking in some essentials.
>
> Ask them, "Would you put used motor oil in the engine of a brand new car?" Of course, they'll say no! We all know that the new car probably would perform fine—for a while! But, in the long run, the poor quality of the oil would shorten the life of the automobile and would lower its performance!
>
> The body is no different! If you put junk food in it, it may perform trouble-free—for a while—but food low in nutrients will have the same long-term effects on the body as used oil does to the automobile—lower performance and greater wear and tear. And, unfortunately, you can't trade in on a new model when this one wears out! Remember, there's lots of "cheap fuel" around today; most packaged foods have many, if not all, of the natural nutrients removed during processing and replaced with chemicals. . . .
>
> Most of your customers will say that they eat three balanced meals a day. Ask them if they are sure they are getting enough of the nutritional elements their bodies require. . . . If there's any doubt, wouldn't they be willing to spend a few pennies a day to be sure?

Even though "nutrition insurance" based such reasoning is seldom more valuable than insurance against a plague of unicorns, many people are willing to spend those "pennies." *Formula IV*, Neo-Life's multiple vitamin-mineral supplement, then cost about 24¢ per day. To potential customers who said they couldn't afford this, distributors were instructed to respond: "Really, the only thing you have to decide is which of these can you afford: healthy cells, or weakened, sluggish cells." Today, *Formula IV* costs about 35¢ a day, at least five times as much as an equivalent drugstore product. For about $1.25 per day, the worried well can buy one of three Uni-Pak formulas "tailored to your individual needs and lifestyle":

- *Active 40+* is offered as "nutritional insurance for the prime of your life."
- *Sports 30* is for "anyone facing extra physical demands daily. Active people of all ages will find *Sports 30* provides extra stamina for a full

day's work. . . . The continuous, even flow of vital nutrients . . . helps keep your energy level high with plenty of reserve endurance."

- *Stress 30* is for "housewives, foremen, students, salesmen—all have deadlines to meet and decisions to make, and that implies some form of stress. Whether brought on by worry, overwork, deadlines, or just daily problems, stress robs the body of valuable nutrients. *Stress 30* replaces them—just the right amounts throughout the day."

Each pack includes two *Formula IV* pills plus five others.

In the early 1980s, prospective customers were invited to take a "stress test" in which they checked off items on a list of forty-three causes of stress, each of which was assigned a point score from 11 to 100. Although this test may have some research applications in the field of psychology, it has nothing whatsoever to do with nutrient needs. But no matter, Neo-Life's Uni-Paks were "designed specifically to help you combat the effects of daily stress," such as marriage (50 points), a mortgage over $10,000 (31 points), and outstanding personal achievement (28 points).

In the mid-1980s, Neo-Life marketed "a program for your heart" that included *Vitamin E*, *Lecithin*, *Lipotropic Adjunct*, and *Herbals, Garlic & Onion*. *Lipotropic Adjunct* and was claimed to help prevent atherosclerosis by helping the body metabolize fats. Neo-Life has also marketed *Toxgard* to "help your body protect itself against heavy metal pollutants in air and water" and to "aid your liver in detoxifying food additives and artificial food colors"; *Liver Plus C*, on a hunch that "nutritionists believe that liver is a rich source of unknown nutritional factors which one day may be better known or appreciated"; and *Pet-Pal* to make your dog or cat less susceptible to "people" diseases. Of course, to become a customer for life, you don't have to fall for all of the deceptions promoted by supplement pushers. Just one.

USA's State-of-the-Art Sales Aids

In 1986, United Sciences of America (USA), Inc., of Carrollton, Texas, began marketing with high-tech videotapes to promote its products. The "Company Introduction" videotape was narrated by William Shatner (Captain Kirk of "Star Trek") and included scenes of a space rocket launching, a giant computer bank, scientific laboratories, prominent medical institutions, and medical journals. Shatner alleged that "our food, water, and air are becoming contaminated" by chemicals ("toxic killers"), that cancer is on the rise, that our soil is being depleted of "vital, life-giving nutrients and important earth minerals," that one out of every three families will be stricken with some form of cancer, and that two out of five people will die of heart disease or stroke. Then he described how company founder Robert Adler had developed a "brain trust of medical and scientific experts who have pioneered one of the most dramatic programs in the history of nutritional science. . . Their mission is clear: to develop a complete nutritional program to protect us from the growing dangers that are threatening the health of our nation." Shatner also suggested that investing in USA's program would result in "looking your best, feeling maximum physical energy and mental well-being, enjoying total health." Another tape related certain ingredients in USA's products to research on the prevention of cancer, heart disease, and other conditions.

USA maintained that its "state-of-the-art nutrition program" had been designed and endorsed by a scientific advisory board that included two Nobel prize winners and several other medical school professors. Eight months after the company began marketing, it had signed up more than 140,000 distributors and was grossing millions of dollars each month. However, it drew a great deal of unfavorable publicity when several advisors denied endorsing the products and Dr. Fredrick J. Stare and other critics challenged the health claims in the videotapes. The resultant scandal plus action by the FDA and three state attorneys-general drove the company out of business. But the use of videotapes as sales tools became standard practice within the MLM industry.

"Diagnosing" and "Prescribing"

Nature's Sunshine Products (NSP), headquartered in Spanish Fork, Utah, markets more than 450 products. The business began in 1972 with herbs, but has expanded into nutritional supplements (some formulated by James Scala, Ph.D., former research director for Shaklee Corporation), homeopathic remedies, skin and hair-care products, water treatment systems, cooking utensils, and a weight-loss plan. NSP's most recent annual report states that in 1993 the company had 144,000 distributors worldwide with total sales of $92 million in the United States and $35 million in other countries.

NSP's distributors, dubbed "Natural Health Counselors," are taught to use iridology (see Chapter 7), muscle-testing (a type of applied kinesiology), and other quack methods to convince people that they need the products. Under state laws, commercial interactions that involve examining people, identifying health problems, and recommending products to solve them, constitute diagnosing and prescribing, which require a license as a health professional. Many NSP distributors are violating these laws.

Many of NSP's products are claimed to "nourish" or "support" various body organs. NSP's distributor kit includes *A Systems Guide to Natural Health*, a wire-bound book with about eighty pages. About half of the book describes various body systems and the products NSP relates to them. For each system, there are "key," "primary," and "complementary" products. Key products combine ingredients to "provide comprehensive nutritional support" for the body system. Primary products are combinations "designed to provide more specialized support for the particular system." Complementary products are single-ingredient items "for individuals who want to round out the systems approach to holistic health." These products include acidophilus, aloe vera, cascara sagrada (a laxative), and magnesium.

The circulatory system's key product is *Mega-Chel*, which contains twelve vitamins, nine chelated minerals, choline, inositol, PABA, bioflavonoids, fish oils, adrenal substance, thymus substance, and spleen substance. The "primary" circulatory products include *CoQ-10 Plus*; *Bugleweed Liquid Herb*; *Capsicum, Garlic & Parsley*; and herbal mixtures that contain from three to fourteen ingredients. The complementary products include butcher's broom root, capsicum, garlic, hawthorn berries, liquid chlorophyll, magnesium, omega-3 fatty acids, and yellow dock root. Each of these products is said to provide "nutritional support" for the circulatory system. Other key products include *Nutri-Calm* ("provides the nutrition the body needs to cope with a busy modern world"), *Master Gland Formula* ("strengthens" the thyroid, adrenals, and pancreas"), and *Immune Maintenance Formula.* Assertions like these violate federal and state laws against marketing products with unsubstantiated health claims.

Most of NSP's homeopathic products are named after a disease or symptom. The product *Parasites,* for example, is said to be for "minor intestinal symptoms associated with parasites such as bloating, abdominal pain, flatulence and diarrhea." The product *Gout* is for "minor pain, heat, redness, and swelling associated with gouty inflammation of the joints." *Incontinence* is for "occasional minor bladder incontinence (involuntary urination) in adults." *Depressaquel* is designed "to assist in the reduction of minor feelings of melancholy, apathy and listlessness by lifting the mood and mental outlook." These claims violate FDA guidelines that forbid the marketing of nonprescription homeopathic remedies for the treatment of ailments that require professional attention (see Chapter 9).

NSP also markets *GlanDiet*, a meal-replacement program based mainly on the book *Dr. Abravanel's Body Type and Lifetime Nutrition Plan* by Elliot B. Abravanel, M.D., and his wife Elizabeth King. The book claims there is a "dominant gland" at the root of every weight problem and that weight can be controlled by soothing the errant gland and moderating its cravings. The book advises that the corrective plan be tailored to the individual's "body type," which is determined by examining the person's shape, body fat distribution, food cravings, sleep patterns, and various other characteristics. Women can be classified as "thyroid," "pituitary," "adrenal," or "gonadal" type, while men can be classified as "thyroid," "pituitary," or "adrenal." The personality traits described for each type resemble those of a typical horoscope. To help distributors design the correct program, NSP provides "a convenient body type questionnaire . . . based solely upon shape and build." *GlanDiet* guidelines list "foods to eat or avoid" and "herbs to use when the urge to snack strikes" for each body type. All dieters are advised to begin with a two- to three-day "cleanse," engage in aerobic exercise, and aim for an overall calorie count of 1,200/day for women or 1,400/day for men. Of course, most people who exercise and restrict calories to such levels will lose weight whether or not they use NSP products.

Enrich International

Enrich International, of Pleasant Grove, Utah, markets more than 150 herbal, homeopathic, and supplement products. It was founded in 1977 as Nature's Labs, sold in 1985, and renamed Enrich soon afterward. In 1993, the company said it had over sixty thousand distributors and projected sales of $80 million. Its president and chief operating officer is Kenneth Brailsford, who launched Nature's Sunshine in 1972 and for several years published a magazine called *The Herbalist.*

Enrich's products have included *Tummy Gum* (for appetite control), *Increase* (a homeopathic product that can correct all types of baldness problems), *Perform* ("which naturally targets impotency and helps naturally to rejuvenate the glands"), *Cataract* ("to aid . . . any eye and vision problems, cataracts being the most severe"), *Endida* ("a nutritional program that works against yeast infections"), and *Co-Q10* (claimed to improve angina pectoris, congestive heart failure, high blood pressure, diabetes, and gum disease). Distributors are given *The Mini Herb Guide*, which specifies products for seventy types of health problems. A disclaimer says that the information "should not be used for diagnosing and prescribing" and "is not intended as a substitute for medical care."

In 1989, Enrich launched a sales aid called "Bionutritional Quest," a one-page document containing thirty-one questions about symptoms, eating habits, and environmental factors. The answers are scored with a "key sheet" purported to tell which body systems need nutritional help. Customers then receive a form

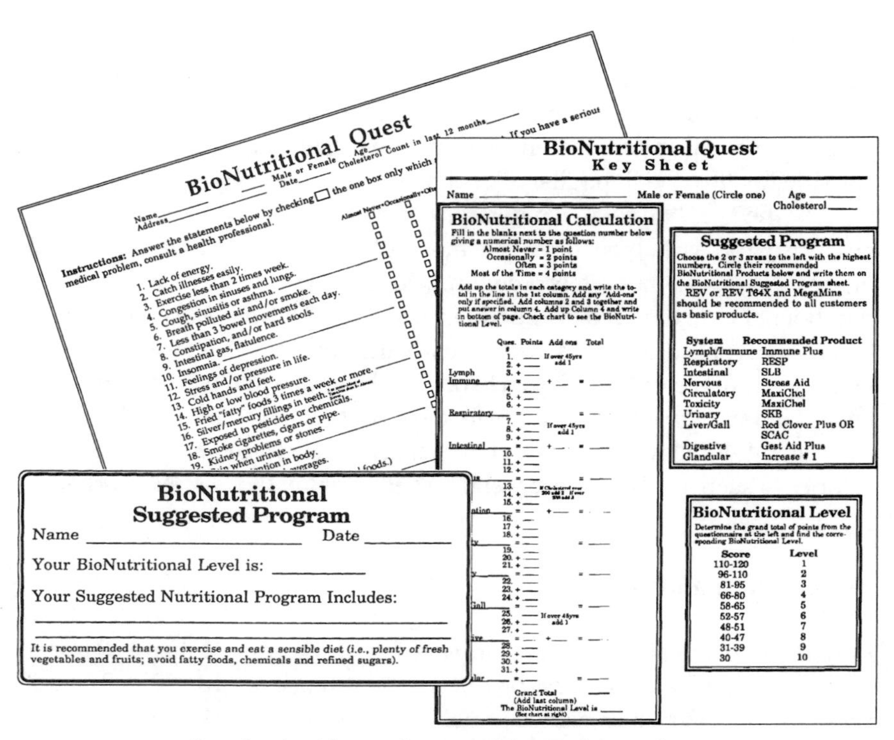

BioNutritional Quest

Name ____ Address ____ Male or Female ____ Date ____ Age ____ Cholesterol Count in last 12 months ____

Instructions: Answer the statements below by checking ☐ the one box only which … If you have a serious medical problem, consult a health professional.

Almost Never • Occasionally • Often

1. Lack of energy.
2. Catch illnesses easily.
3. Exercise less than 2 times week.
4. Congestion in sinuses and lungs.
5. Cough, sinusitis or asthma.
6. Breath polluted air and/or smoke.
7. Less than 3 bowel movements each day.
8. Constipation, and/or hard stools.
9. Intestinal gas, flatulence.
10. Insomnia.
11. Feelings of depression.
12. Stress and/or pressure in life.
13. Cold hands and feet.
14. High or low blood pressure.
15. Fried "fatty" foods 3 times a week or more.
16. Silver/mercury fillings in teeth.
17. Exposed to pesticides or chemicals.
18. Smoke cigarettes, cigars or pipe.
19. Kidney problems or stones.

BioNutritional Quest
Key Sheet

Name ____ Male or Female (Circle one) Age ____ Cholesterol ____

BioNutritional Calculation

Fill in the blanks next to the question number below giving a numerical number as follows:
Almost Never = 1 point
Occasionally = 2 points
Often = 3 points
Most of the Time = 4 points

Add up the totals in each category and write the total in the line in the 1st column. Add any "Add-ons" only if specified. Add columns 2 and 3 together and put answer in column 4. Add up Column 4 and write in bottom of page. Check chart to see the BioNutritional Level.

Ques. # Points Add ons Total

Lymph Immune (1–3; If over 45yrs add 1)
Respiratory (4–6)
Intestinal (7–9; If over 45yrs add 1)
(10–12)
(13–15)
(16–18)
(19–21)
(22–24)
Gall (25–27; If over 45yrs add 1)
(28–31)

Grand Total (Add last column) ____
The BioNutritional Level is ____ (See chart at right)

Suggested Program

Choose the 2 or 3 areas to the left with the highest numbers. Circle their recommended BioNutritional Products below and write them on the BioNutritional Suggested Program sheet.
REV or REV T64X and MegaMins should be recommended to all customers as basic products.

System	Recommended Product
Lymph/Immune	Immune Plus
Respiratory	RESP
Intestinal	SLB
Nervous	Stress Aid
Circulatory	MaxiChel
Toxicity	MaxiChel
Urinary	SKB
Liver/Gall	Red Clover Plus OR SCAC
Digestive	Gest Aid Plus
Glandular	Increase # 1

BioNutritional Level

Determine the grand total of points from the questionnaire at the left and find the corresponding BioNutritional Level.

Score	Level
110-120	1
96-110	2
81-95	3
66-80	4
58-65	5
52-57	6
48-51	7
40-47	8
31-39	9
30	10

BioNutritional
Suggested Program

Name ____ Date ____

Your BioNutritional Level is: ____

Your Suggested Nutritional Program Includes:

It is recommended that you exercise and eat a sensible diet (i.e., plenty of fresh vegetables and fruits; avoid fatty foods, chemicals and refined sugars).

Pseudoscientific test for prescribing Enrich products

stating their "Bionutritional Level" plus recommendations for at least four Enrich products. The entire procedure is utter nonsense.

In 1990, the FDA asked the company to recall nine product-information sheets that contained misleading and unapproved therapeutic claims. Subsequently, Woodland Books, Provo, Utah, which publishes books about herbs and "alternative" health-care methods, sent distributors an envelope with the message: "Here are the tools to help sell your Enrich products." Inside were Woodland's catalog, a similar message from Enrich's president, and a flyer stating that "Woodland's books help create markets for your products." One book was *The Little Herb Encyclopedia,* by Jack Ritchason, who was a leading Enrich distributor.

The Sunrider Story

Sunrider International began operations in 1982 in Orem, Utah, and moved its headquarters to Torrance, California, in 1987. Its board chairman and president is Tei Fu Chen, who was also the company's co-founder. Sunrider markets herbal products with claims that they can help "regenerate" the body. Although some of the ingredients can exert pharmacological effects on the body, there is no evidence they can cure major diseases or that Sunrider distributors are qualified to advise how to use them properly. In 1983, the FDA ordered Sunrider to stop claiming that its *Nutrien Concentrate* was adequate and effective to "produce energy, long life, and lasting health" and that *Calli Tea* was "designed for health and beauty" and helps the user to be "slender, energetic, and full of life." In 1984, the FDA obtained an injunction prohibiting Sunrider from marketing an unapproved sweetener extracted from the herb *Stevia rebaudiana* and sent the company a regulatory letter telling it to stop making more than fifty explicit claims that four of its products could benefit specific organs or were adequate and effective against various disease conditions. In 1989, the company signed a consent agreement pledging to pay $175,000 to the state of California and to stop representing that its products have any effect on disease or medical conditions. The company toned down its literature but continued to make illegal health claims in testimonial tapes included in its distributor kits.

The August 1989 issue of *Longevity* magazine described how the parents of a four-year-old girl with an inoperable brain tumor had put her on a $900-a-month Sunrider regimen with the hope of curing the cancer. When the tumor went into remission (following radiation therapy), Sunrider distributors began telling prospective clients that their products had cured it. Although the child died of her disease several months later, the parents continued to receive phone calls from families of cancer patients inquiring about the "cure."

Until recently, Sunrider glorified the manner in which Chen supposedly learned how to make its formulas and used them to overcome serious obstacles. According to "The Sunrider Story," ancient Chinese temple priests who were leading developers of the martial arts had discovered special plant and herb combinations for increased endurance, energy, and mental alertness and also had discovered a balm to expedite healing of torn or bruised muscles. Chen's great-grandfather was able to obtain manuscripts containing the secrets of five thousand years of research and became a prominent herbal physician. He and Chen's father began teaching them to Chen during his eighth year. Chen subsequently became a Taiwanese national kung fu champion, a medical doctor (in Taiwan), a licensed pharmacist (in the U.S.), a biochemist, and a "world renowned nutritionist."

"At the age of twenty," the story continues, "he became a Senior Research Scientist. He then spent fifteen years in continued research, testing the principles taught in the manuscripts according to modern science and technology. . . . As a young man, Dr. Chen was physically weak. He was small, underweight and overpowered by physical allergies and illness. His own story of transformation was adequate proof of the legitimacy of the secrets on the pages of the manuscripts."

In 1992, a jury in Phoenix, Arizona, concluded that Sunrider Corporation had violated Arizona's racketeering laws. The plaintiff in the case, Debi A. Boling, had charged that Sunrider products had caused her to become very ill. She had also accused the company of making misrepresentations to induce people to buy its products. According to testimony in the case, Ms. Boling had taken products recommended by a local masseuse to reduce the amount of fat on her legs. Soon afterward, she began to lose large amounts of hair from her head, her teeth became discolored, and she experienced severe nausea. To win her case, Boling had to persuade the jury that she had been injured by a criminal act done with fraudulent intent for financial gain. After hearing testimony over a three-month period, the jury awarded her $650,000—$50,000 for actual damages, which were tripled under the state's racketeering law, plus an additional $500,000 for punitive damages.

While preparing for the trial, Boling and her attorney learned that the story about Chen's background was a complete fabrication. Chen's father said in an affidavit that his son was not born into poverty and was not a weak and sickly child. Chen's father also denied having any knowledge that Chen spent much time with his grandfather, studied herbal manuscripts while he was growing up, or was a national kung fu champion. (During a deposition, Chen claimed he had been a champion but had thrown away his medals and "couldn't remember" the specific location where the tournament was held.)

Additional information obtained during depositions made it clear that Chen had never been a licensed pharmacist and was not a medical doctor or a "world renowned nutritionist." In fact, when asked to name the B-vitamins or to say how many D-vitamins there are, he refused to do so and said he would have to look up the information. Nor could he provide or identify any ancient (or even very old) document from which any Sunrider formula was derived. Nor could he provide any basis for saying that he ever was a "senior research scientist." He was merely a teaching assistant who helped set up lab experiments and grade papers.

The *Km* Story

Matol Botanical International, a Canadian firm, markets *Km*, a foul-tasting extract of fourteen common herbs. The product's development is vividly described in company brochures and videotapes, which provide the following details.

Km was formulated in the 1920s by Karl Jurak, a student of agrobiology and biochemistry at the University of Vienna. In his youth, Karl was interested in flowers and plants and displayed an "unquenchable thirst for knowledge." One day while climbing a mountain he suddenly became weak and "dangerously short of breath." To improve his physical condition, he became "driven to establish a state of optimum health." He reasoned that "if he could find a way to focus his natural body energies, he would then find the key to relieving his problems. He decided to apply his knowledge of science and use the plants he loved . . . to prepare a health formula for himself."

After eight months of work, during which he analyzed his own blood samples daily, he arrived at a formula. But although he noted many benefits, the "key" to the formula was missing—"a factor that would perfectly merge all of the virtues of each plant." Finally, in 1922, the "key" was revealed to him in a dream. He completed the formula and found that taking it led to "remarkable improvement." He based his doctoral thesis on this work and, at the age of nineteen, received a doctorate with honors in agrobiology. In 1925, he was awarded a second doctorate, in biochemistry.

In 1932, the story continues, the Canadian government commissioned Jurak to do research, and he emigrated to Canada. For thirty years he continued to prepare the formula himself. He did not sell it, but gave it to friends and relatives until, in 1962, he was no longer able to satisfy the demand and "destiny intervened." In that year Jurak entrusted the formula to his son, Anthony, who had earned his own doctorate in biochemistry. In 1984, Anthony and a friend launched Matol Botanical International.

Although company literature makes no *direct* therapeutic claims for *Km*, one brochure provides pictures of its fourteen herbs and attributes beliefs about their usefulness to various peoples in the past. For example, it says that Indians of Virginia believed that passion flower could "quiet and soothe the body" and that native Indians on the Pacific coast of North America believed that tea made from saw palmetto berries "soothed and quieted the mind." Another brochure quotes Karl Jurak: "In 60 years, given time, I have never seen this product fail once in helping to do some good for the people using it."

It is clear that Matol distributors have made therapeutic claims. Many have circulated flyers or typed reports associating *Km*'s herbal ingredients with organs and health problems for which each herb can supposedly be of benefit. One such flyer, entitled "Herbal Information," refers neither to Matol nor to *Km*, but bears the handwritten name and phone number of the distributor and makes vague therapeutic claims for the herbs in *Km*. Alfalfa, for example, is described as "excellent for arthritis" and said to contain "many vitamins and minerals." A two-color circular touts *Km* as a "blood purifier" that has been "examined" for more than sixty years in the human body and can provide "energy and vitality" and "a greater hope of longer life." (Alfalfa may actually promote arthritis.)

Km was originally marketed in Canada as *Matol,* which was claimed to be effective for ailments ranging from arthritis to cancer, as well as rejuvenation. Canada's Health Protection Branch took action that resulted in an order to advertise only its name, price, and contents. In 1988, the FDA attempted to block importation of *Matol* into the United States, but the company circumvented the ban by adding an ingredient and changing the product's name. In 1990, the company was reported to have 250,000 distributors and a gross sales of $150 million.

Km has never been proven safe or effective for any health purpose whatsoever. The identity and amounts of its herbal ingredients are not public information. Those who feel or look better after using *Km* are encouraged to attribute any improvement to the product's supposed potency.

The Herbalife Story

Herbalife International, of Inglewood, California, markets weight-control products, dietary supplements, and personal-care products. The company was founded in 1980 by twenty-four-year-old Mark Hughes, who states he was inspired by his mother's unsuccessful struggle to control her weight with amphetamines. Herbalife's 1993 retail sales totaled $247 million in the United States and $693 million worldwide. Its principal products are *Formula #1* (a meal-replacement protein drink mix), *Formula #2* (an herbal tablet), *Formula #3* (a multivitamin/mineral tablet), and *Thermojetics*, a weight-control system that includes herbal tablets. The numbered formula products were originally marketed as components of Herbalife's *Slim and Trim* Program. Today the program is called *Herbalife Cellular Nutrition Health and Weight Management System,* and some of the ingredients are different.

Hughes dropped out of high school after ninth grade and wound up in legal difficulty that resulted in his staying for three years at a residential school for troubled youngsters. When he was nineteen, his mother died of a drug overdose. According to a 1985 issue of the *Herbalife Journal:*

> Mark became aware of the need for a safe, effective way to lose weight . . . when his mother died as a direct result of following years of unwise dieting practices. This event left him with a vital interest in nutrition

> and a fervent desire to find a product that would enhance and build health while allowing an individual to take weight off sensibly and safely. . . .
>
> During his search, he had met Richard Marconi, Ph.D., with whom he shared his dream. . . . After a lot of research and testing, Herbalife *Slim and Trim* was born.

After working for two multilevel companies that sold weight-control products but went out of business, Hughes founded Herbalife with help from Marconi, who had manufactured products for one of these companies. Herbalife publications describe Marconi as a "well-respected nutritional expert" and "the leading authority on nutritional products." His "Ph.D." was obtained from nonaccredited Donsbach University (see Chapter 6) after Marconi hooked up with Hughes. After this fact was brought out at a Congressional hearing (described below), Herbalife's *Journal* stopped referring to Marconi as "Dr."

Herbalife's initial marketing included lengthy cable television programs that were filled with financial and health-related testimonials. Sales were also promoted with buttons and bumper stickers that said "Lose Weight Now, Ask Me How."

In 1982, the FDA sent Herbalife a Notice of Adverse Findings, which stated that certain products were misbranded because of labeling claims that they were effective for treating many diseases, dissolving and removing tumors, rejuvenating, increasing circulation, and producing mental alertness. A 1984 FDA Talk Paper notes that the agency had received many complaints about side effects that had occurred during the use of Herbalife products and had stopped when use of the products was stopped. In fact, said the Talk Paper, "Literature given Herbalife distributors states that up to 25% of product users will have adverse effects but claims that this is evidence of the body's improving itself." Several suits were filed by people who alleged that the products had harmed them. Some of these suits were settled out of court with substantial payment, but the amounts have not been disclosed and the case records are sealed.

By 1985, Hughes claimed that Herbalife had over 700,000 distributors and an annual income approaching half a billion dollars a year. But trouble was brewing. In May 1985, Senator William V. Roth, Jr. (R–DE) held two days of hearings on weight-reduction programs, during which he grilled Hughes about the "research and testing" done prior to marketing Herbalife's products. Hughes said, "We have a lot of scientific data on the herbs," but Roth ascertained that no actual testing of Herbalife products had taken place. The hearing also brought to light a study done by Herbalife of 428 users of its products. About 40 percent had experienced headache, constipation, diarrhea, nausea, lightheadedness, palpitations, and/or other transient symptoms that might be attributable to Herbalife products. The occurrence of side effects came as no surprise because several ingredients in Herbalife products were potent laxatives and one product *(N.R.G.)* contained guarana, which is high in caffeine.

In March 1985, the California Attorney General had charged Herbalife with violating California's consumer protection laws. The suit charged that early editions of the *Herbalife Official Career Handbook* made illegal claims that various herbal ingredients were effective against more than seventy diseases and conditions. Although most of these claims were deleted in subsequent editions of the handbook, the company had not replaced the original pages sent to distributors with the revised pages or asked these distributors to destroy them. Similar testimonial claims had been made in the company's cable television broadcasts. The suit also charged that Herbalife had been operating an illegal pyramid scheme. The case was settled in 1986 when Hughes and the company agreed to pay $850,000 and to abide by a long list of court-ordered restrictions on claims and marketing practices.

Just prior to the Senate hearings, Cable News Network aired a four-part report which revealed that Herbalife's supposed "research laboratory" was a conference room that housed a large table and books on herbs, located at one of Marconi's factories. Marconi told a CNN interviewer, "We employed hundreds . . . even thousands of Ph.D.s in the research program for our products." But when asked who they were, he replied, "Why, the research papers that are published and printed that we have access to on our computer."

The adverse publicity caused Herbalife's income to drop sharply, but the company survived, expanded into many foreign countries, and is now a publicly held corporation. The claims have toned down and several potentially toxic ingredients have been removed.

The company's 1994 distributor kit contains a videotape stressing financial opportunity and an audiotape claiming that America's health is declining due to faulty nutrition and that somehow Herbalife products provide special nutritional help at the "cellular level." Herbalife's official position is that it makes no therapeutic claims for *Thermojetics* products and therefore is not required to obtain FDA approval for their sale. We believe that since the products are obviously intended to aid weight reduction, they should be regulated as drugs and be proven safe and effective in order to remain marketable.

Herbalife's annual 10-K report to the Securities and Exchange Commission indicates that trouble may be brewing. One ingredient in Herbalife's *Thermojetics* system is the herb ma huang. This contains ephedrine, a decongestant that poses risks for individuals with high blood pressure, glaucoma, and several other conditions. The report said that in February 1994, Canadian authorities suspended sales of products containing ephedrine. It remains to be seen whether the FDA will take similar action in the United States. We think that it should.

In May 1994, following reports of several deaths and many cases of serious illness among abusers of products containing ephedrine, the Texas Commissioner of Health banned the sale of Nature's Nutrition™ *Formula One*, a product marketed by Alliance USA, an MLM company headquartered in Richardson, Texas. *Formula One*, which includes ma huang extract, kola nut (which contains caffeine), several other herbs, beet powder (said to "enrich the blood"), and chromium picolinate, is marketed as a weight-control aid. The commissioner's action charged that the product was improperly labeled and contained more than five times the level of ephedrine found in ma huang. A state court lifted the ban against *Formula One*, but the Health Department is pursuing its case in federal court.

Barley Green

American Image Marketing (AIM), of Nampa, Idaho, sells *Barley Green*, a powder made by dehydrating juice squeezed from barley grass. In the late 1980s, AIM's distributor kit featured a videotape claiming that the American food supply is lacking in nutrients and filled with toxins. It also alleged that vegetables are "void of nutrients " and that preservatives, artificial flavors, dyes, emulsifiers, artificial sweeteners, and other "unnatural chemicals may rob the body of energy and vitality. "Fortunately, the tape said, a Japanese researcher named Yoshihide Hagiwara had "produced a cell food to balance the lacking American diet."

One segment of the videotape stated that *Barley Green* contains "16 organic vitamins, 11 major minerals, 18 amino acids, 12 trace minerals, and enzymes" and had "captured the life essence." However, another segment of the tape stated that "barley leaf contains 25 kinds of vitamins, including B_{15}, K, and P." (Actually, there are only eleven vitamins for humans. B_{15} and P are not among them.) *Barley Green* was also claimed to "fight pollutants in the body" and to contain "live enzymes," including many that are found in white blood cells. The fact that these enzymes would be destroyed during digestion and therefore would fail to enter the body of *Barley Green* users was not mentioned; nor was the fact that amounts of most of the nutrients in *Barley Green* were insignificant.

The tape contained many testimonials from users who said that *Barley Green* made them more energetic, enhanced their athletic performance, and remedied various problems. Some didn't specify what the problems were, but just stated that they had recovered. Distributors throughout the United States circulated audiotapes and printed materials claiming that *Barley Green* had cured or helped individuals with cancer, arthritis, diabetes, heart disease, and other serious ailments. One chiropractor, hoping to recruit colleagues as distributors, even claimed that the product "eliminates the biochemical component of the subluxation complex" and therefore is "a must for everybody or any Chiropractic office."

In 1988, the FDA ordered AIM to stop making various unsubstantiated health claims for *Barley Green* and five other products. The FDA also told the company to stop making false statements about the quality of the American food supply. In 1989, the FDA seized quantities of several AIM products because their labeling or promotional material exaggerated the dietary value of the products. The case was settled by a consent decree ordering destruction of one product and the offending labeling for the others. However, many distributors continue to make false claims, including claims that *Barley Green* is effective against cancer.

"The Rexall Tradition"

Rexall Showcase International (RSI), launched in 1990, sells weight-control products, dietary supplements, homeopathic remedies, skin-care products, and water filters. Its total sales to distributors were $7.8 million for the six months ending February 28, 1993. It is a subsidiary of Rexall Sundown, Inc., of Ft. Lauderdale, Florida, whose stock is listed on the NASDAQ National Market System.

RSI is described to prospects as the newest addition to the Rexall Family of Companies, "one of the best known, most successful corporate families in America." In the video *Why Rexall Expands to Network Marketing*, Rexall Division's Chief Executive Officer Armend Szmulewitz describes how "the Rexall concept" was launched in 1903 when pharmacist Louis Liggett began developing patent medicines that pharmacists could prescribe to their customers. According to Szmulewitz, Liggett called his line Rexall Products (short for "Rx to all." As the Rexall name gained recognition, Szmulewitz noted, "the items became stronger than the store" and the stores became Rexall stores. In the mid-1980s, the Rexall name and distribution rights were purchased by RSI's parent company.

"With that name came a great tradition," Szmulewitz asserted. "We asked, 'How do we get back to what Rexall was, bringing it back to the person, to the independent pharmacist?' We can't do that. But the person-to-person concept will work—bringing the Rexall store to somebody's house." Noting that people typically take only a second to decide whether to buy a product on the shelf, Szmulewitz said that RSI's story needs to be told in a different format: "Very similar to how the independent pharmacist told it many times. The consumer came in, 'Doc I got something wrong, what do you think? They [pharmacists] spend the time. 'Tell me what's wrong.' 'This is what you need. This is what I think will help.'" Szmulewitz continued: "If we can explain it to someone, if we can train them on how to sell it, train them how to use it, train on what the benefits are, and have those people explain it to other people, we've now brought back what always worked in the Rexall concept: One person talking to another."

An article in the March 1, 1982 issue of *Business Week* magazine provides a somewhat less glowing perspective. It states that the Rexall name had once appeared on about three hundred company-owned stores and twelve thousand franchised outlets (about 20 percent of the country's drugstores). During the 1970s, however, Rexall was unable to withstand competition from rivals that built modern outlets in high-density shopping areas. In 1977, the chain was sold for $16 million to a group of private investors, which divested itself of the stores, pared its manufacturing capacity, and became primarily a distributor of vitamins, health foods, and plastic products such as toothbrushes. Former franchisees were permitted to keep using the Rexall name, but a former company official said this might not promote Rexall products because some of the stores were "eyesores" that conveyed a negative public image.

Today, although many pharmacies carry Rexall products, few still use the Rexall name. Inspection of twenty recent Yellow Page directories selected randomly at a public library found only three "Rexall" pharmacies out of about a thousand listed. Moreover, the law limits what pharmacists can do when people ask them to recommend products.

In 1985, operating control of the Rexall name and distribution rights were acquired by Sundown Vitamins, Inc., a company founded in 1976 by Carl DeSantis. DeSantis, who had worked in advertising and management for Super X Drug Stores and Walgreen Drug Stores, has been board chairman, chief executive officer, president, and principal stockholder ever since. In April 1993, Sundown Vitamins changed its name to Rexall Sundown, Inc., shortly before raising $32.9 million through a public stock offering.

According to its June 1993 prospectus, Rexall Sundown, Inc., markets approximately 740 products through retailers, mail-order ads and catalogs, and independent distributors. Sundown nutritional products are sold through mass merchandisers, drugstore chains, and supermarkets. Rexall nutritional products are sold through independent drugstores. Thompson products are sold in health-food stores. (Thompson Nutritional Products was founded in 1935 and acquired by Sundown in 1990.) The mail-order sales are made through the company's SDV Vitamins division. Person-to-person sales are made through RSI. Rexall Sundown also sells over-the-counter drug products such as cold remedies under the Rexall trademark. Total sales grew from $24.1 million in fiscal 1988 to $93.1 million in fiscal 1993 (which ended August 31, 1993).

Although no health claims are made for most products in the Thompson and SDV catalogs, a few are questionable. Thompson's *PMS Formula for Women* ("beneficial in reducing the severity of PMS symptoms") contains 200 mg of vitamin B_6, a dose that can produce nerve toxicity if taken for several months. Its *CoQ-10* "may revitalize the immune system, protect and strengthen the heart and cardiovascular system, normalize high blood pressure and assist in controlling periodontal disease." Its *Free Form Lysine 500 MG* is claimed to "reduce the severity and recurrence of Herpes Simplex viral infections and aid in the production of antibodies, hormones, and enzymes." SDV's catalog includes *Memo-Vite*; *eyetamins*; *Hair, Skin, and Nails* ("The nutrients your body needs for healthy, lustrous hair, glowing skin, and strong nails"); *Ginkgo Biloba* ("might be the answer" for depression, poor circulation, lack of energy, swollen and achy legs, dizziness, ringing in the ears, or occasionally forgetting one's address or phone number); *Green Tea Extract* ("support for weight loss diets"); and *Aloe Vera Softgels* ("may possibly help reduce the symptoms of arthritis").

RSI's brochures and meetings contain many references to scientific breakthroughs, space-age technology, and research facts and figures. Its sales pitches warn about nutritional deficiency, pollution, and the effects of stress. Its products are promised to provide weight loss without hunger; to meet special nutritional needs; to relieve insomnia, fatigue, and everyday stress; and to make you rich and your own boss in the process. RSI publishes testimonials in its bimonthly magazine and asks distributors to submit them.

RSI's *Bios Life 2 Weight Management Program* includes *Bios Life 2*, a powdered high-fiber mixture that contains a patented chromium product said to "help control appetite and, in particular, to help to control sugar cravings; *Bios Fruit Bars,* said to provide a high-fiber, low-fat snack that, combined with a glass of water, make you "feel full so that you can resist the foods you should avoid"; and *Metaba-TROL*, a homeopathic remedy claimed "to affect your mental, emotional and metabolic inclinations to eat at inappropriate times. . . . a godsend for people who eat because of stress, anxiety or fear, for binge eaters and nervous nibblers."

RSI's dietary supplements (Showcase Nutritionals) include twelve items

SHOWCASE
INTERNATIONAL
Rexall's Health Remedies
Homeopathy:
Real Medicines
Regulated by FDA
Safe and Non-Toxic
Non-Habit Forming
TIME
ALTERNATIVE
MEDICINE

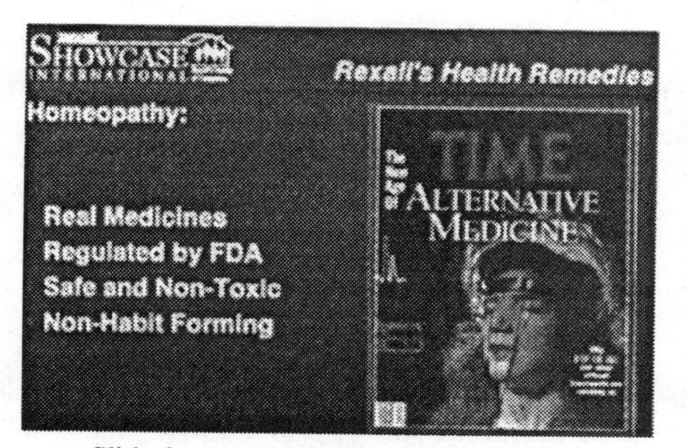

Slide for use at RSI "business briefings"

described in a 1991 brochure as "scientifically correct, break-through products" whose "every ingredient has been thoroughly researched and documented in peer-reviewed literature as having merit in augmenting or otherwise stimulating the functions of certain organs, tissues and systems in the human body." The supplement products include *Workout* ("to aid in your own natural muscular recovery process"), *Energy Essentials* (to "provide the nutrients your body needs to help maximize its natural energy-generating abilities"), and *Essential Bodyguard* (needed because "today's stressful lifestyles can deplete the nutrients your body needs to maintain a healthy immune system"). RSI recommends using one of its multivitamin/mineral products as a base and adding others "to find a combination that suits your diet or lifestyle." Such a program would cost from 18¢ to 96¢ per day, depending on the products chosen.

RSI's homeopathic products include *In•Vigor•Ol* ("a natural tonic, designed for those times when you are troubled with everyday fatigue, general tired feeling and exhaustion"); *Protect•Ol* ("indicated as the initial phase in cleansing the body from many environmental pollutants"); *Calmplex•2000* ("a solution to everyday stress, simple nervous tension and insomnia"); and *Reliev•Ol* lozenges (for "the relief of cough, cold, and allergy symptoms").

RSI's *Aestival* skin-care system is described in company literature as "a natural therapeutic skin-care treatment" that "will absolutely rejuvenate your skin." The products, all for external use, are said to be "enhanced with nourishing botanical extracts, antioxidants, and deep moisturizers so that they beautify and strengthen the fresh skin cells as they clear away the old."

In 1992, a class-action suit was filed against RSI by Patrick J. Hines, a former distributor, who charged that RSI was an illegal pyramid scheme and that the profit potential of becoming a distributor had been exaggerated. The suit papers state: "Of the hundreds of individuals who Hines knew as participating in RSI, almost all are inactive and have sustained the loss of most or all of their investment and have sustained additional economic loss." Similar suits have been filed against Matol Botanical International and against Omnitrition International, Inc., of Carrollton, Texas, which markets supplement products based on formulations by Durk Pearson and Sandy Shaw.

Alga Eaters

Blue-green algae (one of eleven groups of algae) are microscopic plants that grow mainly in brackish ponds and lakes throughout the world. Of the more than fifteen hundred known species, some are useful as food, while others have been reported to cause gastroenteritis and hepatitis. Spirulina entered the limelight in 1981 when *The National Enquirer* promoted it as an "all natural," "safe diet pill" that contains phenylalanine (an amino acid), which "acts directly on the appetite center." The article also said it was "an incredible 65 percent protein, making it the most protein-packed food in the world."

These claims are false. The FDA has concluded that there is no evidence that spirulina (or phenylalanine) is effective as an appetite suppressant. The FDA has also noted that the "65 percent protein" claim is meaningless because, taken according to their label, spirulina products provide only negligible amounts of protein.

In 1982, Microalgae International Sales Corp. (MISCORP) and its founder, Christopher Hills, agreed to pay $225,000 to settle charges that they had made false claims about spirulina. The company had claimed that its spirulina products were effective for weight control and had therapeutic value against diabetes, anemia, liver disease, and ulcers.

Light Force, also founded by Hills, now markets spirulina products with claims that they can suppress appetite, boost immunity, and increase energy. Company sales materials claim that spirulina is a "superfood" and "works to cleanse and detoxify the body." In a 1987 issue of Light Force's magazine, *The Enlightener,* vice president and corporate attorney Steve Kochen spells out the company's "legal guidelines." These include:

- Current regulations . . . prohibit both the company and its Distributors from using any medical research to promote, advertise or sell the products.
- You are free to provide any responsible medical research for the sole purpose of education and information . . . . as long as no mention is made to any specific products, and no attempt is made to sell products at the time the information is made available.

- When using the mail to send research information . . . . any sales information must be provided separately and may not be linked to the medical research.
- You are free to share your personal experience with any of our products, even if that experience involves the alleviation of some health problems or symptoms. However, it is also imperative that you qualify your personal testimonial by saying, "Of course, we cannot make any medical claim for our products or guarantee you will have the same experience."

Despite all this, *The Enlightener* has carried reports about users who lost weight or recovered from arthritis, cancer, multiple sclerosis, and serious injuries while taking Light Force products. None of these reports is accompanied by significant documentation.

In 1982, K.C. Laboratories of Klamath Falls, Oregon, and its president, Victor H. Kollman, began selling *Blue Green Manna* products (derived from another type of alga) with claims that they were effective against a wide range of health problems. In 1983, the FDA began legal action to stop the scheme, but marketing of the products did not stop. Finally, in 1986, at the agency's request, a U.S. District Court judge issued a permanent injunction ordering all parties involved to stop manufacturing, distributing, and selling blue-green algae harvested from Klamath Lake, Oregon. Explaining his decision, the judge said:

> At the trial on January 9, 1986, the government introduced additional evidence of the widespread use of blue-green algae Manna products, and of the therapeutic claims that were made for these products. Victor Kollman denied that he had made therapeutic claims. . . . Nevertheless he continued to claim his product has a beneficial effect on the human body . . . as a food, and not a drug. The government showed that taken at the recommended dosage of 1.5 grams, its value as a nutrient is negligible. Further, the cost of the defendant's products, which exceeds $300 per pound, is so high as compared to other sources of the same nutrients that it is apparent that these products are not intended to be used as a food.

In 1985, the judge had ruled that the products were misbranded and unapproved new drugs, and had issued a preliminary injunction against their sale. His 1986 order cited evidence that more than 2,500 people had been distributing Manna products with therapeutic claims that defied the injunction. He also reported that since the injunction was issued, hundreds of distributors had written or telephoned with claims that Manna products had cured them or members of their families of such problems as Alzheimer's disease, heart trouble, skin disturbances, allergies, prostate problems, lack of sex drive, emotional problems, and alcoholism.

At the 1986 trial, the defendants argued that because other algal products are sold as foods or food supplements, they too should be allowed to sell blue-green algae as food—changing the packaging, trade name, and distribution system if necessary. But the judge ruled that "the demand can no longer be controlled, even if the defendants have a desire to do it." Stating that Kollman had attempted to mislead not only the court but also purchasers of the products, the judge concluded that a permanent injunction was necessary to prevent the defendants from "benefiting from their past violations by meeting the demand they had created for their products." In other words, even if questionable claims

SUPER BLUE-GREEN ALGAE ™

Best of the Green Stuff

- Harvested wild, not artificially cultivated. Grows organically in an unpolluted, snow-fed Oregon lake.
- No synthetic ingredients. Balanced, natural whole food (the lowest on the food chain).
- The highest known source of natural vegetable protein (58%) and chlorophyll in the World!
- *Rich in Beta Carotene (pro-Vitamin A) which helps* prevent cancer (70 times more than carrots, 5,833 times more than yogurt).
- Contains all the essential amino-acids in a perfect balance, almost exactly the same as the human body. (DNA and RNA too).
- An excellent source of Vitamin B-12 (65 times more than kelp, 665 times more than alfalfa, 5.8 times as *much as Chlorella & 19.3 times as much as Spirulina*).
- A natural appetite suppressant. You feel gently satisfied, but not bloated or full.
- Freeze dried (not heat processed), to protect the beneficial enzymes and heat sensitive vitamins.

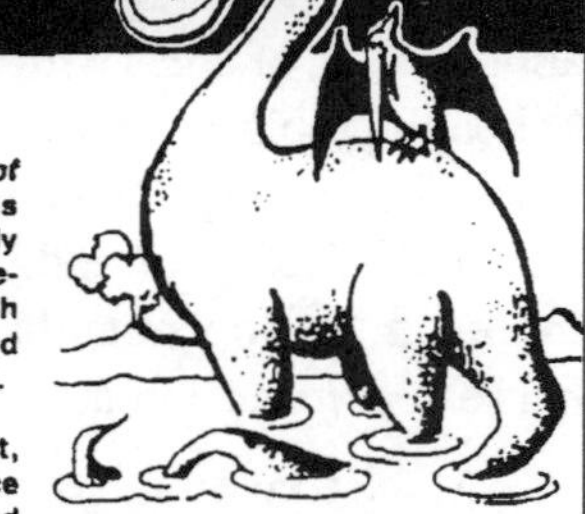

- *A rich source of* neuro-peptides which are quickly absorbed to specifically nourish your brain and nervous system.
- A constant, day-long source *of physical and* mental energy without extreme ups and downs.
- A superb, whole food source of trace minerals and elements (an astonishing 23%), lipids and GLA.
- Ninety-five percent assimilable into the body.
- Commonly reported by satisfied consumers to: Increase physical stamina...improve memory, mental clarity and focus...alleviate stress, anxiety and depression...give relief from fatigue, hypoglycemia and PMS...control excess appetite and cravings...improve digestion and elimination... relieve allergy symptoms...speed recovery from the side effects of medical therapy and heighten anti-pollutant immune functions, and much more!

The Oregon Department of Agriculture has exhibited Super Blue-Green Algae in Korea and Europe. We are listed in the International Trade Journals published by the United States Department of Commerce. *Super Blue Green Products are inspected regularly by nationally recognized laboratories. Cell Tech's powder carries the Kosher Symbol. Ⓚ

Ask too about our Splendid Marketing Opportunity. Serious Income for the Entrepreneur. Earn while you help People become Healthier: $2-5000 a month + within a year.

For a free packet, please call: 1 (800) 99-4-ALGAE (2542) • 1-(818) 993-8215

Ad from 1994 issues of *Health Freedom News*

were stopped, people who believed the previously made claims would still buy the products.

Although the judge's ruling appears to have ended the sale of *Manna* products, a similar line called *Super Blue Green Algae* is still marketed by Cell Tech Inc., a company run by Kollman's brother Daryl. According to a company promotional tape, "By detoxifying your systems and balancing your nutritional levels, Super Blue Green provides your body and spirit with ingredients that result in experiences of increased energy, mental clarity, dietary control and feelings of overall well-being. This can enable people to deal with the many stresses of this modern world."

Cell Tech's literature states that the products do not provide "cures" for diseases and are not intended as a substitute for medical care. Despite this disclaimer, ads placed by several distributors in health-food magazines have made questionable therapeutic claims.

Nu Skin International

Nu Skin International, Inc., of Provo, Utah, was founded in 1984. It markets skin- and body-care products and dietary supplements. Its leading product has been *Nutriol,* a hair-care product said to contain fifty-one amino acids and vitamins. Although no hair-growth claims appeared on the product's label, such claims were made through advertisements and promotional materials. According to an article in *Boston Business*, former president Gerald Ford spoke at the company's 1989 annual convention, where he called Nu Skin "an impressive young company" and said, "I like the attitude they have. The work ethic. The devotion to the basic principles that we love and cherish in America." A few days later, the FDA warned Nu Skin to stop making hair-growth claims. The article noted that when Ford found out, he expressed surprise and embarrassment and terminated his affiliation with Nu Skin. But illegal claims continued in advertisements and promotional materials.

In 1993, Nu Skin and three of its distributors agreed to pay a total of $1,225,000 to settle FTC charges that they made false and unsubstantiated claims for Nu Skin products and exaggerated potential earnings for distributors. Under the agreement, the accused parties are prohibited from making unsubstantiated claims that (1) *Nutriol Hair Fitness Preparation* or any substantially similar product can prevent or remedy hair loss or is as effective or more effective than the prescription drug minoxidil (*Rogaine*), (2) *Face Lift with Activator* or any similar product can permanently remove wrinkles or is equivalent to or better than the prescription drug tretinoin (*Retin-A*), and *Cell-*

Trex or any similar product will promote the healing of third-degree burns. The agreement also specifies how potential earnings must be accurately disclosed.

Motivation: Powerful but Misguided

The "success" of network marketing lies in the enthusiasm of its participants. Many people who think they have been helped by an unconventional method enjoy sharing success stories with their friends. People who give such testimonials are usually motivated by a sincere wish to help their fellow humans. Rarely do they stop to consider how serious it can be to make health recommendations to others. Nor do they realize how difficult it is to evaluate health products on the basis of personal experience. Since we all tend to believe what others tell us about personal experiences, testimonials can be powerful persuaders.

Perhaps the trickiest misconception about quackery is that personal experience is the best way to tell whether something works. When someone feels better after having used a product or procedure, it is natural to give credit to whatever was done. This is unwise, however. Most ailments are self-limiting, and even incurable conditions can have sufficient day-to-day variation to enable bogus methods to gain large followings. In addition, taking some kind of action often produces temporary relief of symptoms (a placebo effect). Financial benefits provide further incentive for giving testimony. For these reasons, scientific experimentation is almost always necessary to establish whether health methods are really effective. Instead of testing their products, multilevel companies urge customers to try them and credit them if they feel better. Some products are popular because they contain caffeine, ephedrine (a stimulant), valerian (a tranquilizer), or other substances that produce mood-altering effects.

Another factor in gaining devotees is the emotional impact of group activities. Imagine, for example, that you have been feeling lonely, bored, depressed, or tired. One day a friend tells you that "improving your nutrition" can help you feel better. After selling you some products, the friend inquires regularly to find out how you are doing. You seem to feel somewhat better. From time to time you are invited to interesting lectures where you meet people like yourself. Then you are asked to become a distributor. This keeps you busy, raises your income, and provides an easy way to approach old friends and make new ones—all in an atmosphere of enthusiasm. Some of your customers express gratitude, giving you a feeling of accomplishment. People who increase their income, their social horizons, or their self-esteem can get a psychological boost that not only can improve their mood but also may alleviate emotionally based symptoms. In *Charismatic Capitalism*, sociologist Nicole Woolsey Biggart observes that "committed distributors see their work as a superior way of life that not only gives them a job, but a worldview, a community of like-minded others, and a self-concept."

Many MLM companies refer to this process as "sharing" and suggest that everyone involved is a "winner." That simply isn't true. The entire process is built on a foundation of deception. *Multilevel marketing provides a powerful financial incentive to spread misinformation.* The main winners are the company's owners and the small percentage of distributors who become sales leaders. The losers are millions of Americans who waste money and absorb the misinformation.

"Nutrition insurance" is promoted with scare tactics. There are enough real things in life to worry about. Who needs imaginary ones? Then there is the matter of money. Who needs to waste hundreds of dollars per year on useless products? Even if people insist on supplementing their diet for "insurance," there is no reason to spend more than a few pennies a day for a multivitamin-mineral supplement. The body cannot tell one brand from another. Nor is there any reason to supplement one's diet with a product that contains more than the U.S. RDA for any nutrient. If all supplement users were to limit themselves to U.S. RDA dosage at the lowest available cost, do you think the health-food industry would survive?

There are also health risks associated with the taking of food supplements. Excess amounts of nutrients can harm people. Do you think that MLM participants—many of whom believe that "more is better"—are qualified to judge how many pills per day their customers should take? Or which of their customers need medical care? Even though therapeutic claims are forbidden by the written policies of each company, the sales process encourages customers to experiment with self-treatment. It may promote distrust of legitimate health professionals and their treatment methods. It may even cause some people to become alienated from their family and friends. Some would argue that the apparent benefits of "believing" in the products outweigh the risks involved. Do you think that people need false beliefs in order to feel healthy or succeed in life? Would you like to believe that something can help you when in fact it is worthless and may be harmful? Should our society support an industry that is trying to mislead us? Can't Americans do something better with the billion or more dollars being wasted each year on multilevel "health" products?

Recommendations

During the past fifteen years, members of our information-gathering network have acquired distributor kits or other materials from more than fifty MLM companies involved with health-related products. We believe that consumers would be wise to avoid such products altogether. The few that have nutritional value (such as multivitamins and low-cholesterol foods) are invariably over-priced and usually not needed. Those promoted as remedies are either un-proven, bogus, or intended for conditions that are unsuitable for self-medica-tion.

Government agencies should police the multilevel marketplace aggres-sively, using undercover investigators and filing criminal charges when wrong-doing is detected. People who feel they have been defrauded by MLM companies should file complaints with their state attorney general and with local FDA and FTC offices. (Chapter 22 tells where to complain.) A letter detailing the events may be sufficient to trigger an investigation; and the more complaints received, the more likely that corrective action will be taken. If you possess a distributor kit that you no longer need, we would be pleased to add it to our collection.

11

How Athletes Are Exploited

More than a hundred companies are marketing phony "ergogenic aids," combinations of various vitamins, minerals, amino acids, and other substances claimed to increase muscle growth and/or enhance athletic performance. Ads for such products often display muscular individuals and/or endorsements from bodybuilding or weightlifting champions. False claims are also spread by word of mouth. *Health Foods Business* estimates that total sales of these products through health-food stores exceeded $130 million in 1993. They are also sold in pharmacies and superstores.

Protein Mythology

Why do many athletes believe that massive amounts of protein are necessary during training? Ellington Darden, Ph.D., former research director for Nautilus Sports/Medical Industries, thinks this belief may have evolved from the ancient Olympic Games. Athletes of that era thought that great strength could be obtained by eating the raw meat of lions, tigers, or other animals that displayed great fighting strength. Today, although few athletes consume raw meat, the idea that "you are what you eat" is still widely promoted by food faddists.

During the early 1900s, as muscles were discovered to contain protein, athletes and coaches mistakenly concluded that protein was the principal component. Muscles actually contain about 70 percent water, 7 percent lipids, and only 22 percent protein, but the belief they are made of protein fit in with the age-old meat-eating practices of athletes.

The protein beliefs of athletes and coaches were further reinforced during the 1930s by Bob Hoffman (1899–1985) and later by Joe Weider (1923–), both of whom published magazines catering to bodybuilders and weightlifters. The first protein supplements were advertised and sold through their magazines. In articles and ads, Hoffman and Weider asserted that athletes have special protein needs, that protein supplements have special muscle-building and health-giving powers, and that the most efficient way to get enough protein is by using supplements. The scientific facts are otherwise:

- Proteins are not absorbed as such by the body. Digestion breaks them down to amino acids that are absorbed and become part of the metabolic pool. Protein or amino acid supplements provide no special nutritional benefit and may even unbalance body biochemistry.
- Amino acids are needed to build or maintain muscles, but muscle-building is not *caused* by eating extra protein. It is stimulated by increased muscular work.
- Energy, vigor, and endurance are related to caloric intake and the availability of adequate energy. Protein is the least efficient source of calories. Athletes will perform better if their extra energy needs are satisfied by extra carbohydrates taken several days before an event takes place.
- Few Americans fail to consume adequate amounts of protein.
- Once basic needs have been met, there is no need for extra protein beyond the Recommended Dietary Allowance. The small additional amount needed during intense training is easily obtainable from a balanced diet.

The Leading Mythmakers

Bob Hoffman, who was a prolific writer, sold supplement products and bodybuilding equipment through his York Barbell Company, of York, Pennsylvania. Joe Roark, a historian for the International Federation of Body Builders (IFBB), estimates that Hoffman wrote more than two thousand articles. Hoffman launched *Strength & Health* in 1932 and *Muscular Development* in 1964. Almost all the ads in these magazines were for York Barbell products. He also wrote columns for *Let's Live* magazine and wrote and published more than thirty books on fitness and nutrition topics.

Jim Murray, who edited *Strength and Health* for several years, revealed recently that Hoffman had formulated his original protein supplement after learning that an advertiser's product had been exceptionally profitable. (Hoffman also stopped accepting ads for the other product.) In the January 1994 *Iron Games History* newsletter, Murray described the "scientific development" of Hoffman's *Hi-Protein*:

> Purely by chance I happened to observe the activities in the "laboratory" as I returned from lunch one day. The "laboratory" was a space in the corner of . . . the ground floor of the York Barbell Company. . . . The sight that met my eyes was Bob Hoffman standing over a fiber drum half full of finely ground soy flour, stirring the contents with a canoe paddle. . . .
>
> Next to the drum was a container of sweet Hershey's chocolate with a scoop thrust into it. After stirring a while, Bob dipped his finger into the mixture . . . and tasted it. With a grimace he exclaimed, "Nobody will buy that!" And he shoveled more scoops of chocolate into the drum and resumed stirring. Eventually he achieved a mix that had a satisfactory taste. . . .
>
> Later, of course, Bob had other suppliers make his nutritional product and I'm sure that quality control improved. The various supplements continued to be highly profitable, however.

For many years, York Barbell marketed certain nutritional products with false and misleading claims. In 1960, the company was charged with misbranding its *Energol Germ Oil Concentrate* because literature accompanying the oil claimed falsely that it could prevent or treat more than 120 diseases and conditions, including epilepsy, gallstones, and arthritis. The material was destroyed by consent decree. In 1961, fifteen other York Barbell products were seized as misbranded. In 1968, a larger number of products came under attack by the government for similar reasons. In the consent decree that settled the 1968 case, Hoffman and York Barbell agreed to stop a long list of questionable health claims for their products. In 1972, the FDA seized three types of York Barbell protein supplements, charging that they were misbranded with false and misleading bodybuilding claims. A few months later, the seized products were destroyed under a default decree. In 1974, the company was again charged with misbranding *Energol Germ Oil Concentrate* and protein supplements. The wheat germ oil had been claimed to be of special dietary value as a source of vigor and energy. A variety of false bodybuilding claims had been made for the protein supplements. The seized products were destroyed under a consent decree.

Despite his many brushes with the law, Hoffman achieved considerable professional prominence. During his athletic career, first as an oarsman and then as a weightlifter, he received over six hundred trophies, certificates, and awards. He was the Olympic weightlifting coach from 1936 to 1968 and was a founding member of the President's Council on Physical Fitness and Sports. *Muscular*

Development is now published by Advanced Research Press, an affiliate of Twin Laboratories, of Ronkonkoma, New York. This company, with a reported income of $88.5 million in 1993, is the number-two marketer of "sports supplements."

Joe Weider began bodybuilding as a teenager and was sixteen when he launched a newsletter called *Your Physique.* According to an article in the December 3, 1989 *New York Times*, Weider acquired many of his initial readers by contacting people whose letters had been published in *Strength & Health,* which he read avidly. Three years later, he persuaded a large magazine distributor to sell *Your Physique* on newsstands, and it quickly reached a circulation of fifty thousand. Soon afterward, Weider started a company that sold bodybuilding equipment and instructional booklets through the mail. In 1946, Joe's brother Ben joined the business and they set up the IFBB, which promotes the sport worldwide and sponsors competitions. Today, Joe runs Weider Health & Fitness, from Woodland Hills, California, while Ben operates the IFBB from Canada. According to press reports, their business empire now grosses over $500 million annually.

Weider Health & Fitness is clearly the dominant player in the sports-

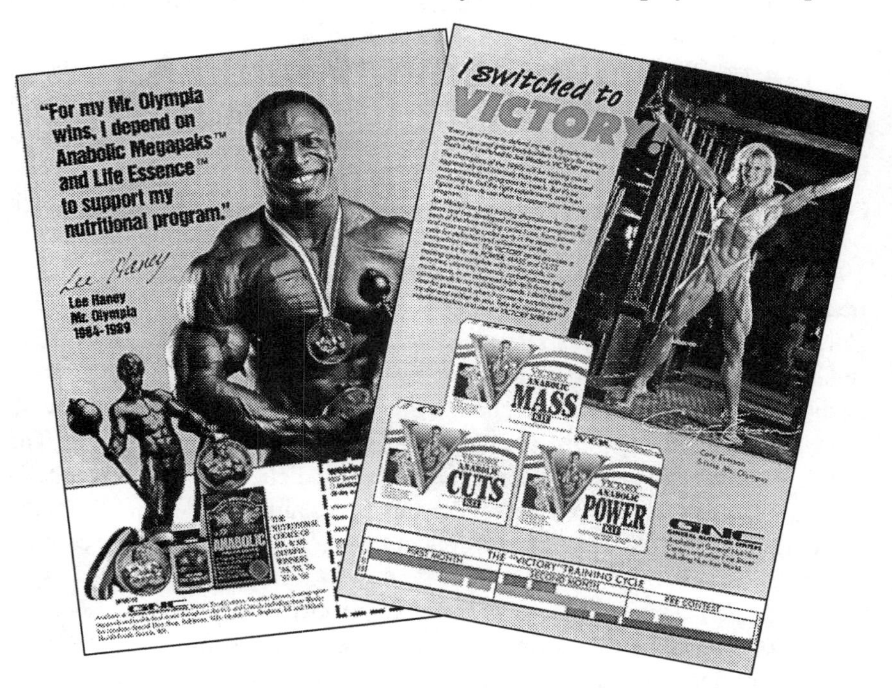

These ads from *Muscle & Fitness* depict bodybuilding champions Lee Haney and Cory Everson, who relate their success to using Weider products.

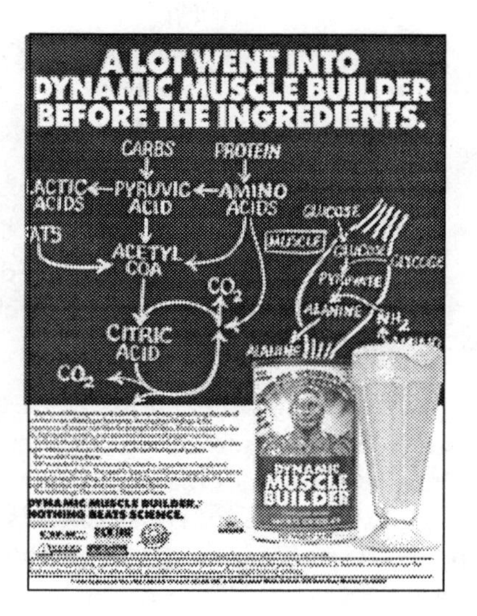

This ad attempts to portray Weider's *Dynamic Muscle Builder* as scientifically formulated and "important for successful weight training." Yet a message near the bottom of the ad admits: "As with all supplements, use of this product will not promote faster or greater muscular gains. The product is, however, a nutritious low-fat food supplement which, like other foods, provides nutritional support for weight training athletes." The biochemical reactions are related to the body's normal energy production. No scientific reason exists for athletes to use this product.

supplement marketplace. It publishes four magazines, sells bodybuilding equipment, broadcasts "Muscle Magazine" on ESPN, and sponsors many athletic and aerobic events throughout the year. The magazines are *Muscle & Fitness* (begun as *Muscle Builder* in 1953), *Shape* (founded in 1981 to cater to women), *Flex* (since 1983), and *Men's Fitness* (since 1987). The supplements include *Anabolic Mega-Pak, Dynamic Life Essence, Dynamic Super Stress-End, Dynamic Power Source, Dynamic Driving Force, Dynamic Fat Burners, Dynamic Liver Concentrate Energizer, Dynamic Sustained Endurance, Dynamic Recupe, Dynamic Body Shaper,* and *Dynamic Muscle Builder.* None of these products appears capable of doing what its name suggests, and none contains any nutrients not readily obtainable from a balanced diet.

In 1984, the FTC charged that ads for Weider's *Anabolic Mega-Pak* (containing amino acids, minerals, vitamins, and herbs) and *Dynamic Life Essence* (an amino acid product) had been misleading. According to the FTC complaint, Weider misrepresented that:

- a typical user of these products would achieve greater muscular development than a nonuser over the course of a few months of weight training;
- a typical user would achieve at least the muscular development of a nonuser, but in a shorter period of time;
- a typical user would achieve results equivalent to those that bodybuilders generally believe are achievable through use of anabolic steroids—rapid and substantial muscular development;

- the products would stimulate greater than normal production or release of human growth hormones, resulting in faster or greater muscular development;
- *Dynamic Life Essence* is unlike any other amino acid source in the world; and
- the *Anabolic Mega-Pak* was developed by a team of the world's most renowned nutritional biochemists, exercise physiologists, and trainers.

The FTC complaint was settled in 1985 when Weider and the company agreed not to falsely claim that these products can help build muscles or are effective substitutes for anabolic steroids. They also agreed to pay a minimum of $400,000 in refunds or (if refunds did not reach this figure) to fund research on the relationship of nutrition to muscle development. Although the claims forbidden by the FTC order no longer appear in Weider ads, similar messages

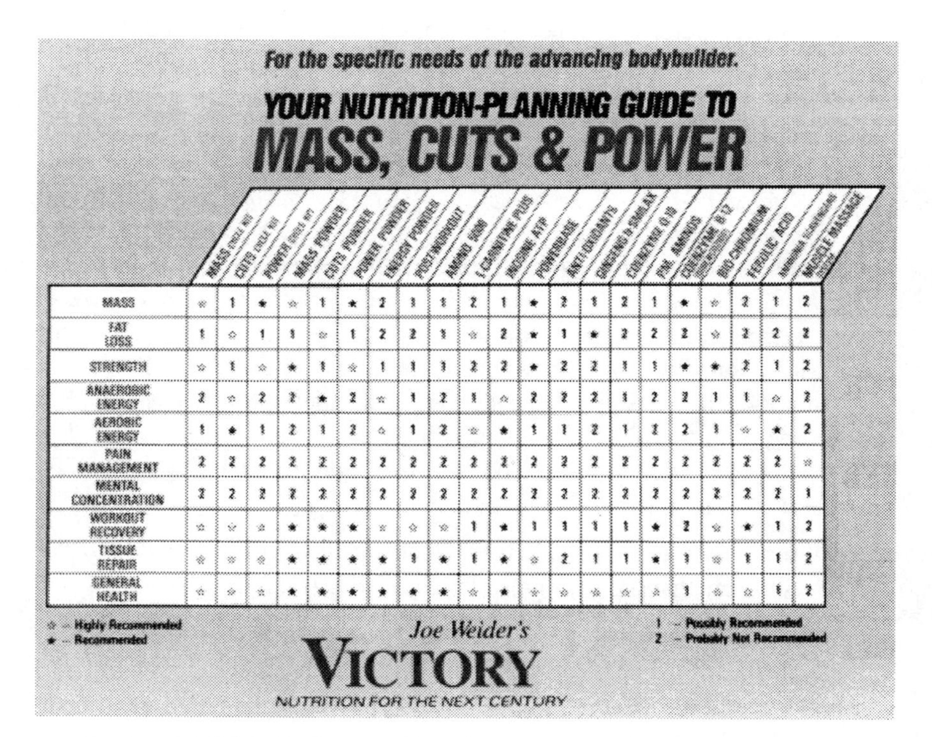
For the specific needs of the advancing bodybuilder.

YOUR NUTRITION-PLANNING GUIDE TO

MASS, CUTS & POWER

	MASS	CUTS	POWER	MASS POWDER	CUTS POWDER	POWER POWDER	ENERGY POWDER	POST-WORKOUT	AMINO 500	L-CARNITINE PLUS	INOSINE ATP	POWERBASE	ANTI-OXIDANTS	GINSENG & SMILAX	COENZYME Q-10	F.M. AMINOS	COENZYME B12	BIO-CHROMIUM	FERULIC ACID		MUSCLE MASSAGE
MASS	☆	1	★	☆	1	★	2	1	1	2	1	★	2	1	2	1	★	☆	2	1	2
FAT LOSS	1	☆	1	1	☆	1	2	2	1	☆	2	★	1	★	2	2	2	☆	2	2	2
STRENGTH	☆	1	☆	★	1	☆	1	1	1	2	2	★	2	2	1	1	★	★	2	1	2
ANAEROBIC ENERGY	2	☆	2	2	★	2	☆	1	2	1	☆	2	2	2	1	2	2	1	1	☆	2
AEROBIC ENERGY	1	★	1	2	1	2	☆	1	2	☆	★	1	1	2	1	2	2	1	☆	★	2
PAIN MANAGEMENT	2	2	2	2	2	2	2	2	2	2	2	2	2	2	2	2	2	2	2	2	☆
MENTAL CONCENTRATION	2	2	2	2	2	2	2	2	2	2	2	2	2	2	2	2	2	2	2	2	1
WORKOUT RECOVERY	☆	☆	☆	★	★	★	☆	☆	☆	1	★	1	1	1	1	★	2	☆	★	1	2
TISSUE REPAIR	☆	☆	☆	★	★	★	★	1	★	1	★	☆	2	1	1	★	1	☆	1	1	2
GENERAL HEALTH	☆	☆	☆	★	★	★	★	★	★	☆	★	☆	☆	☆	☆	☆	1	☆	☆	1	2

☆ – Highly Recommended
★ – Recommended
1 – Possibly Recommended
2 – Probably Not Recommended

Portion of Weider ad indicating which of its products are "highly recommended," "recommended," "possibly recommended," or "probably not recommended" for various purposes.

appear in articles in the magazines and are implied by endorsements and pictures of muscular athletes as well as by names of the products themselves.

False and misleading claims also appear in a series of eighteen booklets published in 1990 by Weider Health & Fitness and marketed through GNC stores. The booklets, thirty-two pages each, were written by Frederick C. Hatfield, Ph.D., with Martin Zucker. Hatfield, a former champion powerlifter, also edited one of Weider's magazines. The first booklet states:

> An increased demand is created for nutrients related to exercise, endurance, muscle breakdown and reconstruction and immunity. . . .
>
> No matter how good you eat, the extraordinary demands you put on your body call for extraordinary nutrition in the form of supplementation.

Several of the booklets list "24 Good reasons why you may need vitamin & mineral supplements," which include many of the misleading claims mentioned in Chapters 2 and 3 of this book. Most of the booklets contain a chart to create your own "designed supplement program." The authors also claim (incorrectly) that "protein deficiencies are common in the American diet" and that supplement formulas "specifically made for athletes" are the best to use. One booklet states:

> Many of these formations are put down by conservative scientists. But they are not using them. It is the athletes, people extremely in touch with their bodies. They will accept or reject a substance based on their own experience.

The Marketplace Expands

During the 1970s, in addition to protein supplements and assorted vitamins, the main products touted to athletes were wheat germ oil and bee pollen. In the early 1980s, Weider Health & Fitness introduced an "Olympians" line "that may well be the key to recuperation, power and sustained endurance." The products, promoted with an endorsement by muscleman Lou ("the Hulk") Ferrigno, were said to have been developed by working closely with "Olympians and nutritional researchers." Most were sustained-release vitamin concoctions that included an exotic ingredient or two. They were marketed through health-food stores as well as through *Muscle & Fitness* and *Shape* magazines.

During the next few years, as public interest in fitness grew rapidly, many other companies entered the market. Several drug companies began claiming that multivitamin or "stress" supplements were just what active people needed. Ayerst, for example, suggested that a two-mile jog was reason to replenish vitamins and minerals with *Beminal Stress Plus*. Revco's *Competition Plus*—"for extra effort sports"—was claimed to "meet the special needs of sports active people." Lederle's *Spartus* was said to be "for the extra demands of physical fitness—a major advance in nutritional support." Ads for *Spartus* stated truthfully that "B-complex vitamins . . . help change the food you eat ...into energy you use" and that zinc and copper are "essential to the body's 'energy generating systems.'" This message was misleading, however, because a person eating normally would get enough of these from food alone.

Spartus was also touted as "the official sports vitamin of the 1984 Winter Olympics." This status is available to companies who pay large sums of money to support the U.S. team and has little to do with the merits of the product itself. This, of course, is not disclosed when products are advertised. Nor has any "official sports vitamin" manufacturer ever disclosed the fact that world-class athletes are among the people least likely to need supplements. Shaklee Corporation and several other companies have sponsored various other teams.

Life Extension, by Durk Pearson and Sandy Shaw, was published in 1982 and followed by appearances by the authors on hundreds of radio and television talk shows. The book claimed that supplements of certain amino acids would cause the body to release growth hormone, which would produce muscle growth and fat loss with little or no effort. These claims were based on faulty extrapolations of experiments in which animals were given large doses of these amino acids by injection. Swallowing amino acids does not cause humans to release growth hormone. But the massive publicity garnered by Pearson and Shaw inspired the health-food industry to market hundreds of new products for athletes and would-be dieters. Many of these products were claimed to be "natural steroids" or "steroid substitutes." In the ensuing years, gamma-oryzanol, inosine, coenzyme Q_{10}, chromium picolinate, germanium, dimethylglycine, boron, L-carnitine, branched-chain amino acids, and many other dubious ingredients have been added to "ergogenic aids." One company has even marketed a "nonsteroidal homeopathic anabolic ...chemical free" product claimed to stimulate muscle growth and increase energy and endurance.

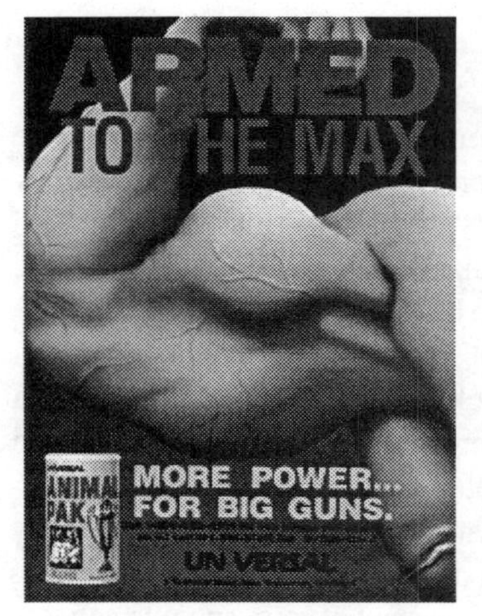

This ad needs no claims because the picture says it all.

Some manufacturers make no claims in their ads but imply them in product names (see table). Many manufacturers use pictures

"Ergogenic" Claims Implied by Product Names

Company	Examples of Products
Bricker Laboratories	Awe-some, Intensity
Good 'N Natural	Anabolic Booster, Super Cut
Makers of KAL	Winners Formula
Nature's Way	Huge, Critical Mass Recovery Formula
Sports Medical Nutrition	Aerobimax, Aminomax, Ligaflex, Staminol
Sports Science	Ultimate Growth Plus Pak, Power Burst Plus
Twinsport	Endurance Athletic Stress Formula
Universal	Genesis Steroid Replacement Kit
Vitol	Russian Lion, Great Workout

of athletes to convey their messages. Some manufacturers make explicit claims in their ads or product literature, while others use simple puffery. Twinsport's *Endurance* products—endorsed by Robert Haas, author of *Eat to Win*—have been claimed to help realize your potential "whether you're a world-class athlete or a weekend recreationalist." Solgar Company, Inc., has said its *Joggers* tablets were formulated "to give an edge to the serious competitor and endurance athlete." Dash Products has offered *Natural Fuel,* "the anabolic nutrient discovery you've been waiting for," and *Smilax Gold*, which "naturally enhances your body's testosterone levels safely, without the harmful effects of steroids." Strength Systems USA Labs, Inc., has promised that its *Super Man* would provide "energy . . . vitality, longevity. The desires of each and every active man"—plus a free condom in each bottle.

In 1983, General Nutrition Corporation published a thirty-six-page booklet called "Fitness Now! Everybody's Guide to Getting in Shape." After suggesting that athletes should be concerned about insufficient nutrient intake, the booklet outlined "beginner," "intermediate," and "advanced" fitness supplement programs. Beginners were advised to take a multivitamin and use a protein supplement. Intermediates were advised to add brewer's yeast and supplements of zinc, beta-carotene, vitamin C (for which "an additional 500–1,000 mg should do for most people"), and vitamin E. Advanced trainees were advised to take protein powder plus GNC's *Power Pak* (a vitamin and mineral supplement "formulated specifically with training and bodybuilder needs in mind") and *Rapid Body Builder Pak*. Regarding the latter, the booklet said:

> This is a special interest formulation that includes items of special interest to fitness-oriented people: Glandular preparation including adrenal, brain, heart, kidney, liver, pancreas, spleen, thymus and pituitary; octacosanol. a special compound found in wheat germ oil that has been shown to improve endurance in trained individuals; bee pollen, a food that is gaining popularity as an energy booster; ginseng, an herb used historically as an aid to endurance; and a mineral electrolyte mixture for replacement of electrolytes lost in sweat.

These GNC recommendations have no rational basis for athletes—or for anyone else.

Several companies have published charts suggesting which products are good for specific purposes. Uni-Pro, of Freemont, California, has marketed a

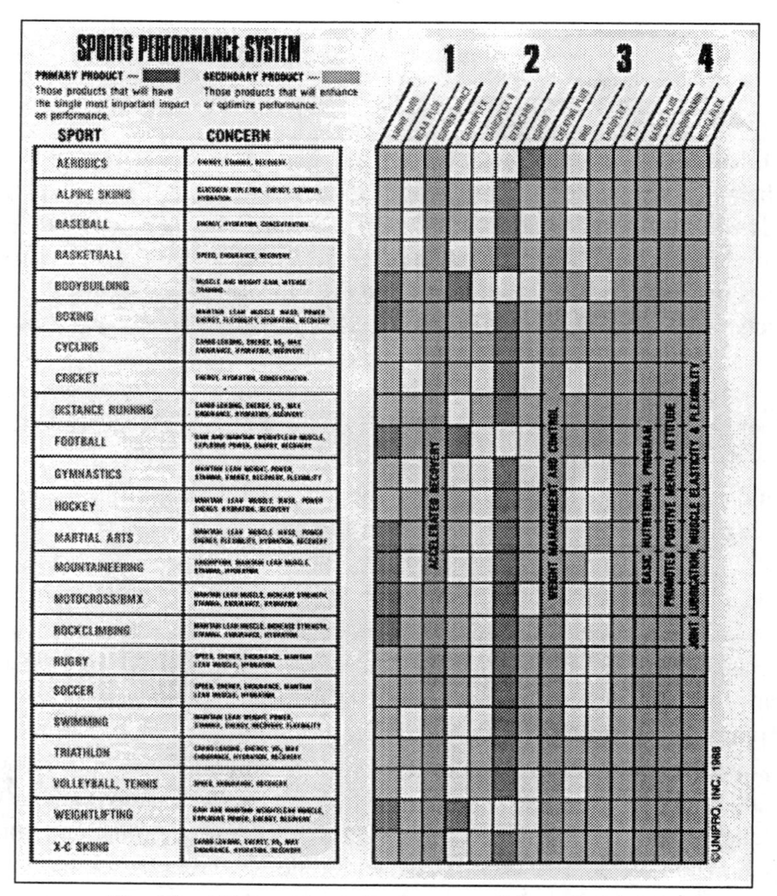

Chart from Unipro Sports Performance System brochure

"Sports Performance System" with four product categories: "anabolic/recovery," "energy/endurance," "metabolic enhancers," and "functional optimizers." A flyer was filled with biochemical tidbits and hype about each product and its supposed benefits for athletes. An accompanying chart, pictured here, listed twenty-three sports, nutritional "concerns" for each sport and the Unipro, Inc., products that supposedly address these concerns. One product, *Endorphamin,* was described as a "futuristic formula that combines the latest scientific advances with those of amino acids, vitamins, minerals, and other nutrients that have been demonstrated to exert a positive influence on an athlete's feelings of well-being, reward, and euphoria." It contained four amino acids, two vitamins, three minerals, octacosanol, inositol, and choline—nothing, we believe, that would alter an athlete's performance or mood.

In 1988, RichLife, of Costa Mesa, California, began marketing a Sports Fitness System composed of *Balanced Electrolyte Replacer, Ultimate Body*

RICHLIFE SPORTS NUTRITION

	Balanced Electrolyte Replacer	Ultimate Body Formula	Muscle Endurance Formula	Chewable Power Tabs	Growth Factor Anabolic	Carbohydrate Muscle Loader
Aerobics	N	N	N	N	R	N
Backpacking	N		R	N		R
Basketball	N		N	N		N
Bicycling	N	R	N	N		N
Body Building	N	N	N	N	N	N
Boxing	N		R	R	R	N
Football	N		N	N	N	N
Gymnastics	N	R	R	R	R	R
Handball	N		N	N		R
Hockey	N		N	N		R
Jogging	N	R	R	N		N
Judo	N		N	N	N	R
Karate	N		N	N	N	N
Marathons	N		N	N	R	N
Racquetball	N		N	N		N
Skiing—Cross Country	N		N	N	R	N
Skiing—Downhill	N		N	N		N
Soccer	N		N	N	R	N
Speed Walking	R		N	R		
Swimming	N	R	R	R	R	N
Tennis	N		N	N		N
Track	N		N	N	R	N
Triathalons	N		N	N	R	N
Volleyball	N		N	N		N
Weight Lifting	N	N	N	N	N	N
Wrestling	N		N	N		R

N = NECESSARY R = RECOMMENDED

Chart from RichLife brochure

Definition, Muscle Endurance Formula, Chewable Power Tablets, Growth Factors Anabolic Formula, and *Carbohydrate Muscle Loader.* The program's brochure contained a table showing which products were "necessary" or "recommended" for each of twenty-six sports. Four or more products were advised for each one. During the same year, Nature's Way, of Springville, Utah, launched its PurePower Sports Nutrition System, which it described as "the only major sports line that uses herbal supplement extracts to help sports-minded people reach their athletic goals." The products included *Huge* (a weight-gain drink), *Revive, Carbocharge, Metamax, Final Cut, Critical Mass, Power Up*, and six other items. The brochure featured an endorsement of "the natural approach to bodybuilding" from Arnold Schwartzenegger.

Muscle Masters Bodybuilding System, marketed by Nature's Plus, of Farmingdale, New York, is promoted with a booklet called "Master the Art of Bodybuilding." The introductory package includes an audiotape, "supplements to potentiate anabolic function," plans for weight-training and muscle-building, and information on the dangers of anabolic steroids. Described as a "natural approach," the system includes "beginner," "intermediate," and "advanced" supplement programs. The "advanced" program includes twenty-three products—with a total of eighty-nine daily doses of various tablets, capsules, powders, wafers, and liquids.

Perhaps the most brazen promotion was the campaign for Schiff's "Ergogenic Pro-Formance System"—a product line that included *Formula 420 Daily Base* ("unsurpassed bodybuilding energizing fuels"), *Formula 560 Ergogenic Organizer* ("antistress, energizing formula to help the body increase endurance"), and *Formula 300 Daily Annex* ("to give the extra . . . edge for ultimate endurance and performance"). According to Schiff, these formulations were "far more advanced than any previously available to the public."

Promotion of these products began during the summer of 1988 with colorful full-page ads in health-food-industry trade publications. The ads stated: "THE BIGGEST NAMES IN FITNESS JOIN FORCES. The National Academy of Sports Medicine [NASM] and Schiff Sports Nutrition create the most advanced fitness program on earth." The program included a "self-guiding System Manual containing over 100 pages of vital information on a balanced fitness plan and realistic goals for performance." Participants were invited to send a completed questionnaire to NASM in order to receive a ten-page computer-generated diet-and-exercise plan. There was also a toll-free number for answering consumer questions. Participants who completed the initial program would receive "an attractive completion certificate" and be encouraged to continue "maintenance level of supplements." Retailers were promised that Schiff would spend more than $5 million on a campaign that would include

THE BIGGEST NAMES
IN FITNESS JOIN FORCES.
The National Academy of Sports Medicine and Schiff Sports Nutrition create the most advanced fitness program on earth.
Schiff
The Ergogenic Pro·Formance System sells sports nutrition and fitness for you.
Again and again.
Schiff Sports Nutrition and the National Academy of Sports Medicine are working hard to make your sports nutrition sales easier and will bring new customers into your store.
The new advertising campaigns will help sell Ergogenic Pro·Formance System to more than 20 million prime target consumers in the second half of 1989 and into the 90's. Fitness, sports and bodybuilding enthusiasts are all targeted in the campaigns, with Schiff committed to print, TV and radio spending at a $5 million national rate.
The product's effectiveness is clearly demonstrated by actual research which was conducted by the National Academy of Sports Medicine. (See charts in ad at right.) And backed by a consumer money-back guarantee.
What's more, each sale triggers additional sales. Buyers return to you for open-stock purchases every month they continue on the program. You're their source of supply. The system is ongoing, with continuing follow-up by the Academy.
Remember, we are doing it all. Just have enough stock on hand. Get in touch with your local Schiff distributor. Or call us, toll-free, at 1-800-526-6251.

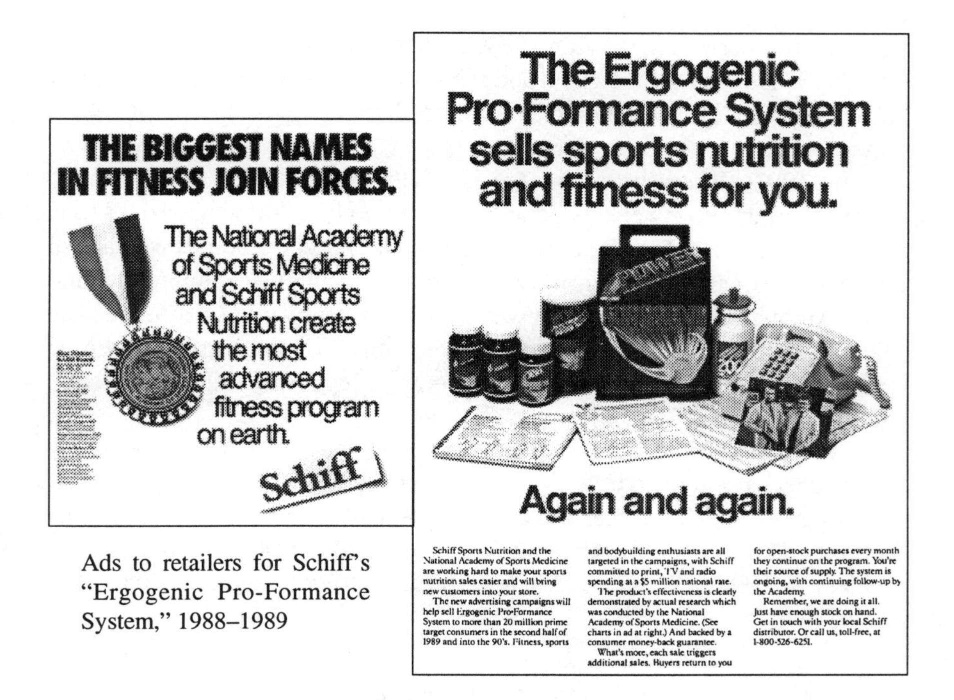

Ads to retailers for Schiff's "Ergogenic Pro-Formance System," 1988–1989

ads in *Sports Illustrated, New Woman, Omni, Longevity, American Health, Let's Live,* and American Airlines' *Vis à Vis.*

The initial ads and product brochures listed a "Blue-Ribbon NASM Board" composed of five prominent professionals, including Donald Cooper, M.D., a member of the President's Council on Physical Fitness. Curious about this, Dr. Stephen Barrett obtained a copy of NASM's incorporation papers and contacted the "Board" members for comment. His investigation revealed that NASM was not a professional organization but a private corporation chartered in October 1988 for "research, education, new product development, exploration and explanation of new technology [and] consulting." All five "Board" members said they had they agreed to be listed in NASM literature, but they had neither endorsed the products nor given Schiff permission to use their names. In fact, said Cooper, "I think the products are of no real value. A well balanced diet can supply all the nutrients and energy that an athlete needs. The only way to reach your maximum potential as an athlete is through hard work and practice. There are no safe shortcuts or miracles in capsules or tablets." Schiff is now a Weider subsidiary.

In the April 1985 issue of *Health Foods Business*, a retailer described how the managers of several gyms and a fitness center referred members to his store.

Once a customer was in the store, he would ask, "Do you want to maintain or optimize?" He then would spend about an hour with each customer and elicit an average sale of $79. (Repeat sales are more lucrative, of course, because they require much less customer attention.)

In 1991, Researchers from the U.S. Centers for Disease Control and Prevention surveyed twelve popular health and bodybuilding magazines (one issue each) and found ads for eighty-nine brands and 311 products with a total of 235 unique ingredients. The most frequent ingredients were amino acids and herbs. Among the 221 products for which an effect was claimed, fifty-nine were said to produce muscle growth, twenty-seven were said to increase testosterone levels, seventeen were said to enhance energy, fifteen were said to reduce fat, and twelve were said to increase strength.

The "sports nutritionals" market has become so lucrative that many pharmacies have entered it. A 1993 report in *Drug Store News* described how the Walgreens, Eckerd, and PayLess chains have set up sports nutritional sections and that GNC was making franchise arrangements with independent retailers. A 1993 GNC ad in *Muscle & Fitness* provides an interesting bit of double-talk:

> no hype. no bull. no phony promises. . . .
>
> If you think that any product is going to do the work for you . . . you're fooling yourself!
>
> Unless you're willing to bust your butt, no supplement alone is going to turn a 98-pound weakling into one of the "Lords of the Bench."
>
> But if you have the drive, determination, and desire to put in the effort, then fuel your body with Pro Performance Amino 1000 Soft Gels . . . . You'll reach your full potential.
>
> Amino 1000 Soft Gels were designed by the pros and created on the principle that liquids can be used by the body faster than tablets. Each soft gel capsule gives you 21 amino acids, Peptide bonded.
>
> Remember . . . you've got to put in the effort and give your body the right fuel. Pro Performance Amino 1000 Soft Gel Caps will give you the edge.

Simple Truths

Do athletes who eat a balanced diet need to concern themselves with extra protein or vitamins? The answer is no. In *The Complete Sports Medicine Book for Women,* sportsmedicine specialist Gabe Mirkin, M.D., and gynecologist Mona Shangold, M.D., explain why:

> You don't need much extra protein even to enlarge your muscles. For example, 1 pound of muscle contains only about 100 grams of protein, since it is composed of more than 72 percent water. So if you are gaining 1 pound of muscle every week in an excellent strength training program, you are adding only about 100 grams of protein each week, or about 15 grams of protein each day. Two cups of corn and beans will meet this need—far less than you would expect. . . .
>
> Requirements for only four vitamins increase with exercise: thiamin, niacin, riboflavin, and pantothenic acid. These vitamins are used up minimally in the breakdown of carbohydrates and, to a small degree, protein for energy. But you will find them abundantly in food. . . . Furthermore, deficiencies of these vitamins have never been reported in athletes.

What about other products?

Two pharmacists have analyzed the claims for nineteen "natural" substances claimed to help build muscles, increase stamina, enhance energy, or facilitate weight loss. Claims for these substances were gathered from ads in bodybuilding magazines, product labels, and fact sheets for health-food retailers. In a report in the May 1993 *Annals of Pharmacotherapy*, the authors concluded: (1) "anabolic" claims for Argentinean bull testes, boron, cyclofinil, dibencozide, gamma-oryzanol, *Menispermum conadense*, plant sterols (diosgenin, smilagenin, hecogenin), and saw palmetto berries were unfounded; (2) certain claims for chromium picolinate, clenbuterol, guarana, inosine, kola nut, and ma huang have scientific support, but products containing these substances are marketed in a misleading manner; (3) claims that yohimbe bark is an anabolic agent are supported by studies in animals but not humans; and (4) claims for carnitine and arginine/ornithine combinations have some scientific support but should still be regarded as unproven.

The most thorough investigation has been conducted by David Lightsey, an exercise physiologist and nutritionist who coordinates the National Council Against Health Fraud's Task Force on Ergogenic Aids. During the past four years, he has telephoned more than eighty companies that market "ergogenic aids." In a recent interview, Lightsey told Dr. Barrett:

> In each case, I told a company representative that I had been asked to collect data on the company's product(s) and issue a formal report. After they described the alleged benefits, I would ask how data supporting these claims were collected. As my questions became more specific, their responses became more vague. Some said they could not be more specific because they did not wish to reveal trade secrets.
>
> I ended each interview with a request for written documentation.

> Fewer than half sent anything. Most of the studies they sent were poorly designed and proved nothing. The few that were well designed did not support product claims but were taken out of context.
>
> Some companies claimed that one team or another was using their products. In each such case, I contacted the team management and learned that although one or more players used the company's products, the management had neither endorsed the products nor encouraged their use.

Lightsey believes there are two reasons why many athletes believe that various products have helped them: (1) use of the product often coincides with natural improvement due to training, and (2) increased self-confidence or a placebo effect inspires greater performance. Any such "psychological benefit," however, should be weighed against the dangers of misinformation, wasted money, misplaced faith, and adverse physical effects—both known and unknown—that can result from megadoses of nutrients. Moreover, how many people who are involved in fitness programs or recreational sports *need* a placebo for inspiration?

More Enforcement Action Is Needed

Until recently, little government effort has been made to protect consumers from wasting money on "sports nutrient" products. In 1975, the FTC began a rulemaking proceeding for protein supplements that resulted in a staff recommendation to ban therapeutic and "fat-burning" claims in ads. However, although the commission concluded that protein supplements offered no benefit to athletes, it decided to carry out enforcement on a case-by-case basis rather than attempting to regulate the industry as a whole. This decision, made in 1984, typified the antiregulatory philosophy of the Reagan Administration and was an invitation to more widespread fraud.

The FTC took the action noted above against Weider Health & Fitness, the market leader. In 1986, the agency also acted against A.H. Robins and its subsidiary, the Viobin Corporation, which had been making false claims for wheat germ oil products for more than fifteen years. During this time, Viobin had falsely advertised that *Viobin Wheat Germ Oil* (liquid), *Promtabs* (tablets), and *Prometol* (capsules) would increase endurance, stamina, vigor, and total body reaction time, and would help overcome fatigue. The company also claimed that these benefits were backed by "more than 18 years of University research." The case was settled with a consent agreement prohibiting representations that the oil could help consumers improve endurance, stamina, vigor, or other aspects of athletic fitness, or that its active ingredient "octacosanol" is related in any way to body reaction time, oxygen uptake, oxygen debt, or athletic performance.

In 1992, the New York City Department of Consumer Affairs (DCA) published a report called *Magic Muscle Pills!! Health and Fitness Quackery in Nutrition Supplements.* DCA investigators found that manufacturers they contacted for information about their products were unable to provide a single published report from a scientific journal to back the claims that their products could benefit athletes. The investigators also noted that one supplement program recommended in *Muscle & Fitness* would cost more than $11 *per day.*

Along with its report, DCA issued "Notices of Violation" to six of the companies whose products it had investigated. The companies cited for "deceiving or misleading consumers by falsely representing and/or exaggerating the benefits, qualities or effects" of their products were:

- Metabolic Nutrition, Inc., Miami, Florida, whose *Optigenetics Advanced Cell Growth Formula* was claimed to "stimulate muscle growth even while you sleep"
- Cybergenics, a subsidiary of L & S Research, Lakewood, New Jersey, whose *Cyberblast, Cybertrim, Cybergain,* and *Vortex* were claimed to do such things as "speed up the metabolization of body fat" and cause "depletion of body fat"
- Universal Nutritional Systems, New Brunswick, New Jersey, whose *Hot Sauce* was described as "an anabolic inferno" and "the most efficient muscle-building supplement," which would allow the user to "watch . . . muscles explode with incredible strength, massive size and pure energy"
- ROM Research, Baltimore, Maryland, whose *Ultra Pro* could "pack on the muscle" and "produce huge gains in record time"
- Champion Nutrition, Concord, California, which advertised *Metabolol* with the claim that "nothing is more powerful at adding muscle without fat"
- Mega-Pro International, St. George, Utah, whose *Meg-Amino 1500* was said to be "the most powerful muscle-building amino acid" and whose *Smilax Spray* was said to be "designed to enhance your body's natural production of testosterone."

DCA warned consumers to beware of terms like "fat burner," "fat fighter," "fat metabolizer," "energy enhancer," "performance booster," "strength booster," " ergogenic aid," "anabolic optimizer," and "genetic optimizer." Calling the bodybuilding supplement industry "an economic hoax with unhealthy consequences," DCA officials urged the FDA and FTC to stop the "blatantly drug-like claims" and false advertising used to promote these products. We share these sentiments.

In April 1994, the FTC announced that it had reached a consent agreement under which General Nutrition Corporation would pay $2.4 million dollars to settle charges that it had falsely advertised forty-one products, most of which had been packaged by other manufacturers (see Chapter 21). The products included *Cybergain, Amino 1500*, Weider's *Super Fat Burners*, ten other "muscle builders," and four other phony "ergogenic aids."

In July 1994, the FTC announced that L&S Research and its founder and chief executive officer Scott Chinery had agreed to pay $1.45 million to settle charges that they had made numerous false and unsubstantiated claims in the advertising and sale of *Cybergenics Total Body Building System, Cybergenics for Hard Gainers, Cybertrim, Quicktrim*, and *Mega-Fat Burner Tablet* (also called *Super Fat-Loss Tablet*). The FTC had also charged that "before-and-after" photos used in the ads were deceptive because they did not reflect the typical or usual experience of users. The consent agreement prohibits claims that these or similar products can cause a user to gain more muscle or lose more fat than a nonuser of such a product, unless there is reliable scientific evidence to support such an assertion. The agreement also bans unsubstantiated claims that the inclusion of chromium picolinate in a product or program will cause a user to build muscle, lose weight, or lower blood cholesterol.

The FTC has not indicated whether it plans to take action against other manufacturers, but its legal staff is well aware that the "sports nutrition" marketplace needs further cleaning up.

12

Dubious Doctoring

This chapter covers a broad range of dubious nutrition-related practices, some of which are the exclusive province of physicians, others of which are not. The health-food industry promotes these practices through its publications and through networking with the practitioners involved.

"Fad" Diagnoses

Years ago, many nervous or tired people were said to have "adrenal insufficiency." The vast majority of these people were not only misdiagnosed but were also treated with adrenal gland extract, a substance that the FDA later banned because it was too weak to treat the actual disease. "Low thyroid" (hypothyroidism) was likewise unjustifiably diagnosed in many cases of fatigue and/or obesity. Today's "fad" diagnoses—each used to explain various common symptoms—are chronic fatigue syndrome, "Gulf War syndrome," "hypoglycemia," "environmental illness," "candidiasis hypersensitivity," "food allergies," "Wilson's syndrome," "parasites" (discussed in Chapter 6), and "mercury amalgam toxicity."

Chronic fatigue syndrome (CFS) originally was thought to be related to infectious mononucleosis. Other viruses are now suspected, but some physicians feel the condition is merely a label placed on symptoms that may not have a single cause or may reflect bodily reactions to tension or chronic depression. Assuming that chronic fatigue syndrome is an actual disease, only a small percentage of chronically tired people have it. According to criteria developed by the U.S. Centers for Disease Control and Prevention, the diagnosis should never be made unless fatigue persists or recurs for at least six months and is severe enough to reduce the patient's activity level by more than half. In addition, the fatigue should be accompanied by several other symptoms, such as severe headaches, low-grade fever, joint or muscle pain, general muscle weakness, sleep disturbance, and various psychological symptoms. Other likely causes of fatigue must be carefully ruled out. Testing for antibodies to the Epstein-Barr virus (the usual cause of mononucleosis) is not useful for evaluating severe fatigue because 80 percent of healthy adults have positive antibody tests, presumably from mild or inapparent infection at an earlier age. No treatment has been proven effective for CFS, although antidepressant drugs may help relieve certain symptoms.

Consumer Reports advises conservative measures: a balanced diet, adequate sleep, avoidance of excess stress, gradually increasing exercise without overdoing it, and—above all—patience. Calling CFS "a magnet for quacks," the magazine warns that "some practitioners create CFS patients by finding the syndrome in people who clearly don't have it." In 1990, its medical writer visited three "CFS specialists" and said he had been tired for eight months. The first said the reporter's system was "sluggish" and needed to be "detoxified." He charged $185 and recommended blood tests costing $922.50. The others ordered Epstein-Barr tests, among others, and said the results were abnormal. One prescribed a drug used to treat heroin addiction and the other recommended vitamin injections to "bolster the immune system." Experts said that neither the tests, the diagnosis, or the recommended treatments were appropriate.

"Gulf War syndrome" is a term being applied to many ailments that occurred among military personnel during or after they served in the campaign against Iraq. The symptoms of this supposed condition include aching muscles, irritability, fatigue, thickened saliva, weight loss, weight gain, hair loss, sore gums, diarrhea, nausea, memory loss, skin rashes, and headaches. Careful studies have shown that the patterns of illness among Gulf War veterans and veterans who served elsewhere are similar except for symptoms related to stress. It is clear that many who believe they have "Gulf War syndrome" have ailments that would have developed anyway, and many others have symptoms that are stress-related. Some of these individuals are being told they suffer from "multiple chemical sensitivity," a fad diagnosis discussed below.

Real cases of adrenal insufficiency, hypoglycemia, and hypothyroidism definitely exist, *but they are rare* and should be carefully checked by laboratory testing before the diagnosis is made. The diagnosis of hypoglycemia, for example, should be reserved for patients who get symptoms two to four hours after eating, develop blood glucose levels below 45 mg per 100 ml whenever symptoms occur, and are immediately relieved of symptoms when blood sugar is raised. The glucose tolerance test is not reliable for evaluating most cases of suspected hypoglycemia. Low blood sugar levels without symptoms have no diagnostic significance because they occur commonly in normal individuals fed large amounts of sugar. The only way to reliably diagnose hypoglycemia is to prove that blood sugar is low whenever symptoms occur during the patient's usual living pattern. The most practical way to do this is probably with a home testing device.

Doctors who overdiagnose hypothyroidism often base their diagnosis on "low" temperature readings determined by placing the thermometer under the armpit. This is not a valid test of thyroid function. Proper diagnosis requires blood tests that measure thyroid hormone levels.

"Environmental illness"—sometimes referred to as "multiple chemical sensitivity" or "allergy to everything"—is based on the notion that when the total load of physical and psychological stresses exceeds what a person can tolerate, the immune system goes haywire and hypersensitivity to tiny amounts of common foods and chemicals can trigger a wide range of symptoms. Doctors advocating this notion call themselves "clinical ecologists" or specialists in "environmental medicine." Their treatment approach involves elimination of exposure to foods and environmental substances to which they consider the patient hypersensitive. Extreme restrictions can involve staying at home for months or living in a trailer designed to prevent exposure to airborne pollutants and synthetic substances. In many cases, the patient's life becomes centered around the treatment.

The American Academy of Allergy and Immunology, the nation's largest professional organization of allergists, has warned:

> Although the idea that the environment is responsible for a multitude of health problems is very appealing, to present such ideas as facts, conclusions, or even likely mechanisms without adequate support is poor medical practice.

Clinical ecologists base their diagnoses primarily on the results of "provocation" and "neutralization" tests, which are performed by having the patient report symptoms that occur within ten minutes after suspected substances are administered under the tongue or injected into the skin. If any symptoms occur, the test is considered positive and lower concentrations are given until a dose is found that "neutralizes" the symptoms. Researchers at the University of California have demonstrated that these procedures are not valid. In a double-blind study, eighteen patients each received three injections of suspected food extracts and nine of normal saline over a three-hour period. The tests were conducted in the offices of clinical ecologists who had been treating them. In nonblinded tests, these patients had consistently reported symptoms when exposed to food extracts and no symptoms when given injections of saline (dilute salt water). But during the experiment, they reported as many symptoms following saline injections as they did after food-extract injections, indicating that their symptoms were nothing more than placebo reactions. "Neutralizing" doses were equally effective whether they were food extracts or saline. The symptoms included nasal stuffiness, dry mouth, nausea, fatigue, headaches, and feelings of disorientation or depression.

In 1991, a jury in New York State awarded $489,000 in actual damages and $411,000 in punitive damages to the estate of a man who committed suicide after several years of treatment by Warren M. Levin, M.D., a clinical ecologist. Testimony at the trial indicated that although the man was a paranoid schizophrenic who thought "foods were out to get him," Levin had diagnosed him as a "universal reactor" and advised that, to remain alive, he must live in a "pure" environment, follow a restrictive diet, and take supplements. During the trial, Levin admitted that since 1974, when he began practicing clinical ecology, he had diagnosed every patient who consulted him as environmentally ill. State licensing authorities have concluded that Levin's license should be revoked, but he remains in practice during the appeals process.

Rejection by the scientific community has not dampened the enthusiasm of clinical ecologists, about four hundred of whom belong to the American Academy of Environmental Medicine. Clinical ecologists also play a significant role in the American Academy of Otolaryngic Allergy (AAOA), which was founded in 1941 by Theron Randolph, M.D., and others who espoused diagnostic and treatment procedures that responsible allergists regarded as invalid. AAOA has about two thousand members, most of whom are board-certified otolaryngologists. The percentage who espouse the practices of clinical ecology is unknown, but some AAOA seminars are taught by leading clinical ecologists. AAOA has endorsed the use of provocation and neutralization testing.

"Candidiasis hypersensitivity" is an alleged condition whose symptoms are said to be multiple and include fatigue, depression, inability to concentrate, hyperactivity, headaches, skin problems (including hives), abdominal pain and bloating, constipation, diarrhea, respiratory symptoms, and problems of the urinary and reproductive organs. The main promoters of "candidiasis hypersensitivity" have been C. Orian Truss, M.D., of Birmingham, Alabama, author/publisher of *The Missing Diagnosis,* and William G. Crook, M.D., of Jackson, Tennessee, who wrote and published *The Yeast Connection.* According to Crook, "If a careful checkup doesn't reveal the cause for your symptoms, and your medical history [as described in his book] is typical, it's possible or even probable that your health problems are yeast-connected." He also claims that lab tests, such as culturing to determine the presence of the yeast, don't help much in diagnosis because "Candida germs live in every person's body. . . . Therefore the diagnosis is suspected from the patient's history and confirmed by his response to treatment."

Crook claims that the problem arises because "antibiotics kill 'friendly germs' while they're killing enemies, and when friendly germs are knocked out, yeast germs multiply. Diets rich in carbohydrates and yeasts, birth control pills, cortisone, and other drugs also stimulate yeast growth." He also claims that large numbers of yeasts weaken the immune system, which is also adversely affected by nutritional deficiencies, sugar consumption, and exposure to environmental molds and chemicals. To correct these alleged problems, he prescribes allergenic extracts, antifungal drugs, vitamin and mineral supplements, and diets that avoid refined carbohydrates, processed foods, and (initially) fruits and milk.

The health-food industry has responded to Crook's ideas by marketing such products as *Candi-Care, Candida-Guard, Candida Cleanse, Candistat, Cantrol, Yeast Fighters, Yeast Guard, Yeastop, Yeasterol*, and *Yeast•Trol.* Manufacturers have also marketed lines of "yeast-free" supplements claimed to be "safer" than ordinary ones. The existence of "anti-Candida" products has enabled health-food retailers, chiropractors, naturopaths, and bogus "nutritionists" to jump on the "Candida" bandwagon.

Crook's book contains a seventy-item questionnaire and score sheet to determine how likely it is that health problems are yeast-connected. Shorter versions of this questionnaire have appeared in magazine articles and in ads for products sold through health-food stores. The one pictured on the following page is from an ad that accompanied a promotional article in the April 1986 issue of *Redbook* magazine. The article's author believed she suffered from the condition and accepted Crook's ideas as gospel. The ad—for Nature's Way's *Cantrol*—contained a toll-free number for ordering the product or obtaining further information. According to a company official, more than one hundred thousand people responded. Before the article was published, Nature's Way notified retailers that its ad would "specifically instruct the consumer to go to their local health food store to purchase Cantrol."

Cantrol is a conglomeration of capsules containing acidophilus, evening primrose oil, vitamin E, linseed oil, caprylic acid, pau d'arco, and several other substances. In 1989, the Federal Trade Commission charged that the "Yeast Test" was invalid and there was no reasonable basis for claiming that *Cantrol* was effective against yeast problems. In 1990, Nature's Way and its president,

Kenneth Murdock, signed a consent agreement to stop making unsubstantiated claims about *Cantrol* and to pay $30,000 to the National Institutes of Health to support research on yeast infections.

The American Academy of Allergy and Immunology regards the concept of candidiasis hypersensitivity as "speculative and unproven" and notes that everyone has some of its supposed symptoms from time to time. In a strongly worded position paper, the academy warned that some patients who take the

Take the Yeast Test.

Do you have a yeast problem?
Here's what it is and how to fight it.

We call the type of yeast normally found in our bodies "Candida colonies." Normally they are harmless. However, they can sometimes grow rapidly due to a variety of conditions. When this happens they are no longer friendly microorganisms, but have developed into a "Candida albicans" problem. Worse, they have an adverse effect on our health.

Nature's Way, the makers of Cantrol™, a total nutritional plan designed to help control Candida albicans, has developed a simple test to help you determine if you have a yeast problem.*

Y N
☐☐ 1. Do you feel tired most of the time?
☐☐ 2. Do you suffer from intestinal gas, abdominal bloating or discomfort?
☐☐ 3. Do you crave sugar, bread, beer or other alcoholic beverages?
☐☐ 4. Are you bothered by constipation, diarrhea, or alternating constipation and diarrhea?
☐☐ 5. Do you suffer from mood swings or depression?
☐☐ 6. Are you often irritable, easily angered, anxious or nervous?
☐☐ 7. Do you have trouble thinking clearly, suffer occasional memory losses or have difficulty concentrating?
☐☐ 8. Are you ever dizzy or lightheaded?
☐☐ 9. Do you have muscle aches or stiffness with normal activity?
☐☐ 10. Have you had an unexpected weight gain without a change in diet?
☐☐ 11. Are you bothered by itching or burning of the vagina or prostate or a loss of sexual desire?
☐☐ 12. Have you ever taken antibiotics?
☐☐ 13. Are you currently or have you ever used birth control pills?
☐☐ 14. Have you ever taken steroid drugs, such as cortisone?

***This quiz is provided for general information only and is not intended to be used for self-diagnosis without the advice and examination of a qualified health professional. Some of the symptoms could indicate a more serious condition which could require the assistance of a health professional.**

If you answered 6 or more questions with a "yes," you may have a yeast problem. Read about how Cantrol can help. that helps to control Candida. These ingredients come in portion-controlled packages for added convenience and freshness.

Portion of 1986 magazine ad for *Cantrol*

inappropriately prescribed antifungal drugs will suffer side effects, and that overuse of these drugs could lead to the development of resistant germs that endanger everyone. In 1990, a double-blind trial found the antifungal drug nystatin no better than a placebo for relieving systemic or psychological symptoms of "candidiasis hypersensitivity syndrome."

"True believers" in "candidiasis hypersensitivity" and "environmental illness" are diagnosing and treating them in most or even all of the people who consult them. Some of these doctors are also diagnosing "hypoglycemia" and/or "chronic fatigue syndrome" excessively. We believe they are unfit to practice medicine and should have their medical license revoked.

Other Dubious Allergy Practices

Many dubious practitioners claim that food allergies may be responsible for virtually any symptom a person can have. In support of this claim—which is false—they administer various tests purported to identify offending foods.

The most notorious such test is cytotoxic testing. This test—also called cytotoxicity testing, leukocyte antigen sensitivity testing, Bryan's test, the Metabolic Intolerance Test, or sensitivity testing—was vigorously promoted during the early 1980s by storefront clinics, laboratories, nutrition consultants, chiropractors, and medical doctors. Advocates claimed it could determine sensitivity to food, which they blamed for asthma, arthritis, constipation, diarrhea, hypertension, obesity, stomach disorders, and many other conditions.

To perform the test, about 10 cubic centimeters of a patient's blood are placed in a test tube and centrifuged to separate the white cells (leukocytes). These are mixed with plasma and sterile water and applied to a large number of microscope slides, each of which has been coated with a dried food extract like that used by allergists for skin testing. The cells are then examined under a microscope at various intervals over a two-hour period to see whether they have changed their shape or disintegrated—supposedly signs of allergy to the particular food. Typically, the test results are used to explain the patient's symptoms and to design a "personalized diet program" that includes vitamins and minerals—sold by those administering the test.

Controlled studies have never shown cytotoxic testing to be reliable, and some studies have found it to be highly unreliable. For example, one study found that white cells from allergic patients reacted no differently when exposed to substances known to produce symptoms than when exposed to substances to which the patients were not sensitive. Several medical associations and even the American Chiropractic Association have denounced cytotoxic testing.

The most aggressive marketer of cytotoxic testing was probably Bio-Health Centers (BHC) of Huntington Beach, California, which charged $350 to test for 186 common foods and additives. One of its ads—headlined "DISASTER LINKED TO THE FOOD YOU EAT"—claimed that "if you currently suffer from any health difficulties, this test is worth taking." A brochure from the company suggested that cytotoxic testing can be useful in solving the problems of overweight, headaches, stomach and intestinal problems, depression, stress, confusion, sinus problems, asthma, arthritis, and hypoglycemia. BHC teams composed of a "nutritionist" and a nurse traveled around the country, holding evening meetings during which they could service about thirty people per night—for a gross intake of about $10,000. Testing could also be obtained by mailing a blood specimen to the lab. One person who took the test was Alberta Slavin, a consumer reporter whose husband had been president of the American Academy of Allergy and Immunology. Although Mrs. Slavin had no allergies, her test report listed twenty-five substances she should avoid.

In 1985, BHC was ordered to stop marketing its cytotoxic services in New York State. After a woman's blood sample was mailed by an investigator for the New York Attorney General, BHC incorrectly reported that the woman was sensitive to many foods. When an FDA investigator submitted a sample of cow blood as his own, BHC claimed that allergy was present to twenty-two substances, including cow milk, cottage cheese, and yogurt. Other enforcement actions were taken by authorities in California, Pennsylvania, and the state of Washington. These actions plus unfavorable publicity have almost driven cytotoxic testing from the health marketplace. But a few practitioners still perform it, and some use similar "food sensitivity" tests.

Another test claimed to locate "hidden allergies" is the ELISA/ACT™, developed by Russell Jaffe, M.D., Ph.D., and performed by Serammune Physicians Lab (SPL), of Reston, Virginia, which Jaffe directs. According to an SPL brochure:

> When we think of allergies, we immediately think of an allergy whose symptoms occur within minutes of ingesting a food or chemical. The symptoms include hives and itching. . . .
>
> "Hidden" or "delayed" allergies are more difficult to identify because the onset of symptoms is delayed from 2 hours to 5 days and the symptoms range from physical pain to unexplained fatigue. Scientific estimates are that as much as 60% of all illness is due to hidden allergies.

The brochure states that any of the following may indicate the presence of hidden allergies: chronic headaches, migraines, difficulty sleeping, dizziness, runny or stuffy nose, postnasal drip, ringing in the ears, earaches, blurred vision, irregular or rapid heartbeat, asthma, nausea and vomiting, constipation, diarrhea, irritable bowel syndrome, hives, skin rashes (psoriasis, eczema), muscle aches, joint pain, arthritis, nervous tension, fatigue, depression, mental dullness, and difficulty in getting your work done.

The ELISA/ACT™ is performed by culturing the patient's lymphocytes and seeing how they react to up to three hundred foods, minerals, preservatives, and other environmental substances. After the test is completed, the practitioner (typically a chiropractor) recommends dietary modification and supplements. SPL maintains a referral list of practitioners who perform the test and suppliers who can provide "special combinations of the suggested supplements to reduce the number of 'pills' you may have to take." The complete (300-item) profile plus interpretation costs $695.

Although the ELISA/ACT™ test can assess the levels of certain immune responses, these are not necessarily related to allergy and have nothing whatsoever to do with a person's need for supplements. Moreover, many of the symptoms listed in SPL's brochure are unrelated to allergy and are not appropriately treated with supplement products.

The correct way to assess a suspected food allergy or intolerance is to begin with a careful record of food intake and symptoms over a period of several weeks. Symptoms such as swollen lips or eyes, hives, or skin rash may be allergy-related, particularly if they occur within a few minutes (up to two hours) after eating. Diarrhea may be related to a food intolerance. Vague symptoms such as dizziness, weakness, or fatigue are not food-related.

If significant symptoms occur, the next step should be to see whether avoiding suspected foods for several weeks prevents possible allergy-related symptoms from recurring. If so, the suspected foods could be reintroduced one at a time to see whether symptoms can be reproduced. However, if the symptoms include hives, vomiting, swollen throat, wheezing, or other difficulty in breathing, continued self-testing could be dangerous, so an allergist should be consulted.

Proper medical evaluation—done best by an allergist—will include careful review of your history and intradermal skin testing with food extracts to see whether an allergic mechanism is involved in your symptoms. In cases where skin testing might be dangerous, a radioactive allergy sensitivity test (RAST) may be appropriate. The RAST is a laboratory test in which the technician mixes a sample of the patient's blood with various food extracts to see whether antibodies to food proteins are present in the blood. It is not as reliable as skin testing and is more expensive. If testing appears to confirm the presence of a genuine food allergy, a food-challenge test can be done in the doctor's office to clinch the diagnosis.

In addition to cytotoxic testing and ELISA/ACT™, the following procedures are not valid for the diagnosis or treatment of food allergies: provocative testing (in which substances are injected under the skin rather than into the skin); sublingual testing (in which suspected foods are placed under the tongue); neutralization (in which progressively smaller doses of substances are administered until the patient no longer reacts); other food immune complex and IgG tests (which assess immune reactions that are common but not necessarily related to allergy); and desensitization (in which progressively larger doses of a food are injected). While desensitization may work for hay fever and other allergies related to inhaled substances, they are worthless for foods and can be dangerous.

"Wilson's Syndrome"

"Wilson's Syndrome" was named in 1990 by E. Denis Wilson, M.D., who claims to have discovered a type of abnormally low thyroid function in which routine blood tests of thyroid are often normal. Its supposed manifestations include fatigue, headaches, PMS, hair loss, irritability, fluid retention, depression, decreased memory, low sex drive, unhealthy nails, low motivation, easy weight gain, and about sixty other symptoms. Wilson claims the condition is "especially brought on by stress" and can persist after the stress has passed. He claims that the main diagnostic sign is a body temperature that averages below 98.6°F (oral), and that the diagnosis is confirmed if the patient responds to treatment with a "special thyroid hormone treatment." He states that "Wilson Syndrome" patients may feel better when taking vitamin supplements, but their symptoms return when the supplements are stopped. He also claims that his syndrome is more common than heart disease or cancer.

In 1991, a fifty-year-old woman died after excessive amounts of thyroid hormone prescribed by Wilson had caused rapid heartbeat that led to a heart attack. In 1992, the Florida Board of Examiners reprimanded Wilson, fined him $10,000, and suspended his license for six months. In order to resume practice, he must undergo psychological testing, serve three years' probation, and take courses each year in endocrinology, the scientific method, and medical ethics. He is also barred from prescribing or administering thyroid preparations for any patient unless the board determines that the medical community has accepted the existence of "Wilson's Syndrome" and Wilson's methods for diagnosing and treating it.

As far as we know, Wilson has not resumed practice. He has, however, established a Wilson's Syndrome Foundation in Summerfield, Florida. Callers to the foundation's toll-free number (800-457-3237) can order his book and doctor's manual and, for $3 extra, can obtain the name of a doctor who treats the condition. (The recorded message states that there are two hundred such doctors.) Wilson has also established a $1.99-per-minute "support line" for doctors and patients, supervised by "a member of the medical staff who has worked closely with Dr. Wilson." Since a health-food magazine recently carried an article about "Wilson's Syndrome" written by a "holistic" physician who is also a radio talk-show host, this fad diagnosis appears to be making inroads into the "alternative" medical community.

Note: Don't confuse "Wilson's Syndrome" with Wilson's disease, a *real* (though rare) disease caused by a defect in the body's ability to metabolize copper.

Megavitamin Therapy

During the early 1950s, a few psychiatrists began adding massive doses of nutrients to their treatment of severe mental problems. The original substance used was vitamin B_3, (nicotinic acid or nicotinamide), and the therapy was termed "megavitamin therapy." Since that time the treatment regimen has been expanded to include other vitamins, minerals, hormones, and diets, any of which may be combined with conventional drug therapy and/or electroconvulsive therapy. Today this approach is called "orthomolecular psychiatry," a term meaning "treatment of mental disease by the provision of optimum molecular environment for the mind, especially substances normally present in the human body." In practice, the word "optimum" always seems to mean "more."

Proponents suggest that abnormal behavior is caused by molecular imbalances correctable by administration of the "right" nutrient molecules at the right time (*ortho* is Greek for "right"). The orthomolecular approach is now used to treat many other diseases. It is described in such books as *Orthomolecular Psychiatry: A Treatment Approach*, by Linus Pauling and David Hawkins, M.D.; *Mega-Nutrition*, by Richard Kunin, M.D.; and *Dr. Pfeiffer's Total Nutrition,* by Carl C. Pfeiffer, M.D., Ph.D. Dr. Kunin's book claims that a balanced diet is a practical impossibility and that "the nutrition-prescription movement is . . . a new direction toward which all of medicine is moving." Both he and Dr. Hawkins are psychiatrists who have served as president of the Orthomolecular Medical Society.

Dr. Pfeiffer, who died in 1989, was director of the Princeton Brain Bio Center (now called the Princeton Bio Center), in Skillman, New Jersey, a facility that offered "nutritional" treatment for:

> the schizophrenias and biochemical deficiencies associated with aging, alcoholism (must be in AA and not drinking), allergies, arthritis,

> autism, epilepsy, hypertension, hypoglycemia, migraine, depression, learning disability, retardation, mental and metabolic disorders, skin problems, and hyperactivity.

Its fee for an initial evaluation has been about $300, including $100 for consultation with a doctor and the rest for laboratory tests that most physicians would not consider necessary or useful for diagnosing the above disorders. (Nor would most doctors agree that the disorders are associated with nutrient-related biochemical deficiencies.) The evaluation fee does not include the ten or more nutrients typically prescribed.

A special task force of the American Psychiatric Association has investigated the claims of the megavitamin and orthomolecular therapists. Its 1973 report notes that orthomolecular psychiatrists use unconventional methods not only in treatment, but also in diagnosis. The report's conclusion, perhaps the most strongly worded statement ever published by a scientific review body, states:

> This review and critique has carefully examined the literature produced by megavitamin proponents and by those who have attempted to replicate their basic and clinical work. It concludes in this regard that the credibility of the megavitamin proponents is low. Their credibility is further diminished by a consistent refusal over the past decade to perform controlled experiments and to report their new results in a scientifically acceptable fashion.
>
> Under these circumstances this Task Force considers the massive publicity which they promulgate via radio, the lay press and popular books, using catch phrases which are really misnomers like "megavitamin therapy" and "orthomolecular treatment," to be deplorable.

The Research Advisory Committee of the National Institute of Mental Health reviewed pertinent scientific data through 1979 and agreed that megavitamin therapy is ineffective and may be harmful. After the U.S. Defense Subcommittee looked into this therapy, it was removed as a treatment covered under the CHAMPUS insurance program for military dependents.

Various claims that megavitamins and megaminerals are effective against psychosis, learning disorders, and mental retardation in children were debunked in reports by the nutrition committees of the American Academy of Pediatrics in 1976 and 1981 and the Canadian Academy of Pediatrics in 1990. Both groups have warned that there is no proven benefit in any of these conditions and that megadoses can cause serious toxic effects. The 1976 report concluded that a "cult" had developed among followers of megavitamin therapy.

One study that received considerable attention from the news media compared thirty Welsh children who received a multivitamin/mineral tablet with thirty who received a placebo and thirty who were untreated. The authors claimed, in an article published in 1988 in the British journal *Lancet*, that the vitamin group showed a significant increase in intelligence, as measured by an I.Q. test. However, the study was poorly designed. Researchers who followed through with well-designed tests found no difference between treated and untreated groups.

Chelation Therapy

Chelation therapy is a series of intravenous infusions containing a synthetic amino acid (EDTA) and various other substances. Proponents claim it is effective against atherosclerosis, coronary heart disease, peripheral vascular disease, arthritis, multiple sclerosis, Parkinson's disease, psoriasis, Alzheimer's disease, and problems with vision, hearing, smell, muscle coordination, and sexual potency. However, none of these claimed benefits has been demonstrated by well-designed clinical trials.

The primary organization promoting chelation therapy is the American College of Advancement in Medicine (ACAM), which was founded in 1973 as the American Academy of Medical Preventics. The group conducts courses, sponsors the *American Journal of Advancement of Medicine,* and administers a "certification" program that is not recognized by the scientific community. The 1992–93 edition of the *Encyclopedia of Medical Organizations and Agencies* states that ACAM has 450 members.

ACAM's protocol states that the number of chelation treatments to achieve "optimal therapeutic benefit" for patients with symptomatic disease ranges from twenty ("minimum"), thirty (usually needed), or forty ("not uncommon before benefit is reported") to as many as one hundred or more over a period of several years. "Full benefit does not normally occur for up to three months after a series is completed," the protocol states, and "follow-up treatments may be given once or twice monthly for long-term maintenance, to sustain improvement and to prevent recurrence of symptoms." The cost, typically $75 to $100 per treatment, is not covered by most insurance companies. Some chelationists, in an attempt to secure coverage for their patients, misstate on their insurance claims that they are treating heavy-metal poisoning or giving "intravenous medication."

Between 1963 and 1985, independent physicians published at least fifteen separate reports documenting the case histories of more than seventy patients who had received chelation treatments. They found no evidence of change in the atherosclerotic disease process, no decrease in the size of atherosclerotic plaques, and no evidence that narrowed arteries opened wider. More recently, two randomized, controlled, double-blind studies of chelation therapy were published in peer-reviewed German medical journals. One involved forty-five patients with intermittent claudication, a condition in which impaired circulation causes the individual to develop pain in the legs upon walking. The other involved sixteen patients with coronary heart disease. In both experiments, those who received chelation therapy did no better than those who did not.

Chelation therapy is not risk-free. Cases of fatal kidney damage and other complications have been reported.

In October 1989, an article in *FDA Consumer* listed chelation therapy as one of "The Top Ten Health Frauds." Three issues later, a letter from a proponent complained that the listing was inappropriate because the FDA had approved the protocol of a clinical trial that was underway. The letter was followed by "an apology for the error," which stated that the editor had not been aware that chelation therapy had been approved for a study.

The FDA should not have backed down. Mere permission for a clinical trial is not proof that a method works. Nevertheless, for several years, proponents trumpeted the *existence* of the study as evidence that their claims were justified. The study was not completed, however. Proponents claim that a drug company involved in funding the study changed its mind, leaving them without the resources to complete it. Even if the study had been completed and had demonstrated benefit in intermittent claudication, it would not have proven that chelation is safe or effective for anything else.

In 1992, a group of cardiovascular surgeons in Denmark published results of a well-designed study of EDTA treatment for severe intermittent claudication. A total of 153 patients in two groups received twenty infusions of EDTA or a placebo for five to nine weeks. The changes seen in pain-free walking distances were similar for the EDTA-treated and the placebo group, and there were no long-term therapeutic effects noted in three-month and six-month follow-ups. These investigators concluded that chelation was not effective against intermittent claudication.

For many years, proponents claimed that chelation therapy was a "chemical Roto Rooter" that cleaned out atherosclerotic plaque from the body's arteries. This claim was based on the notion that chelation removes calcium deposits in the plaque and that, without calcium, the plaque disintegrates. This is incorrect, however, because calcium deposits don't form in the early stages of atherosclerosis; and even if they did, EDTA would be unable to pass through artery cell membranes to reach the deposits. More recently, proponents have claimed that chelation therapy blocks production of free radicals involved in a chain of reactions that result in atherosclerosis. Saul Green, Ph.D., a research biochemist, exploded this theory in the September/October 1993 issue of *Nutrition Forum*, in which he explained that EDTA actually combines with iron in the blood to *increase* the number of free radicals produced. Green concluded:

> If chelation therapists practiced in a scientific manner, their publications would show an interest in obtaining objective proof that chelation could alter the progress of the atherosclerosis, that occluded blood vessels could be cleared, that plaque deposits could be reduced, and that hardened arteries could be "softened." Their data would include carefully documented case reports with long-term follow-up, comparisons of angiograms or ultrasound tests before and after chelation, and data from autopsies of former patients. But chelationists have published no such data.
>
> The few well-designed studies that have addressed the efficacy of chelation for atherosclerotic diseases have been carried out by "establishment "medical scientists." Without exception, these found no evidence that chelation worked. . . .
>
> These same conclusions have been reached by the FDA, National Institutes of Health, National Research Council, California Medical Society, American Medical Association, Centers for Disease Control and Prevention, American Heart Association, American College of Physicians, American Academy of Family Practice, American Society for Clinical Pharmacology Therapeutics, American College of Cardiology, and American Osteopathic Association. . . .
>
> The chelation "establishment" is not being victimized by a prejudiced and arrogant medical orthodoxy, but by its own unwillingness to mount a rigorous, placebo-controlled, double-blind clinical trial and stand by the results.

"Metabolic Therapy"

"Metabolic therapy" is a loosely defined approach whose proponents claim to diagnose abnormalities at the cellular level and correct them by normalizing the patient's metabolism. According to its proponents, cancer, arthritis, multiple sclerosis, and other "degenerative" diseases are the result of metabolic imbalance caused by a buildup of "toxic substances" in the body. Proponents claim that scientific practitioners merely treat the symptoms of the disease while they treat the cause by removing "toxins" and strengthening the immune system so the body can heal itself. Of course, the "toxins" are neither defined nor objectively measurable.

"Metabolic" treatment regimens can include diets, coffee enemas, vitamins, minerals, glandulars, enzymes, and various nostrums that are not legally marketable in the United States. The regimens for cancer also include laetrile, a quack cancer remedy made from apricot pits. No scientific study has ever shown that "metabolic therapy" or any of its components is effective against cancer or any other serious disease.

The most visible proponent of "metabolic therapy" was Harold Manner, Ph.D., a biology professor who entered the public spotlight in 1977 by announcing that he had cured cancer in mice with injections of laetrile, enzymes, and vitamin A. (Actually, he digested the tumors by injecting them with digestive enzymes, which cannot cure cancer that has spread to another part of the body.) During the early 1980s, Manner left his teaching position and became affiliated with a clinic in Tijuana, Mexico, which was later renamed the Manner Clinic. Although he claimed a 74 percent success rate in treating cancers, there is no evidence that he kept track of patients after they left his clinic.

Manner marketed his methods to chiropractors, naturopaths, and physicians. At a 1988 seminar, he said there were nearly six hundred "qualified metabolic physicians" worldwide. Those who joined Manner's Metabolic Research Foundation were promised $200 for each patient referred to Manner's clinic. Although Manner died in 1988, the clinic is still operating.

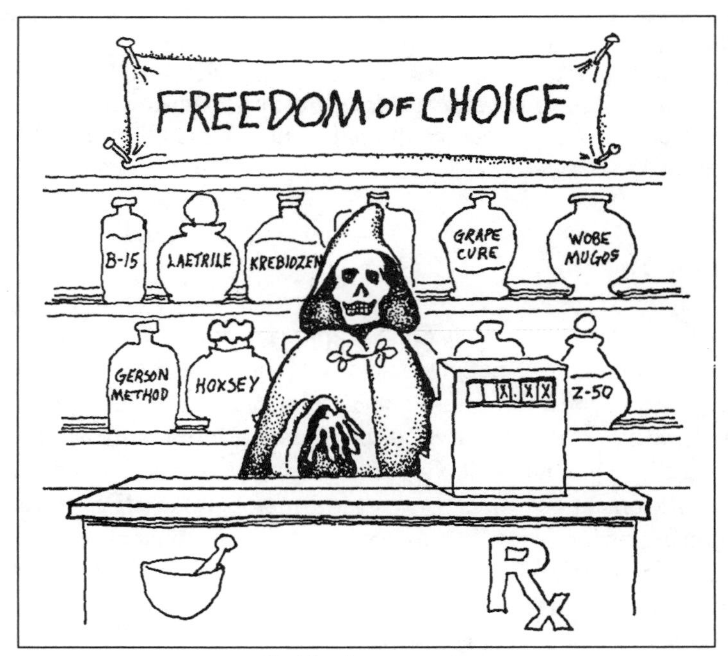

Cashing in on cancer.

Most "alternative" practitioners believe that insurance companies should cover their care. Many encourage their patients to file insurance claims and even to sue if claims are denied. During the 1988 Manner seminar, Ronald King, a claims supervisor for North American Health Insurance Coordinators, of Dallas, Texas, described how his company filed insurance claims for "alternative health care" facilities. King said that by using persistence and filling out claim forms with the "right" procedure codes, his company was able to collect on most of the claims it filed. He indicated that instead of revealing what actually took place, his company would enter code numbers for standard treatment. King said that North American kept 16 percent of the amount collected on behalf of its clients—one of which was the Manner Clinic. Manner added that his clinic billed insurers for this commission by calling it "administrative costs."

In 1994, after a lengthy investigation by the FBI, a federal grand jury indicted King along with North American's president Cameron Edward Frye and its vice president Gary Paul Stankowski, on fourteen counts of conspiracy, mail fraud, wire fraud, and laundering of monetary instruments. The grand jury charged that North American's "principal business was the filing of false and fraudulent claims" for health-insurance benefits. According to the indictment, the trio obtained payment of health insurance claims for unorthodox treatments provided at Mexican facilities by pretending that the claims covered conventional therapies administered within in the United States. The indictment also alleges that fraudulent claims inflated the fees for services rendered, billed for services never provided, utilized false dates of service, and falsified diagnoses. The FBI estimates that claims submitted by North American had caused insurance companies to pay out more than $43 million during the previous seven years, mostly for treatment at Mexican clinics. The indictment papers identified six such clinics whose services were fraudulently described on claims submitted by North American.

Chinese Medicine

Chinese medicine—also called oriental medicine and traditional Chinese medicine (TCM)—is said to be based on notions of "harmony" and "balance," in which a healthy person is someone in "complete harmony, both internally and with nature." It is based on mystical concepts and notions about the body that date back more than two thousand years.

TCM practitioners define health as a balance of *yin* and *yang*, which the ancient Chinese regarded as "complementary but opposing qualities" that make up everything in the natural world. TCM holds that the organs of the body (some of which do not correspond to anatomical structures recognized by scientific medicine) may suffer from "deficiency" or "excess" of yin or yang, which can be corrected with herbs or foods that have the appropriate yin/yang characteristics. TCM also speculates that the body's vital energy ("*chi*" or "*qi*") circulates through hypothetical channels called "meridians," which have branches connected to bodily organs and functions, and that disease is caused by "imbalance" or interruption of *chi*. Some practitioners claim they use both scientific medicine and TCM in their practice.

The diagnostic methods used by TCM practitioners differ significantly from those of scientific physicians. They include:

- Inspection of the patient's complexion, general demeanor, body language, and tongue. Certain areas of the tongue are said to correspond to specific organ systems in the body.
- Questioning about symptoms, medical history, diet, lifestyle, and reactions to environmental variables such as the weather
- Listening to the tone and strength of the voice
- Smelling body excretions, the breath, and body odor
- Using pulse diagnosis. Whereas scientific practitioners take one pulse at either wrist to determine rate and rhythm, TCM practitioners check six alleged pulses at each wrist and identify more than twenty-five alleged pulse qualities such as "sinking," "slippery," "soggy," "tight," and "wiry." TCM's "pulses" supposedly reflect the type of imbalance, the condition of each organ system, and the status of the patient's "*chi*."
- Palpation of "acupuncture points," which are said to be located along the meridians. Originally there were 365 such points, corresponding to the days of the year, but some proponents maintain there are more than two thousand.

TCM's treatment modalities include medicinal herbs, "food therapy," acupuncture, massage, and exercise, all of which are claimed to restore yin/yang balance and increase the body's resistance to illness. Herbal prescriptions contain many ingredients. The basis for selecting foods is not nutrient content but "hotness" or "coolness," general effect on the body, and flavor. Different flavors are said to have an affinity for specific organs.

Those who espouse the traditional Chinese view of health and disease consider acupuncture and its variations valid for the gamut of disease; they say that acupuncture removes blocks and balances the flow of *chi* throughout the body. Others who practice acupuncture reject these trappings and claim that it offers a simple way to achieve pain relief. Traditional acupuncture, as now practiced, involves the insertion of stainless steel needles into various body areas. Low-frequency current may be applied to the needles to produce greater stimulation. Other procedures used separately or together include: moxibustion (burning of floss or herbs applied to the skin); injection of sterile water, procaine, morphine, vitamins, or homeopathic solutions through the inserted needles; applications of laser beams; placement of needles in the external ear (auriculotherapy); and acupressure (use of manual pressure). Some practitioners place needles at or near the site of disease, while others select points on the basis of symptoms. Practitioners of Qigong dispense with needles and allegedly influence their patients' *chi* directly to bring about "stress reduction." Some TCM practitioners state that the electrical properties of the body may become imbalanced weeks or even months before health problems become apparent on a physical level. These practitioners claim that acupuncture can be used to treat conditions when the patient just "doesn't feel right," even though no disease condition is apparent.

Acupuncture was introduced to the United States in about 1825 but generated little interest until President Richard M. Nixon's 1972 visit to China. Since then, it has been promoted for the treatment of pain and a wide variety of other problems. Although many articles claiming benefit have been published, the quality of most research studies has been poor. There is no evidence that acupuncture influences the course of any disease. Acupuncture needles are considered "investigational" devices by the FDA and are not approved for the treatment of any disease.

TCM originated long before modern knowledge of anatomy, biochemistry, physiology, and pharmacology developed. Its theories are too nebulous and its practices too voluminous to be testable. Its herbal remedies have not been studied systematically. Although effective ingredients may exist in some of them, harmful ones may also be found. TCM's practitioners include medical and osteopathic doctors (who can legally administer almost anything they consider "treatment"), chiropractors (who are licensed in all states and essentially unregulated), naturopaths (who are licensed in a few states and permitted to practice in others), and laypersons (who acquire an acupuncture license or simply set up shop as an acupuncturist or herbalist).

Would you like your *chi* balanced? Or your meridians unblocked? Do you crave foods that will "tonify" your stomach? Would you enjoy drinking herbal teas with fifteen ingredients to "cool your liver fire" and/or treat the "root" of your disease? Or swallowing handfuls of herbal pills to dispel the "dampness" of your spleen? Would you like to consult someone who thinks such mumbo jumbo makes more sense than scientific medicine? If so, your local TCM practitioner will be pleased to accommodate you.

Dubious Dental Practices

Many dentists are promoting unscientific "nutritional" methods that can be quite lucrative. A 1985 article in a dental trade journal stated: "Are you interested in doubling your net practice income? We almost did it last year. . . . We used nutritional counseling as the vehicle." The increased income would be produced by charging high consultation fees and/or selling dietary supplements that are unnecessary and overpriced. The "counseling" may be based on fraudulent diagnostic methods such as hair analysis, lingual vitamin C testing, or dubious tests for "food allergies." Some dentists are distributors for multilevel companies that market supplements and herbal preparations with suggestions that everyone should use them.

In 1988, an article in another dental trade journal stated: "With the success of fluoridation, many dentists are having problems filling appointment books. A substantial number of open appointments could be filled with giving clinical nutritional advice." The suggested fees were $250 for the first visit and $50 for follow-up visits. The article was accompanied by a sample "breakfast nutritional prescription" that included a mixture of *Cheerios*, wheat bran, and oat bran, to which wheat germ, lecithin granules, raisins, skim milk, and half a banana, are added. The concoction was to be eaten "slowly, while thinking of a pleasant day at the shore (or at the mountains)."

Some dentists espouse "balancing body chemistry," which they claim can prevent a wide variety of "degenerative" diseases. These dentists use inappropriate laboratory tests (such as hair analysis) to determine the biochemical state of the patient and recommend diets and expensive food supplements to achieve "balance." Some dentists use computers to analyze the diets of their patients and recommend supplement concoctions, usually by brand name. While computer analysis of diet can be valuable when done properly, it is not a valid basis for recommending supplements.

Promoters of "holistic dentistry" typically claim that disease can be prevented by maintaining "optimum" health, or "wellness." John E. Dodes, D.D.S., president of the New York Council Against Health Fraud, has noted that "'Wellness' is something for which quacks can get paid when there is nothing wrong with the patient. In the dental office, these schemes usually involve the purchase of expensive dietary supplements or a plastic bite appliance."

Practitioners of "dental kinesiology" may consider muscle testing useful in locating diseased teeth, determining sensitivity to tooth filling materials, restricting orthodontic treatment, constructing oral devices, and more. Typically they test muscle strength by pushing or pulling the patient's arm before and after vitamins or other substances are placed under the patient's tongue.

"Treatment" then consists of expensive vitamin supplements or a special diet. Dental kinesiology is a variant of applied kinesiology (discussed in Chapter 15), which is not a legitimate approach.

Some dentists use pendulums to test for "food compatibility." Some perform dental procedures under pyramid-shaped structures that they believe will reduce the incidence of infection. Some employ what they call Chinese medicine—including herbalism, acupuncture, vitamin therapy, and whatever else they wish to throw in. Others are dabbling with iridology, reflexology, body "auras," Kirlian photography, black box devices, and other occult practices. If a dentist you consult advocates any of the methods described in this chapter, switch to another dentist.

"Mercury-Amalgam Toxicity"

One of the simplest ways to bilk people is to tell them something they have is no good and sell them something else. During the past decade, a small but vocal group of dentists, physicians, and various other "holistic" advocates have been doing exactly that—by claiming that mercury-amalgam ("silver") fillings are toxic and cause a wide range of health problems including multiple sclerosis, arthritis, headaches, Parkinson's disease, and emotional stress. They recommend that mercury fillings be replaced with either gold or plastic ones and that vitamin supplements be taken to prevent trouble during and after the process.

These dentists typically use an industrial mercury detector to indicate that "toxic" amounts of mercury are being released. To use the device, the dentist asks the patient to chew vigorously for ten minutes, which may cause tiny amounts of mercury to be released from the fillings. Although this exposure lasts for just a few seconds and most of the mercury will be exhaled rather than absorbed by the body, the machines give a falsely high readout, which the anti-amalgamists interpret as dangerous. The most commonly used device multiplies the amount of mercury it detects in a small sample of air by a factor of 8,000. This gives a reading for a cubic meter, a volume far greater than the human mouth. The proper way to determine mercury exposure is to measure blood or urine levels, which indicate how much has been absorbed into the body. Scientific testing has shown that the amount of mercury absorbed from fillings is only a tiny fraction of the average daily intake from food and is insignificant.

The false diagnosis of mercury-amalgam toxicity is potentially very harmful and reflects extremely poor judgment on the part of the practitioner. The American Dental Association Council on Ethics, Bylaws and Judicial Affairs considers the unnecessary removal of silver amalgam fillings "improper and unethical." We believe that dentists who engage in this practice should have their license revoked.

The leading advocate of "balancing body chemistry" and "mercury-amalgam toxicity" is Hal A. Huggins, D.D.S., a dentist from Colorado Springs, Colorado. Huggins is also crusading against root canal therapy, which he claims can make people susceptible to arthritis, multiple sclerosis, amyotrophic lateral sclerosis, and other autoimmune diseases. As is the case with mercury-amalgam fillings, there is no objective evidence that teeth treated with root canal therapy produce any adverse effect on the immune system or any other part of the body.

Holistic Philosophy

The term "holistic" (also spelled "wholistic") is frequently used in both scientific and nonscientific circles. However, considerable confusion surrounds its use. Scientific practitioners regard holistic medicine as treatment of the "whole patient," with due attention to emotional and spiritual factors as well as the patient's lifestyle. But most others who label their approach holistic use unscientific methods of diagnosis and treatment. These practitioners typically say they "treat the whole body" rather than treating any one organ or body system, the patient's symptoms, or the disease. Douglas Stalker, Ph.D., and Clark Glymour, Ph.D., who have studied the holistic movement closely, consider it "a pablum of common sense and nonsense offered by cranks and quacks and failed pedants who share an attachment to magic and an animosity to reason."

Many "holistic" practitioners see disease as primarily caused by stresses and "imbalances." Although stress is a factor in many ailments, it has not been demonstrated that stress-reduction techniques advocated in the name of holism are actually effective in preventing disease. The concept of "imbalances" is even more fanciful. Acupuncturists claim to balance "life forces"; chiropractors

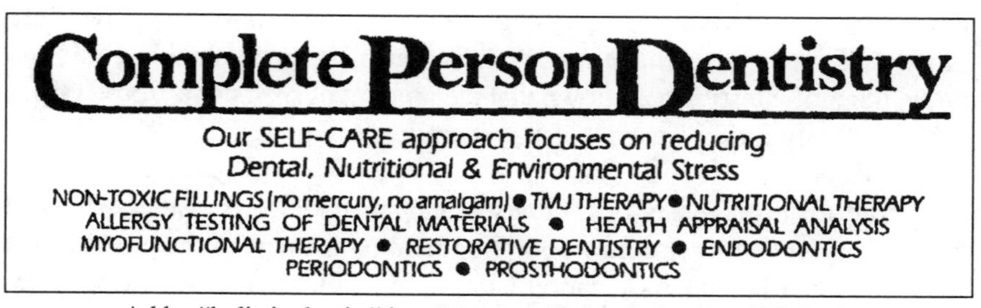

Ad by "holistic dentist" in a "resource directory for natural living"

claim to balance spines; some unorthodox dentists claim to balance "body chemistry"; applied kinesiologists claim to balance muscles; and various other healers claim to balance people's spiritual, mental, and physical "systems" to bring them "into harmony with nature." A common goal is a state of "wellness" that goes far beyond the absence of disease.

Holistic proponents make a serious error by pretending that all of medical science is one system and then listing various others as separate but equal systems. They may call modern medicine "Western medicine" to distinguish it from "Eastern medicine." Or they may call it "allopathic medicine," a term coined almost two centuries ago by Samuel Hahnemann, the founder of homeopathy. In Hahnemann's day, allopathy included cupping, bloodletting, and many other primitive methods then considered orthodox. These methods were abandoned long ago as medical scientists learned how to determine what works and what doesn't. Scientific medicine now includes all methods of treatment that are sensible, reliable, and reproducible from one practitioner to another. Holistic advocates attempt to reduce its significance by defining it as "one approach." Dozens of unscientific approaches are then promoted as "alternatives."

Many holistic promoters purport to find "the amounts of nutrients that will provide the utmost in health." Many use hair analysis and other questionable diagnostic tests. Most recommend high dosages of vitamins and minerals for the prevention and treatment of disease. There is no doubt that diet plays a role in the production of some diseases. Overweight is certainly a widespread problem, and some aspects of diet are related to the development of cardiovascular disease and cancer. But holistic promoters go far beyond what is scientifically valid.

Chiropractors have been particularly active in organizing "holistic" and "wellness" centers that offer "natural" treatments and "preventive" services, but the methods recommended usually include unnecessary vitamin supplements, unnecessary spinal adjustments, and exercise programs of questionable value. In contrast, wellness programs run by responsible physicians and other scientific practitioners stress attention to risk factors. These programs offer help in stopping smoking, dietary counseling to promote weight control and nutrient balance, and exercise methods that increase heart strength and endurance.

At one time in the past, the holistic label had a valuable and specific meaning. Today, however, it has become a banner around which all manner of questionable practitioners are rallying. It appears to us that the concept of holism has been irretrievably corrupted by confused practitioners and promoters of quackery. The word "holistic" and its associated slogans should be abandoned by scientific practitioners.

Questionable Groups

Practitioners engaged in unscientific practices tend to support one another politically and emotionally, and many have banded together in professional groups. Some of these groups admit health-care providers who are not physicians. Some publish a journal, and some have set up a "specialty board" that "certifies" applicants but lacks standing within the scientific community. Some are seeking passage of laws that would prevent state licensing boards from disciplining their members for unprofessional (unscientific) practices.

The International Academy of Preventive Medicine (IAPM) was founded in 1971 "to create an atmosphere conducive to open discussion of preventive medical practices among physicians, dentists, Ph.D.'s and health-related professions." Subsequently it merged with a similar group, the International College of Applied Nutrition, to form the International Academy of Nutrition and Preventive Medicine (IANPM). IANPM, which has about four hundred members, publishes the *Journal of Applied Nutrition* and operates the International Association of Clinical Nutritionists. The journal's largest financial supporters during the past few years have been the National Nutritional Foods Association and a few supplement manufacturers.

The American Holistic Medical Association (AHMA) was founded in 1978 by physicians who supposedly wished to use nontraditional methods as adjuncts to traditional ones. AHMA's 1989–1990 directory describes it as "an organization of physicians dedicated to medicine for the whole person." The directory lists about 350 members, most of whom are medical or osteopathic physicians. Other holistic groups include the Holistic Dental Association (about two hundred members), American Holistic Nurses Association (about 1,500 members), and American Holistic Veterinary Medical Association (about four hundred members).

AHMA sponsors conferences and publishes a bimonthly magazine called *Holistic Medicine.* AHMA is closely affiliated with the American Holistic Medical Foundation, whose primary purpose is to raise funds to support AHMA research and educational projects. However, it appears to have raised little money and sponsored no significant research. The topics covered at AHMA conferences have included acupuncture theory, anthroposophic medicine, ayurvedic medicine, balancing body chemistry, homeopathy, nontraditional methods of diagnosis, "nutritional therapy," and many other approaches not recognized as valid by the scientific community. Many exhibitors at the meetings are promoters of questionable products and services. Thomas Chalmers, M.D., who evaluated the issues of AHMA's *Journal of Holistic Medicine* from 1980 through 1982, found only two well-designed studies among their forty-seven articles. The journal ceased publication in 1986. AHMA's 1987 "Nutritional Guidelines" booklet recommends that everyone take vitamin and mineral supplements "because even the best diet will rarely contain an optimum amount of nutrients." This statement has no basis in reality.

AHMA would like to protect its members from legal difficulty when they use questionable methods. Years ago, an attorney suggested that if AHMA "were to establish a sound membership base and establish official positions on various types of treatment modalities, this provision might come into play and be used to the benefit of physicians who were employing alternative therapy sanctioned by the Association." In 1988, its president wrote to the state attorneys general urging that AHMA be permitted to provide peer review of holistic physicians under investigation by their licensing boards.

Most professional members of these groups prescribe or recommend megavitamins and/or questionable dietary practices for a wide variety of ailments. Megavitamin proponents have also formed the American Association of Orthomolecular Medicine, which has about three hundred members. The American College of Advancement in Medicine is composed mainly of medical and osteopathic physicians who have a special interest in chelation therapy. "Clinical ecologists" have banded together in the American Academy of Environmental Medicine and the American Academy of Otolaryngic Allergy. The International Association of Dentists and Physicians, formed in 1991, is open to all types of licensed or "certified" health-care providers. Described as a "minority trade association," it hopes to set "standards" for unconventional methods that will be recognized by insurance companies, regulatory agencies and the courts. The Foundation for the Advancement of Innovative Medicine (FAIM) was formed in 1986 to foster public awareness of methods "outside the mainstream of conventional medicine." Its activities are detailed in Chapter 20.

The American Quack Association (AQA) was founded in 1985 and grew to about 350 members, most of whom were health professionals. Its dues were $6 a year. Its main purposes appeared to be providing emotional support to its members, poking fun at their critics, and stimulating positive public feelings toward unconventional practitioners. Noting that "Discrimination, legal investigation, persecution, prosecution, and even imprisonment have variously been the fate of those few physicians and others who have publicly counseled alternative means of health care," AQA's "Articles of Health Freedom" demanded that "no law or regulations shall be made prohibiting the right of people to freely assemble for healing of any type." They also opposed "any penalty whatsoever against anyone employing any form of treatment for cancer or any other disease for him or herself or others, except in cases of fraud, deception or the use of force." AQA's logo depicted a stressed but smiling duck flying through the "Q" of AQA. The group quietly stopped operating in 1989.

AQA's founder and vice president was Roy Kupsinel, M.D., a "holistic" practitioner in Ovieda, Florida. Kupsinel publishes *Health Consciousness*, a bimonthly magazine with articles on "holistic" health care, cosmic philosophy, conservative causes, and the "persecution" of his beloved colleagues. It also contains ads for questionable products and services. While AQA remained active, the last few pages of *Health Consciousness* were printed upside down as the *Journal of the American Quack Association,* which was edited by AQA president and cofounder Jonathan V. Wright, M.D. (see Chapter 17). In a 1987 issue of *Health Consciousness*, Kupsinel described how he was expelled from his county and state medical societies following charges related to his "nutritional/hypoglycemia practice." He also stated that he had suffered from hypoglycemia; mercury-amalgam toxicity; allergies to foods, chemicals and inhalants; hypothyroidism; and eight other "common denominators of degenerative disease."

If professionals who believe in science could campaign half as persistently as the "unscientific community" described throughout this book, nutritional quackery would be much more difficult to sell and consumers would be much better protected.

13

Nutrition-Related Cultism

The *American Heritage Dictionary* defines "cult" as "a religion or religious sect generally considered to be extremist or false, with its followers often living in an unconventional manner under the guidance of an authoritarian, charismatic leader" and "a usually nonscientific method or regimen claimed by its originator to have exclusive or exceptional power in curing a particular disease." We regard "nutrition cults" as systems of dietary practices based on dogma set forth by their promulgators rather than on nutritional facts. They typically involve rigid beliefs that: (1) certain foods have special ability to cure specific diseases; (2) certain foods are harmful and should be eliminated from the diet; and (3) "natural foods" are best.

This chapter discusses three systems that fit this description: macrobiotics, naturopathy, and Natural Hygiene. Each of these is rooted in *vitalism*, the concept that bodily functions are due to some sort of "vital force" that is not explainable by the laws of physics and chemistry or measurable by any scientific method.

Vitalistic proponents maintain that diseases should be treated by stimulating the body to heal itself rather than by "treating symptoms." Homeopaths, for example, claim that illness is due to a disturbance of the body's "vital force," which they can correct with very dilute remedies (see Chapter 9), while naturopaths speak of the power of "nature," which they can augment by "detoxification." Some vitalists assert that food can be "dead" or "living" and that "live" foods contain a dormant or primitive "life force" that humans can assimilate. Jack Raso, M.S., R.D., author of *"Alternative" Healthcare: A Comprehensive Guide,* has noted that "although vitalists often attempt to gain status by making a pretense of being scientific, deep down they reject the scientific method."

Macrobiotics

Macrobiotics (which means "way of long life") is a quasireligious philosophical system founded by George Ohsawa (1893–1966). Ohsawa claimed to have cured himself of serious illness by changing from the modern refined diet then sweeping Japan to a simple diet of brown rice, miso soup, sea vegetables, and other traditional foods. He wrote that refined sugar and excess animal protein are two main causes of all illness, including cancer and mental illness. He outlined a ten-stage Zen macrobiotic diet in which each stage became progressively more restricted, with the "highest" level consisting of just grains. The diet was claimed to enable individuals to overcome all forms of illness, which Ohsawa attributed to dietary excesses.

In 1966, the Passaic (New Jersey) Grand Jury reviewed three cases of death and two cases of near-death from malnutrition among Zen macrobiotic adherents and concluded that the diet "constitutes a public health hazard." In 1967, the *Journal of the American Medical Association* reported how one of these adherents had developed scurvy within ten months of starting the diet. These cases set the tone for scientific medicine's view of macrobiotics. In 1971, the AMA Council on Foods and Nutrition stated that followers of the diet, particularly the highest level, stood in "great danger" of malnutrition.

Current macrobiotic proponents espouse a diet that is less restricted but still can be nutritionally inadequate. They recommend whole grains (50 to 60 percent of each meal), vegetables (25 to 30 percent of each meal), whole beans or soybean-based products (5 to 10 percent of daily food), nuts and seeds (small amounts as snacks), miso soup, herbal teas, and small amounts of white meat or seafood once or twice weekly. The optimal diet is said to be achieved by balancing "yin" and "yang" foods. The yin/yang classification is not related to nutrient content but is based on the food's color, pH, shape, size, taste, temperature, texture, water content, and weight; the region and season in which the food was grown; and how it is prepared and eaten.

Today's leading proponent is Michio Kushi, a former student of Ohsawa, who founded and is president of the Kushi Institute in Brookline, Massachusetts. He also established *East West Journal*, a monthly magazine now published independently and called *Natural Health*. Institute publications state that the macrobiotic way of life should include chewing food at least fifty times per mouthful (or until it becomes liquid), not wearing synthetic or woolen clothing next to the skin, avoiding long hot baths or showers (unless you have been consuming too much salt or animal food), having large green plants in your house to enrich the oxygen content of the air, and singing a happy song every day. *Natural Health* promotes a wide variety of "alternative" methods and tends to be critical toward scientific medicine and various public health measures. Books and magazines, special food items, macrobiotic cooking classes, and other macrobiotic products and services are obtainable through local health-food stores and regional macrobiotic teaching centers ("East West Centers"). General bookstores also carry books by Michio Kushi and other proponents.

Macrobiotic diets have been promoted for maintaining general health and for preventing and "relieving" cancer, AIDS, and other diseases. Kushi's books

YOU CAN REGAIN YOUR HEALTH

CANCER
HEART DISEASE
DIABETES
ARTHRITIS

FOR COMPLETE INFORMATION
CALL TOLL FREE 1-800-523-7799
IN PA. CALL 215-337-1935
OR WRITE: MARTY KALAN
KUSHI MACROBIOTIC
HEALTH CENTER
Valley Forge Hilton Hotel
Valley Forge, Pa. 19406

In the midst of the growing trend of life-threatening illnesses, many people are realizing that the human body has the ability to recover. The Kushi Macrobiotic Health Center offers the unique opportunity to acquire the knowledge and understanding to unlock this tremendous potential.

Our purpose is to provide all the resources necessary to care for such degenerative illnesses as cancer, heart disease, diabetes, arthritis and others, or simply to insure good health, happiness and longevity.

The Center, under the personal supervision of Michio Kushi, world's foremost authority on macrobiotics and natural healing, features a complete staff of skilled dietary counselors, massage therapists, physical therapists and medical professionals.

The location of the Center, within the luxurious Valley Forge Hilton Hotel is just outside Philadelphia.

We have established the Kushi Macrobiotic Health Center to assist you in making the most positive transformation of your life.

KUSHI MACROBIOTIC HEALTH CENTER

Local newspaper ad from the early 1980s

contain case histories of people whose cancers supposedly disappeared after they adopted macrobiotic eating. However, there is no objective evidence of any such benefit, and the diet itself can cause cancer patients to undergo serious weight loss and die sooner. Studies of children living in macrobiotic communities in The Netherlands and in New England have found that they tended to be smaller, shorter, and to weigh less than children fed normal diets. Deficiencies of vitamin B_{12}, iron, and vitamin D have also been reported. Macrobiotics received a great deal of favorable publicity in the early 1980s due to Anthony J. Sattilaro, M.D., who claimed that the macrobiotic diet had cured him of prostate cancer. Sattilaro had undergone conventional therapy but credited macrobiotics for his improvement. His story was published in *East West Journal* and two books that he wrote: *Recalled by Life* and *Living Well Naturally.* Despite his claims that he had been pronounced cured, he died of the disease in 1989. Several lawsuits have claimed that cancer patients who relied on macrobiotic methods instead of proven therapy met with disaster. As far as we know, however, no such case has come to trial.

In 1986, *Health Foods Business* published an article called "Capture the Macrobiotic Market Share," which stated:

> The good thing about macrobiotic shoppers is that they are one-store shoppers who average more per purchase than other customers. . . .
>
> Let's look at what turns an otherwise normal human being into a macrobiotic. . . .
>
> The majority . . . suffer from a degenerative illness and are attempting to cure themselves. They've read some macrobiotic literature, frequently *Recalled By Life* . . . or have had a consultation from one of Michio Kushi's students. . . .
>
> Show these new customers how (and what) to buy in bulk. . . . Offer to special order items you don't normally carry. If a shopper is convinced that he/she can cure his/her melanoma by eating a macrobiotic diet, which included shiitake mushrooms, you'd best get those mushrooms, or you'll lose that shopper to a competitor who will!

In 1989, Jack Raso attended a five-day seminar for professionals given at the Kushi Institute, which is located on six hundred acres in Becket, Massachusetts. In *"Alternative" Healthcare* he described how participants were encouraged to make "diagnoses" based on such things as astrological conditions, weather conditions, the patient's "aura" and "vibrations," acupuncture meridians, and other nebulous attributes not recognized by medical science.

Lawrence Lindner, executive editor of the *Tufts University Diet and Nutrition Letter,* had a private consultation with a certified senior macrobiotics counselor at the Kushi Institute as part of an assignment for *American Health* magazine. In the May 1988 issue, Lindner reported being told: (1) his heart was somewhat enlarged because he ate too much fruit, (2) his kidneys were weak, (3) he was slightly hypoglycemic, (4) deposits of fat and mucus were starting to build up in his intestines, (5) cold drinks could freeze the deposits and cause kidney stones, and (6) he should avoid eating chicken because it is linked with pancreatic cancer and melanoma. The consultation cost $200. Lindner concluded: "The macrobiotic lectures, courses, books and tapes . . . besides running into hundreds or thousands of dollars, teach a philosophy of life, not nutrient interactions." In a subsequent interview, he added, "Some people are attracted to macrobiotics because, like a typical cult, it seems to offer simple solutions to a variety of life's problems."

Naturopathy

Naturopathy, sometimes referred to as "natural medicine," is a system of "healing" said to rely solely on "nature." Naturopaths claim to remove the underlying cause(s) of disease and to stimulate the body's natural healing processes. They assert that diseases are the body's effort to purify itself, and that cures result from increasing the patient's "vital force" by ridding the body of waste products and "toxins." The American Association of Naturopathic Physicians (AANP) states: "Naturopathic medicine has its own unique body of knowledge, evolved and refined for centuries." Although naturopaths say they "emphasize prevention," they tend to oppose immunization procedures.

Before 1961, the doctor of naturopathy (N.D.) degree could be obtained at a number of chiropractic schools; now it is available only from three full-time schools of naturopathy and several correspondence schools. Training at the full-time schools follows a pattern similar to that of chiropractic schools: two years of basic science courses and two years of clinical naturopathy. Two years of preprofessional college work are required for admission. In 1987, the U.S. Secretary of Education approved the Council on Naturopathic Medical Education (CNME) as an accrediting agency for the full-time schools. As with acupuncture and chiropractic schools, this recognition is not based upon the scientific validity of what is taught but upon other criteria.

The leading naturopathy school, Bastyr University, in Seattle, Washington, is accredited by the CNME. Besides its N.D. program, Bastyr offers a B.S. degree program in Natural Health Sciences with majors in nutrition and Oriental medicine, and M.S. programs in nutrition and acupuncture. Bastyr also provides health-food retailers and their employees with home-study programs that promote "natural" approaches for the gamut of disease (see Chapter 6). The other four-year schools are the National College of Naturopathic Medicine in

Portland, Oregon, and the recently opened Southwest College of Naturopathic Medicine and Health Sciences in Scottsdale, Arizona. Much of these schools' funding has come from companies that market dietary supplements, homeopathic products, and/or herbal remedies.

Naturopaths are licensed as independent practitioners in seven states and Washington, D.C., and can legally practice in a few others. A directory in the January/February 1992 issue of *East West Natural Health* lists nearly four hundred naturopaths with practices in twenty-seven states, the District of Columbia, and Puerto Rico. The total number of practitioners is unknown but includes chiropractors and acupuncturists who practice naturopathy. In 1993, an AANP official said that his group represented more than eight hundred naturopaths and that licensure efforts were underway in sixteen states. Naturopathic services are not covered by Medicare or most insurance policies.

Most naturopaths allege that virtually all diseases are within the scope of their practice. They offer treatment at their offices and at spas where patients may reside for several weeks. Their current methods include fasting, "natural food" diets, vitamins, herbs, tissue minerals, homeopathic remedies, cell salts, manipulation, massage, exercise, colonic enemas, acupuncture, Chinese medicine, natural childbirth, minor surgery, and applications of water, heat, cold, air, sunlight, and electricity. Radiation may be used for diagnosis, but not for treatment.

Naturopaths assert that their "natural" methods, when properly used, rarely have adverse effects because they do not interfere with the individual's inherent healing abilities. This claim is utter nonsense. Any medication (drug or herb) potent enough to produce a therapeutic effect is potent enough to cause adverse effects. Drugs should not be used (and would not merit FDA approval) unless the probable benefit is significantly greater than the probable risk. Moreover, medically used drugs do not usually interfere with the healing processes.

The most comprehensive naturopathic publications are *A Textbook of Natural Medicine* (for students and professionals) and the *Encyclopedia of Natural Medicine* (for laypersons). The text, which has forty-three contributors and more than a thousand pages, was edited by Joseph E. Pizzorno, N.D., president of Bastyr University, and Michael T. Murray, N.D., a faculty member. The pair also wrote the 630-page encyclopedia. Both books recommend questionable dietary measures, vitamins, minerals, and/or herbs for more than seventy health problems ranging from acne to AIDS. For many of these conditions, daily administration of ten or more products is recommended—some in dosages high enough to cause toxicity.

Because these books refer to hundreds of references with which we are unfamiliar, a complete analysis of their ideas would be extremely time-consuming. But even a brief look reveals serious gaps in the authors' knowledge and presentation of the subject matter. In many instances, findings applicable to small numbers of people are cited as though they apply to everyone. In some cases, treatments are recommended even though the authors indicate that the evidence supporting them is preliminary, speculative, or even conflicting. Dubious diagnostic tests are also discussed as though they have validity.

The *Encyclopedia of Natural Medicine* claims that "in most instances, the naturopathic alternative offers significant benefits over standard medical practices." For the few illnesses where the authors acknowledge that medical treatment is essential (because otherwise the patient may die), they propose naturopathic treatment in addition. In more than a few passages, the authors describe prevailing medical practices inaccurately. The book claims, for example, that medical treatment of hypothyroidism involves the use of desiccated thyroid or synthetic thyroid hormone, but that naturopaths prefer desiccated thyroid. The authors recommend supplements of iodine, tyrosine (an amino acid), vitamins A and C (in potentially toxic dosages), zinc, vitamin E, riboflavin, niacin, and pyridoxine (in unsafe amounts). This advice is ridiculous. Scientific physicians consider desiccated thyroid (made from dried animal glands) inferior because its potency can vary from batch to batch. Synthetic thyroid hormone does the job efficiently. The supplements are a waste of money. The book also claims (incorrectly) that taking one's armpit temperature upon awakening is a reliable test for thyroid function. The chapter on "Candidiasis" espouses Dr. William Crook's unsubstantiated notions (see Chapter 12) and even includes Crook's three-page questionnaire for determining the probability that "yeast-connected problems are present." The questionnaire does not have the slightest validity. The chapter on allergies says that there is "much controversy" over cytotoxic testing and that in order for electroacupuncture and muscle-testing (applied kinesiology) to gain wider acceptance, more research will have to be done and a satisfactory explanation of their mode of action will have to be developed. Since none of these quack procedures makes the slightest sense, no amount of research can prove them valid.

Murray is also a strong proponent of "juicing" (see Chapter 8). In *The Complete Book of Juicing*, he recommends juices for treating scores of ailments. He also advises everyone to use supplements because "even the most dedicated health advocate . . . cannot possibly meet the tremendous nutritional requirements for optimum health through diet alone." This is nonsense.

In 1968, the U.S. Department of Health, Education, and Welfare (HEW) recommended against coverage of naturopathy under Medicare. HEW's report concluded:

> Naturopathic theory and practice are not based upon the body of basic knowledge related to health, disease, and health care which has been widely accepted by the scientific community. Moreover, irrespective of its theory, the scope and quality of naturopathic education do not prepare the practitioner to make an adequate diagnosis and provide appropriate treatment.

Although some aspects of naturopathic education have improved in recent years, we believe this conclusion is still valid.

Natural Hygiene

Natural Hygiene, an offshoot of naturopathy, is a philosophy of "natural living" that advocates a raw-food diet of vegetables, fruits, and nuts; denounces most medical treatments; and promotes periodic fasting and "food combining" (avoiding food combinations it considers detrimental). Although its followers do not espouse the use of dietary supplements, they trumpet the health-food industry's philosophy about "natural foods" and its antagonism toward scientific methods. According to an American Natural Hygiene Society (ANHS) brochure:

> Natural Hygiene rejects the use of medications, blood transfusions, radiation, dietary supplements, and any other means employed to treat or "cure" various ailments. These therapies interfere with or destroy vital processes and tissue. Recovery from disease takes place in spite of, and not because of, the drugging and "curing" practices.

The brochure also states:

> A thoroughgoing rest, which includes fasting, is the most favorable condition under which an ailing body can purify and repair itself. Fasting is the total abstinence from all liquid or solid foods except distilled water. During a fast the body's recuperative forces are marshalled and all of its energies are directed toward the recharging of the nervous system, the elimination of toxic accumulations, and the repair and rejuvenation of tissue. Stored within each organism's tissues are nutrient reserves which it will use to carry on metabolism and repair work. Until these reserves are depleted, no destruction of healthy tissue or "starvation" can occur.

Regular ANHS membership costs $25 and includes a subscription to *Health Science,* the group's thirty-two-page bimonthly magazine. Natural Hygiene is said to have been founded during the 1830s by Sylvester Graham. An article in *Health Science* stated that Natural Hygiene enjoyed considerable popularity, but then declined until it was "resuscitated" from being "almost dead" by Herbert M. Shelton (1895-1985). ANHS was founded in 1948 by Shelton and several associates and is now headquartered in Tampa, Florida. The group has about eight thousand members and has vigorously promoted certification of "organic foods" and opposed compulsory immunization, fluoridation, and food irradiation. *Health Science* lists twenty practitioners in the United States on its "professional referral list." Most are chiropractors, but a few hold medical, osteopathic, or naturopathic degrees.

In a 1978 interview in *Health Science*, Shelton described his educational background: "I postgraduated from the University of Hard Knocks and left before I got my diploma. I went through the usual brainwashing process of the school system in Greenville, Texas, and revolted against the whole political, religious, medical and social system at the age of sixteen." During the next several years, he obtained a "Doctor of Physiological Therapeutics" degree from the International College of Drugless Physicians, a school established by Bernarr Macfadden, and took a postgraduate course at the Lindlahr College of Natural Therapeutics in Chicago. Then he went to New York where, "after nine months of brainwashing," he acquired degrees in chiropractic and naturopathy. In 1920, after further study and apprenticeship at various institutions, Shelton published the first of his forty books, *Fundamentals of Nature Cure.* In 1928, he founded Dr. Shelton's Health School in San Antonio, which operated at seven different locations until 1981.

In 1982, a federal court jury awarded over $800,000 to the survivors of William Carlton, a forty-nine-year-old man who died after undergoing a distilled water fast for thirty days at Shelton's Health School. An article in the *Los Angeles Times* stated that Carlton had died of bronchial pneumonia resulting from a weakened condition in which he lost fifty pounds during his last month of life. The article also noted that he was the sixth person in five years who had died while undergoing treatment at the school. Shelton and his chiropractic associate claimed in their appeal that Carlton had persisted in fasting even though the chiropractor had advised him to stop. However, a court of appeals upheld the verdict and the U.S. Supreme Court declined further review.

Several advocates of Natural Hygiene have produced best-selling books. *The Beverly Hills Diet* (1981) by Judy Mazel, recommends eating just fruit for the first ten days, then adding other types of foods in various combinations. The book lost most of its luster when three cases of severe diarrhea, muscle weakness, and dizziness among its followers were reported in the *Journal of the American Medical Association. Fit for Life* (1985), by Harvey and Marilyn Diamond, calls for eating fruit only in the morning and mostly vegetables during the rest of the day. A third book, *Unlimited Power* (1986), by Anthony Robbins, confines similar misinformation to a single chapter. Robbins is known best for his advocacy of firewalking and other techniques said to build self-confidence.

One reason for *Fit for Life*'s commercial success—until the media caught on—was Harvey Diamond's "Ph.D. in nutritional science" from the American College of Health Science, in Austin, Texas. This entity, which was founded in 1982 and subsequently called the College of Life Science, not only lacked accreditation but also lacked authorization from the Texas Department of Higher Education to grant degrees. Its proprietor was T.C. Fry, a high-school dropout whom Diamond described as "today's most eminent, active proponent of Natural Hygiene." During the mid-1980s, Fry's catalogs claimed "you can become an expert nutritionist in less than a year" by taking the school's 111-lesson correspondence course. Students could acquire a certificate of proficiency after thirty-two lessons, a "bachelor of science degree" after fifty-eight lessons, a "master of science degree" after eighty-four lessons, and a "doctor of philosophy degree" in nutrition science at the end. He also promised that graduates could earn $500 to $1,000 weekly as a "nutrition or health specialist . . . . even if you're not a high school graduate." In 1986, however, state authorities obtained a permanent injunction barring Fry from representing his enterprise as a college or granting any more degrees or academic credits without authorization from the Texas Department of Higher Education. Fry, doing business as the Life Science Institute (and later as Health Excellence Systems), continued to market his voluminous writings and correspondence courses. As far as we know, however, he has not violated the injunction.

Fit for Life contains more silly ideas than any other "nutrition" book we have ever seen. It states that when certain foods are combined in the body, they "rot" and "putrefy," creating digestive cesspools that somehow poison the system and make a person fat. To avoid this, the authors recommend that fats, carbohydrates, and protein foods be eaten at separate meals, concentrating on fruits in the morning and vegetables in the afternoon. They favor fruits and vegetables because foods high in water content can "wash the toxic waste from the inside of the body" instead of "clogging" the body. Actually, digestion is a process of controlled disintegration in which digestive juices break down the foods into smaller chemical components so they can pass through the intestinal wall. Contrary to the Diamonds' assertion, the process is completed within a few hours. Their ideas are on a par with the notion that the moon is made of green cheese. So, for that matter, are the vitalistic notions of macrobiotics and naturopathy.

14

Maharishi Ayur-Ved: TM Goes "Health Food"

Do you walk quickly? Are you a slow eater? Do you like to travel? Do you have trouble making decisions? Are your veins quite visible? Do you have long, thick eyelashes? Do you have soft, melting eyes? Do your dreams frequently involve fear, anxiety, being chased, running, jumping, flying, or falling?

According to the ad from Maharishi Ayurveda Products International, (MAPI) Inc., pictured on the next page, your answers to these and sixty other questions would reveal which of ten "body types" you have. "When you understand your own body type," the ad stated, "you are able to see how different foods, seasons of the year, behavior patterns and other influences affect your natural balance. That gives you much more control over the way you feel, and it allows you to compensate for imbalances long before there is a chance of falling sick." The ad also explained that "body types"—identified as *vata, pitta, kapha,* and "mixed"—"are part of a scientifically tested all-natural approach to health and happiness that can make a major difference in the quality of your life." By filling out the questionnaire and sending it with $14.95, you would receive:

> 1) Your Ayurveda body type evaluation, 2) Personalized dietary recommendations, 3) Recommendations for the special Maharishi Ayurveda herbal supplements, 4) An audiocassette tape and color brochure explaining the principles of the Maharishi Ayurveda Program.

When Dr. Stephen Barrett responded to the ad, he learned that his body type was "Kapha-Pitta." To achieve "balance" and thereby enhance his health,

The Maharishi Ayurveda program for health and happiness

What Is Your Body Type?

"Determining your Ayurvedic body type is a key step in gaining more complete control of your own health and well-being." —***Donn Wiedershine, MD***

Are you a quick-moving, restless sort of person? If so, you may be classified as a "Vata" type according to the world's most complete scientific system of natural medicine—Maharishi Ayurveda.

If you are fiery and aggressive, you are probably a "Pitta" type. If you are strong and steady, you might be a "Kapha" type. Or you may be a mixed type—there are ten possibilities in all.

These classifications are part of a scientifically tested all-natural approach to health and happiness that can make a major difference in the quality of your life.

The special power of the Maharishi Ayurveda approach is its ability to pinpoint exactly how every kind of influence affects each person's own special balance.

For example, salty food can be upsetting for a Pitta or Kapha physiology, but it can be helpful for a Vata type.

According to Donn Wiedershine, MD, a leading Maharishi Ayurveda specialist, "When you understand your own body type, you are able to see how different foods, seasons of the year, behavior patterns and other influences affect your natural balance. That gives you much more control over the way you feel, and it allows you to compensate for imbalances long before there is a chance of falling sick."

To take advantage of this valuable program, just fill out the questionnaire below. For a fee of $14.95, you will receive: 1) Your Ayurveda body type evaluation. 2) Personalized dietary recommendations. 3) Recommendations for special Maharishi Ayurveda herbal supplements. 4) An audiocassette tape and color brochure by leading doctors explaining the principles of the Maharishi Ayurveda program.

Your satisfaction is guaranteed.

Instructions: *For each item, circle the number that indicates how well the statement describes you. Circle "0" if it does not describe you at all. Circle "6" if it describes you fully. If it describes you somewhat, circle a number between "0" and "6" to show how much it describes you. This information will be kept confidential.*

Section 1

1. Quick about doing things, walks quickly 0 1 2 3 4 5 6
2. Poor memory 0 1 2 3 4 5 6
3. Enthusiastic and vivacious 0 1 2 3 4 5 6
4. Thin physique, don't gain weight easily 0 1 2 3 4 5 6
5. Learn new things very quickly 0 1 2 3 4 5 6
6. Veins quite visible 0 1 2 3 4 5 6
7. Have difficulty making decision 0 1 2 3 4 5 6
8. Digestion not too strong, tendency to have gas or constipation 0 1 2 3 4 5 6
9. Cold hands and feet 0 1 2 3 4 5 6
10. Tendency towards anxiety and worry 0 1 2 3 4 5 6
11. Sensitive to cold weather 0 1 2 3 4 5 6
12. Easily influenced by environment 0 1 2 3 4 5 6
13. Talkative, rapid in speech 0 1 2 3 4 5 6
14. Joints make cracking and popping sounds 0 1 2 3 4 5 6
15. Not much tolerance for physical exercise or work 0 1 2 3 4 5 6
16. Teeth are either very large or very small and somewhat irregularly space or crooked 0 1 2 3 4 5 6
17. Emotional 0 1 2 3 4 5 6
18. Difficulty in falling asleep or light and interrupted sleep 0 1 2 3 4 5 6
19. Dry skin 0 1 2 3 4 5 6
20. Dreams frequently involve fear, anxiety, being chased, running, jumping, flying, falling 0 1 2 3 4 5 6
21. Easily become afraid 0 1 2 3 4 5 6
22. Like to travel 0 1 2 3 4 5 6
23. Lean body type 0 1 2 3 4 5 6

Section 2

1. Very sharp intellect 0 1 2 3 4 5 6
2. Strong digestion—can eat anything you like 0 1 2 3 4 5 6
3. Perspire easily 0 1 2 3 4 5 6
4. Aversion to hot weather—prefer weather that is too cold rather than too hot 0 1 2 3 4 5 6
5. Become uncomfortable if a meal is delayed or missed 0 1 2 3 4 5 6
6. Become irritable or angry easily 0 1 2 3 4 5 6
7. Very orderly and precise in your activities 0 1 2 3 4 5 6
8. Presence of any of these: early graying of hair, balding, sandy blond or red hair color, early wrinkling 0 1 2 3 4 5 6
9. Large capacity for food 0 1 2 3 4 5 6
10. Stubborn, stick to your own ideas 0 1 2 3 4 5 6
11. Outspoken in your ideas 0 1 2 3 4 5 6
12. Bold and adventurous 0 1 2 3 4 5 6
13. Chivalrous and courteous 0 1 2 3 4 5 6
14. Complexion which is red or yellowish in color 0 1 2 3 4 5 6
15. Two or more bowel movements per day which tend to be somewhat loose 0 1 2 3 4 5 6
16. Prefer cold foods and drinks 0 1 2 3 4 5 6
17. Sharp or abrupt in speech 0 1 2 3 4 5 6
18. Anger comes easily but is short lived 0 1 2 3 4 5 6
19. Sharp, intelligent or penetrating eyes 0 1 2 3 4 5 6
20. Impatient 0 1 2 3 4 5 6
21. Sensitive to the sun—prefer the shade 0 1 2 3 4 5 6
22. Perfectionist 0 1 2 3 4 5 6
23. Medium body build and weight 0 1 2 3 4 5 6

Section 3

1. Tend to be slow and easy about doing things 0 1 2 3 4 5 6
2. Larger body build, strong muscles 0 1 2 3 4 5 6
3. Tend to gain weight easily 0 1 2 3 4 5 6
4. Easily able to miss a meal without discomfort 0 1 2 3 4 5 6
5. Peaceful mind, not easily disturbed 0 1 2 3 4 5 6
6. Tendency toward excess mucous, phlegm, respiratory problems, allergies, or sinus problems 0 1 2 3 4 5 6
7. Thick, dark, healthy, wavy hair 0 1 2 3 4 5 6
8. Happy appearance 0 1 2 3 4 5 6
9. Sleep deeply—need 8 hours or more 0 1 2 3 4 5 6
10. Soft, smooth skin 0 1 2 3 4 5 6
11. Strong, white, regular teeth 0 1 2 3 4 5 6
12. High tolerance for physical work or exercise 0 1 2 3 4 5 6
13. Slow eater 0 1 2 3 4 5 6
14. Soft, pleasing, attractive appearance 0 1 2 3 4 5 6
15. Slow, stable gait when walking 0 1 2 3 4 5 6
16. Speech tends to be sweet and soft in nature 0 1 2 3 4 5 6
17. Slow to get irritated 0 1 2 3 4 5 6
18. Excellent memory 0 1 2 3 4 5 6
19. Tendency towards plumpness 0 1 2 3 4 5 6
20. Athletic physique 0 1 2 3 4 5 6
21. Long, thick eyelashes 0 1 2 3 4 5 6
22. Large, soft, melting eyes 0 1 2 3 4 5 6

Name ____________

Address ____________

City/State/Zip ____________

Evaluation Fee: $14.95 ❑ Check enclosed

❑ Visa ❑ MC Acct. # ____________ Exp. Dt.

Cut out this page and send to: Maharishi Ayurveda Products Int'l, Inc. Lake Shandelee Rd., Dept. V, Livingston Manor, NY 12758

©1988 Maharishi Ayurveda Products International, Inc.

Tear out this entire page

Ad from March 1988 *Vegetarian Times* magazine.

he was advised to follow a "pitta-pacifying diet" in the late spring and a "kapha-pacifying diet" in early spring, and also to include various Maharishi Ayur-Veda herb teas and spices. In addition, he was advised to take *Maharishi Amrit Kalash* (herbal tablets and fruit concentrate), investigate transcendental meditation (TM), and consult an ayurvedic physician for a more detailed evaluation. Instead of following this advice, however, he collected a large number of source materials in order to see what this mumbo jumbo was all about. One of these was a MAPI booklet that claimed: "The value of Maharishi Ayur-Veda is that it does not treat superficial symptoms. It corrects the underlying imbalance which is the root cause of any health problem."

"Ancient Roots"

According to Maharishi proponents, ayurvedic medicine originated several thousand years ago (published estimates vary from two thousand to six thousand years), but much of it was lost until reconstituted in the early 1980s by the Maharishi Mahesh Yogi, the founder of TM. The "revived" version has been termed Maharishi Ayurveda, Maharishi Ayur-Veda and, more recently, Maharishi Ayur-Ved. Maharishi Ayur-Veda (now called Maharishi Ayur-Ved) is also the trademarked name of products sold by the Maharishi's followers. However, these names are often used interchangeably.

Ayur comes from the Sanskrit *ayus*, meaning "life" or "life span." *Veda* has been interpreted as "knowledge" and "science." Thus, ayurveda is supposedly the science of life or longevity. Ayurvedic medicine is rooted in four Sanskrit books called the *Vedas*—the oldest and most important scriptures of India, shaped sometime before 200 B.C.E. These books attributed most disease and bad luck to demons, devils, and the influence of stars and planets. Ayurveda's basic theory states that the body's functions are regulated by three "irreducible physiological principles" called *doshas*, whose Sanskrit names are *vata, pitta,* and *kapha*. Like astrologic "signs," these terms are used to designate individuals as well as the traits that typify them.

• *Vata* is said to represent motion and flow and to control breathing, circulation, and neuromuscular activity. Its dominant characteristic is said to be "changeable." Its attributes are said to be "dry, light, cold, rough, subtle, mobile, clear, and dispersing." The problems caused by *vata* "imbalance" are said to include short attention span, fatigue, insomnia, dry skin, constipation, intestinal gas, and menstrual cramps. To "balance" *vata*, people should eat more sweet, sour, and salty foods.

• *Pitta* is said to control metabolism, energy exchange, and digestion. Its dominant characteristic is "intense." Its attributes are said to be "oily, penetrating, hot, light, mobile, liquid, and sour smell." The problems caused by *pitta* "imbalance" allegedly include impatience, tyrannical behavior, hot flashes, skin diseases, high blood pressure, and peptic ulcers. To "balance" *pitta*, people should eat more sweet, astringent, and bitter foods.

• *Kapha* is said to control body structure, cohesion, and balance. Its dominant characteristic is "relaxed." Its attributes are said to be "heavy, slow, cold, oily, slimy, dense, soft, and static." *Kapha* "imbalance" allegedly causes clumsiness, depression, high cholesterol, drowsiness, cysts and allergies, overweight, procrastination, possessiveness, and greed. To "balance" *kapha*, people should eat more bitter, astringent, and pungent foods.

Like astrologic writings, ayurvedic writings contain long lists of supposed physical and mental characteristics of each constitutional type. For example, *Ayurveda: The Science of Self-Healing,* by Vasant Lad, M.D., tabulates twenty for each type, some of which are listed in the table on the following page. Lad notes, however:

> These descriptions reflect the pure aspect of each constitutional element; however, no individual constitution is made up solely of any

Body-Mind Characteristics
(From *Ayurveda: The Science of Self-Healing*)

Feature	Vata	Pitta	Kapha
Frame	Thin	Moderate	Thick
Hair	Black, dry, kinky	Soft, oily, yellow, early gray, red	Thick, oily, wavy, dark or light
Teeth	Protruded, big and crooked. Gums emaciated	Moderate in size. Soft gums. Yellowish	Strong. White
Physical activity	Very active	Moderate	Lethargic
Pulse	Thready, feeble, moves like a snake	Moderate, jumping like a frog	Broad. Slow. Moves like a swan
Financial status	Poor. Spends money quickly on trifles	Moderate. Spends on luxuries	Rich. Moneysaver. Spends on food

> one element. Rather, each person is a combination of all three elements, with a predominant tendency toward one or more. These characteristics must be further adjusted according to racial tendencies and cultural preferences, since different races and cultures have native proclivities for specific body and lifestyle characteristics.

He further states:

> The symptoms of disease are always related to derangement of the balance of the [three doshas]. Once we understand the nature of the imbalance, balance may be reestablished through treatment.
>
> Ayurveda teaches us very precise methods for understanding the disease process before any overt signs of the disease have manifested. . . . Day to day observations of the pulse, tongue, face, eyes, nails and lips provide subtle indicators. Through these, the student of Ayurveda can learn what pathological processes are occurring in the body, which organs are impaired, and where the *dosha* and toxins have accumulated. Thus . . . pathological symptoms can be detected early and preventative measures taken.

Maharishi Ayur-Veda proponents claim that pulse-reading is "like a window giving a complete view of your psychophysiology at any given time." A MAPI booklet states:

> In Western medicine, where physicians "take your pulse," they simply count the number of beats per minute. But Ayurvedic pulse diagnosis

> is a sophisticated science. Ayurvedic doctors are trained to detect specific qualities . . . that indicate a state of balance or imbalance in Vata, Pitta and Kapha. They can even tell what area of the body has accumulated an imbalance and what type of symptoms are likely to develop if the imbalance is not corrected. . . . Pulse diagnosis is an extremely valuable technique because it allows the physician to detect the specific imbalance that is the root cause of any health problem.

In the videotape "Introduction to Maharishi Ayurveda Consultation Program," Richard Averbach, M.D., vice president of the Maharishi Ayurveda Association of America, states that the "root cause of disease" can be found in "the relationship between mind and body."

TM Comes East

Transcendental meditation (TM) is a technique in which the meditator sits comfortably with eyes closed and mentally repeats a Sanskrit word or sound (mantra) for fifteen to twenty minutes, twice a day. Although the teacher supposedly chooses the mantra to fit each individual, investigators have noted that people with similar sociocultural characteristics often receive the same mantra.

TM is alleged to help people think more clearly, improve their memory, recover immediately from stressful situations, reverse their aging process, and enjoy life more fully. Proponents also claim that "stress is the basis of all illness" and that TM is "the single most effective thing you can do to improve all aspects of health and to increase inner happiness and learning ability." Meditation may temporarily relieve stress—as would many types of relaxation techniques—but the rest of these claims have no scientific basis.

The TM movement was launched in India in 1955 by the Maharishi Mahesh Yogi, who had studied mysticism for many years. According to *TM: Discovering Inner Energy and Overcoming Stress* (1975), by Harold H. Bloomfield, M.D., and associates, in 1958 the Maharishi "proclaimed the possibility of all humanity's attaining enlightenment" and inaugurated a "World Plan" intended to encompass "every individual on earth." Shortly thereafter, he embarked upon a world tour to spread his teachings.

Eric Woodrum, a sociologist who spent a year as a participant-observer of TM activities, has divided the early TM movement into three phases. From 1959 to 1965, TM was promoted as the most important component of a program of spiritual evolution and mental detachment (nirvana). During the late 1960s, the movement expanded rapidly as it won major publicity by identifying with aspects of the counterculture. Since 1970, the movement has emphasized alleged practical, physiological, material, and social benefits of TM for conventional persons, with few other-worldly references. Woodrum concluded that average meditators regarded TM as a useful mental exercise and paid little or no attention to its quasireligious belief system. Members of the inner movement, however, think in metaphysical terms and state that TM can transform the world. TM leaders maintain that large groups of people meditating together produce "the Maharishi Effect," which can reduce the incidence of crime and auto accidents. This claim has been debunked by investigators who checked statistics in cities where the phenomenon had allegedly occurred.

In the mid-1970s, the Maharishi began professing he could teach advanced meditators to levitate (rise and float in apparent defiance of gravity). Although thousands of people paid $3,000 each for lessons, the best they could demonstrate was cross-legged "hopping" to an altitude of about a foot.

In 1987, a federal court jury awarded $137,890 to an ex-devotee who contended that TM organizations had falsely promised that he could learn to levitate, reduce stress, improve his memory, and reverse the aging process. In 1988, an appeals court ordered a new trial. In 1991, the *Des Moines Register* reported that the case had been settled out of court for about $50,000.

Ayurveda Is "Enlivened"

A MAPI brochure states that in 1980, the Maharishi "gathered around him the foremost . . . renowned scholars and physicians of Ayur-Ved, to enliven the age-old knowledge of Ayur-Ved in its completeness and original purity." The result, according to MAPI, was "a new breakthrough in natural medicine which offers a scientifically validated and truly holistic approach to health." Maharishi Ayurveda's goal, another brochure states, "is to prevent disease and promote perfect health and longevity, creating a disease-free individual and a disease-free society." According to proponents, about six hundred American physicians subsequently became members of the American Association of Ayurvedic Medicine (AAAM), with one hundred of them "fully trained in Maharishi Ayur-Veda techniques and practices."

AAAM was founded in 1985 by Deepak Chopra, M.D., an endocrinologist who became director of the Maharishi Ayurveda Health Center in Lancaster, Massachusetts, as well as president of AAAM. Chopra has written seven books and gained considerable public exposure through appearances on the "Donahue" and "Oprah Winfrey" shows. One of his books, *Ageless Body, Timeless Mind,* is reported to have sold over a million copies. The April 11, 1994, issue of *Forbes* magazine called Chopra "the latest in a line of gurus who have prospered by blending pop science, pop psychology, and pop Hinduism."

Chopra promises "perfect health" to those who—with the help of Maharishi Ayur-Veda—can harness their consciousness as a healing force. Chopra claims that "remaining healthy is actually a conscious choice." He states:

> If you have happy thoughts, then you make happy molecules. On the other hand, if you have sad thoughts, and angry thoughts, and hostile thoughts, then you make those molecules which may depress the immune system and make you more susceptible to disease.

Chopra's audiocassette program, "Magical Mind, Magical Body," is marketed by Nightingale-Conant with promises that it will help you "achieve a brilliantly blissful life." On the "Donahue" show, Chopra maintained that people who are happy not only have fewer colds but are less likely to get heart disease or cancer. Elsewhere he has said that the herbs prescribed in ayurvedic treatment "take the intelligence of the universe and match it with the intelligence of our own body."

In 1993, Chopra left the Lancaster clinic, ceased his formal affiliation with the TM organization, and became executive director of the Sharp Institute for Human Potential and Mind Body Medicine in San Diego, California. In this capacity, he expects to lecture and do research related to ayurvedic methods. He is also a consultant to the Center for Mind Body Medicine, which charges $1,125 to $3,200 for its weeklong "purification" program.

TM Goes the Health-Food Route

MAPI has advertised in health-food magazines that in 1986 three ayurvedic physicians revived an ancient herbal formula called *Maharishi Amrit Kalash*. The ads state that the formula "brought perfect health to the Vedic civilization thousands of years ago" and can "restore balance and order to the entire physiology by enlivening the connection between mind and body." Since that time, MAPI has offered an expanding line of herbal formulas and teas, "designer foods," personal-care products, cough syrups, mineral supplements (with herbs), books, audiocassettes, and CDs, variously promised to "nourish," "cleanse," "balance," "protect," "energize," "vitalize," "invigorate," "enliven," "soothe," "strengthen," "correct," "stabilize," "improve," and/or "regulate" the mind, the body, or a body component. Its herbal formulas include *Mind Plus* ("for aiding mental activity"), *Rasayana One* ("for balance"), *Rasayana Two* ("to aid mental clarity"), *Meda Formula* ("for better metabolism of fat"), *Hepata Care* ("for aiding liver function"), *Hepata Care, Jr.* ("for children under 12"), and *Rasayana for Students* ("to nourish the full potential of your mind"). MAPI also markets its products through health-food stores. "Perfect Health" Gift Certificates are available in $15, $25, and $50 denominations.

*Maharishi Amrit Kalas*h, "recommended for everyone for daily use," comes as *Ambrosia* herbal tablets and *Nectar* herbal fruit concentrate (a black, foul-smelling powder). People who join the MAPI Continuity Club receive automatic monthly shipments of both products for about $900 a year. A MAPI brochure states:

> Maharishi Amrit Kalash is a highly sophisticated herbal complex that strengthens, balances, and awakens the full potential of mind and body in a way no ordinary supplement can. . . .
>
> In a recent survey, 78% of the people interviewed said Maharishi Amrit Kalash was the most beneficial supplement they had ever taken. The majority also reported:
>
> - more energy, stamina, and freedom from fatigue
> - improved mental clarity
> - greater happiness and well-being
> - more calmness and reduced stress.

One recent ad claims that *Maharishi Amrit Kalash* is "up to 1,000 times more potent in fighting free radicals than vitamins C and E." Another claims that it is "1,000 times more effective than vitamin C or E" as an antioxidant and is "the most effective substance ever tested for eliminating excess free radicals and the damage they cause." We don't believe these statements can be substantiated or even tested.

Many other herbal preparations have been available through ayurvedic physicians who can purchase them at a 30 percent discount for resale to their patients. A catalog from the late 1980s refers to these products as "food supplements" but states which ones are useful ("as a dietary complement") for cancer, epilepsy, poliomyelitis, schizophrenia, tuberculosis, and more than eighty other ailments. Another publication, marked "confidential," lists "indications according to disease entities" for about seventy products identified by number. Practitioners may also select remedies with "Maharishi Ayurveda Treatment and Prevention Programs," a computer program that generates reports for both the doctor and the patient. The data entered include disease codes and body types. Another service that has been available from practitioners is "Blissfully Thin: The Maharishi Ayurveda Approach to Effortless Weight Loss,"

Proponents claim that Maharishi Ayur-Ved offers "the most powerful technology of prevention in the world today" and provides a "solution to the health care crisis." Its full program for "creating healthy individuals and a disease-free society" has twenty components: development of higher states of consciousness through advanced meditation techniques, use of primordial sounds, correction of "the mistake of the intellect," strengthening of emotions,

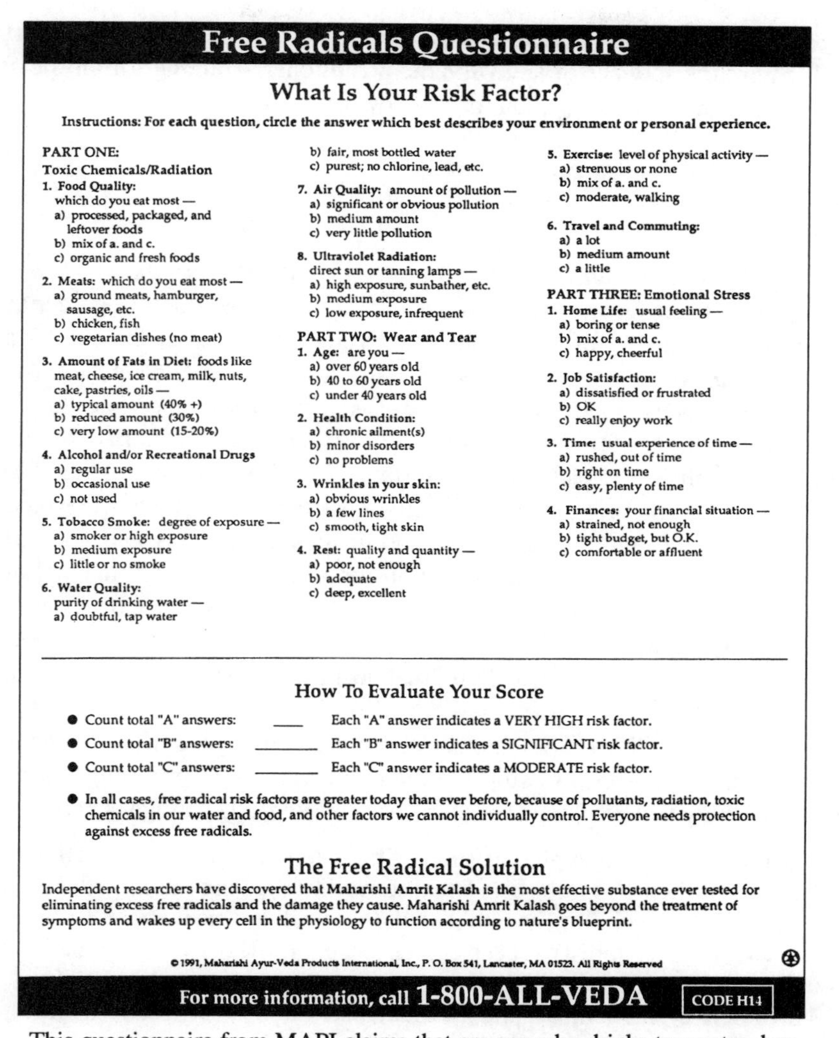

Free Radicals Questionnaire

What Is Your Risk Factor?

Instructions: For each question, circle the answer which best describes your environment or personal experience.

PART ONE:
Toxic Chemicals/Radiation

1. **Food Quality:** which do you eat most —
   a) processed, packaged, and leftover foods
   b) mix of a. and c.
   c) organic and fresh foods

2. **Meats:** which do you eat most —
   a) ground meats, hamburger, sausage, etc.
   b) chicken, fish
   c) vegetarian dishes (no meat)

3. **Amount of Fats in Diet:** foods like meat, cheese, ice cream, milk, nuts, cake, pastries, oils —
   a) typical amount (40% +)
   b) reduced amount (30%)
   c) very low amount (15-20%)

4. **Alcohol and/or Recreational Drugs**
   a) regular use
   b) occasional use
   c) not used

5. **Tobacco Smoke:** degree of exposure —
   a) smoker or high exposure
   b) medium exposure
   c) little or no smoke

6. **Water Quality:** purity of drinking water —
   a) doubtful, tap water
   b) fair, most bottled water
   c) purest; no chlorine, lead, etc.

7. **Air Quality:** amount of pollution —
   a) significant or obvious pollution
   b) medium amount
   c) very little pollution

8. **Ultraviolet Radiation:** direct sun or tanning lamps —
   a) high exposure, sunbather, etc.
   b) medium exposure
   c) low exposure, infrequent

PART TWO: Wear and Tear

1. **Age:** are you —
   a) over 60 years old
   b) 40 to 60 years old
   c) under 40 years old

2. **Health Condition:**
   a) chronic ailment(s)
   b) minor disorders
   c) no problems

3. **Wrinkles in your skin:**
   a) obvious wrinkles
   b) a few lines
   c) smooth, tight skin

4. **Rest:** quality and quantity —
   a) poor, not enough
   b) adequate
   c) deep, excellent

5. **Exercise:** level of physical activity —
   a) strenuous or none
   b) mix of a. and c.
   c) moderate, walking

6. **Travel and Commuting:**
   a) a lot
   b) medium amount
   c) a little

PART THREE: Emotional Stress

1. **Home Life:** usual feeling —
   a) boring or tense
   b) mix of a. and c.
   c) happy, cheerful

2. **Job Satisfaction:**
   a) dissatisfied or frustrated
   b) OK
   c) really enjoy work

3. **Time:** usual experience of time —
   a) rushed, out of time
   b) right on time
   c) easy, plenty of time

4. **Finances:** your financial situation —
   a) strained, not enough
   b) tight budget, but O.K.
   c) comfortable or affluent

How To Evaluate Your Score

- Count total "A" answers: ____ Each "A" answer indicates a VERY HIGH risk factor.
- Count total "B" answers: ________ Each "B" answer indicates a SIGNIFICANT risk factor.
- Count total "C" answers: ________ Each "C" answer indicates a MODERATE risk factor.
- In all cases, free radical risk factors are greater today than ever before, because of pollutants, radiation, toxic chemicals in our water and food, and other factors we cannot individually control. Everyone needs protection against excess free radicals.

The Free Radical Solution

Independent researchers have discovered that **Maharishi Amrit Kalash** is the most effective substance ever tested for eliminating excess free radicals and the damage they cause. Maharishi Amrit Kalash goes beyond the treatment of symptoms and wakes up every cell in the physiology to function according to nature's blueprint.

© 1991, Maharishi Ayur-Veda Products International, Inc., P. O. Box 541, Lancaster, MA 01523. All Rights Reserved

For more information, call **1-800-ALL-VEDA** CODE H14

This questionnaire from MAPI claims that anyone who drinks tap water, has strained finances, travels or commutes a lot, or engages in strenuous exercise is at very high risk for free radical damage.

Vedic structuring of language, music therapy, enlivening of the senses, pulse diagnosis, psychophysiological integration, neuromuscular integration, neurorespiratory integration, purification (to remove "impurities due to faulty diet and behavioral patterns"), dietary measures, herbal food supplements, other herbal preparations, daily behavioral routines, religious ceremonies, nourishing the environment, and promoting world health and world peace.

Most of these programs cost several hundred dollars, but some cost thousands and require the services of an ayurvedic practitioner. Training for physician practitioners costs about $4,000 for coursework.

JAMA Reacts

In May 1991, the *Journal of the American Medical Association (JAMA)* published a letter from by Chopra and two others, which described certain theories and practices of Maharishi Ayur-Veda. Shortly after the letter was published, *JAMA*'s editors learned that the authors had violated *JAMA*'s conflict-of-interest policy by failing to reveal various connections to TM enterprises. This triggered a report by *JAMA* associate news editor Andrew A. Skolnick, published in October, which stated: "An investigation of the [TM] movement's marketing practices reveals what appears to be a widespread pattern of misinformation, deception, and manipulation of lay and scientific news media." The American Association for Ayur-Vedic Medicine and the Lancaster Foundation (a nonprofit foundation that supports TM and Maharishi Ayur-Veda research) responded with a lawsuit accusing Skolnick and *JAMA*'s editor (George M. Lundberg, M.D.) of making false and defamatory statements in the article.

In August 1992, a U.S. District Court judge denied plaintiffs' motion for a preliminary injunction to stop Skolnick and Lundberg from engaging in further activity that disparages Maharishi Ayur-Veda. The judge stated:

> Because we find that plaintiffs have little likelihood of success on the merits of their claim . . . and because we find that the public will be harmed by the chilling of public debate regarding a health care issue in which keen interest has been evidenced, plaintiff's motion is denied.
>
> . . . .We find that the statements made by defendants must be afforded protection, despite the fact that they have caused some damage to plaintiffs' reputation.

In 1993, the judge dismissed the suit "without prejudice," which means it can be filed again. Do you think it will be? Do you think that "balancing" your "doshas" will lead to perfect health? Do you believe that Maharishi Ayur-Ved can solve America's healthcare crisis? We do not.

15
"Chiropractic Nutrition"

In 1979, a chiropractor in Peoria, Illinois, prescribed massive doses of vitamin A for nine-year-old Lynne Cramton and her four-year-old brother Dale II. Their mother had sought help for their ichthyosis, a congenital disorder in which the skin is scaly and resembles that of a fish. Claiming that his treatment would strengthen their immune system, the chiropractor advised vitamin regimens that included daily vitamin A dosage of 750,000 International Units (IU) for Lynne and 675,000 IU for Dale. These amounts were more than two hundred times the RDA and over twenty times the level at which the body's stores of vitamin A are likely to build up to toxic levels.

Within a few months, both children developed symptoms of vitamin A poisoning. Lynne experienced headaches (caused by swelling of the brain), musculoskeletal pain and tenderness, hair loss for two months, and damage to the growth centers of several of her bones. Dale developed bone pain and enlargement of his liver and spleen. Although their acute symptoms subsided after the vitamin A was stopped, both children were permanently damaged. One of Lynne's legs is several inches shorter than the other, which has caused her to develop scoliosis. Dale has permanent damage to his liver and spleen. Suits on their behalf against the chiropractor and two vitamin A manufacturers were eventually settled for a total of about $900,000. But, of course, no amount of money can repair the health problems caused by the excessive vitamin A.

The chiropractor's "treatment" was not only senseless but took place a month after the FDA had issued a monograph and proposed rule on vitamin and mineral products for over-the-counter use. Based on the advice of an expert advisory panel, the document described the toxic effects of high-dose vitamin A and said that vitamin A had not been proven safe or effective against ichthyosis.

Survey Results

The percentage of chiropractors engaging in unscientific nutrition practices is unknown, but several reports suggest that it is substantial. In 1980, 84 percent of 2,715 chiropractors who responded to a survey by the California Board of Chiropractic Examiners said they provided nutrition supplements to their patients. In 1988, 74 percent of about 2,400 respondents to a survey by the leading chiropractic newspaper, *Dynamic Chiropractic,* reported using nutrition supplements in their practices.

Not long afterward, researchers from San Jose State University's Department of Nutrition and Food Science mailed a survey to 438 members of the San Francisco Bay Area Chiropractic Society. Of the one hundred who responded, 60 percent said that they routinely provide nutrition information to their patients, 38 percent said they provide it on request, 60 percent claimed that they treat patients for nutritional deficiencies, 19 percent said they use hair analysis, and 9 percent indicated that they use "applied kinesiology" for nutritional assessment.

In 1989, a spokesperson for Douglas Laboratories (a company that sells nutrition products only to chiropractors) stated that "roughly 65 percent of all chiropractors are dispensing nutrition products, and more of them are doing it every day." A 1992 promotion said that Douglas's nutrition program was "the fastest, easiest way for chiropractors to build their practices" and that the company produced more than 460 nutritional products for over three thousand healthcare professionals worldwide.

A 1991 survey by the National Board of Chiropractic Examiners (NBCE) also found high percentages: 83.5 percent of 4,835 full-time practitioners who responded said they had used "nutritional counseling, therapy or supplements" and 37.2 percent said they had used applied kinesiology within the previous two years. Neither hair analysis nor applied kinesiology techniques are valid for nutrition assessment of patients.

In 1993, Paul A. Brown, M.D., telephoned one hundred chiropractic offices in Minnesota and was informed that seventy-eight of them sold vitamin supplements. Brown also inspected the vitamin/supplement section at the bookstore of Northwestern College of Chiropractic, in Bloomington, Minnesota. The section contained ninety-six linear feet of shelf space, which held 284 different products. The products included homeopathic remedies, Chinese medicinals (labeled mostly in Chinese), and a wide variety of concoctions containing vitamins, minerals, glandular substances, herbs, and/or enzymes. Most products appeared to be therapeutically worthless.

Typical Chiropractic Beliefs

Chiropractic is based upon the belief that most ailments are the result of spinal problems. The "discovery" of chiropractic was announced in 1895 by Daniel David Palmer, a grocer and "magnetic healer" who practiced in Davenport, Iowa. Palmer believed that he had restored the hearing of a partially deaf janitor by "adjusting" a bump on his spine. Not long afterward he decided that the basic cause of disease is "nerve interference" caused by misaligned spinal bones that could be adjusted back into place by hand.

Today's 45,000+ chiropractors can be divided into two main types: "straights" and "mixers." Straights tend to cling to Palmer's doctrine that most illness is caused by misaligned vertebrae ("subluxations") that can be corrected by "spinal adjustment." Mixers acknowledge that germs, hormones, and other factors play a role in disease, but they tend to regard mechanical disturbances of the nervous system as the underlying cause (through "lowered resistance"). In addition to spinal manipulation, mixers may use nutritional methods and various types of physiotherapy (heat, cold, traction, exercise, massage, and ultrasound). About three hundred chiropractors have joined the National Association for Chiropractic Medicine (NACM), a reformist group that has renounced Palmer's basic theories. Its members limit their practice to musculoskeletal problems and have denounced the unscientific methods used by other chiropractors. NACM is merging into the newly formed Orthopractic Manipulation Society of North America, a group based on similar principles but open to physicians and physical therapists as well.

Many chiropractic communication channels promote the questionable claims of food faddists described throughout this book. Articles in many chiropractic publications exaggerate what nutrients can do. Many of their magazines, newspapers, and journals contain ads by companies that market irrational supplement formulations intended for treating health problems for which they have not been proven safe and/or effective. The American Chiropractic Association (ACA), which is the largest chiropractic organization, has sponsored seminars featuring such speakers as Emanuel Cheraskin and the late Carlton Fredericks (see Chapter 17). Seminars sponsored by food supplement companies and by various "chiropractic nutritionists" advocate many highly questionable nutritional methods. A few seminars have even recommended quack cancer remedies. Logan College of Chiropractic and the ACA Council on Nutrition sponsor twelve-hour seminars on "The Subluxation Complex: Neurological and Nutritional Considerations." The course's purpose is to "describe how diet and nutritional supplementation can inhibit the production of the chemical irritants [that perpetuate subluxations]. . . . Nutrition applied to our patients in this fashion constitutes a nutritional or biochemical adjustment."

Although some aspects of scientific nutrition are taught in chiropractic schools, many ideas that chiropractors absorb—before, during, and after their schooling—are as unscientific as their basic theory of disease. Chiropractors who give nutritional advice typically recommend vitamin supplements that are unnecessary or are inappropriate for treating health problems. Some chiropractors charge thousands of dollars for programs involving "diagnostic" evaluations, vitamins, adjustments, and/or massage over a period of several months.

Some chiropractors who prescribe supplements but don't sell them refer their patients to health-food stores. David Singer, D.C., who teaches chiropractors how to build their practice, suggests setting up a relationship in which: (1) patients referred to the store get a discount, (2) store employees get a 50 percent discount on chiropractic services, (3) the store distributes "stress surveys" that encourage consultation with the chiropractor, (4) customers who complain of health problems are given a "courtesy card" for a free chiropractic examination, and (5) the chiropractor conducts "stress evaluations" at the store, which will draw in passersby who shop before or after the test.

ACA Council on Nutrition

The American Chiropractic Association's Council on Nutrition, founded in 1974, has about three hundred members. It holds symposiums and seminars and publishes a quarterly journal (*Nutritional Perspectives*) and a monthly newsletter. The journal states that the council is "dedicated to the health of mankind on the premise that proper nutrition is a major factor in promoting and maintaining good health and preventing disease." During the past two years, the journal has contained editorials, letters to the editor, abstracts of scientific reports, book reviews, reprints from *FDA Consumer* and other publications, and a few skimpy case reports. One issue contained an article claiming that hypothyroidism is rampant and telling how chiropractors should diagnose it (with an unscientific test) and treat it (inappropriately) with supplements. Typical issues contain twenty-eight to thirty-two pages, of which about 35 percent are ads by supplement manufacturers. The title page states that ads "are initially screened" by a committee of the council, but that neither the council nor its personnel are responsible for the advertising and that publication of the ads does not imply approval or endorsement by the journal or the council.

Recent issues of the council's newsletter have supported the (bogus) idea that mercury-amalgam fillings are dangerous and opposed pending legislation to strengthen the FDA. One issue was accompanied by a form letter asking the FDA to lift its ban on L-tryptophan supplements.

The Council on Nutrition also appoints the American Chiropractic Board of Nutrition, which sets standards and administers a certifying examination for chiropractors. To become certified, chiropractors must take three hundred hours of approved courses and pass an examination in basic and clinical nutrition. The 1994 ACA membership directory lists thirty-five chiropractors who were board-certified as of October 1993. To maintain certification status, the chiropractor must submit evidence each year of active involvement in chiropractic education at an approved college or must submit detailed case histories or a paper on nutrition for publication. However, *Nutritional Perspectives* contains few case reports or research studies by council members.

In 1991, the ACA passed the following resolution, which was co-authored by the executive director of its Council on Nutrition:

> The ACA's Council on Nutrition holds the position that it is appropriate for doctors of chiropractic to recommend the use of vitamins, minerals, and food supplements for their patients, to the extent this is not in conflict with state statutes and regulations. The recommendation of nutritional supplements should include a nutritional assessment of the patient. The practitioner shall record the rationale for the supplements in the patient's chart. The doctor should attempt to determine that the products being recommended are not experimental.

[Translation: Chiropractors may recommend anything they call a food supplement as long as some reason for its use is recorded in the patient's chart and an *attempt* is made to figure out whether the product works. Whether the reason makes sense or the product actually works is besides the point.]

A similar resolution was passed regarding weight-control programs. Commenting on these resolutions, the newsletter's editor said:

> Save and memorize these resolutions! Their importance cannot be overstated. Before these resolutions were passed, there was no official "opinion" or direction by the ACA regarding this area. With these resolutions, we have, for the first time, something in writing; a part of the American Chiropractic Association that says YES WE CAN use nutrition. . . . Now we have the clout and the backing of the American Chiropractic Association behind us.

Marketing Strategies of Supplement Companies

Many companies market supplements exclusively or primarily through chiropractic offices, where they typically are sold for at least twice their wholesale cost. Thousands of these products are intended for the treatment of disease, even though they are questionable and lack FDA approval for this use. Since federal law prohibits unproven health claims on the labels of nutritional products marketed in interstate commerce (see Chapters 5 and 19), the manufacturers seldom state openly what their products are for. Instead, claims are conveyed through product literature distributed at chiropractic meetings, company-sponsored seminars, by mail, and by "independent" regional distributors who handle products for one or more companies. Some companies provide their own product literature, which may or may not provide complete directions for use. Some companies provide copies of articles from the popular press or health-food magazines that promote substances contained in their products. A few distribute elaborate manuals listing the diseases their products can supposedly treat. In 1987, for example, Seroyal Brands, Inc., published *Bioregulation Therapy Guide*, which tells which products to prescribe for more than a hundred diseases and conditions. Some companies give similar advice by telephone. Other companies stress quality or price advantage and let chiropractors figure out for themselves what the products are for. Many products are simply named after an organ (e.g., *Ora-Brain*), bodily function (*Anabolic MegaPak, Gluco-Stabil*), or health problem (*ArthEase, Candidaforte Pack*). Other products have code names or numbers that the company explains elsewhere.

During the past two years, Dr. Stephen Barrett has surveyed catalogs, ads, and product literature from more than fifty companies that market "supplement" products to chiropractors. Vita-Herbs, of St. Louis, Missouri, even markets a product called *Spine Align,* a "biologically active concentrate of freeze-dried raw whole spinal column." Literature for the product states it can "repair," "regenerate," "correct," and "normalize" the spine and "activate the body's own Innate." (This refers to "Innate Intelligence," the metaphysical term used by fundamentalist chiropractors to describe the body's self-healing capacity.) The table opposite illustrates illegal claims made by ten other companies. (Each box represents one company.)

Regional distributors may mail information or visit chiropractic offices in much the same way that drug "detailers" attempt to inform physicians. However, the information delivered by legitimate drug company representatives is strictly regulated by the FDA and must be complete and based on well designed scientific tests. The information delivered to chiropractors has neither of these characteristics and is transmitted through channels that are intended to be hidden from the FDA. It is clear that much of the communication system between supplement manufacturers and distributors and their chiropractic clients is intended to avoid government prosecution by "distancing" illegal claims from product labels.

Several chiropractors and naturopaths have written manuals suggesting specific products for large numbers of diseases. Those that we have collected within the past few years contain a disclaimer that nothing should be construed as a claim or representation that any of the products mentioned constitutes or is intended for use as a cure, palliative, or ameliorative for any of the conditions noted. One of the books, *The Unauthorized Guide to Nutritional Products & Their Uses,* by David Williams, D.C., states that its information was "compiled from specific recommendations made by various manufacturers." The fifty-eight-page guide specifies which products from three manufacturers can be used to treat diabetes, epilepsy, glaucoma, "most cardiovascular problems," multiple sclerosis, and more than two hundred other health problems.

Illegal Claims Made for "Nutritional" Products

Products	Claims in Catalogs or Product Literature
Super Fat Burner Formula	Accelerates fat loss and enhances muscle definition
Immune Life	Promotes thymosin, trophic hormones, natural killer cells, interferon, and T-cells
Hypoglycil PressureLo	The perfect product for people who feel tired and unwell Brings together the minerals, vitamins, herbs, and other key factors that address a major health concern
Astra Essence	Promotes longevity useful in our society where many show signs of premature aging or kidney deficiency from fast-paced lifestyles
Parasidal	Destroys parasites
Stress Buster	Contains . . . vital nutrients that will help you fight the "burn-out" of stress
Adrenogen The Mind System	For glandular systems overtaxed by stress or stimulants Specifically formulated to help fuel the brain's production of mental energy
Cardio-Care	Nutrition for a healthy heart — supplies all the nutrients known to benefit the heart and circulatory system
Orchic Test Infusion	Increases testosterone production to promote muscle mass and strength gains in both men and women
Yeast Protection and Defense Formula	Nutritional support for individuals experiencing candidiasis and related yeast infections

Although it advises readers to use the book as a guide, with the help of a physician, it tells how to order the products from a mail-order discount house.

In December 1991 *The Chiropractic Journal* (a newspaper distributed free-of-charge to chiropractors) published an ad from Physiologics, of Boulder, Colorado, which said:

> Are you ignoring a major income source? Spend 5 seconds per patient and increase your gross profits $53,000 or more per year. According to national studies, over 50 percent of the population could benefit from some type of nutritional support therapy. Of those individuals who use supplements, the average purchase is 1.5 supplements per visit. That means if you see an average of 30 patients per day, you will have the opportunity to provide 15 of them with nutritional supplements. Our studies show your average profit margin per patient equals $13.75 . . . = $53,625 gross profit per year.

Promotion through Seminars

Many companies (and/or their "independent" distributors) sponsor seminars at which chiropractors are taught pseudoscientific nutrition concepts—including the use of supplement products to treat disease. These seminars enable manufacturers and distributors to provide information on alleged therapeutic uses that would not be legal to place on product labels.

During the 1970s, for example, a fifteen-hour course called The Doctor's Seminar on Nutrition was conducted by Richard Murray, D.C., and John Courtney. Brochures for the seminar described them as "the two most knowledgeable men in nutrition available on the American scene today." Murray was said to practice "more nutrition than any other doctor in America," using "in excess of $200,000 of Standard Process products each year." (Whether this was a wholesale figure or the amount paid by patients was not specified.) Courtney was identified as a vice president of Standard Process Laboratories and "the most knowledgeable man in nutritional research today."

This company, a division of Vitamin Products Company, Milwaukee, Wisconsin, was founded by the late Royal Lee, a nonpracticing dentist who was described in 1963 by a prominent FDA official as "probably the largest publisher of unreliable and false nutritional information in the world." Brochures for the seminar also said that Mr. Courtney "worked closely with Dr. Lee for more than 30 years" and that in 1978, "nearly a thousand doctors listened to Dr. Murray in seminar." One of the seminar's subjects was "successful handling of multiple sclerosis, muscular dystrophy, impotency and mental disorders." Food supplements have no legitimate role in the treatment of these conditions—but no matter. One of Lee's principles, listed in Standard Process Laboratory's booklet "Applications of Nutritional Principles for the Chiropractic Profession" is: "A fact need not be 'proved' to be useful."

In recent years, Murray has been affiliated with Nutri-West, a company in Douglas, Wyoming, owned and operated by chiropractor Paul A. White. Nutri-West's distributors include Berman Chiropractic Supply (BCS), which markets supplements and homeopathic products to chiropractors and other practitioners in nine northeastern states. In 1987, a *Consumer Reports* editor on assignment to *Nutrition Forum* gained entrance to a BCS-sponsored seminar advertised by BCS as "the kickoff of Nutri-West's new therapeutic food manual." The 164-page manual, distributed at the seminar, described how to use Nutri-West products for 142 diseases and conditions including epilepsy, heart disease, and whooping cough. The cost of a regimen for a patient whose case was presented at the meeting was over $5 per day. In addition to talking about products, the speaker (who wrote the manual) described how chiropractors could send him a completed questionnaire and a sample of the patient's blood and receive a computerized "personalized therapeutic report" describing which nutrients to prescribe. The speaker also described "creative" ways to bill insurance companies so they would pay for certain tests without realizing that the tests had been misused.

Following publication of the *Nutrition Forum* article, a lawyer representing Nutri-West sent Dr. Barrett a letter stating that the manual had not been published or distributed by Nutri-West and that the speaker had "no ties whatsoever" to the company, had not helped to formulate any of its products, and had "never written or participated in the writing of any product literature that Nutri-West distributes." The letter also stated:

> Since Nutri-West has no relationship whatsoever to [the speaker] and the distributor sponsoring the seminar is totally independent, your article's assertion that Nutri-West is responsible for what transpired at the seminar is totally erroneous. . . .
>
> To avoid any further damage to Nutri-West, it is absolutely essential that Nutrition Forum . . . . issue a statement, acceptable to Nutri-West, correcting the factual inaccuracies and false implications set forth in the article. . . .
>
> If I do not receive a response to this communication within that time, I shall assume that no amicable resolution of this matter is possible and shall proceed accordingly.

Nutrition Forum's attorney replied that it would be possible to publish the attorney's assertions (with appropriate replies from Barrett) in a future issue of the newsletter. But he warned:

> It is obvious that the intended use of Nutri-West's products goes beyond what appears on their labels. The fact that a manual and associated literature which describe therapeutic uses of Nutri-West's products was given out at a meeting of potential prescribers of these products by an exclusive regional distributor of these products establishes the "intended use" rather clearly.
>
> As you know, should this case be litigated, the discovery process would enable my client to fully explore and inspect all communications between Nutri-West, its distributors, its chiropractic customers, and their patients, as well as [the seminar speaker] and his clients. We would also endeavor to inspect patient records to determine how the products are actually used. Full discovery of Nutri-West's operations is not an unappealing prospect.

This reply was accompanied by documents supporting the *Nutrition Forum* report, including a flyer promoting evening primrose oil published as "a research information service" by Nutri-West. The contents of the flyer had also been published, word-for-word, as an article in *The American Chiropractor*—co-authored by Dr. White and the seminar speaker. Nothing further was heard from either Nutri-West or its attorney.

In 1992, Jack Raso, M.S., R.D., attended a BCS-sponsored ten-hour seminar promoting Nutri-West products. The speaker was Murray—retired from practice but described in the seminar flyer as "the dean of contemporary clinical nutrition," an "internationally acclaimed researcher, teacher, and consultant," and a lifelong friend and colleague of Royal Lee. Among other things, Murray recommended that people in perfect health take six supplement products each day, a "preventative" regimen that would cost about $36 per month. Some of the products had been formulated by him for Nutri-West. Raso's observations are detailed in the chapter on "chiropractic nutrition" in *Mystical Diets* (Prometheus Books, 1993).

Promotion through Newsletters

Several individual chiropractors publish newsletters that promote questionable nutrition practices.

• Bruce West, D.C., who publishes the monthly *Health Alert,* also markets supplement products to his readers. In a recent mailing he plugged *Cardio-Plus* ("to protect against heart attacks, angina, and stroke"), *Chlorophyll Complex Perles* (a "super longevity product" to make you "look younger and feel more energetic"), *Catalyn* ("to improve your immune function and beat fatigue"), and *Min-Tran* (to "easily combat stress" and help avoid kidney stones and cataracts). The products, for which West charges $64 for a month's supply, are manufactured by Standard Process Laboratories, which still supplies many unconventional practitioners. According to West:

> Catalyn is the most time-honored product ever made by Standard Labs. Like the company that produces it, it has been proven effective by withstanding the test of time. First produced in 1930, it has been utilized MILLIONS OF TIMES. In fact, more physicians who practice nutrition have utilized this product over ANY OTHER.

West's mailing did not specify the basis for this statement. Nor did it mention that it is illegal to claim that *Catalyn* boosts immunity. Nor did it reveal that the FDA had twice ordered the manufacturer (then doing business as Vitamin Products Company) to stop making false claims for *Catalyn* and later obtained a criminal conviction against the company for marketing 115 products with illegal claims (see Chapter 20).

In another mailing, West urged his readers to buy a special filter to remove chlorine from their shower water in order to protect themselves and their children from skin difficulties and various other health problems. According to the flyer, "people who have suffered precancerous keratotic lesions on their skin for decades. . . . say their lesions clear up within a matter of weeks once the chlorine is removed from their shower." In yet another mailing, West made explicit (and illegal) therapeutic claims for more than fifty Standard Process products that could be purchased from him by mail.

Although some chiropractors give rational nutrition advice to their patients, chiropractic journals contain little or no discussion of what should be advised. Although patients have been seriously harmed by toxic doses of vitamin A prescribed by chiropractors, I have seen no case reports in chiropractic journals or warnings that high doses can be toxic. Nor has any prominent chiropractor or major chiropractic organization ever openly suggested that there is anything wrong with the way chiropractors "practice nutrition." The March 1993 issue of *ACA Journal of Chiropractic* even contains an article called "The Subluxation Complex: Nutritional Considerations," which states:

> Chiropractors can . . . greatly influence the production of chemical irritants through nutritional intervention. . . . Such an approach could significantly reduce the . . . reflexogenic activity that initiates/perpetuates the development of the subluxation complex.

• David Beaulieu, M.S., D.C., operates Preventics, Inc., which markets supplements and promotes them through its newsletter, *VitalSigns*. Purchasers of the supplements receive a free subscription. A biographical sketch in the newsletter states that Beaulieu has a master's degree in biology-nutrition from the University of Bridgeport, has been a board member and secretary of the

International Academy of Preventive Medicine, and has hosted a radio talk show.

• David Williams, D.C., claims that his monthly newsletter *Alternatives* reveals "secrets . . . you can use to increase your lifespan and dramatically improve your health." Each issue is filled with tips and tidbits boosting nutritional products and other "natural therapies." A 1989 report contained in his solicitation brochure states that "*Alternatives* details the latest methods from around the world to preserve or regain your health without the use of drugs or surgery." The brochure also describes Williams as "America's #1 expert in natural healing therapies" and states that he is "a foremost consultant to some of the world's most prominent health institutions dealing with preventive medicine." The brochure states that over 130,000 people subscribe to *Alternatives* and that "over 130,000 people have been helped by the special all-natural healing techniques we've uncovered, verified and presented in every issue." (How Williams determines that readers have been helped is not specified.)

Treatment Systems

Many chiropractors espouse elaborate systems of diagnosis and treatment that are represented as nutrition-related but are not recognized as valuable by the scientific community.

• *Applied kinesiology (AK)* was initiated in 1964 by George J. Goodheart, Jr., D.C. It is based on the claim that every organ dysfunction is accompanied by a specific muscle weakness, which enables diseases to be diagnosed through muscle-testing procedures. Its practitioners—most of whom are chiropractors—claim that nutritional deficiencies, allergies, and other adverse reactions to foods or nutrients can be detected by having the patient chew or suck on them or by placing them on the tongue so that the patient salivates. Some practitioners advise that the test material merely be held in the patient's hand or touched to other parts of the body. Proponents claim that nutrients tested in these various ways will have an immediate effect: "good" substances will make specific muscles stronger, whereas "bad" substances will cause weaknesses that "indicate trouble with the organ or other tissue on the same nerve, vascular, nutrition, etc., grouping." A leading AK text, for example, states:

> If a patient is diagnosed as having a liver disturbance and the associated pectoralis major [chest muscle] tests weak, have the patient chew a substance that may help the liver, such as vitamin A. If . . . the vitamin A is appropriate treatment, the muscle will test strong.

Testing is also claimed to indicate which nutrients are deficient; if a weak muscle becomes stronger after a nutrient (or a food high in the nutrient) is chewed, that supposedly indicates "a deficiency normally associated with that muscle."

Goodheart states that AK techniques can also be used to evaluate nerve, vascular, and lymphatic systems; the body's nutritional state; the flow of "energy" along "acupuncture meridians"; and "cerebro spinal fluid function." AK "treatment" may include special diets, food supplements, acupressure (finger pressure on various parts of the body), and spinal manipulation.

The leading publisher/distributor of AK educational materials for chiropractors and their patients appears to be Systems DC, of Pueblo, Colorado. Its pamphlet on infections and child health states:

> When an infection develops, have your child examined by your doctor using applied kinesiology. He can evaluate the energy patterns and usually find the reason that the infection developed in the first place. By correcting the energy patterns within the body and paying specific attention to nutritional supplements and dietary management, the infection which your child (using natural health care) does develop will be adequately taken care of in most cases.

Although the claims of applied kinesiology are so far removed from scientific reality that testing them might seem a waste of time, competent researchers have subjected the muscle-testing procedures to well-designed controlled tests. One investigator found no difference in muscle response from one substance to another, while others found no difference between the results with test substances and with placebos.

The International College of Applied Kinesiology (ICAK) has set "standards" based on the work of Goodheart and his followers who allege they have subjected AK to "extensive scientific study." Certification by its board (which is not recognized by chiropractic's official accrediting body) requires a minimum of 300 hours of study under an ICAK diplomate, 5,000 hours of practical experience, authorship of two research papers, and passage of written and practical examinations. According to ICAK's 1992 status statement:

> Applied kinesiology examination should enhance standard diagnosis, not replace it. . . .
>
> There are both lay persons and professionals who use a form of manual muscle testing without the necessary expertise to perform specific and accurate tests. Some fail to coordinate the muscle testing findings with other standard diagnostic procedures. These may be sources of error that could lead to misinterpretation of the condition present, and thus improper treatment, or failure to treat the appropriate condition.

It appears to us, however, that the nutrition-related claims and practices of chiropractors affiliated with ICAK are no less looney than those of other muscle-testers who are not ICAK-affiliated.

• *The Morter HealthSystem* is described in its literature as "a complete alternative healthcare system" that has grown out of the Bio Energetic Synchronization Technique (B.E.S.T.) developed by chiropractor M.T. Morter, Jr., of Rogers, Arkansas. A recent brochure states that Morter "has been one of the world's leading pioneers in MindBody Healing for more than 25 years " and served as president of two chiropractic colleges. His system is said to have a following of "thousands" and to correct physical (biomagnetic), nutritional, and emotional stresses.

B.E.S.T. is based on the idea that "stress-induced energy imbalance will cause the body to become divided into areas of North and South energy." According to a recent booklet:

> Morter B.E.S.T. doctors renormalize the body's energy field so that it can become revitalized. . . . In a healthy body there is no polarization of north or south energy. . . .
>
> Through (1) correct interpretation of body language, (2) complete switching with every treatment, (3) the correct transfer of energy, (4) the exact synchronization of body pulsation, (5) the correct nutritional program, and (6) sufficient time, health can be restored.

The booklet also states that development and repair of the body is controlled by its electromagnetic field. Followers of B.E.S.T. postulate

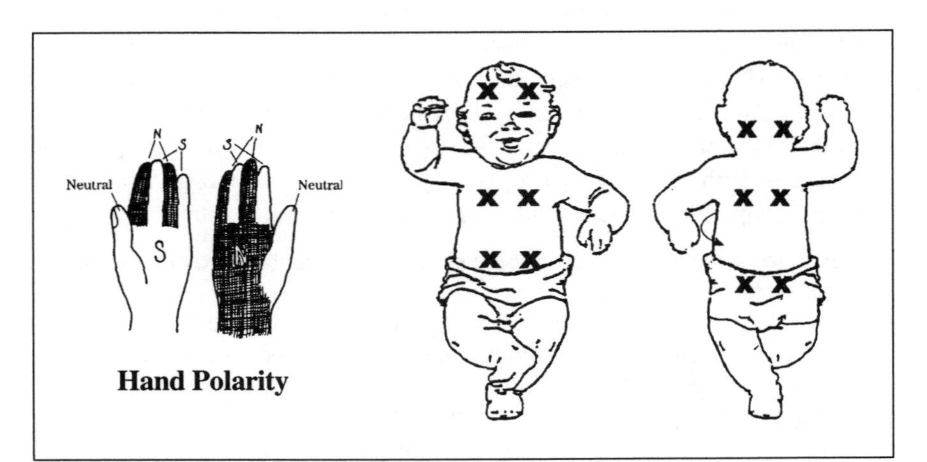

Drawings from the booklet "Baby B.E.S.T.: Infant Adjusting / Care" indicate "polarity" of the fingers and the "contact points" where they are applied while the infant lies face up.

that an imbalance in the patient's electromagnetic field causes unequal leg length, which the chiropractor can instantly correct by applying his own electromagnetic energy to proper points on the body. According to this notion, two fingers on each of the chiropractor's hands are North poles, two are South poles, and the thumbs are electromagnetically neutral. When imbalance is detected, the hands are held for a few seconds at "contact points" on the patient's body until "pulsation" is felt and the patient's legs test equally long. Proponents recommend that such testing be started early in infancy and continued at least monthly throughout life. According to a 1989 mailing, "it is possible for a single doctor to collect over $300,000/year using only B.E.S.T."

The "nutritional" component is based on the belief that "patients can maintain life and vitality by consuming four times as much alkaline-forming as acid-forming foods." Proponents claim that testing saliva pH [degree of acidity or alkalinity] can determine whether a person's symptoms are nutritionally or emotionally based and indicates whether the most effective method of care should be nutritional supplementation and/or adjustive. According to Morter literature:

> The two principal sources of physiological toxins affecting patients are: (1) Over-consumption of Protein and (2) Imbalance of the body's timing system, caused by stresses such as trauma, toxicity and [negative] thoughts.

The recommended supplements include *Alka•Green* (a 100% barley juice concentrate recommended as the best "overall body alkalizer"), *Alka•Slim* ("the only weight reduction formula designed to alkalize and energize at the same time"), *Alka•Pan* (a pancreatic enzyme formula "designed to reduce stress in the body and aid digestion"), and several other products containing herbs not specified in a flyer "for doctors only." For babies, a mixture of raw goat milk, carrot juice, and distilled water is said to be "an excellent replacement for infant formulas."

Fortunately for the untreated masses, there is no reason to be concerned about the "acidity" or "alkalinity" of either the diet or the body. In the absence of serious disease, digestive and metabolic mechanisms maintain the cells of the body at their appropriate pH regardless of which foods are eaten. Unfortunately for babies, raw (unpasteurized) goat milk is unsafe because it can harbor dangerous bacteria.

• *Contact Reflex Analysis (CRA)* is an elaborate pseudoscientific system that resembles aspects of applied kinesiology and B.E.S.T. Its codeveloper and leading proponent is Dick A. Versendaal, D.C., of Holland, Michigan.

Versendaal claims that CRA can "test every conceivable condition in the human body . . . help that patient, and know how long it will take for that patient to get well." Testing is done by pulling on the patient's outstretched arm while placing one's finger or hand on one of about seventy-five "reflex" points on the patient's body. (Versendaal states that the front of the hand is electrically "positive," the back is "negative," and the fingers are "neutral.") If the arm is weak and can be pulled downward, the reflex "blows," indicating that disease corresponding to the reflex is present. "Nutritional" products—most manufactured by Standard Process Laboratories—are then prescribed to correct the alleged problems. His 1993–94 schedule lists twenty-seven seminars "given under the auspices of Parker College of Chiropractic" at locations throughout the United States.

A flyer for Versendaal's 260-page "textbook," *Contact Reflex Analysis and Designed Clinical Nutrition*, describes it as "a reference manual for over 1000 syndromes and their treatments." But his flyer for patients states:

> CRA is not a method of diagnosis. It is a means by which a doctor uses the body's reflexes to accurately determine the root cause of a health problem.
>
> CRA is also a marvelous preventative technique, used to find a problem before it becomes a full-blown health issue. Find it early and correct it.

Doctors who contact Versendaal about his work may receive a stack of testimonials, including one from a chiropractic client who states:

> I no longer feel a need to distinguish between a medical and Chiropractic patient. Every patient (with a few exceptions), now falls into the realm of Chiropractic Care being the most appropriate efficient, and least invasive approach to rectifying the cause of their disease. . . .
>
> I am *successfully treating* chronic acne, Staph. & Strep. infections, infertility, vision loss, dental problems, paroxysmal atrial tachycardia, obesity, allergies, anemia, etc., on a daily basis and with tremendous results.

Versendaal claims his method is so efficient that it can generate a million dollars a year working only fifteen hours a week. At a 1992 seminar he stated that he saw a patient every three minutes in his office at a cost of $35 for the initial visit, $25 for weekly follow-up visits, and $10 for additional weekly visits if a patient was seen more than once per week. His writings and seminars are loaded with bizarre statements about the body in health and disease. For example:

> Eighty percent of diseases are due to allergy.
>
> The two main causes of disease are gallbladder disease and staph infections.
>
> People can only get fat from prostate and ovarian hormones going bad.

The most common cause of hair loss in men and women is poor blood.
The kidneys are controlled by the thyroid gland.
The uterus stores every hormone the body needs.
Doctors don't know this: The most common cause of juvenile diabetes is parasites.
Yeast infections cause fibroids of the uterus and breast.
Most of the skin is made up of calcium (not protein).
The most common cause of chronic constipation is parasites. Constipation means that the lymphatics have dried up.
The heart rarely wears out unless you are born with a weak heart.
Subluxation of the ankle can cause a stiff neck.
Rheumatism (rheumatoid arthritis) has three causes: too much calcium in the body, too little calcium in the body, and infection.

During the seminar Versendaal tested a parade of patients and recommended a Standard Process product for each problem he alleged, typically six or twelve per day of each one. He explained that, "Standard has a product for practically everything that can happen to a man." Since most patients had multiple problems, the typical regimen ranged from twenty to forty pills per day, which would cost the patient from five to twenty-eight cents each. The highest number prescribed was seventy-three, which would have cost about $14

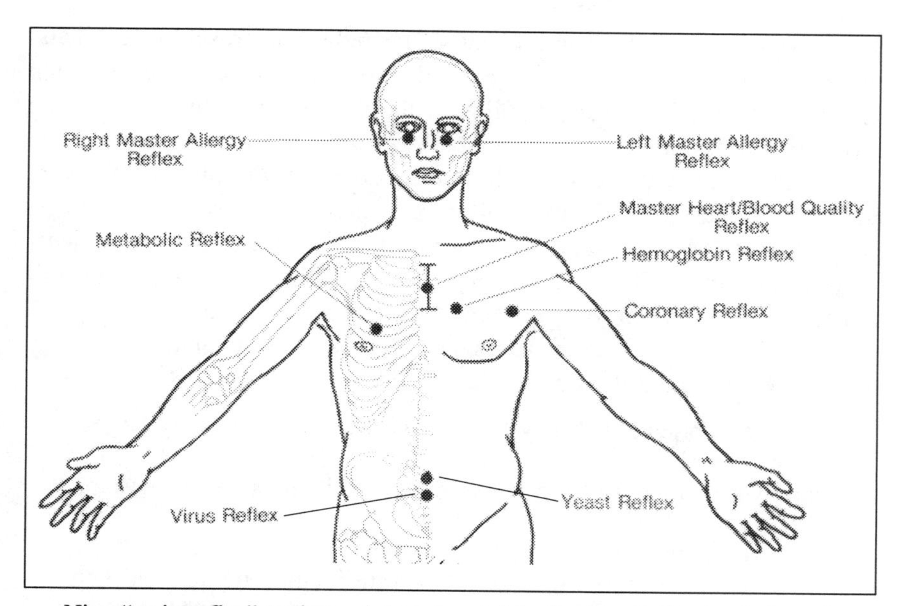

Nine "main reflex" testing points as located in *Contact Reflex Analysis and Designed Clinical Nutrition, 2nd edition* (1993).

per day. Most of the magic pills are made of dehydrated vegetables and animal organs.

In no case did Versendaal obtain a detailed history of a patient's problem or perform any standard type of physical examination. When one woman he examined said she had neurofibromatosis, he asked her what it was. (It is a group of hereditary disorders in which multiple noncancerous tumors appear in the skin and/or elsewhere in the body.) After she displayed some tumors, he tested her reflexes and concluded they were "almost the same thing as fatty tumors" and were caused by "staph." When a woman who smoked asked him to check whether her lungs were damaged, he found a slightly weak "lung reflex," concluded that she had only "slight damage," and advised taking one *Pneumotropin* pill daily to repair the damage. (He did not suggest that she stop smoking!) When a woman described pain in her hip and leg, Versendaal said it was sciatic nerve pain caused by a "ruptured disk" pinching a nerve in her *neck.* (The sciatic nerve runs from the lower part of the spine down each leg.) When a teenage girl complained of bronchitis and stomachaches, Versendaal told her the cause was "parasites." When a woman complained of discomfort in her knee and fingers, he diagnosed "carpal tunnel syndrome" in both wrists, concluded that she had rheumatism, and said: "You have adrenal failure, and that's causing your rheumatism. Your body is filling up with poisons from poor circulation from weak adrenals."

In other cases, Versendaal diagnosed heart disease, prostate disease, and "infections" of the eye, ear, liver, lung, and knee without examining any of the body parts involved—merely by pulling on the patient's arm while touching the corresponding "reflex" points.

After several patients said to have recovered from disabling illness were presented, Versendaal said, "In my office, miracles are the norm. When you get started with CRA, God starts sending you patients. He sends you patients nobody can help. . . . There are special people that God chooses—gives the gift of healing. The reason you are here now is because God sent for you." Versendaal also advised seminar attendees on strategies to maintain credibility and stay out of legal difficulty. These included:

Don't tell patients that they have a disease. Tell them they have a syndrome.

Don't write a lot of stuff [in the patient's chart]—the less you have the better.

Don't find more than two or three things at a time to treat. If more problems are present, start treating some for three months and then switch to others. That way patients won't be faced with too much expense at one time.

The 1994–95 *National Directory of Chiropractic* lists 37,540 chiropractors and some of the techniques they use. If the book accurately reflects what chiropractors are doing, at least one hundred in the United States are using CRA, 800 are using B.E.S.T., and 4,400 are using applied kinesiology.

• *NUTRI-SPEC* is a system of pseudoscientific nonsense marketed by Guy R. Shenker, D.C., of Mifflintown, Pennsylvania. According to ads in the *Digest of Chiropractic Economics:*

> How can you rise straight to the top of the clinical nutrition field? With a scientific testing system to determine the specific nutritional needs of every patient in your own office in five minutes; and the supplements to fulfill those needs immediately – with NUTRI-SPEC. . . .
>
> Your patients will fully appreciate your professionalism as you scientifically uncover the causes underlying their health problems, instead of taking a shot in the dark at their symptoms.

Interested chiropractors can purchase a 372-page manual and can borrow or purchase a videotape showing how the system is used with seven patients. According to the book, "there is no patient whose health problem does not have a nutritional component. . . . That makes nutrition a clinical tool with universal application and with almost unlimited potential." Brochures for patients assure that NUTRI-SPEC tests tell the chiropractor "in what ways your body chemistry tends to slip off balance" and reveal "exactly which foods and nutritional supplements you need and which you should avoid."

During the first visit, the chiropractor determines the patient's respiratory rate, body temperature, blood pressure, pulse (standing or lying down), breath-holding ability, pupil size, degree of thickness or coating of the tongue, several characteristics of the patient's saliva and urine, and various reflexes. Saliva and urine samples can also be sent together with other data to obtain a "NUTRI-SPEC PROFILE" that provides additional information.

Using NUTRI-SPEC's unique scoring system, the chiropractor then determines whether the patient is in or out of "water/electrolyte balance," "anaerobic/dysaerobic balance," "acid/alkaline balance," and "sympathetic/parasympathetic balance." The test findings also enable the chiropractor to diagnose "sex hormone insufficiency," "myocardial insufficiency," "pineal stress," "thymus stress," and about twenty-five other fanciful conditions. Based on all these findings, the chiropractor makes dietary recommendations and prescribes supplements (available only from NUTRI-SPEC) to correct the alleged imbalances. The supplements would cost patients like those shown in the video from 80¢ to about $3 per day, half of which is profit to the chiropractor. If follow-up visits—"repeating just the tests that were abnormal"—fail to show "improvement," the dosage of these products is adjusted.

• *Biomagnetic therapy* is a pseudoscientific approach championed by Richard Broeringmeyer, D.C., N.D., of Murray, Kentucky, who claims:

> Magnetic analysis can determine functional state of an organ, nerve, or tissue. When it has been determined whether the organ is in a state of hypo or hyper function, the clinician can then determine the proper magnetic and nutritional treatment.

Flyers for Broeringmeyer's Nutrition and Biomagnetic Seminar have described him as "a recognized world leader in the fields of nutrition, preventative medicine and biomagnetics" and have stated that the seminar would provide "a complete background in basic nutrition, all that is needed by a doctor with no experience in Clinical Nutrition." *Principles of Magnetic Therapy*, a booklet Broeringmeyer published in 1991, states that "when the body is in balance electromagnetically and all nutrition are available [sic] disease cannot exist." He also claims that "all disease begins with energy loss," that a healthy cell spins counterclockwise while its nucleus spins clockwise producing energy, and that diseased cells spin the opposite way, "drawing energy from the body to the disease." Among other things, his seminars teach how to use magnetic and nutritional procedures for "normalizing organs and systems."

The Bottom Line

Although some chiropractors may give rational nutrition advice to their patients, it is clear that a substantial percentage of them do not. Chiropractic journals contain little or no discussion of scientific nutrition or how chiropractors can do appropriate nutrition counseling. Although we know of several people who were seriously harmed by vitamin megadoses prescribed by chiropractors, we have seen no case reports in chiropractic journals or warnings that high doses can be toxic. As far as we know, however, despite the many problems described in this chapter, no prominent voices within the chiropractic mainstream have openly suggested there is anything wrong with the way their colleagues "practice nutrition."

16

"Passive Greed": The Pharmacy Connection

Much of this book describes how the health-food industry uses misinformation to push its products. This chapter examines how pharmacists and so-called "ethical" manufacturers add to public confusion and share the loot. Our analysis is based on information from pharmacy-school educators plus twenty-years' worth of pharmacy journals and trade publications.

When we speak of the "health-food industry," we refer mostly to promoters who greatly exaggerate the value of nutrients or use blatant scare tactics associated with a basic rejection of scientific facts. Drug companies that promote "nutritional insurance" with more subtle scare tactics are equally guilty of profiteering, although most of their other activities are rooted in science. Some distinction should also be made between owner-operated and chain-operated drugstores. The latter are far more likely to be unprincipled in their vitamin promotions.

Supplement sales in drugstores have risen sharply in recent years. The 1993 total, according to a report in *Drug Store News,* was $880 million, with multivitamins as the leading category. Although a large percentage of supplements sold through pharmacies are unnecessary or irrationally formulated, pharmacists don't seem to mind selling them. Herbal, homeopathic, and aromatherapy products are also being sold through pharmacies.

The "Education" of Pharmacists

Pharmacy schools correctly teach their students that people who eat a balanced diet rarely need supplements. But after they graduate, pharmacists are seldom reminded of this fact. The subject of inappropriate vitamin use is rarely mentioned in their scientific journals, and their trade publications talk mainly about vitamin promotion. Moreover, most of the trade publications actually encourage pharmacists to utilize many of the sales techniques used by health-food retailers!

A 1978 article in *Drug Topics*, for example, told pharmacists how to exploit public interest in food supplements:

> One way to stay ahead of consumer buying patterns is to keep tabs on what customers are reading—health food magazines, nutrition articles in women's magazines or any of the more popular paperback vitamin books.... By keeping track of what is happening in the health food store trade right now, you can get the jump on what might be happening in drugstore vitamin sales six months from now....
>
> A trend that underscores the need for a complete vitamin line is the continuing segmentation of the market into target categories. First came special formulations for women containing iron; now there are special vitamins for men containing zinc (said to aid prostate problems). Today there are vitamins tailored for different age groups, stress formulas for the anxious, and energy compounds for the athletes—especially joggers. Just now appearing on the shelves are vitamins aimed specifically at strengthening the hair, and another new product advertises itself as a beauty formula.

"The vitamin business is not unlike the fashion industry," said one expert who was interviewed in the article. "What sells depends upon what is in vogue. The difference is that while manufacturers and designers set the styles in fashions, in vitamins it's the customers with the latest scientific findings in hand who determine sales trends." (To keep pharmacists abreast of these trends, trade publications have frequent articles about what sells well.) The marketing director of a private label manufacturer suggested that "the smart merchandiser is going to stock what people want." Another vitamin marketing specialist advised pharmacists to convey the idea that their drugstores had a "total" vitamin department so that the customer doesn't have to shop elsewhere. He also advised selling health-related paperbacks and magazines next to the vitamin section. (The ones that promote supplements, of course.)

William H. Lee, a pharmacist aligned with the health-food industry, has given similar advice:

> Even if you do not carry health-related paperbacks as a rule, you must put in and sell health-related titles. They will be your best salesman. People will read about the use of various vitamins and minerals. You as a pharmacist may not be able to recommend a certain combination

> for a certain condition. The law forbids you to do it. But if a person chooses to follow a path because he believes it will do him some good, then he has a right to buy and try what he wishes.

(Translation: You can't lie, so let the books lie for you.)

Lee has actively promoted the types of products sold in health-food stores by writing books, booklets, and articles in health-food magazines and newspapers. The biographical sketch in one of his booklets states he is a "master herbalist with a doctorate in nutrition" and "a consultant to the direct marketing industry on nutritional matters." His letterhead has further identified him as a nutritional consultant working by appointment.

During the mid-1980s, Lee promoted supplements in a monthly nutrition column in *American Druggist*, which drew protests from scientifically oriented pharmacists. In correspondence with critics, Lee stated that he was "on the cutting edge of nutrition" and that his column was "intended to put pharmacists on an equal footing with health food stores when it comes to advice and sale of supplements." He also wrote that he is a graphologist, that his doctoral degree is in pharmacognosy from the University of Amsterdam, and that he had taken nutrition courses at New York University, the New School, Union University, and Donsbach University (see Chapter 6).

Lee's thirty-page booklet, "The Question & Answer Book of Vitamins . . . plus a Dictionary of Nutrition," was published in 1984 and distributed free to health-food stores by Barth's, of Valley Stream, New York, a company that sells supplement products through health-food stores and by mail. About half of the fifty answers in the booklet either contained significant errors or were misleading. Several months after a detailed critique and other pertinent information were sent to *American Druggist,* Lee's column stopped appearing.

In the early 1980s, Lee marketed a mail-order "Personal Computerized Nutrition Profile," which cost $24.95. Prospective buyers were told that their answers to 266 questions would indicate "the way your body communicates its nutritional adequacies or inadequacies, including mild, moderate or severe deficiencies, and the amount of supplemental nutrients to be included in your daily regimen." This test resembled Kurt Donsbach's "Nutrient Deficiency Test" and was just as invalid.

In 1982, *Drug Store News* carried a thirty-two-page insert called "Nutrition Centers: A how-to manual for setting up, maintaining, merchandising, servicing and getting rich (and maybe famous) from this hot new department." The booklet's apparent purpose was to suggest how pharmacies could compete with health-food stores "to capitalize on the fitness and nutrition trend sweeping the country." Its suggestions, "designed to give retailers a running jump," included: (1) luring clerks away from health-food stores, (2) attending the annual convention of the National Nutritional Foods Association (NNFA), and (3) not diagnosing or prescribing. Regarding the latter, the article stated:

> What if a customer complains of headaches and asks your health center manager "What should I take?" According to Bob Grenoble, executive director of NNFA, the answer must be worded *very* carefully: "You can explain what the product is traditionally used for. You can refer the customer to the shelf area where the product is. We also recommend that retailers refer customers to books and literature. There's a very fine line between prescribing and explaining."

To make things easy, the insert included suggestions about books, magazines, and booklets that the health-food industry uses to convey "authoritative knowledge."

A recent article in *American Druggist* contains additional advice about beating the competition:

> To make sure your customers buy their vitamins from you and not from the mass merchandisers or specialty outlets like GNC, you must convince them that you know vitamins and that you have what they need at a price they expect.
>
> How do you make sure that vitamin consumers will come to you and not the local warehouse club? One way is to reinforce the pharmacist's advisory role by conveying a level of awareness consumers won't find at supermarkets. You need to stay current. Important vitamin studies on antioxidants have emerged . . . identifying health benefits linked to vitamin consumption.
>
> While the Food & Drug Administration may not let manufacturers mention health benefits of their vitamins, they can't censor pharmacists (at least, not yet). Consumers who missed the studies' results in *Time, Newsweek,* and TV news shows should learn from their pharmacists what benefits might be gained from vitamins A or B, or calcium.

One pharmacist quoted in the article expressed hope that manufacturers would provide copies of vitamin-promoting articles from consumer magazines to give to customers. In-store merchandising material, the pharmacist said, should include language that says, "Ask your pharmacist for a recommendation." In another article, the co-owner of Nat-rul Health Products (a pharmacist) advises laminating such articles and attaching them to the shelves or the counter where vitamins are displayed. This article concludes:

> How should consumers determine whether they should take antioxidants or other vitamins? And how can they choose one antioxidant over another? By consulting with their pharmacists first. Counseling and sales opportunities don't come any easier.

Ask Your Pharmacist?

Many drug company ads suggest that consumers seek advice about vitamins from their doctor or their pharmacist. Curious about what pharmacists might say, Dr. Stephen Barrett designed a study to find out. The first phase was a visit to ten pharmacies in Allentown, Pennsylvania, by a young woman who complained of either tiredness or fatigue and asked whether a vitamin would help. Eight out of the ten pharmacists sold her vitamin products and one sold her a bottle of L-tryptophan (an amino acid).

For nervousness, one pharmacist recommended B-complex "to help rebuild your nervous system." Another recommended *Stresstabs* because "what you burn up is your B and C vitamins if you're under a lot of stress." Another, asked about nervousness, said he didn't recommend vitamins or going to a doctor who might prescribe tranquilizers. But he sold the investigator stress vitamins when she mentioned that she sometimes feels tired. The pharmacist who recommended L-tryptophan tablets said, "I know they are good because people buy them all the time."

For tiredness, one pharmacist recommended a multivitamin with iron even though advising that "you're taking a needle in a haystack chance that it's iron causing the tiredness." A second recommended a stress formula, while a third recommended a multivitamin. Another recommended a stress formula with zinc, indicating that "zinc helps build body tissue." Another suggested *Stresstabs* as a "tonic" and said, "That's what they have for when you burn the candle at both ends."

To explore how pharmacists are taught to handle such situations, Barrett sent questionnaires to the deans of all seventy-two pharmacy schools in the United States. All but one of the fifty-one who responded said this situation is covered in such courses as pharmacy practice. Almost all thought that pharmacists should attempt through questioning to identify possible causes of tiredness or nervousness and should ask whether a doctor had been consulted. More than half said that pharmacists should advise that vitamins are unlikely to help either condition. Yet not one of the pharmacists consulted in Allentown did any of these things.

Intrigued by these findings, *Consumer Reports* enlisted reporters to visit ten more stores in Missouri and ten in California. Nine of the twenty pharmacists recommended products and fewer than half recommended that a doctor be consulted. One who recommended a product said, "It might be a vitamin deficiency, particularly if you're not eating a balanced diet." When the reporter asked whether vitamins might help even if his diet were balanced, the pharmacist replied, "Yes. You might not be absorbing the food."

In the early 1980s, Edith Kalman, a registered dietitian, received inappropriate advice from three out of four pharmacists she consulted in New York City. When she complained of *severe* fatigue and expressed concern about anemia, one pharmacist guaranteed that Kalman would feel better within a week if she took a B-complex supplement plus a daily multivitamin. When she complained of fatigue and loss of stamina during long-distance runs, another pharmacist advised taking vitamins E, C, and B-complex. When Kalman asked for a recommendation for acne, the pharmacist said that vitamin A was a preventive and could "clear the blood of impurities." When Kalman complained that her gums bled heavily after brushing and asked whether the problem could be a vitamin deficiency, the pharmacist correctly insisted that she consult a physician or dentist.

In 1991, Kenneth Smith, a student at Kent State University, visited twenty-five pharmacies in Ohio and posed the same questions to pharmacists or retail clerks. In all but four instances he was advised to make a purchase. Two years later, Donna Mitchell, another KSU student, asked ten pharmacists whether a vitamin would help her feel less tired. Eight suggested that she buy a vitamin product.

Sundown Vitamins
Committed to A Healthy America
Dick Clark sells Sundown, and your customers will buy.
America wants to look and feel as young as Dick
Independent market research shows that consumers who are the heaviest purchasers of vitamins immediately recognize Dick Clark–and regard him as a symbol of youthfulness. Dick is now Sundown's national spokesman on radio, t.v. and point-of-purchase. Typical consumer reactions: "If I could look as young as he looks, I'd take the same brand of vitamins too." And, "I'm switching. That man does not age, and if he's taking those vitamins, I'm going to take them."

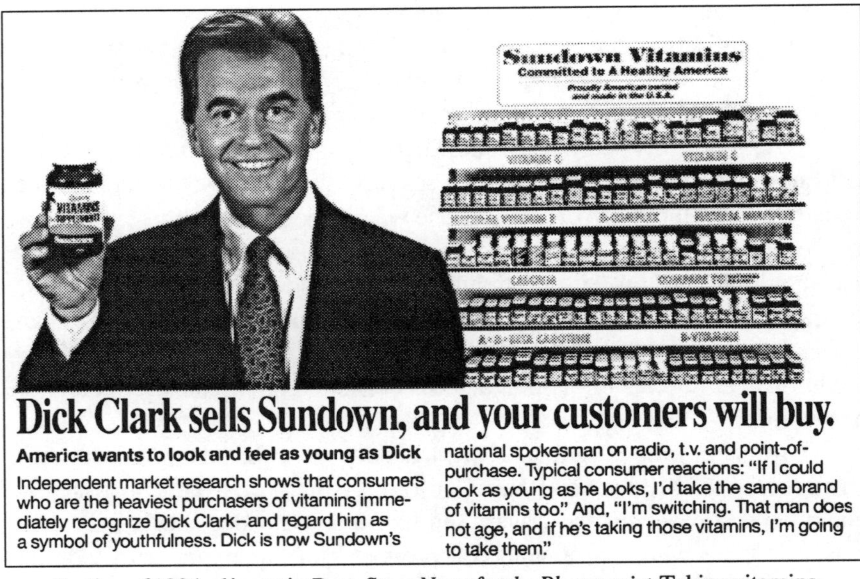

Portion of 1994 ad insert in *Drug Store News for the Pharmacist.* Taking vitamins will not make people look younger. Should this type of advertising induce pharmacists to carry products?

A few years ago, two pharmacy school professors sent a questionnaire on supplement-related activities and "alternative methods" to one thousand pharmacists in the Detroit metropolitan area and received 197 responses. Among the 116 who identified their five most common reasons for recommending vitamins or minerals, sixty-six (56 percent) listed fatigue and fifty-seven (49 percent) listed stress.

What do you think these findings mean?

Advertising Tactics

Health-food-industry propaganda is not the only reason why vitamin sales are booming. Advertising by so-called "ethical" manufacturers is also a big factor. Some of this advertising is done to persuade drugstores to stock their brands. Much of it, however, is done to persuade the public—*and pharmacists themselves*—that everyone should take supplements. When a manufacturer plans a major advertising campaign, it typically will be announced in trade publications so that druggists can stock up on the products promoted.

Hoffmann-La Roche, Inc., which produces most of the bulk nutrients repackaged by other vitamin manufacturers, advertises heavily to physicians, pharmacists, and the general public. Roche's Vitamin Nutrition Information Service distributes reports that quote scientific literature but are heavily biased toward vitamin supplementation—exaggerating the need and minimizing the risks by omitting adverse facts. Roche also generates press coverage by sponsoring scientific meetings.

During the early 1980s, Roche engaged in blatant scare tactics to stimulate vitamin sales. Two ads questioned whether people were getting enough vitamin E but failed to mention that in the United States, no case of vitamin E deficiency based on faulty diet had ever been reported. Another ad asked "How much vitamin C gets lost on the way to the table?" and (falsely) suggested that food processing places people at risk of dietary deficiency. Roche's campaign to plug biotin included a brochure entitled, "Is BIOTIN missing in your vitamin supplement?" The brochure described biotin's importance for good health and what happened when biotin deficiency was induced in laboratory animals. The brochure failed to note that biotin is made by bacteria within the human intestine and that deficiency does not occur in humans on a dietary basis (unless they gorge themselves on raw eggs); thus there is no reason whatsoever for people to worry about not getting enough biotin in food. Advertising to doctors spotlighted "vitamin underachievers" and described how Roche was telling the public (dishonestly) about the risk of deficiency. And a booklet for children ages

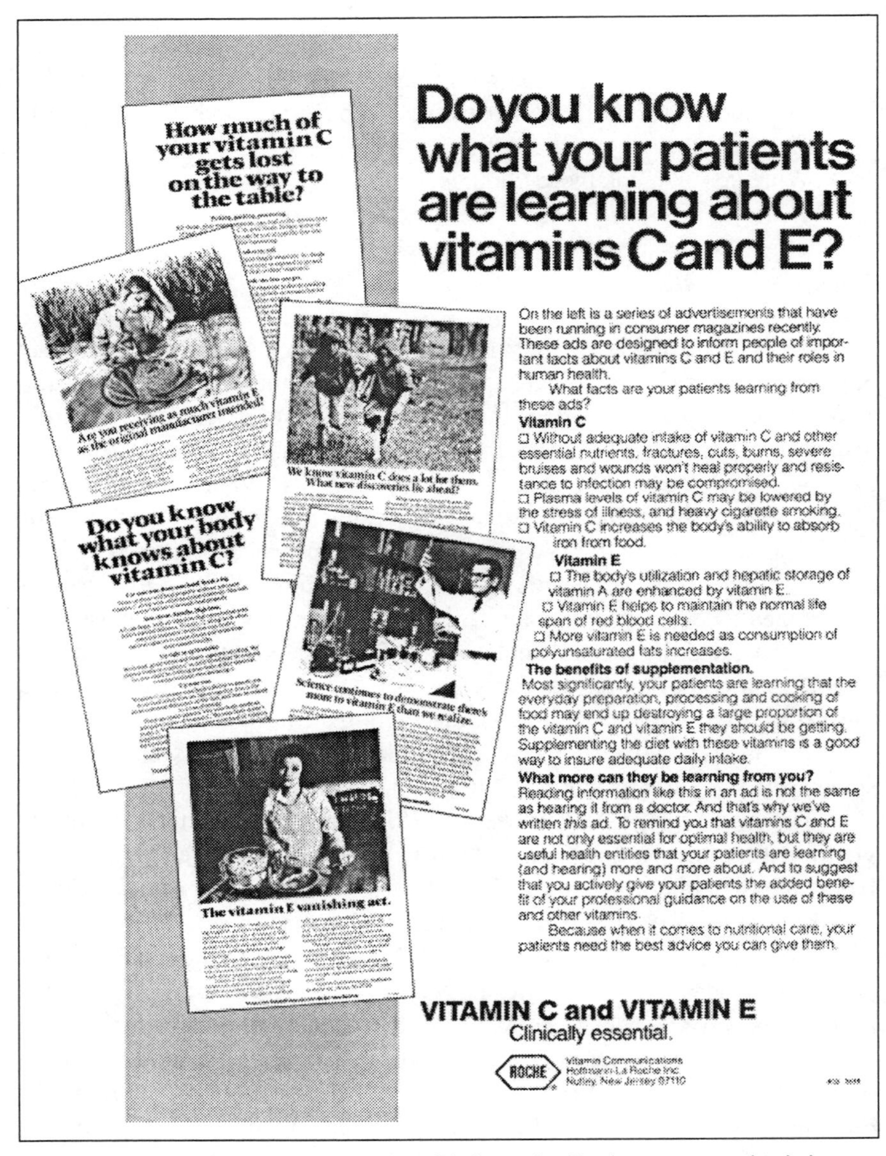

This 1981 ad to doctors repeated the misinformation Roche was presenting in its ads to the public. The ad exaggerated the likelihood that patients would become deficient in vitamins C and E and urged doctors to reinforce its message that supplementing the diet was a good way to ensure adequate intake.

thirteen to seventeen stressed the importance of getting enough nutrients and warned that "many people are not getting the full amount."

In 1983, Roche ran a series of ads with the theme "Don't Take Chances, Take A Supplement" (see Chapter 3). According to an article in *Drug Store News,* the main thrust of this campaign was directed at pharmacists who—Roche assumed—would relay the information to customers. The article also noted that Roche planned a training program "so that pharmacists will more readily engage in nutrition counseling."

Roche's more recent ads have been more subtle and include all or most of the following themes: (1) nutrient or nutrient group X does such-and-such in the body; (2) X is abundant in such-and-such foods, (3) some people don't get enough of X, (4) while not substitutes for eating a variety of foods, supplements can be an important addition to your diet, and (5) research is under way to determine whether supplementation with X can protect against cancer (or another disease). Some ads don't mention supplementation and merely advise eating foods rich in antioxidant nutrients. Do you think these ads are intended to encourage dietary improvement or to stimulate supplement sales?

In the early 1980s, Hudson Pharmaceutical Corporation advertised to pharmacists that it was "committed to helping you sell more vitamins [and] to bringing pre-sold customers into your store." Stores that carried its products were provided with free "educational" materials (see Chapter 3) and offered "in-store vitamin sales training for your people to help them sell vitamins more knowledgeably." In 1980, in an interview in *Drug Topics,* company president Ed Samek said that "health-food stores and supermarkets have stolen a great many customers from drugstores, and now is the time for drugstores to take that business back." At that time, Hudson was using radio commercials geared toward "seasonal trends" in vitamin sales. In January and February 1980, vitamins were suggested to counter the supposed effects of stress. Fun and fitness were featured in March and April. May and June used a "natural" theme, and September related vitamins to going back to school.

In 1981, Hudson began "Nutra-Phone," a daily "educational" message on nutrition and health that could be heard by dialing a telephone number in New York City. Not surprisingly, many of its messages used scare tactics to promote the sale of unnecessary supplements. Research associates of the American Council on Science and Health (ACSH) studied the contents of thirty-four taped messages related to nutrition and found significant errors or omissions in about half of them. They also objected to the fact that many of the tapes ended with a message to take supplements "for extra protection." In a report to Samek, ACSH's Kathleen Meister stated:

> "Extra protection" implies that taking more than the recommended amounts of vitamins will provide an extra benefit. There is no good evidence of this, and the suggestion is harmful, since it may lead people to take dangerously large amounts of supplements.
>
> It is clear . . . that your tapes are designed to serve [your] interests as sellers of supplements, and not . . . the interests of the public. Your tapes are a form of advertising, not a consumer education service. We are disturbed that they have been presented to the public as an educational device, rather than an advertising device.

In October 1986, *Consumer Reports* took issue with the American Association of Retired Persons, which operates the largest nonprofit mail-service pharmacy in the world. (Its gross sales are over $200 million per year.) To promote *Activitamins,* AARP's Pharmacy Service catalog had claimed: "A vigorous lifestyle puts extra demand on your body. So if you play golf or tennis or swim, walk, jog or bike, you should know about our formula." Calling this claim "bunkum," *Consumer Reports* also criticized AARP for selling bee pollen, royal jelly, bone meal, several amino acids, kelp, alfalfa, rutin, and biotin "despite lack of any scientific evidence that using such substances as supplements serves any nutritional need."

After Dr. Barrett filed a complaint with the National Advertising Division of the Council of Better Business Bureaus, AARP announced that it would stop publishing the misleading claims for *Activitamins,* but it continued to sell them as well as the other items criticized by *Consumer Reports*. In 1987, AARP Pharmacy Service appointed a nutrition advisory board to offer advice and consumer messages about vitamin, mineral, and supplement products. Following the board's appointment, products with potentially toxic doses of vitamin A were reformulated, misleading claims were stopped, and most dubious products were withdrawn from the pharmacy service's catalog. However, some of the consumer messages in the catalog have been written in double-talk that encouraged inappropriate use of supplements.

Lederle, the leading promoter of misinformation on stress supplements (see Chapter 3), is now misleading the public about antioxidants. Its recent ads for *Protegra* state:

> Alert your customers to the importance of antioxidant nutrients.
>
> • Free radicals, normal byproducts of cellular metabolism, can attack cells and damage them.
>
> • Antioxidants help neutralize free radicals and stop them from damaging cells.
>
> • Antioxidant nutrients are found primarily in fruits, vegetables, nuts and grains.

• 2 to 4 servings of fruit and 3 to 5 servings of vegetables per day are recommended to maintain good health.

• However, studies show that only 1 out of 10 Americans actually eats enough of the right foods to meet these recommendations.

• PROTEGRA is specially balanced to supplement dietary antioxidant nutrient intake.

• PROTEGRA can be taken by itself or with a multiple vitamin.

Although most of these statements are true, the ad as a whole is misleading. *Protegra* contains megadoses of vitamins E and C plus moderate amounts of five other nutrients. It is not necessary to eat five or more portions of fruits and vegetables each day to ingest an adequate supply of antioxidant nutrients. More important, as we note in Chapter 8, it has not been proven that megadoses of vitamin E or C are beneficial. A recent Roche ad in *Drug Topics* headed "Antioxidant Vitamin Protection...Why you should make it your business" provided essentially the same message.

In-Store Promotion

A recent survey by Hearst Business Publishing Research found that 109 (49.5 percent) of 220 druggists said that they offered their customers literature about vitamins. Most literature we have seen includes a table of vitamin functions and symptoms of deficiency.

The table of "vitamins" posted by Drug Emporium includes choline, inositol, para-aminobenzoic acid (PABA), and "P" (bioflavonoids), none of which are vitamins for humans. One column of the table is a ridiculous list of "Factors Working Against Vitamins" that includes sugar as "working against" niacin, thiamin, and choline, and stress as "working against" B-complex vitamins, riboflavin, folic acid, and vitamin C. Accompanying the table is a list of "Robber Barons" that supposedly increase vitamin needs. One such item is "the stress of living."

The "CVS Quick Reference Guide To Vitamins And Minerals," a flyer distributed in the vitamin section of CVS drugstores, includes a table of functions and food sources of vitamins plus lists of other nutrients with which they supposedly are "more effective." The accompanying text states:

> You know how important vitamins and minerals are. But did you know that factors such as pollution, stress, and physical activity can rob your body of the nutrients it needs to maintain good health?
>
> Sometimes a balanced diet just isn't enough, and supplements are necessary.

> This handy guide will help you evaluate your situation. . . . You'll simply find general information about what various vitamins and minerals do, where they can be found in nature, how they can get depleted from your body and how you can make them more effective.

Not quite. The flyer contains at least seven scare statements that are false or misleading. The most blatant are that "smoking in general can cause a vitamin C insufficiency" and that "over-exerting or not getting quite enough exercise" can "deplete your body's natural resources."

The Issue of Homeopathy

In 1992, the British Pharmaceutical Conference backed the promotion and sale of homeopathic remedies by pharmacies. This took place when a large majority of pharmacists who attended a debate rejected a motion to cease involvement in such activities. The motion's sponsor, Brian Harrop, said that since homeopathy had no scientific basis, pharmacists who condoned the sales of homeopathic remedies were not living up to their reputation as "experts" on medicines and were collectively guilty of hypocrisy.

One pharmacist who favored the motion said that medical doctors and other professionals would not sell or prescribe a medicine they did not believe worked. One pharmacist who opposed the motion said it would result in other motions, casting doubt on other products, and soon the shelves in pharmacies would be depleted of stock. Pharmacists might not be able to sell vitamins, slimming preparations, or diabetic foods. It was hypocritical to attack homeopathy while turning a blind eye to other products that may not have a proven effect. Another pharmacist reported that when she sold a homeopathic product, she informed the buyer that she did not endorse it on a scientific basis. This approach, she said, provided a way out for pharmacists who were unhappy selling homeopathic products.

As far as we know, no similar debate has taken place in the United States. Most pharmacy educators ignore the topic, and professional organizations and their journals do likewise. Trade publications, on the other hand, provide a steady stream of promotional articles and ads. Among the 197 Detroit-area pharmacists who responded to the vitamin/alternative survey, 27.4 percent said homeopathy was "useful," 18.3 percent judged it "useless," and 54.3 percent "didn't know." The researchers thought that if more questionnaires had been returned, the percentage of unfavorable answers would have been higher. Regardless, most pharmacists appear to know very little about homeopathy.

Meanwhile, homeopathic products are being promoted vigorously through ads and articles in pharmacy trade publications. The most outrageous of these promotions is a sixteen-page supplement to *U.S. Pharmacist,* a magazine that normally is quite scientific. The program was supported by a grant from a homeopathic manufacturer and is approved for continuing education credit by the University of Wisconsin School of Pharmacy. The material covers the history and theories of homeopathy, "prescribing basic homeopathic remedies," and "the need to become involved in homeopathy." The course material concludes: "The pharmacist who has knowledge of allopathic as well as natural medicine will provide the ultimate in pharmaceutical care."

An insert from Nature's Way Products, Inc., in *Drug Store News for the Pharmacist*, states: "It is predictable that American consumers today are more receptive than ever to alternatives such as homeopathic medicines given the high cost, limitations and dangers associated with conventional medicines." Sunsource Health Products, Inc., of Kilei, Hawaii, recently announced a multimedia campaign that would create "an incredible 300 million impressions weekly throughout the entire year." The campaign will include ads in health and fitness magazines, sixty-second radio ads on more than two thousand stations, and TV ads during "Wheel of Fortune," "The Price is Right," and the talk shows hosted by Phil Donahue, Maury Povich, and Sally Jesse Raphael. An article in the same publication described how a pharmacist in New York City saw homeopathic medicines as "a niche he could capitalize on." The article noted that the store used more than thirty feet of shelf space for homeopathic products and that a manufacturer's representative made regularly scheduled visits to the pharmacy to consult with patients and recommend products.

Ethical Questions

Almost all drugstores carry a large assortment of vitamin products, including many "natural" ones. While most chain stores promote them vigorously, most individually owned ones do not. Some pharmacies use deceptive tactics (like placing vitamin C products among cold remedies or vitamin A with eye-care products), while others display their vitamins inconspicuously.

Profiting from vitamins is not difficult. A *Drug Store News* survey of 455 heads of households found that 70 percent believed that vitamins and mineral supplements could help prevent illness and disease. The conditions that they thought supplements could help protect against were common colds (67 percent of those surveyed), anxiety (37 percent), heart disease (32 percent), cancer (29 percent), and insomnia (21 percent).

If asked point blank, most pharmacists will admit that few of their customers need supplements and that megadoses of vitamins should be taken only under medical supervision. Why, then, do they stock and sell them willingly? Many pharmacists claim that if they try to discourage vitamin purchases, most customers will get angry and shop elsewhere. Do you think this is true? (Would these pharmacists be willing to post signs stating: "You don't need supplements, but if you've been talked into them, we'll be happy to sell them to you."?) Or do you think the bottom line is money? According to an article in *Drug Topics*, "the vitamin category is one of the drugstore's top money-makers. For the space it requires, nothing equals the vitamin section for fast turnover (typically 5–7 times a year) and large profits." *Drug Store News* states: "Vitamins are a valuable trip generator for drug stores. Respondents [to a survey] said they buy vitamins about once a month and spend an average of $80 a year." Other reports have noted that even though prescription drugs are more costly, the profit per transaction is often higher on supplement products.

Do you think that pharmacists—whom the public believes have expert knowledge of the products they sell—should take advantage of customers who are confused by health-food-industry propaganda? *We believe that pharmacists have as much of an ethical duty to discourage inappropriate use of vitamin and mineral supplements as physicians do to advise against unnecessary surgery or medical care.* Do you know of any pharmacists who do so?

Merlin Nelson, Pharm.D., M.D., while working as an assistant professor of pharmacy practice at Wayne State University School of Pharmacy, wrote a hard-hitting article called "Promotion and Selling of Unnecessary Food Supplements: Quackery or Ethical Pharmacy Practice?" In the October 1988 issue of *American Pharmacy*, he stated:

> Why do pharmacists continue to promote and sell food supplements to healthy individuals who do not need them? I have concluded that the most common reason is greed. Advertising creates a demand that the pharmacist can supply and make a profit. . . . Pharmacists are apparently more interested in a sale than in the patient's welfare.
>
> Some pharmacists may be influenced by misleading advertising as much as consumers are. Some pharmacists may "believe" in certain supplements because of personal experience or testimonial evidence from friends, colleagues, or patients, while others promote "nutrition insurance." . . .
>
> Suggesting vitamins and minerals for such nonspecific symptoms as stress, tiredness, and nervousness is outright fraud. The most common response I have heard to this statement is, "Well, if they *think* it will help them, it just might." We have an ethical responsibility to tell the truth. The placebo response can be elicited with reassurance without the use of tablets, capsules, syrups, or any other . . . nostrum.

Nelson believes that pharmacists who advise patients not to waste money on vitamins might generate respect rather than antagonism. His article noted: "Patients are impressed when a pharmacist discourages the purchase of an unneeded item and dispenses sound advice. Patients feel personally helped by such unselfish behavior and often respond with long-term loyalty."

Has any pharmacist, pharmacy school professor, or professional pharmaceutical organization ever made a sustained effort to warn the American public that food supplements are promoted fraudulently? Is there a conspiracy of silence? Is there any reason why the pharmaceutical profession should not make a determined effort to protect Americans from being misled by major pharmaceutical manufacturers, as well as by the health-food industry? Are educators silent about supplements because drug companies donate money to their schools and research projects? Are trade-publication editors merely mouthpieces for their advertisers? Can't pharmacies exist without selling products to people who don't need them?

And what about homeopathic products? Why aren't pharmacy students being taught that they don't work? Why aren't pharmacy-school educators and journal editors attacking them as frauds? Why does a profession based on science tolerate the sale of homeopathic products through drugstores?

The American Pharmaceutical Association (APhA), which is the largest professional organization of pharmacists, sets standards, promotes professional education, publishes *American Pharmacist* and other scientific publications, and provides information to members as well as to the public. In 1988, the association adopted a policy advocating programs that "address the public health implications of the misuse and/or abuse" of nutritional supplements. The policy also encouraged pharmacists "to provide health education regarding unsubstantiated and/or misleading health claims" for supplements.

Though well intended, this action did not address the problems we discuss in this chapter. For one thing, the policy background document states: "The one-a-day type of vitamin product that more than 40% of the public takes as a 'legitimate food supplement' is not the problem." More important, the policy fails to criticize the *advertising* or *selling* of products that are useless or irrationally formulated.

The Tenth Edition of APhA's *Handbook of Nonprescription Drugs* contains a chapter titled "Nutritional Products." The chapter correctly states:

> In most cases, the typical American diet does not need supplementation. Nutrition experts agree that foods, not supplements, are the preferred source of vitamins and minerals and that most individuals can easily meet their requirements by eating a balanced diet.

Pharmacists and their customers have millions of conversations per year about dietary supplements and related products. Can you imagine what would happen to quackery in America if pharmacists discouraged inappropriate purchases of these products? Do you think that will ever happen?

17

The Endless Parade of Gurus

In a 1910 book called *Stover at Yale,* a fictional character called Ricky Rickets told his friend Dink Stover how to become a millionaire within ten years:

> First, find something all the fools love and enjoy, tell them it's wrong, hammer it into them, give them a substitute, and sit back, chuckle, and shovel away the ducats. Why, in the next 20 years, all the fools will be feeding on substitutes for everything they want . . . and blessing the name of the foolmaster who fooled them.

Ricky was commenting on the patent medicine craze of his day. But his remarks accurately reflect how "nutrition" gurus have penetrated the American mind. Although the development of science has the potential to curb faddism, the parallel development of mass communication has enabled faddists to reach vast audiences of unsuspecting people.

"Nature Salesmen"

Sylvester Graham (1794–1851) mixed religious fanaticism with a zeal for the natural, "uncomplicated" life. He was one of the first American "health reformers" to reach large audiences. His initial focus on the evils of alcohol soon expanded to other health concerns. "The simpler, plainer, and more natural the food," he said, "the more healthy, vigorous, and long-lived will be the body." Among the prohibited foods were salt and other condiments (these and sexual excesses caused insanity), cooked vegetables (against God's law), and chicken pies (caused cholera). His most vigorous attacks were against "unnatural" substances such as meat, white flour products, and water consumed at mealtime. Although Graham's health petered out at the age of fifty-seven, his spirit remains with us in the cracker that bears his name.

John Harvey Kellogg (1852–1943) supposedly ate his way through medical school on a diet of apples and graham crackers. He belonged to a Seventh-day Adventist group that had founded a religious colony and health sanitarium at Battle Creek, Michigan. It has been said that he and his brother Will were the first men to make a million dollars from food faddism. Under Dr. Kellogg's leadership, the Battle Creek Sanitarium attracted hordes of wealthy clients whose intestines he "detoxified" with enemas and high-fiber diets. In an effort to provide a dried bread product upon which his clients could exercise their teeth without breaking them, he hit upon the idea of a wheat flake. By 1899, the flakes had evolved into a cereal-based company that soon had many competitors. One was Charles W. Post, a former Kellogg patient, who ground up wheat and barley loaves, called his new product "grape nuts," and marketed it as a cure for appendicitis, malaria, consumption (tuberculosis), and loose teeth. Such were the humble beginnings of two of today's giant cereal producers: the Kellogg Company and the Post Division of General Foods (now part of Philip Morris).

Horace Fletcher (1849–1919) was one of the few faddists to achieve some scientific recognition for his work. Grossly overweight and in poor health at the age of forty, he retired from business and sought "cures" throughout the world. After reading books "only to find that no two authors agreed," he finally "determined to consult Mother Nature herself for direction." Reasoning that "if Nature had given us personal responsibility it was not hidden away in the dark folds and coils of the [intestines] where we could not control it," he decided that the mouth held the key to the whole situation. Extremely thorough chewing—later termed "Fletcherizing"—was the key to good health. Using this method, he lost more than sixty pounds and (because of the weight loss) felt much better.

Although he didn't look it, Fletcher had always been exceptionally strong. When he demonstrated his prowess at Yale University and elsewhere, people attributed his strength to his dietary habits. Fletcherizing, which was quite tedious, actually helped some people to eat less and therefore suffer less from the effects of overeating. (Today we call such maneuvers to eat less "behavior modification.") But as Fletcher's enthusiasm for his own theories increased, he gradually cut down further on the amount of food he ate and sometimes fasted for several days at a time. He died at Battle Creek Sanitarium, probably as a result of malnutrition.

Bernarr Macfadden (1868–1955) was the first faddist to use mass media techniques to amass a fortune. At age eighteen, well-muscled as a result of a three-year exercise program, he launched his career as a teacher of "physical culture." Pupils were sparse, but he survived by selling bodybuilding gadgets and posing (almost nude) for pictures. *Physical Culture* magazine, which he began publishing in 1896, was a great success. The number of subscribers reached 100,000 within two years and eventually passed one million.

Two themes ran through almost every article in the magazine. One was that medical care (which he steadfastly avoided) should be rejected in favor of "natural" methods. The other was a special dietary program which included fasting. Within the next two decades, Macfadden published more than twenty books, including a five-volume *Encyclopedia of Physical Culture* containing "complete instruction for the cure of all diseases through physcultopathy." He also began other magazines—including *True Story, True Experiences* and *True Detective*—all of which promoted eccentric health schemes and allowed advertisements for questionable methods of healthcare. As medical science developed, Macfadden's influence gradually faded away. But Macfadden Holdings, Inc., his corporate descendant, now publishes the *National Enquirer, Weekly World News,* and several monthly romance magazines.

One "Expert" After Another

Gayelord Hauser (1895–1984) promised to add years to your life with wonder foods: skim milk, brewer's yeast, wheat germ, yogurt, and blackstrap molasses. He lectured frequently and was a partner in Modern Products, Inc., of Milwaukee, Wisconsin, a company that markets products bearing his name. Hauser wrote a syndicated newspaper column and more than a dozen books reported to have sold close to fifty million copies in the United States and abroad. One book, *Look Younger, Live Longer,* led the bestseller list in 1951. That same year, the FDA seized copies of the book, claiming they were being used to promote sales of blackstrap molasses as a cure-all. The court readily agreed that the molasses was misbranded by many false claims in the book.

D.C. Jarvis, M.D. (1881–1966) wrote that body alkalinity was the principal threat to American health and that honey and apple cider were the antidotes. False claims in his book were the basis for an FDA seizure of a product called "Honegar." Melvin Page, D.D.S., who warned that milk was an underlying cause of cancer, persuaded many of his followers to stop drinking it or giving it to their children. William Howard Hay warned against eating protein and white bread and urged frequent use of laxatives. Thus came one faddist after another, each with his own brand of fear and magic.

Adolphus Hohensee (1901–1967) began his training in nutrition by taking a job as a soda jerk. After dabbling in real estate (with time in jail for mail fraud) and the field of transportation (during which time he was arrested for passing bad checks), Hohensee resumed his education. In 1943, he acquired an Honorary Degree of Doctor of Medicine from a nonaccredited school and followed this with Doctor of Naturopathy degrees from two schools that he did not attend. In 1946, he acquired a chiropractic license in the state of Nevada.

A master showman, Hohensee could lecture for hours about the terrible American diet that would stagnate the blood, corrode blood vessels, erode the kidneys, and clog the intestines. He said that most people had intestinal worms, which, fortunately, could be cured by his special cleansing. He promised a long life to those who consumed his wonder products. Repeated prosecution by the FDA made him more cautious about selling his products during lectures, but his promotion of the gamut of food myths sent his audiences flocking to nearby health-food stores whose shelves just happened to be well-stocked with his product line. In 1955, alert reporters caught Hohensee eating a meal of forbidden foods after one of his lectures. In 1962, he began serving an eighteen-month prison term for selling honey with false claims. But neither of these setbacks dampened his enthusiasm or that of his loyal followers.

Lelord Kordel (1904–), who wrote about twenty books, recommended high-protein foods, lecithin ("the miracle nutrient"), and high-dosage vitamin and mineral supplements for everyone. According to court records, he began producing and marketing supplements in 1941, operating under various trade names. In 1946, he was convicted of misbranding and fined $4,000. One product in the case was *Gotu Kola*, an herbal tablet said to restore youth and "produce erect posture, sharp eyes, velvety skin, limbs of splendid proportions, deep chests, firm bodies, gracefully curved hips, flat abdomens" and even "pleasing laughter." Thirteen other products were falsely claimed to be effective against various conditions including heart disease, liver troubles, tuberculosis, bone infections and impotence.

Kordel had a brush with the FTC in 1957 and two more with the FDA in 1961. In 1963, when he was president of Detroit Vital Foods, Inc., products shipped by the company were found to be misbranded because they were accompanied by Kordel publications which falsely claimed that nutritional products could treat practically all diseases. After the appeals process was ended in 1971, Kordel was fined $10,000 and served one year in prison. Current catalogs from Vital Foods, Inc., describe him as "America's leading vitamin and diet expert" and claim that he has never been ill.

The Consultant

Carlton Fredericks (1910–1987) was described on the covers of some of his books as "America's Foremost Nutritionist." He considered himself an expert and gave copious advice in books and in articles for health-food publications. According to the FDA, however, Fredericks had virtually no nutrition or health science training. He graduated from the University of Alabama in 1931 (under his original name: Harold Frederick Caplan) with a major in English and a minor in political science. His only science courses were two hours of physiology and eight hours of elementary chemistry. He had various jobs until 1937 when he began to write advertising copy for the U.S. Vitamin Corporation and to give sales talks, adopting the title of "nutrition educator."

Records of the Magistrates' Court of New York City show that Fredericks began diagnosing patients and prescribing vitamins for their illnesses. After agents of the New York State Department of Education investigated, Fredericks was charged with unlawful practice of medicine. In 1945, after pleading guilty, he paid a fine of $500 (rather than spend three months in jail) and joined the rolls of those with criminal convictions in connection with nutrition frauds. One investigator reported that Fredericks had pulled several times on her left arm and diagnosed poor circulation in the arm due to "nerve pressure" in her shoulder.

Fredericks then enrolled in New York University's School of Education and received a master's degree in 1949, and a night-school Ph.D. in communications in 1955, without having taken a single course in nutrition. The title of his doctoral thesis was "A Study of the Responses of a Group of Adult Female Listeners to a Series of Educational Radio Programs." These were his own radio programs—broadcast on New York City's WOR and distributed at times to other stations. The WOR broadcasts alone—which spanned thirty years—were reported to generate thousands of letters a week. Fredericks's thesis analyzed how much of certain things he said on his program was retained by its listeners and how it affected their food-buying habits.

According to an article in *The Reporter* magazine, Fredericks was listed as "Chief Consultant" to Foods Plus, Inc., a vitamin company that ran into trouble with the FDA. In 1960, more than 200,000 bottles of the firm's food-supplement preparations were seized as misbranded because literature accompanying them contained false claims that the preparations were useful in treating dozens of diseases. In 1961, the Federal Communications Commission concluded that Fredericks had a contract with Foods Plus to turn over all mail received as a result of public appearances so that the company could use the names for marketing purposes. Fredericks terminated his relationship with Foods Plus in 1962, shortly after the FDA again charged the company with misbranding products. The judge who decided this case in 1965 concluded that Fredericks had been telling a vast radio audience that vitamins and minerals could be used to treat more than fifty problems, including arthritis, epilepsy, multiple sclerosis, and even "lack of mental resistance to house-to-house salesmen." Fredericks' former contract with Foods Plus, the court ruled, made his questionable claims part of the company's product labeling. As an expert witness in the court case, Dr. Victor Herbert described Fredericks as a "charlatan." The defense attorney's objection was overruled after Dr. Herbert read aloud the *Random House Dictionary* definition of charlatan: "one who pretends to more knowledge than he possesses; quack."

Fredericks was one of the originators of the crusade to discredit sugar. He deftly channeled this single theme into a number of variations that reflected and exploited public concerns about alcoholism, emotional disorders, and hypoglycemia (low blood sugar). Once, after being introduced on the Merv Griffin Show as a "leading nutritional consultant," Fredericks was asked to estimate the number of Americans suffering from hypoglycemia. His reply, "twenty million," had no basis in fact. True hypoglycemia, as a disease, is rare.

For many years, Fredericks wrote a column for *Prevention* magazine. In 1976, *Prevention* invested $100,000 to sponsor a series of radio programs distributed free-of-charge to stations throughout the United States. Robert Franklin, the show's producer, said that the programs generated large numbers of letters from desperately ill people, many of whom seemed to think that Fredericks was a medical doctor. (This is not surprising because generally he was introduced as "Dr. Fredericks.") Franklin was so disgusted by the mail that he decided to syndicate a program that gave reputable advice, and the Harvard University School of Public Health agreed to sponsor it for three years. In a subsequent column in *Let's Live* magazine, Fredericks stated that he would not do individual consultations by mail, but he would send "nutritional therapy" protocols to physicians who wrote on their professional stationery. Toward the end of his career, he did "nutrition consultations" for $200 each at the offices of Dr. Robert Atkins.

In his books and broadcasts, Fredericks attacked the medical profession and the FDA, cited questionable advice, and attributed a myriad of therapeutic qualities to foods and food supplements. He often used humor to illustrate his points and to ridicule those with whom he disagreed. Overall, he encouraged unsafe degrees of self-diagnosis and self-treatment. A heavy smoker, he died of a heart attack at the age of seventy-six.

New Strategy

In 1961, the FDA dismantled what was probably the largest organized health scam up to that time—the promotion of "Nutri-Bio" by more than seventy-five thousand full- and part-time sales agents. Directly and indirectly, the product was being recommended as the answer to practically all health problems. Company literature containing misleading claims also included the book *Stay Young and Vital* by Hollywood actor Bob Cummings, a Nutri-Bio vice president. Huge quantities of other sales literature were involved in the case. In the Chicago area alone, Nutri-Bio agents turned in close to fifty tons of it for destruction.

The prosecutions of Nutri-Bio, Foods Plus, Lelord Kordel, and Adolphus Hohensee were part of a vigorous FDA campaign in the late 1950s and early 1960s. During this period, more than two hundred successful actions for misbranding were carried out, several prominent faddists were sentenced to prison, and the courts ruled that any false message given in the context of a sale could be considered part of a product's labeling. The 1962 Kefauver-Harris Amendment to the Food, Drug, and Cosmetic Act, which made it illegal to market a drug until it is proven effective, added still another weapon against quackery.

By 1965, it must have been clear to leaders of the health-food industry that marketing products labeled with false claims was a risky business. But the industry soon reorganized to get around the law. Most supplement manufacturers stopped labeling their products as effective against specific diseases. Industry emphasis shifted somewhat from "miracle" drugs to "nutritional insurance," an approach that tends to attract little attention from federal prosecutors. "Specialization" developed whereby most publicists of misleading nutritional claims would no longer have a direct financial tie to the sale of specific products. And common substances—vitamins, minerals, herbs and the like—would be promoted through the media without reference to brand names.

Thus, instead of claiming that his vitamin X preparation would cure cancer or flat feet, a manufacturer could rely upon books, magazine articles, and talk shows to publicize the supposed benefits of vitamin X or the supposed difficulty of getting enough of it in one's diet. In effect, the media became the label!

Although the health-food industry was well established by the mid-1960s, it had not yet penetrated the average consumer's mind. Most of its customers were considered cultists. Two developments changed this, however. The first was the explosive growth of mass communication—particularly television. The second was a growing public concern about pollution. Rachel Carson's *Silent Spring,* though filled with errors, increased public concern about pesticides and decreased public confidence in governmental protection. The concept of "organic farming" enabled faddists to arouse the interest of many people who weren't looking for miracle foods, but just wanted to feel that their food was safe. Sales pitches like "Make sure you have enough" and "Beware of chemicals in your food" converted the majority of Americans into at least occasional "health food" customers.

The High Priestess

Adelle Davis was the first "health authority" among modern food faddists who had any formal professional background. She was trained in dietetics and nutrition at the University of California at Berkeley, and got an M.S. degree in biochemistry from the University of Southern California in 1938. Despite this training, she promoted hundreds of nutritional tidbits and theories that were unfounded. At the 1969 White House Conference on Food and Nutrition, the panel on deception and misinformation agreed that Davis was probably the most damaging source of false nutrition information in the nation. Most of her ideas were harmless unless carried to extremes, but some were very dangerous. For example, she recommended magnesium as a treatment for epilepsy, potassium chloride for certain patients with kidney disease, and megadoses of vitamins A and D for other conditions.

Davis's most popular book was *Let's Eat Right to Keep Fit*. George Mann, M.D., Sc.D., of Vanderbilt University School of Medicine undertook the fatiguing task of documenting the book's errors and found an average of one mistake per page. In *Let's Get Well,* Davis listed 2,402 references to "document" its thirty-four chapters. However, experts who checked the references have reported that many of them contain no data to support what she said in the chapter. In Chapter 12, for example, a reference given in her discussion of "lip problems" and vitamins was an article about influenza, apoplexy, and aviation, with mention of neither lips nor vitamins. Gordon Schectman, a researcher at Columbia University's Institute of Human Nutrition, compared 201 statements in Chapter 5 with the publications cited to back them up. He concluded that only thirty (27 percent) of these statements were supported by the references and that 112 (56 percent) were either contradicted or not related.

During the early 1970s, Edward Rynearson, M.D., emeritus professor of medicine at the Mayo Clinic, observed:

> *Let's Get Well* is "dedicated to the hundreds of wonderful doctors whose research made this book possible." There are thousands of references in it (on one of her television appearances she said "jillions"). . . . One could guess that a large corps of helpers, each armed with scissors, read large quantities of literature, most of it published in the English language. It is credible that when a reference was encountered to vitamins, minerals, hormones, cancer, and so forth, the reference

> was snipped out and placed with hundreds of others . . . which were then used to support her often uncritical and unscientific assumptions.
>
> On page 9 she says, "The hundreds of studies used as the source material for this book have been conducted almost entirely by doctors, perhaps 95 percent of whom are professors in medical schools." . . . I doubt if 10 percent were.

When Rynearson contacted eighteen experts whose work had been cited in the book, all said they disliked the book and many said their views had been misquoted or taken out of context. Dr. Victor Herbert noted that in each instance where she referred to a scientific paper written by him, she misrepresented what he had written.

In 1971, a four-year-old victim of Davis's advice was hospitalized at the University of California Medical Center in San Francisco. The child appeared pale and chronically ill. She was having diarrhea, vomiting, fever, and loss of hair. Her liver and spleen were enlarged, and other signs suggested she had a brain tumor. Her mother, "a food faddist who read Adelle Davis religiously," had been giving her large doses of vitamins A and D plus calcium lactate. Fortunately, when these supplements were stopped, the little girl's condition improved.

Little Eliza Young was not so fortunate. During her first year of life she was given "generous amounts" of vitamin A as recommended in *Let's Have Healthy Children.* As a result, according to the suit filed in 1971 against Davis and her publisher, Eliza's growth was permanently stunted. The estate of Adelle Davis settled in 1976 for $150,000. Two-month-old Ryan Pitzer was even less fortunate. According to the suit filed by his parents, Ryan was killed in 1978 by the administration of potassium chloride for colic as suggested in the same book. The suit was settled out of court for a total of $160,000—$25,000 from the publisher, $75,000 from Davis's estate, and $60,000 from the potassium product's manufacturer. After the suit was filed, the book was recalled from bookstores, but it was reissued after changes were made by a physician allied with the health-food industry.

Davis's recommendation of potassium for colic (illustrated on the next page) was based on misinterpretation of a 1956 article in *Nutrition Reviews* about potassium metabolism in *gastroenteritis*. The article referred to a previous study of 653 hospitalized infants which found that the incidence of abdominal bloating and intestinal paralysis were higher among sixty-seven who had low levels of potassium. The article noted that although potassium might improve these symptoms, giving it to a dehydrated infant could cause cardiac arrest. (This is what killed Ryan Pitzer.) The article had nothing whatsoever to do with colic and did not state that "most babies needed 3,000

> **In a study of 653 sick babies, every infant with colic had low blood potassium. "Improvement was dramatic," and the colic disappeared immediately, when physicians gave 500 to 1,000 milligrams of potassium chloride intravenously or 1,000 to 2,000 milligrams by mouth. These doctors found that most babies needed 3,000 milligrams of potassium chloride (⅔ teaspoon) before colic was corrected. They suggested that potassium be given to prevent colic, especially during diarrhea, when much of this nutrient is lost in the feces. Potassium is also lost when too much salt (sodium) is allowed a baby, and/or when pantothenic acid is so deficient that the adrenals become exhausted.**

This is the passage in the 1972 paperback edition of *Let's Have Healthy Children* that led to Ryan Pitzer's death. The "study" was largely a figment of Adelle Davis's imagination.

milligrams of potassium chloride" to recover. The dosage was 1,000 to 2,000 milligrams administered over a twenty-four-hour period, not all at once. The "immediate and dramatic improvement" to which Davis referred was in one infant (not 653) and took about a week. The potassium loss was caused by persistent vomiting and diarrhea, not "too much sodium."

In 1972, a group of distinguished nutritionists had an opportunity to ask Davis to indicate what scientific evidence backed up many of her speculations. Like most food faddists, she did not base her ideas on such evidence. To question after question, she answered, "I will accept your criticism," "I could be wrong" or "I'm not saying it does." But she never told her followers that many of her claims had no factual basis or could be harmful.

Adelle Davis used to say that she never saw anyone get cancer who drank a quart of milk daily, as she did. She stopped saying that when she died of cancer in 1974, leaving behind her a trail of ten million books and a following that was large, devoted, and misinformed.

The Theoretician

The widespread public belief that high doses of vitamins are effective against colds and other illnesses is largely attributable to Linus Pauling, Ph.D., winner of the Nobel Prize for chemistry in 1954 and for peace in 1962. In 1968, he postulated that people's needs for vitamins and other nutrients vary markedly and that to maintain good health, many people need amounts of nutrients much greater than the Recommended Dietary Allowances (RDAs). And he speculated that megadoses of certain vitamins and minerals might well be the treatment of choice for some forms of mental illness. He termed this approach "orthomolecular," meaning "right molecule." Since then, he has steadily expanded the number of illnesses he believes can be influenced by "orthomolecular" therapy and the number of nutrients that are suitable for such use. No responsible medical or nutrition scientists share these views, but Pauling's prestige has elevated megavitamins from mere flimflam to a controversial issue.

In 1970, Pauling announced in *Vitamin C and the Common Cold* that taking 1,000 mg of vitamin C daily will reduce the incidence of colds by 45 percent for most people but that some people need much larger amounts. (The RDA for vitamin C is 60 mg.) The 1976 revision of the book, retitled *Vitamin C, the Common Cold and the Flu*, suggested even higher dosages. A third book, *Vitamin C and Cancer* (1979) claims that high doses of vitamin C may be effective against cancer. Yet another book, *How to Feel Better and Live Longer* (1986), states that megadoses of vitamins "can improve your general health . . . to increase your enjoyment of life and can help in controlling heart disease, cancer, and other diseases and in slowing down the process of aging." Pauling himself reportedly takes 12,000 mg daily and raises the amount to 40,000 mg if symptoms of a cold appear. In 1993, after undergoing radiation therapy for prostate cancer, Pauling said that vitamin C had delayed the cancer's onset for twenty years. This is not a testable claim.

Scientific fact is established when the same experiment is carried out over and over again with the same results. To test the effect of vitamin C on colds, it is necessary to compare groups which get the vitamin to similar groups which get a placebo (a dummy pill which looks like the real thing). Only in this way is it possible to determine whether the effect of vitamin C is greater than the effect of doing nothing. Since the common cold is a very variable illness, proper tests must involve hundreds of people for significantly long periods of time. At least sixteen well-designed, double-blind studies have shown that supplementation with vitamin C does not prevent colds and at best may slightly reduce the symptoms of a cold. Slight symptom reduction may occur as the result of an antihistamine-like effect, but whether this has practical value is a matter of dispute. Pauling's views are based on the same studies considered by other scientists, but his analyses are flawed.

The largest clinical trials, involving thousands of volunteers, were directed by Dr. Terence Anderson, professor of epidemiology at the University of Toronto. Taken together, his studies suggest that extra vitamin C may slightly reduce the severity of colds, but it is not necessary to take the high doses suggested by Pauling to achieve this result. Nor is there anything to be gained by taking vitamin C supplements year-round in the hope of preventing colds.

Another important study was reported in 1975 by scientists at the National Institutes of Health who compared vitamin C pills with a placebo before and during colds. Although the experiment was supposed to be double-blind, half the subjects were able to guess which pill they were getting. When the results were tabulated with all subjects lumped together, the vitamin group reported fewer colds per person over a nine-month period. But among the half who hadn't guessed which pill they had been taking, no difference in the incidence or severity was found. This illustrates how people who think they are doing something effective (such as taking a vitamin) can report a favorable result even when none exists.

In 1976, Pauling and Dr. Ewan Cameron, a Scottish physician, reported that a majority of one hundred "terminal" cancer patients treated with 10,000 mg of vitamin C daily survived three to four times longer than similar patients who did not receive vitamin C supplements. However, Dr. William DeWys, chief of clinical investigations at the National Cancer Institute, found that the study was poorly designed because the patient groups were not comparable. The Vitamin C patients were Cameron's, while the other patients were under the care of other physicians. Cameron's patients were started on vitamin C when he labeled them "untreatable" by other methods, and their subsequent survival was compared to the survival of the "control" patients after they were labeled untreatable by their doctors. DeWys reasoned that if the two groups were comparable, the lengths of time from entry into the hospital to being labeled untreatable should be equivalent in both groups. However, he found that Cameron's patients were labeled untreatable much earlier in the course of their disease—which means that they entered the hospital before they were as sick as the other doctors' patients and would naturally be expected to live longer.

Nevertheless, to test whether Pauling might be correct, the Mayo Clinic conducted three double-blind studies involving a total of 367 patients with advanced cancer. The studies, reported in 1979, 1983, and 1985, found that patients given 10,000 mg of vitamin C daily did no better than those given a placebo.

Science aside, it is clear that Pauling is politically aligned with the promoters of unscientific nutrition practices. He says his initial interest in vitamin C was aroused by a letter from biochemist Irwin Stone, with whom he subsequently maintained a close working relationship. Although Stone was often referred to as "Dr. Stone," his only credentials were a certificate showing completion of a two-year chemistry program, an honorary chiropractic degree from the Los Angeles College of Chiropractic, and a "Ph.D." from Donsbach University, a nonaccredited correspondence school.

In a little-publicized chapter in *Vitamin C and the Common Cold,* Pauling attacked the health-food industry for misleading its customers. Pointing out that "synthetic" vitamin C is identical with "natural" vitamin C, he warned that higher-priced "natural" products are a "waste of money." And he added that "the words 'organically grown' are essentially meaningless—just part of the jargon used by health-food promoters in making their excess profits, often from elderly people with low incomes." But *Vitamin C, the Common Cold and the Flu,* issued six years later, contained none of these criticisms. This omission was not accidental. Pauling informed Dr. Barrett that, after his first book came out, he was "strongly attacked by people who were also attacking the health-food people." His critics were so "biased," he decided, that he would no longer help them attack the health-food industry while another part of their attack was directed at him.

The Linus Pauling Institute of Medicine, founded in 1973, is dedicated to "orthomolecular medicine." Many of the institute's fundraising brochures have contained questionable information. They have falsely claimed, for example, that no significant progress has been made in cancer treatment in the past twenty years. This viewpoint, which is frequently expressed by promoters of unproven cancer therapies, is simply untrue. The institute's largest corporate donor has been Hoffmann-La Roche, the pharmaceutical giant that is the dominant factor in worldwide production of vitamin C. Many of the Institute's individual donors were solicited with the help of Rodale Press (publishers of *Prevention* magazine) and related organizations that publicized the Institute and allowed the use of their mailing lists.

During the mid-1970s, Pauling helped lead the health-food industry's campaign for passage of the Proxmire Amendment, which weakened FDA protection of consumers against misleading nutrition claims (see Chapter 20). In 1977 and 1979, Pauling received awards and presented his views on vitamin C at the annual conventions of the National Nutritional Foods Association (the major trade association of health-food retailers, distributors and producers.) In 1981, he accepted an award from the National Health Federation (NHF) for "services rendered in behalf of health freedom" and gave his daughter a life membership in this organization. NHF, as detailed in Chapter 20, promotes the gamut of quackery. Pauling has also appeared as a speaker at a Parker School for Professional Success Seminar, a meeting where chiropractors were taught highly questionable methods of building their practices. An ad for the meeting invited chiropractors to pose with Pauling for a photograph (which presumably could be used for publicity when the chiropractors returned home).

In 1983, Pauling and Irwin Stone testified at a hearing on behalf of Oscar Falconi, a vitamin promoter charged by the Postal Service with making false claims for several products. Pauling supported Falconi's contentions that vitamin C was useful not only in preventing cancer, but also in curing drug addicts and destroying both viruses and bacteria. Pauling also testified in 1984 before the California Board of Medical Quality Assurance in defense of Michael Gerber, M.D., who was accused of improperly administering to patients. One was a fifty-six-year-old woman with treatable cancer who—the Board concluded—had died as a result of Gerber's neglect while he treated her with herbs, enzymes, coffee enemas, and chelation therapy. The other patients were three-year-old twin boys with ear infections for which Gerber had prescribed 70,000 or more units of vitamin A daily and coffee enemas twice daily for several weeks. Gerber lost his license to practice medicine as a result of the hearings. In 1992, Pauling testified in behalf of "clinical ecologist" Warren M. Levin, M.D., during hearings that culminated in a recommendation by New York State authorities that Levin's license should be revoked for "gross negligence," "fraudulent practice," and "moral unfitness."

A flyer distributed in 1991 by the Linus Pauling Institute recommends daily doses of 6,000 to 18,000 mg of vitamin C, 400 to 1,600 IU of vitamin E, and 25,000 IU of vitamin A, plus various other vitamins and minerals. These dosages have no proven benefit and can cause troublesome side effects.

Although Pauling's megavitamin claims lack the evidence needed for acceptance by the scientific community, they have been accepted by large numbers of people who lack the scientific expertise to evaluate them. After all, he's a distinguished Nobel Prize winner. And that's good enough for John Q. Public, who naively assumes that Pauling's prestige as a chemist makes his health and nutritional claims valid.

The "Internationally Recognized Nutritionist"

Paavo Airola's publications have described him as "an internationally recognized nutritionist, naturopathic physician, award-winning author, and renowned lecturer," "a world-leading authority on nutrition and holistic medicine," "America's foremost nutritionist," and "America's #1 bestselling health author." He was said to have studied nutrition, biochemistry, and biological medicine in Europe; spent many years studying ancient, herbal, and alternative healing methods during worldwide travels; and directed biological medical clinics in Europe and Mexico. But no details of his educational background were provided.

Airola touted a diet that stressed fresh, raw, organically grown fruits, vegetables, and grains. Animal proteins were out, except for farm-fresh-fertilized eggs, and unpasteurized cow or goat milk. He claimed that meat caused cancer and that protein requirements could be met from plant sources if they were eaten raw. Enzymes, he said (incorrectly), made the protein in these foods complete. He recommended vitamins, minerals, herbs, and fermented foods, and "revealed" health and beauty "secrets" from all over the world.

Airola died in 1983, but most of his books are still distributed by Health Plus Publishers of Scottsdale, Arizona, and sold through health-food stores. In 1985, to encourage retailers to stock up, Health Plus mailed this message:

> Take just one of our books, *How to Get Well*, by Dr. Paavo Airola (800,000 copies sold to date—mostly in health-food stores). That book recommends vitamins, minerals and other supplements, herbs, juices, and natural foods for more than sixty common ailments, as well as equipment such as juicers, seed grinders, and flour mills.
>
> For example: for osteoporosis . . . you have the potential of selling: 14 vitamins and supplements, modestly estimated at $5.00/product; 5 herbal products @ $3.00 each; groceries . . . $20; possibly a piece or two of equipment such as a juicer or seed grinder ($200). TOTAL: $305.00 . . . And your customer will most likely return for replenishment of supplements and foods.
>
> These figures might not be accurate, but you get the picture. Now multiply these figures times hundreds of customers and 60+ ailments, and you can see what far-reaching effects one book such as *How to Get Well* can have on your overall sales volume.

Are You Confused? (1971), said to have over 700,000 copies in print, covered Airola's basic philosophy with each of his health "secrets" described at length. To help readers decide what information is "absolutely reliable, objective and scientifically correct," he suggested that "laboratory research and animal tests are only of limited value as compared to the thousands of years of actual human experience with nutrition capable of producing superior health."

How to Keep Slim, Healthy, and Young with Juice Fasting (1971), said to have 500,000 copies in print, described how to fast for up to forty days on juices made from raw fruits and vegetables. The book told how Airola supposedly cured patients of arthritis, cancer, asthma, obesity, diabetes, and abnormal heart rhythms, all with juice fasting. Prolonged fasting is dangerous because it causes breakdown of proteins in vital organs such as the heart and kidneys. But Airola claimed (incorrectly) that the body decomposes only dead, dying and damaged cells, tumors, and abscesses, and that all vital organs are spared. He said raw juices were "youthifying" and called juice fasting "the oldest and most effective healing method known to man." His recommendations included string bean skin tea for diabetes, carrot juice for emphysema, and apple juice for nervousness.

But he also attempted to disclaim responsibility by stating (in boldface type): "The information in this book is not intended as diagnosing or prescribing; it should be used in cooperation with your doctor to solve your health problems. In the event you use the information yourself, you are prescribing for yourself, which is your constitutional right, but the author and publisher assume no responsibility."

How to Get Well (1974) offered "a complete therapeutic program" for more than sixty health problems, including arthritis, bladder infection, cataracts, diabetes, emphysema, heart disease, impotence, multiple sclerosis, paralysis (from a stroke) and stomach ulcers. For each of these he recommended "foods, vitamins, food supplements, juices, herbs, fasting, baths and other ancient and modern nutritional and biological modalities." The vitamin guide listed twenty-three "vitamins," even though the scientific community recognizes only thirteen.

Everywoman's Book (1979) suggested that headstands might make the breasts firmer and that eating lots of salty foods prior to conception would increase the odds of having a boy, while eating calcium-rich foods would increase the odds of having a girl.

Worldwide Secrets for Staying Young (1982) covered "proven and effective ways to halt and reverse the aging processes and live a long and healthy life." Each of the first thirteen chapters provided "health and longevity secrets" from one part of the world. Claiming that "one of the true fountains of youth is optimum nutrition," the book also claimed that humans should live to the age of 120 unless they "kill themselves prematurely by violating the basic laws of health and life."

Despite all this, Airola was only sixty-four when he suffered a fatal stroke.

The Magazine Salesmen

> Man has been a creature of fallacy ever since time began. It seems to be inherent in his nature to believe in false things. . . . In the field of medicine, especially, man seems to delight in being completely taken in.

J.I. Rodale, who wrote this in 1954, seemed to understand how gullible people can be. Like Carlton Fredericks, Rodale had changed his original name (Jerome Irving Cohen) to one that was more promotable. Rodale was a shrewd businessman. His financial success attracted considerable attention in the early 1970s, and the publicity he received boosted his profits even more. He died in 1971, leaving a publishing empire to his son Robert. In 1991, Rodale Press's reported gross income was $289 million and the circulation of its leading magazine, *Prevention,* was over three million. Robert remained head of the company until 1990, when he was killed in a traffic accident while visiting the Soviet Union.

For many years, *Prevention* was the leading magazine promoting the health-food industry's viewpoints. It attacked ordinary foods and recommended supplements and "health foods" with claims that often were ludicrous. J.I. Rodale imagined many dangers lurking in our food supply. He accused sugar of "causing criminals," and blamed bread for colds, stomach irritation, bronchitis, pneumonia, conjunctivitis, rickets in children, and steatorrhea in adults. He warned that "coke" drinkers would become sterile. Even roast beef, pickles, ice cream, and bagels aroused his concern. An article in the *New York Times Magazine* reported that each day, J.I. took seventy food-supplement tablets and would spend ten to twenty minutes under a shortwave machine "to restore his body electricity." He would live to one hundred, he told the reporter, unless he was run down by "a sugar-crazed taxi driver." But a few weeks later, at age seventy-two, he died of a heart attack while taping a TV interview for the Dick Cavett show.

Before J.I. Rodale's death, *Prevention* was filled with nonsense promoting dietary supplements for everyone—and ads from mail-order companies offering them for sale. (In fact, a recent Rodale Press film states that J.I.'s plan for *Prevention* was to "write all kinds of articles that would help the advertisers sell products so they would take more advertising.") Readers were told that our food supply was depleted of nourishment. News of nutritional "discoveries" was slanted to suggest that people who take food supplements are likely to benefit from discoveries which are just around the corner. Many articles contained therapeutic claims that would be illegal on product labels. Each issue contained two dozen or so letters from readers telling how nutritional remedies had supposedly helped them. A 1973 survey reported that families that subscribed to *Prevention* spent an average of $190 per year for vitamin supplements and health foods—which was five to ten times as much as it would have cost to supply an average family with a well balanced multivitamin/mineral product.

Although water fluoridation is an extremely valuable and real way to use dietary supplementation to prevent disease (tooth decay), J.I. Rodale was adamantly opposed to it. Before his death, most issues of *Prevention* contained vicious attacks on fluoridation in articles, editorials, and letters to the editor. Communities around Rodale's headquarters in Emmaus, Pennsylvania, were subjected to an even greater amount of antifluoridation propaganda. In 1961, for example, Rodale Press spent more than $10,000 on a scare campaign which defeated a fluoridation referendum in nearby Allentown. The fears Rodale aroused still prevent Allentown's water supply from being fluoridated today. Following J.I.'s death, *Prevention* stopped attacking fluoridation and making ridiculous claims for dietary supplements. But it continued to recommend supplements for everyone.

During the 1980s, *Prevention* shifted toward the scientific mainstream. In 1985, it dropped Carlton Fredericks and Jonathan Wright as columnists. During the next two years it acquired a prominent editorial advisory board and began sending many of its articles to experts (including Dr. Stephen Barrett) for prepublication review. Partly in response to these changes, ads for vitamins and other supplements dropped from forty to fifty pages per issue to perhaps four or five, and some health-food-industry writers even complained that *Prevention* had "sold out to the establishment." Today *Prevention* emphasizes healthy food choices, appropriate exercise programs, and other health-promoting activities. However, although its advice on most topics is accurate, it still tends to encourage unnecessary use and undue experimentation with dietary supplements. Unlike most other nutrition-related articles in *Prevention*, vitamin-pushing editorials by top editor Mark Bricklin have little prepublication review by experts. Although the magazine no longer glorifies unscientific practitioners, it rarely criticizes what they do—thus leaving its readers to fend for themselves in the marketplace. And ads for dubious products and/or services still appear in every issue—particularly in the classified section—despite efforts by Barrett to persuade Bricklin to screen them out.

Rodale Press has published several booklets that give ambiguous and conflicting advice about dietary supplements. "Prevention's Guide to Vitamins and Minerals" (1987) states that "the preferred source of vitamins and minerals is your food," but it adds: "While it's possible to obtain recommended amounts of vitamins and minerals entirely from food, many people do not." The booklet's longest section is filled with speculations that encourage supplementation. One passage states, for example, that "there's a hint of a chance that folic acid may help with behavior problems that come with some forms of mental retardation." Another passage states: "There have also been speculations that [vitamin] C helps ward off cancer." The Rodale booklet "The Healing Power of Nutrition" (1989) follows a similar pattern. Its section on vitamin C describes supplementation to prevent colds as a "does-it-or-doesn't-it controversy." Rather than simply saying it doesn't, the passage provides a jumble of data about vitamin C's role in immunity.

In recent years, Rodale's book division and the Prevention Book Club have marketed some books that are authoritative and others that espouse quack ideas. Ads for the books are even more blatant than the books themselves. For

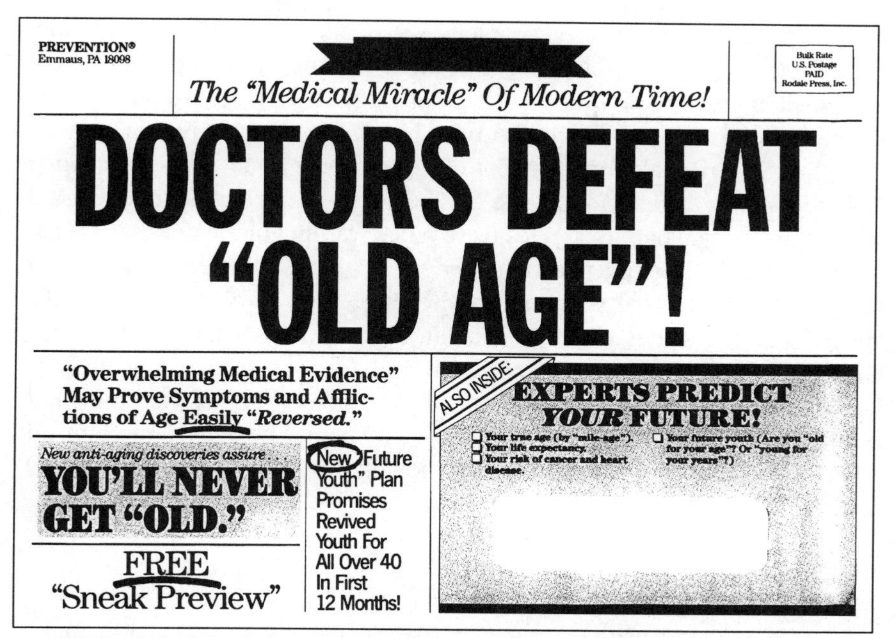

Mail solicitations for Rodale's health-related books are typically written in the style of a tabloid newspaper. This book, *Future Youth: How to Reverse the Aging Process,* offers a jumble of advice and speculation that does not deliver what the mailer promises.

example, a mailer for *The Doctor's Vitamin and Mineral Encyclopedia*, by Sheldon Saul Hendler, M.D., was headlined "The World's Most Powerful Healing Vitamins and Minerals" and promised information on "a substance that reverses the aging process," a "heavy duty smart pill" that "stops the aging process and dramatically improves your memory," and a one-a-day supplement that "could dramatically reduce your chances of breast cancer." The pertinent passages in the book reported unwarranted speculations based on preliminary or anecdotal evidence.

Understanding Vitamins and Minerals (1988), part of the "Prevention Total Health System" series, was promised to provide "the latest reports on over 100 illnesses and health problems, and the vitamins and minerals that have cured or prevented them." The book was also touted as "what we believe is the most dependable book ever on vitamins and minerals." Unfortunately for readers, the book is loaded with poor advice, and many "experts" whom the book quotes are prominent promoters of quackery. Chapter 2 ("Why You Need Food Supplements") states that "almost everyone falls into one or more of the categories of people who need supplements." Chapter 11 ("Personal Supplement Program") contains eight pages of charts that suggest using high doses of eleven vitamins and four minerals for fatigue, stress, depression, and "looking ten years older than you should." Advice like this is completely loony.

In 1989, Rodale Press sent *Prevention* readers an ad for *Nutrition Prescription,* by Brian Morgan, Ph.D. The ad promised that the book would provide "a 'crystal ball' that gives us advance warning of the diseases we are most vulnerable to" plus a nutritional program "specifically designed to defeat the disease, reverse the symptoms and change your medical future for the better." The ad also described Dr. Morgan as "America's leading authority on nutrition." Calling the book "an inseparable mixture of good and poor advice," Dr. Barrett urged the National Advertising Division (NAD) of the Council of Better Business Bureaus to ask Dr. Morgan whether he considered himself "America's leading authority." After reviewing Dr. Morgan's resumé, NAD concluded that he was not.

Attacks on Additives

Many school-age children have been labeled "hyperactive" or "hyperkinetic." In 1973, Benjamin Feingold, M.D., a pediatric allergist from California, proposed that salicylates, artificial colors, and artificial flavors were causes of hyperactivity. To treat or prevent this condition, he suggested a diet that was free of these chemicals. Feingold's followers now claim that asthma, bedwetting, ear infections, eye-muscle disorders, seizures, sleep disorders, and stomach aches may respond to the Feingold program and that sensitivity to synthetic additives and/or salicylates may be a factor in antisocial traits, compulsive aggression, self-mutilation, difficulty in reasoning, stuttering, and exceptional clumsiness. The 1986 *Feingold Handbook* even states that "sensitivity to synthetic chemicals in the food or environment, or to some natural salicylates" can cause *adults* to suffer from nervous habits, chronic fatigue, impulsiveness, poor self-image, poor coordination, mental and physical sluggishness, temper flare-ups, headaches, depression, erratic sleep patterns, and a "tendency to interrupt." This is sheer nonsense.

Adherence to the Feingold diet requires a drastic change in family lifestyle and eating patterns. Homemade foods prepared "from scratch" are necessary for many meals. Feingold strongly recommended that the hyperactive child help prepare the special foods and encouraged the entire family to participate in the dietary program. *The Feingold Cookbook* states: "A successful response to the diet depends on 100 percent compliance. The slightest infraction can lead to failure: a single bite or drink can cause an undesirable response that may persist for seventy-two hours or more."

Many parents who have followed Feingold's recommendations have reported improvement in their children's behavior. In fact, many families have banded together into cultlike local groups and a national association to promote the dietary program. But carefully designed experiments have failed to support the idea that additives cause hyperactivity. Improvement, if any, appears related to changes in family dynamics such as paying more attention to the children. Experts have also pointed out that the foods recommended by Feingold's book, *Why Your Child is Hyperactive* (1975), included some that were high in salicylates and excluded others that were low in salicylates.

Because the Feingold diet does no physical harm, it might appear to be helpful therapy in some instances. However, the potential benefits should be weighed against the potential harm of teaching children that behavior and school performance are related to what they eat rather than what they feel. There is additional potential for harm in creating situations in which a child's eating behavior is regarded as peculiar by other children. We felt sorry for the youngster who, years ago, announced on a "Donahue" show that he had misbehaved because he had "slipped" off his diet and eaten a candy bar.

Additional Feingold-related mischief may loom on the horizon. The September 1992 issue of the Feingold Association's newsletter, *Pure Facts,* claimed that teachers and children have been noted to suffer from the effects of chemicals used in construction, furnishing, housekeeping, maintenance, renovation, pest control, food service, and classroom activities at their schools. An article titled "The Sick Building Syndrome" stated that one child was repeatedly disciplined for reacting to his teacher's perfume, another child became abusive toward his mother because of the school's newly painted lunchroom, and that yet another child required tutoring because of a very bad reaction to a leak in the school's oil furnace. Claims like these are similar to those made by clinical ecologists (see Chapter 12). Although exposure to chemical fumes in poorly ventilated buildings can make people ill, the idea that perfume causes misbehavior is nonsensical.

In 1970, a team of "Nader's Raiders" led by attorney James Turner published *The Chemical Feast,* a blistering attack on the FDA. The book stated that the FDA would not acknowledge "the relationship between deteriorating American health and the limited supply of safe and wholesome food." During the following year, other Nader associates formed the Center for Science in the Public Interest (CSPI) to investigate and report on a variety of food and chemical issues.

CSPI said it intended to "improve the quality of the American diet through research and public education." It promised to "watchdog" federal agencies that oversee food safety, trade, and nutrition. It also launched an annual National Food Day to call public attention to food issues. What issues? A 1975 Food Day brochure claimed: "Chemical farming methods create environmental havoc." A 1976 brochure stated: "Every few months, it seems, another common food additive is found to be harmful. . . . And agricultural chemicals have polluted everything from the nation's water supply to mother's milk." CSPI has campaigned vigorously for government certification of "organically grown foods" and sponsored annual conferences on this subject. In 1986, it launched Americans for Safe Foods (ASF), a coalition of more than forty consumer, environmental, and rural groups. ASF charged that much of the nation's food supply was riddled with pesticides, bacteria, drugs, and other hazards.

CSPI, which now has more than 400,000 members, is headed by one of its cofounders, Michael F. Jacobson, Ph.D., whose doctoral degree is in microbiology. Its monthly newsletter, *Nutrition Action, a*dvises everyone to consume less salt, to avoid fat-laden foods, to increase the fiber content of their diet, and to take vitamin supplements even with a well-balanced diet. Almost every issue chides the products of food companies that CSPI believes are "more concerned with big profits than with good nutrition."

Unlike the traditional attackers of chemicals, Jacobson and his colleagues don't stress magical ideas about foods and are not obviously outlandish. Nor do they appear to be motivated by personal financial gain. They have stimulated several valuable government actions to protect consumers against misleading claims in food and vitamin advertising. They have campaigned vigorously to maintain and strengthen FDA regulation of food supplements, which the health-food industry wants to weaken. (Industry leasders reacted by denouncing CSPI.) However, CSPI's many unjustified attacks have undermined public confidence in our food supply and lent credibility to what the faddists have been saying all along. If CSPI were truly interested in public health, it would wage the same kind of warfare against alcohol and tobacco as it has against food processors.

Unfortunately, many of our country's largest and most respected food companies have also jumped on the "back-to-nature" bandwagon. Today the words "natural" and "additive-free" appear on almost every type of edible product. Even beer and candy bars (the so-called "health bars") bear these magic words. Food companies that exploit the unfounded public fear of additives may profit financially while ignoring their responsibility to the American public. An educational campaign aimed at promoting sound nutrition and exposing food faddism would be a much more commendable course of action.

A Leading "Pioneer"

Robert Atkins, M.D., refers to himself and like-minded colleagues as "the pioneers of Nutrition Medicine who risked their professional standing to develop the methodology that led the Nutrition Breakthrough." Atkins condemns the medical profession as "pill poppers," and drug pushers, but he does not hesitate to recommend megadoses of nutritional supplements for a wide variety of diseases and conditions. His books include *Dr. Atkins' Diet Revolution* (1971), *Dr. Atkins' Superenergy Diet* (1977), *Dr. Atkins' Nutrition Breakthrough* (1981), *Dr. Atkins' Health Revolution* (1988), and *Dr. Atkins' New Diet Revolution* (1992).

Atkins founded and directs The Atkins Center for Complementary Medicine, which is located in a modern six-story building he owns in New York City. According to an article in *Newsday,* Atkins heads five corporations, including the Robert Atkins Professional Corp., which grossed $3.8 million in 1991, the Atkins Center, which grossed $5.3 million, and his private practice, which grossed $320,000 that year. He also publishes a monthly newsletter (*Health Revelations)* and hosts "Design for Living," a nightly radio talk show on station WOR. The former host of the program was Carlton Fredericks who, in the mid-1980s, performed "nutritional consultations" at Atkins's offices. *Dr. Atkins' Health Revolution* is dedicated to Fredericks, whom Atkins identified as his "mentor."

Patients who consult Atkins typically undergo hair analysis and/or various other tests that are not recognized as valid by the scientific community. Early in 1993, Atkins was consulted by a forty-year-old investigator for the "Geraldo" show who told Atkins she was concerned about her weight and was worried because her thirty-five-year-old brother had recently had a heart attack. Atkins (incorrectly) diagnosed hypoglycemic and multiple food allergies. The diagnosis of "hypoglycemia" was based on a glucose tolerance test, which is not an adequate test for hypoglycemia. Even if it were, her lowest recorded value was 69 mg per 100 ml, which is not a subnormal level. The "allergies" were diagnosed with cytotoxic testing, which is not a valid test for allergies (see Chapter 7). She was also told (incorrectly) that she had a yeast infection that required treatment with a carbohydrate-restrictive diet. The total bill came to about $1,100 for two visits and laboratory tests plus $129 for supplement products. When a reference was made to his income as reported in the *Newsday* article, Atkins replied, "We don't have a profit margin. What we charge our patients enables us to break even."

The supplements are sold at a counter in the lobby of Atkins's office building and are also available by mail. A 1991 brochure describes "Dr. Atkins'

Targeted Nutrition Program" as a regimen in which "building blocks" are added to a "basic formula" to "help the body create its own cures." The seventeen "building blocks" included *Anti-Arthritic Formula*, *Cardiovascular Formula*, *Diabetes Mellitus Formula*, *Heart Rhythm Formula*, *Hypoglycemia Formula*, and *Urinary Frequency Formula*. (The labels of some of these products do not contain the full name of the product but merely a code—such as *CV* for *Cardiovascular Formula* and *DM* for *Diabetes Mellitus Formula.)* The brochure states that the formulas evolved over twenty-five years of Atkins's experience in using nutrition to treat more than forty thousand patients. The full name and ingredients of most of the formulas are stated in the Appendix of *Dr. Atkins' Health Revolution* .

It is a federal crime to market a product intended for the treatment of disease unless it is generally recognized by experts as safe and effective for its intended purpose. In his testimony in the Levin case, Atkins denied that the products were intended to treat medical conditions and said they were merely convenient formulations for "managing nutritional deficiencies."

It appears that Atkins has also issued misleading receipts that patients could use to seek reimbursement from their insurance companies. In 1993, a reporter noted the following announcement posted on the cashier's cage in the lobby of his building:

As of May 18, 1993 the receipts/superbills you will be receiving will

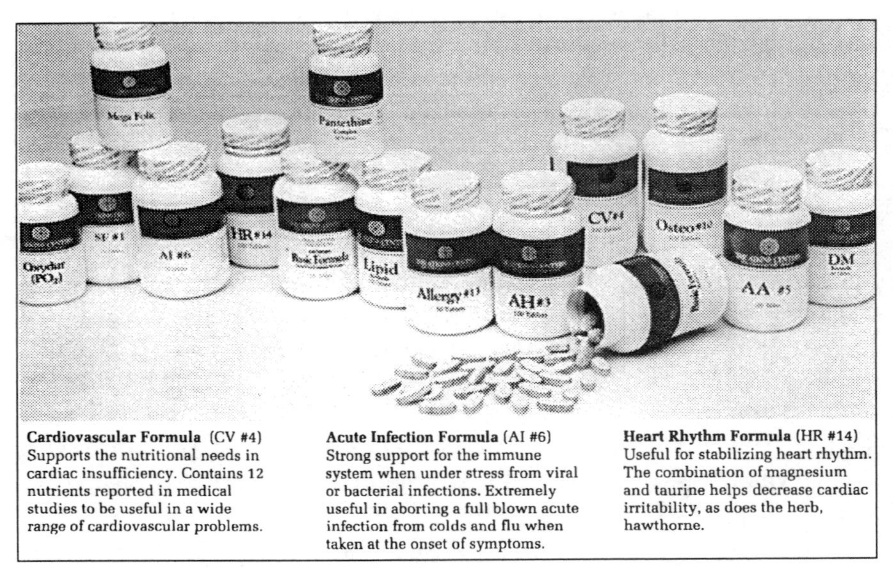

A portion of Atkins's 1991 brochure for supplements.

> no longer state "Prescribed Medicine. Instead they will state: "Vitamin Mineral/Herbal Supplements." This is due to the fact that insurance companies are asking us to be more specific than we have been in the past. . . . UNLESS YOUR POLICY SPECIFICALLY STATES THAT VITAMINS ARE COVERED, THEN YOU MAY ASSUME THAT THEY ARE NOT. We recommend that you do not submit the vitamins to your insurance carrier for reimbursement. It may effect your ability to collect on the rest of your claim.

In July 1993, based on the 1991 brochure, an FDA report charged that six of Atkins's products were being marketed with unsubstantiated claims: *Pantethine Complex, Acute Infection Formula, Anti-Arthritic Formula, Anti-Hypertension Formula, Lipid Formula,* and *Diabetes Mellitus Formula.* The report was based on the 1991 brochure. His current brochure makes unsubstantiated claims for at least seventeen of the twenty-three products it describes. The full names for *Acute Infection Formula, Anti-Arthritic Formula, Anti-Hypertension Formula,* and *Diabetes Mellitus Formula* no longer appear in the brochure, but the products, claims, and labeling (with code names) continue.

In 1991, Atkins testified in behalf of Warren M. Levin, M.D., at a disciplinary hearing held by the New York State Department of Health Board of Professional Conduct. Before the hearing he wrote in his newsletter that he used the "same or equivalent practices" as Dr. Levin. During his testimony, Atkins said that about 40 percent of the patients who consult him have "functional hypoglycemia" and that about one third require treatment for a problem related to *Candida.* He also admitted that he is not certified by the American Board of Internal Medicine because he failed the oral examination and decided not to take it again. (This is a test of the ability to examine patients and make appropriate treatment plans.) In 1992, the licensing authorities judged Levin guilty of "gross negligence," "fraudulent practice," and "moral unfitness" and recommended that his license be revoked.

In August 11, 1993, the authorities suspended Atkins's medical license after investigating a case in which a 77-year-old breast cancer patient used a hand-held pump to inject herself with ozone gas. According to press reports, the suspension was triggered by a complaint from an emergency room physician who had treated the woman for left-sided weakness caused by a brain embolism (blood vessel obstruction). In his newsletter, Atkins stated that the patient had merely "suffered a minor reaction that left her weak-kneed" and that she had returned to him for further therapy. On August 17, a New York State Supreme Court judge ruled that Atkins could resume seeing patients as long as he does not treat them with ozone. The state investigation of Atkins continues.

The "Health Crusader"

Gary Null, whose books bill him as "one of America's leading health and fitness advocates," is one of the nation's leading promoters of dubious treatment for serious disease. He hosts radio and television talk shows, writes books, delivers lectures, and has marketed supplement products. According to an article in *East West* magazine, Null became interested in nutrition during his twenties while working as a short order cook in New York City, where he now resides. He "researched" the subject and wrote *The Complete Guide to Health and Nutrition*, which was published in 1972 and sold briskly after Null appeared on a succession of prominent talk shows. He began hosting radio shows around that time and eventually got his own show on WABC, the flagship radio station of the ABC network. Later he moved to WMCA, which broadcast Null's show on Sunday nights to about two hundred stations across the United States. He now hosts a daily show on WBAI in New York City.

Null is prone to see conspiracies behind many of the things he is concerned about. His favorite target is the pharmaceutical industry, which he says "cannot afford to have an alternative therapy accepted." He has spoken out against fluoridation, immunization, food irradiation, mercury-amalgam fillings, and many forms of proven medical treatment. His series on "The Politics of Cancer," which was published in *Penthouse* magazine in 1979 and 1980, promoted questionable methods that he said were being "suppressed" by the medical establishment. His fourteen-part series, "Medical Genocide," which *Penthouse* carried from 1985 through 1987, began with an article calling our medical care system a "prescription for disaster." The rest of the series promoted chiropractic and homeopathy, claimed that effective nutritional methods for treating AIDS were being suppressed, claimed that chelation therapy was safe and effective for treating heart disease, recommended questionable approaches for arthritis, and endorsed treatments for cancer that the American Cancer Society recommends against.

Null says he holds an associate degree in business administration from Mountain State College in West Virginia, a bachelor's degree from Thomas A. Edison State College in New Jersey, and a Ph.D. in human nutrition and public health sciences from The Union Institute in Cincinnati, Ohio. Edison State, a nontraditional school with neither campus nor courses, awards accredited bachelor's degrees based on career experience, equivalency exams, and courses taken at other schools. Union is also accredited, but its degree requirements and standards are vastly inferior to those of most universities. Students design their own program, form and chair their own doctoral committee, and are required to attend only an introductory colloquium and a few interdisciplinary seminars.

One of the three "adjunct professors" who passed judgment on Null's Ph.D. thesis was a physician who has pinch-hit for Null as a radio host and helped Null develop supplement formulations.

Traditional universities require that the research for a doctoral degree make a genuine contribution to the scientific literature. Null's thesis, entitled "A Study of Psychological and Physiological Effects of Caffeine on Human Health," does not appear to do this. His research project compared the effect of a week of caffeine versus a week without caffeine among small numbers of volunteers, more than half of whom dropped out or were disqualified for noncompliance. Null's thesis purports to compare the "adrenal function" of seventeen people who remained in the study for the full two weeks. But his determination involved measurements of blood pressure and urine characteristics that are not scientifically recognized as valid for that purpose.

The most notable of these tests involved measurement of the specific gravity, pH (acidity), and surface tension of single samples of urine—a test used by Emanuel Revici, M.D. Null notes that the theory behind the test "is still the subject of debate and has not yet gained wide scientific support"—a rather strange way to describe a test that is utterly worthless for any medical purpose whatsoever. (The specific gravity of urine reflects the concentration of dissolved substances and depends mainly on the amount of fluid a person consumes. Urine acidity depends mainly on diet, but varies considerably throughout the day. Thus the acidity of a single sample of urine can provide no useful information about a patient's metabolism. The surface tension of urine has no medically recognized diagnostic value.) Revici, whose unproven methods of cancer treatment triggered a ten-year struggle with New York State licensing authorities, had his medical license revoked in 1993.

Following forty-one pages of findings, calculations, tables, and graphs, Null concludes that "chronic caffeine users tend to have diminished adrenal function" which he blames on "exhaustion" of the glands. "Fortunately," he adds, "there are non-drug nutritional programs which have the ability to repair or rebalance weakening adrenal glands toward normal." His recommended program includes lifestyle changes plus supplementation with five vitamins and three other products.

The supplements marketed by Null have included *Guard-Ion* (an "antioxidant" formula claimed to help protect athletes from free radicals the body can't control), *Gary Null's AM-PM Vitamin-Mineral Formula* (a "revolutionary breakthrough in vitamin preparation" that provides the nutrients needed at the best times for the body's anabolic and catabolic activities), *Candida Complex* (to bolster the body's defenses against yeast infection), *Endurance Factor* (containing "all the nutrients and enzymes that have made Bee Pollen famous"), *Energy Plus* (a royal jelly tablet), *Rebalancer* (a "cleansing formulation" for adults exposed to air pollutants, pesticides, or preservatives, or who have "internal metabolic imbalances"), *CoEnzyme* Q_{10} ("may reverse deficiencies and improve organ function, especially in the heart), *Sport DMG* (an N,N-dimethylglycine product to "improve cardiovascular function and to enhance the body's natural immune response system), and *Gary Null's Immune Nutrients* ("to nourish and stimulate immune function, not merely at a marginal level of preventing disease and degeneration, but a positive level of striving for wellness and excellence, for optimal health"). Claims made for some of these products are illegal.

In 1992, an Arizona company and its owners agreed to pay $200,000 to settle Federal Trade Commission charges of falsely claiming that bee pollen products could produce weight loss, permanently alleviate allergies, reverse the aging process, and cure, prevent, or alleviate impotence or sexual dysfunction (see Chapter 8). They were also charged with falsely stating that bee pollen products cannot result in an allergic reaction. Some of the false claims were made in "infomercials" that were misrepresented as news or documentary programs, even though they were paid ads. One such program ("TV Insiders") featured an interview "by satellite" with "Dr. Gary Null . . . *the* authority on health and nutrition." Null said that the human body ages because it doesn't produce enough enzymes, and that "you can't get any better food than bee pollen" because it is "loaded" with enzymes and contains a nutrient that "can help the inside of your body prevent the capillaries from aging." Records from The Union Institute indicate that Null "graduated" on August 31, 1989, which, according to an FTC document, was at least three months after broadcasting of the infomercial began. However, Null was not charged with wrongdoing.

The "Persecuted" Doctor

Jonathan V. Wright, M.D., a Harvard graduate who obtained his medical degree at the University of Michigan, began practicing in 1973 in Kent, Washington, a few miles southeast of Seattle. In *Dr. Wright's Book of Nutritional Therapy* (Rodale Press, 1979), he labels his approach "nutritional biochemistry" and describes how he treats a wide range of health problems with vitamins, minerals, other "natural" substances, and/or dietary measures. He and Alan Gaby, M.D., of Baltimore, give seminars on "Nutrition as Therapy," which present their theories in detail. In 1985, Wright cofounded and became president of the American Quack Association, a support network for "holistic" practitioners (see Chapter 12). In 1993, he became chairman of the board of governors of the National Health Federation, a militant lobbying group whose activities are described in Chapter 20.

During the past few years, Wright has achieved considerable notoriety battling the FDA. The dispute surfaced in July 1991 when law enforcement officers seized 103 bottles of L-tryptophan from the For Your Health Pharmacy, adjacent to Wright's clinic. The FDA had banned the marketing of L-tryptophan after it was implicated in an outbreak of eosinophilia-myalgia syndrome, but Wright continued to prescribe it. In August 1991, he filed suit, asserting that the outbreak was due to a contaminant and that his tryptophan was safe and therefore legal to dispense. The suit also asked the court to return the product and bar the FDA from "unreasonably interfering" with his ability to exercise clinical judgment in treating patients.

During the same month, according to an FDA affidavit, FDA investigators observed mold in some glass vials at the pharmacy and were informed that the products had been made at a laboratory adjacent to Wright's clinic. Further investigation indicated that Wright and the pharmacist were co-owners of the laboratory and clinic and that a clandestine manufacturing facility was being constructed in a vacant business next to the pharmacy. When the investigators went to the laboratory, Wright would not permit them to conduct a full inspection. During the next few months, however, illegally marketed products were identified by inspecting trash from the clinic and pharmacy.

In December 1991, an FDA inspector posed as a patient and was diagnosed with an Interro device, a computerized galvanometer that measures changes in the skin's electrical resistance and depicts them on the screen of a monitor. (The reading on the screen is determined by how hard the probe is pressed against the patient's finger; the harder the pressure, the less skin resistance and the higher the reading. The FDA Center for Devices and Radiologic Health has said that the device is "adulterated and misbranded" and can have no legal medical use.) According to his report, the woman who operated the device probed points on one of the inspector's fingers while selecting items on the screen that were said to represent substances to which he might be allergic. The woman explained that the height of a vertical bar that appeared when she probed his finger would indicate whether or not he was sensitive to the item being tested. After the test was completed, a printer next to the monitor printed a list of foods, chemicals, and other substances, with numerical values corresponding to readings on the Interro screen. Then he was given several homeopathic medicines, instructions for using them, and an article saying that they would result in dramatic relief of his allergic symptoms.

In February 1992, Wright's clinic posted a notice claiming that state-licensed physicians are "exempt from the restrictions and regulations of the federal Food and Drug Administration as a matter of federal law." The notice also stated that "no employee, agent or inspector of the FDA shall be permitted on these premises."

On May 4, 1992, a U.S. magistrate issued warrants authorizing the FDA to conduct criminal searches at Wright's clinic and the adjacent pharmacy. The warrants were based on affidavits which concluded that the clinic had been "receiving, using, and dispensing several unapproved and misbranded foreign-manufactured injectable drug products" and that the pharmacy had been dispensing them. Two days later, FDA agents accompanied local police officers who broke down the front door of the Tahoma clinic. Wright and his supporters claim that the search party entered with guns drawn and terrorized the clinic staff. Federal officials state that the police broke down the door because the clinic staff had refused to open it when they knocked, a gun was drawn because the officers suspected that those inside might be hostile, but the gun was never pointed at anyone and was reholstered as soon as the area was deemed safe. The authorities seized products, patient files, computer records, and Interro devices from the clinic and additional materials from the pharmacy. Two weeks later, the state pharmacy board summarily suspended the pharmacy's license, an action taken only when the board feels that public health may be endangered.

Sherman L. Cox, Assistant Secretary for Licensing and Certification for the state of Washington, has stated that the search of Wright's clinic was not an attack by the State or the FDA on "alternative medicine" or "freedom of health care." In a letter he noted that the For Your Health pharmacy "was manufacturing a number of drugs and was distributing these drugs not only to patients on prescription but also to other doctors around the country for use in their offices. . . . In addition, the pharmacy was not properly licensed as a manufacturer and the drugs were being made under unsafe conditions."

Wright and his allies have characterized the search procedure as "the Vitamin-B Bust" and sold videotapes showing part of the raid, the reaction of several clinic employees, and demonstrations staged by Wright supporters. However, Cox noted that the items seized "were not just injectable vitamins but included a number of unapproved drugs." He did concede that the police officers' fear of danger was the result of assuming that the FDA definition of "illegal drugs" was the same as the county's definition (which covered heroin, cocaine, etc.).

During a "Larry King Live" television broadcast, an FDA official said that the agency became interested in Wright's activities after someone complained that he was prescribing L-tryptophan and sending people to the pharmacy to have the prescriptions filled. Wright maintained that he had a right to do this because his supply was not contaminated. When Larry King asked why he thought the FDA ban did not apply to him, Wright replied, "My lawyer said I could use it."

The health-food industry is attempting to arouse public sympathy and fire up its own supporters by claiming that the authorities used excessive force—that Wright "had committed no crime but was only providing his patients with nutritional supplements and non-toxic, natural therapeutics." Wright and his supporters have generated extensive press coverage of their version of the controversy and set up a legal defense fund. The Nutritional Health Alliance, a group campaigning to weaken FDA jurisdiction over vitamins, has given $50,000 to the fund.

In August 1992, Wright signed an agreement consenting to the destruction of the 103 bottles of L-tryptophan that had been seized and agreeing to pay at least $850 to cover court costs and fees associated with the action. But he also filed a suit seeking a court order barring the FDA from regulating what he does. In a recent interview he stated that the pharmacy had given up its license and gone out of business, but that he continued to operate his clinic. For Your Health is now operating as a health-food store. A grand jury convened to determine whether Wright should be criminally prosecuted for violating FDA drug laws has not yet reported its findings.

The "Interpreter"

Jeffrey S. Bland, Ph.D., is undoubtedly the health-food industry's most prolific publicist and interpreter of nutrition-related scientific developments. (His interpretations consistently favor the use of supplements.) A former chemistry professor, he appears frequently at trade shows, writes books and articles, produces audio and video tapes, markets nutritional products and home study courses, conducts seminars for health professionals and health-food retailers, and serves as a consultant to several organizations that share the supplement industry's views. Bland is president of HealthComm (originally called J.S.B. and Associates), which he formed in 1984 "to educate doctors about nutrition." He has also been a research associate at the Linus Pauling Institute of Medicine and has directed its nutrient analysis laboratory. He has a B.S. in biology from the University of California at Irvine and a Ph.D. in chemistry from the University of Oregon.

Bland's advice to the health-food retailers was vividly described in *Nutrition Forum* in an article by science writer Odom Fanning, who attended a seminar called "Nutritional Selling: A Powerful Customer Service," at a trade show held in 1985 in Washington, D.C. The seminar, led by Bland, included several skits in which he played storekeeper and three retailers played customers. Members of the audience were also invited to act as customers and pose their "toughest question" to the four panelists acting as clerks. Bland's delivery was rapid-fire, with frequent use of biochemical concepts and "emerging" research findings that he considered relevant and encouraging.

Much of the seminar concerned how product information might be communicated without "prescribing," which would be practicing medicine without a license. Bland said he would try to make it clear to customers that he is concerned about their medical management, that they have been seeking good care, and that he was not practicing medicine but "trying to support them with nutritional information adjunct to traditional medical care." He also warned that requests for specific product information should be handled cautiously to avoid being "nailed for prescribing." When a retailer asked about the limits of advice, he replied:

> If a client asks a question that specific, you need to decide whether he is a client or a friend, and how well you know him. If he is a friend, then I would take him out to lunch, away from your store and talk to him as a friend. Don't talk as the store proprietor because that would be

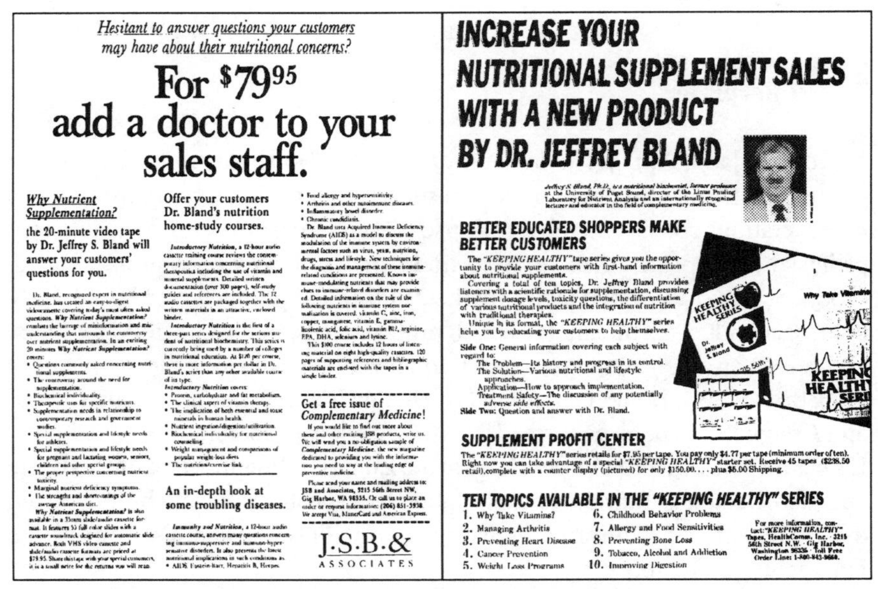

In 1986, Bland advertised in *Natural Foods Merchandiser* that his educational materials would boost supplement sales.

> diagnosis and treatment. No matter what you think you are offering as a service, you are really, by the letter of the law, doing things that could be interpreted as diagnosis and treatment. However, if, as a friend, you anecdotally talk about your experience as a human being, there's no law that prevents freedom of speech.

When asked what retailers should become knowledgeable about, Bland rattled off a long list of biochemical terms and tidbits related to amino acids—"things you should have in the back of your mind even though you're not going to prescribe for treatment." At another point, he described how to question a customer who asks about a breast lump in order to assess whether it might be amenable to nutritional intervention.

One of Bland's products is "Why Nutrient Supplementation?"—a twenty-minute videotape or slide/audiocassette program intended for in-store customer viewing. In it Bland claims that: (1) "marginal deficiencies" are common in the United States; (2) many people who are under the presumption that they are healthy because they are not diseased would actually benefit from higher levels of health if they were taking a regular nutritional supplement; (3) if you eat a balanced diet, the need for supplementation may be reduced; and (4) "prudent nutritional supplementation" can "optimize nutrient quality" to help augment health and prevent disease. Bland also lists ten situations where supplements are supposedly needed, but says nothing about how individuals can determine whether they fit these supposed categories. (Presumably, those listening to the tape will either "play it safe" by buying a supplement or ask the retailer for advice on "optimization.")

Bland's other informational products are so voluminous and complex that we don't have the time to evaluate them. Regardless of their accuracy, however, we doubt that most retailers, unconventional physicians, chiropractors, and naturopaths can utilize the information they contain in a rational and responsible way.

Bland is also president of Nu-Day Enterprises, which markets a diet program. In 1991, the FTC charged Bland and Nu-Day with falsely claiming that their program could cause weight loss by "tuning up the body's heat-producing machinery." The program, which cost $59.95 for a two-week supply, contained a meal-replacement formula; *Nu-Day Herbulk* (said to be a "natural appetite suppressant" that provides fiber and "cleanses the digestive system"); an instructional booklet; and an audiocassette. It was promoted with a thirty-minute television infomercial entitled "The Perfect Diet," which offered "amazing true stories of people like yourself losing twenty, thirty, fifty pounds or more, safely, quickly and naturally." Without admitting wrongdoing, Bland signed a consent agreement to pay $30,000 for redress and to refrain from making unsubstantiated claims that the Nu-Day Diet Program, or a similar program, would cause weight loss by altering the body's metabolism.

The Bible Maven

Earl Mindell, R.Ph., helped found the Great Earth chain of health-food stores, which, numbering about 130 stores, is now the nation's third largest. His books include *Earl Mindell's Vitamin Bible Earl Mindell's Vitamin Bible for Your Kids, Earl Mindell's Pill Bible, Earl Mindell's Quick & Easy Guide to Better Health, Earl Mindell's Shaping Up with Vitamins, Unsafe at Any Meal, Earl Mindell's Herb Bible,* and *Earl Mindell's Food as Medicine*. In 1993, he began editing a monthly newsletter called *Joy of Health.*

Total sales of Mindell's *Vitamin Bible* are said to be more than six million copies in fifteen languages. The book was written while he was working toward a "Ph.D." at the University of Beverly Hills, a nonaccredited school that lacked a campus or laboratory facilities. His adviser for the project was James Kenney, Ph.D., R.D., a genuine expert who is now a nutritionist at the Pritikin Longevity Center in Santa Monica, California. Kenney reviewed the manuscript and told Mindell that it contained over four hundred errors, more than one hundred of which were important. Kenney says that most of the errors remain in the published edition. The acknowledgments section of the book recognizes Kenney for his help and also thanks the American Medical Association, the National Academy of Sciences, the National Dairy Council, the American Academy of Pediatrics, and the Nutrition Foundation, "without whom a project of this scope could never have been completed." However, the fact that all these prestigious organizations would strenuously disagree with information in the book is not mentioned. *Shaping Up with Vitamins* thanks these groups plus the American Dietetic Association, which Mindell surely must know disagrees with his views on supplementation. The book's jacket refers to Mindell as "America's #1 Vitamin Expert."

In a section entitled "The Whole Truth," *Vitamin Bible* tells what each vitamin and mineral can supposedly do for you and gives advice for self-treatment with supplements of many of them. For example, it suggests pantothenic acid for tingling hands and feet, vitamin D for conjunctivitis, and calcium for menstrual cramps. This section also promotes substances that Mindell incorrectly calls "vitamins" B10, B11, B13, B15, B17, P, T, and U. There is no evidence that any of these substances are essential to humans or that supplements of any of them are beneficial. Furthermore, B15 (pangamic acid) and B17 (laetrile) pose health risks. Another section of the book recommends self-treatment with supplements for more than fifty ailments and conditions including acne, bad breath, baldness, headaches, measles, mumps, prostatitis, syphilis, gonorrhea, and warts. None of these recommendations is valid.

In *Vitamin Bible for Kids,* Mindell advises parents who suspect that their child is deficient in any nutrient to consult a "nutritionally oriented doctor" or (if mineral deficiency is suspected) to obtain a hair analysis. Among other things, the book recommends vitamin supplements for acne, bronchitis, athletes foot, canker sores, chicken pox, clumsiness, colitis, dandruff, diabetes, forgetfulness, impetigo, insect bites, prickly heat, poison ivy, stomachaches, tonsillitis, and warts. For multiple sclerosis, it recommends orotic acid, which Mindell refers to as vitamin B13. And for children "whose little white lies are growing darker," he recommends eliminating sugars, refined starches, and junk foods from the diet and supplementing with B-complex vitamins.

Earl Mindell's Quick & Easy Guide to Better Health claims twenty-eight substances are vitamins. It provides a "basic vitamin-mineral program for beginners" and suggests five additional supplements "as you become more sophisticated in nutrition."

Earl Mindell's Herb Bible is full of inaccuracies and unproven claims. In a review in *Nutrition Forum,* herb expert Varro Tyler, Ph.D., noted that the book misidentified many of the plants it discussed.

Earl Mindell's Food as Medicine presents Mindell's views on the possible benefits of more than a hundred foods. The claims are more conservative than those in his other writings, and readers are advised to follow the USDA's Food Guide Pyramid system. However, the book still contains exaggerations, errors, and dubious advice,

Mindell is co-editor of Keats Publishing Company's "Good Health Guides," a large series of booklets promoting dozens of questionable supplements. His fellow editor is Richard A. Passwater, whose "Ph.D." is from Bernadean University, a nonaccredited correspondence school that was never legally authorized to grant any degrees.

Mindell has also written information sheets that for many years were distributed as educational material in health-food stores. More than sixty were issued between 1980 and 1984. Although all of them warned that the information they contain was "not intended as medical advice but only as a guide in working with your doctor," it is clear that health-food stores used them to boost product sales by making claims that would be illegal on product labels. Some describe how various vitamins, minerals, and amino acids function in the body and provide tidbits on research involving these substances. Others promote such products as ginseng, bee pollen, chelated minerals, kelp (to help the thyroid gland), yucca extract tablets (for arthritis), papaya (to help digestion), octacosanol ("the amazing energy sustainer"), and golden seal root (for stomach and liver troubles).

Most of the information sheets are misleading, and many contain errors. In #63, for example, Mindell stated that research done at Temple University in Philadelphia found that rats fed dehydroepiandrosterone (DHEA) lost weight. What actually happened, however, was that rats who received dosages fifty times greater than those marketed for humans did not lose weight but merely gained less than expected. Great Earth was one of many companies selling DHEA pills as a "fat fighter" until the FDA ordered all DHEA products off the marketplace in the spring of 1985.

Flyer #44B suggested that supplements of glucomannan (a plant fiber) are an effective appetite suppressant—which they are not. A previous version of this flyer claimed that studies conducted by Judith Stern, D.Sc., of the University of California at Davis, showed that subjects taking glucomannan lost more weight than control subjects. Actually, no significant differences were found between the two groups, and mention of Dr. Stern was deleted after she threatened to take legal action.

Flyer #4B suggested that supplementation with lecithin can prevent heart disease, aid anemia, strengthen weak muscles, reverse psoriasis, improve memory and balance, and even "appears to help multiple sclerosis." (Mindell has called lecithin "the Roto-Rooter of the nutritional world" because "it cleans out blood vessel walls.")

Flyer #31 claimed that superoxide dismutase (SOD) is an "anti-aging enzyme" which may be effective against arthritis, atherosclerosis, cancer, and senility. Even if this were true, SOD in pill form could not possibly be effective. Tests on animals have shown that oral supplementation does not affect tissue SOD activity—a finding easily predictable from the fact that SOD, like all other proteins, would be digested rather than absorbed intact into the body.

Flyers #9A and #9B endorsed the theory of Benjamin Frank, M.D., that increasing intake of RNA and DNA through dietary measures or supplements will "reverse the aging process." (*Dr. Frank's No-Aging Diet,* popular fifteen years ago, recommended eating sardines, yeast, and other foods rich in these nucleic acids.) Nucleic acids, found in all living matter, are basic to cell reproduction. Like SOD, however, those that are eaten are digested and never reach the cells intact. Moreover, nucleic acids are like specific blueprints. If DNA and RNA from sardines or yeasts could actually work in human cells, they would turn people into sardines or yeasts.

Mindell says that everyone should take supplements. He claims that foods from the grocery store are depleted of vitamins and minerals and, therefore, are nutritionally inadequate. He says that smokers need extra vitamin C, those who drink alcohol need extra B-vitamins, and that women taking birth-control pills need extra B_6. During a lecture in Tucson several years ago, Mindell said he personally took "twenty-odd" supplements twice daily. He also said that "natural" vitamins, such as natural vitamin C with rose hips, are better than synthetic ones. Even Linus Pauling, whom Mindell frequently quotes, has pointed out that there is no difference between the two in nutritional value.

Mindell's lecture included advice that was potentially dangerous. He said, for example, that vitamin A is safe in amounts up to 100,000 IU per day and that any potentially toxic doses carry warnings. Neither of these statements is true. Cases have been reported in which daily dosage with 25,000 IU of vitamin A

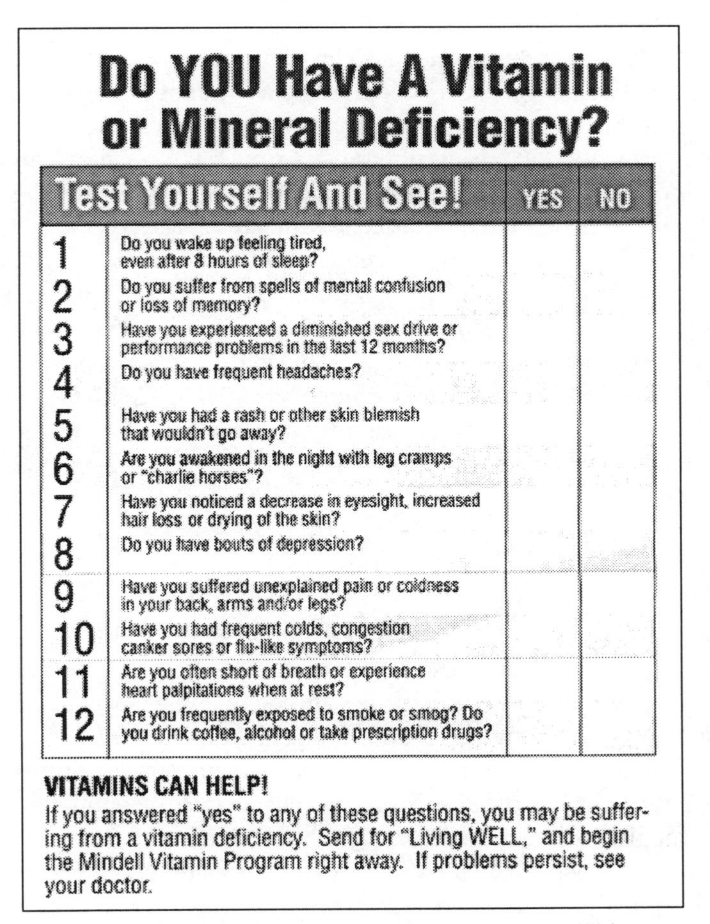

Do YOU Have A Vitamin or Mineral Deficiency?

Test Yourself And See!		YES	NO
1	Do you wake up feeling tired, even after 8 hours of sleep?		
2	Do you suffer from spells of mental confusion or loss of memory?		
3	Have you experienced a diminished sex drive or performance problems in the last 12 months?		
4	Do you have frequent headaches?		
5	Have you had a rash or other skin blemish that wouldn't go away?		
6	Are you awakened in the night with leg cramps or "charlie horses"?		
7	Have you noticed a decrease in eyesight, increased hair loss or drying of the skin?		
8	Do you have bouts of depression?		
9	Have you suffered unexplained pain or coldness in your back, arms and/or legs?		
10	Have you had frequent colds, congestion canker sores or flu-like symptoms?		
11	Are you often short of breath or experience heart palpitations when at rest?		
12	Are you frequently exposed to smoke or smog? Do you drink coffee, alcohol or take prescription drugs?		

VITAMINS CAN HELP!

If you answered "yes" to any of these questions, you may be suffering from a vitamin deficiency. Send for "Living WELL," and begin the Mindell Vitamin Program right away. If problems persist, see your doctor.

Quiz from brochure for Mindell's newsletter. "Living Well" is a twenty-four-page booklet filled with questionable advice.

has caused toxic levels to build up in the body over periods of months or years. And supplements of this strength do not contain warning labels. At one point during his talk, Mindell tried to persuade a member of the audience to follow his advice rather than that of his doctor by claiming that medical doctors are ignorant about vitamins.

Mindell's newsletter has been promoted with a twenty-page brochure which states:

> Dr. Earl Mindell—the world's expert on dietary supplements and nutrition—has helped more people live better with vitamins than any man alive. For 28 years Dr. Mindell has led a personal crusade to help people all over North America heal themselves the healthy way nature intended.

According to the brochure, vitamins can "lift your mood, boost your brain power, raise your energy levels, strengthen your eyesight and hearing, pump up your immune system, and protect you for many, many years of healthy living!" They can also "REVERSE heart disease and slow the growth of tumors." To reassure doubters, the brochure states: "ALL RECOMMENDATIONS MADE BY DR. MINDELL MEET STRICT CRITERIA FOR SAFETY AND EFFECTIVENESS."

Now retired from active management of his stores, Mindell spends much of his time writing, lecturing, and appearing on talk shows (more than three hundred a year, according to the newsletter brochure). A recent letter listing his credentials states that he has a "Ph.D." from Pacific Western University and a "master herbalist" degree from Dominion Herbal College. Despite these nonaccredited credentials and the astonishing number of inaccuracies he has promoted, his nonsense is rarely questioned by members of the media who encounter him.

"America's #1 Pediatrician"

Pediatrician Lendon H. Smith, M.D., contends that nutrition plays a major role in behavior and that nutritional remedies are helpful in a wide range of diseases and conditions. He claims, for example, that allergies, alcoholism, insomnia, hyperactivity in children, and a variety of other ailments are the result of enzyme disturbances which can be helped by dietary changes. He recommends a variety of food supplements and avoidance of white sugar, white flour, pasteurized milk, and other foods that are not "natural." For many years, his ideas were promoted widely on his own syndicated TV program and through guest appearances on other shows. During Smith's heyday, a "Donahue" show executive said, "Unlike other M.D.s, Smith presents well on the air and has a special rapport with parents. He's funny, interesting and makes people feel good about themselves and their children."

Smith's books include: *The Children's Doctor, Feed Your Kids Right, Improving Your Child's Behavior Chemistry, Encyclopedia of Baby and Child Care, Feed Yourself Right, Foods for Healthy Kids, Dr. Smith's Low Stress Diet,* and *Dr. Smith's Diet Plan for Teenagers.* Most were published by the trade division of McGraw-Hill, a leading publisher of college textbooks.

In *Improving Your Child's Behavior Chemistry,* Smith writes, "It is amazing how children's behavior can be turned around 180 degrees by a vitamin C and B injection. Overnight, they sleep better, begin to eat, and are cheerful, calm and cooperative the next day." (We suspect that the reason for any such behavior change is not nutritional but fear of having more shots.)

In *Feed Your Kids Right,* Smith suggested that a daily dose of 15,000 to 30,000 units of vitamin A is "about right for most of us." He also recommended a stress "formula" with up to 10,000 mg of vitamin C and 50,000 units of vitamin A each day for a month. These dosages, of course, are dangerous—particularly to children. For pregnant women, he recommended daily supplements of 20,000 to 30,000 units of vitamin A, a dosage high enough to cause birth defects. The book's jacket calls Smith "one of the nation's foremost pediatricians."

According to McGraw-Hill's "Tip Sheet" for interviewers, *Feed Yourself Right* gives "nutritional" advice to combat allergies, alcoholism, depression, diabetes, cancer, hypoglycemia, and "the stresses undergone during the different decades of adulthood." The Tip Sheet also said that Smith was prepared to reveal "the secret of long life" and whether the medical establishment will think *Feed Yourself Right* is "another quack book." The book advises people troubled by recurrent infections to "eat no food more frequently than once every four to five days."

In 1973, the Oregon State Board of Medical Examiners placed Smith on probation for prescribing medication that was "not necessary or medically indicated" for six adult patients, one diagnosed as hyperactive and the other five as heroin addicts. He was also ordered to confine his practice to pediatrics. According to a report in *The Washington Post*, Smith, like many pediatricians, had prescribed *Ritalin* to calm hyperactive children. While working in a free clinic for drug addicts, he theorized that many heroin addicts had been hyperactive children and prescribed *Ritalin* for them also. However, trouble arose when some of the addicts sold his prescriptions to buy heroin. *Ritalin* is a controlled substance, and Smith did not have federal approval to run a program for addicts. In 1974, the Oregon Board agreed to allow Smith to write prescriptions for narcotic drugs under certain conditions, but in 1975 he was again restricted because the Board felt he was prescribing *Ritalin* for too many children. His probation lasted until 1981.

Shortly after the Board's action in 1973, Smith turned to "nutritional therapy" and allied himself with naturopaths, homeopaths, and chiropractors. Later he became the first physician named to the board of the Portland-based National College of Naturopathic Medicine. He has been a frequent speaker at health-food-industry seminars and has also lectured at dental meetings.

In June 1977, *Oregon Times* magazine published a lengthy interview with Smith that included the following remarks:

> Q. How does the rest of the medical community react to your diet theories?
> A. I get flack from my medical peer group who think I'm completely nuts.
> Q. At least they are reluctant to buy your ideas on hyperactivity.
> A. Most doctors are people that are academically oriented. They did well in high school and college. And in medical school, in order to get through they had to be still. They are not restless and hyperactive in general.
> Q. Were you restless and hyperactive?
> A. Sure!
> Q. How did you get through medical school, then?
> A. I was just bright enough that I could do it. I would sit in the back of the class in medical school and write letters to girl friends and do crossword puzzles. And if it really got bad I would pick my nose.

In 1987, Smith permanently surrendered his medical license rather than face Board action on charges of insurance fraud. According to press reports, the trouble arose because he had signed documents authorizing insurance payments for patients he had not seen. The patients had actually been seen by chiropractors, homeopaths, and others whose treatment was not covered at "nutrition-oriented" clinics in which Smith had worked.

Since this trouble occurred, Smith has been far less visible in both the general and "alternative" media. He has written columns for health-food and chiropractic publications and has published a newsletter called *The Facts*. In the November 1989 issue of the latter, he advises readers to smell the vitamins and minerals they take. (This "really works," he says. "No one over- or underdoses.") According to Smith's theory, if a multivitamin obtained in a health-food store becomes malodorous, "it means the customer has taken enough of the tablets and his body is now saying he had had enough." In a column in *Total Health,* he advised parents that if a child who has a good self-image shows symptoms of depression, they should consider inappropriate diet as an explanation: "My rule is, if a person likes something and they must have it every day, it is probably causing the symptoms. If depression comes and goes, then diet is surely the inciting agent."

In 1993, Video Remedies Inc. of Davie, Florida, began marketing "Homeopathic Care of Infants and Children," a videotape that portrays Smith as a practicing physician (see Chapter 9). The videotape shows Smith in what appears to be a medical office, with four framed certificates behind him. During the tape he advises a mother whose toddler sits on her lap with a stethoscope draped around her neck. He explains what homeopathy is about and suggests that vaccinations do more harm than good. The tape is intended to guide the use of a homeopathic remedy kit that has Smith's picture on its case. One piece of advice that is particularly horrendous is that if an acute earache does not respond within twenty-four hours to a homeopathic remedy, another should be selected from the brochure accompanying the tape. At the end of the "appointment," Smith quips, "Now go pay your bill." In 1994, Video Remedies invited retailers to meet "America's #1 Pediatrician" at its booth at the Natural Products Expo West.

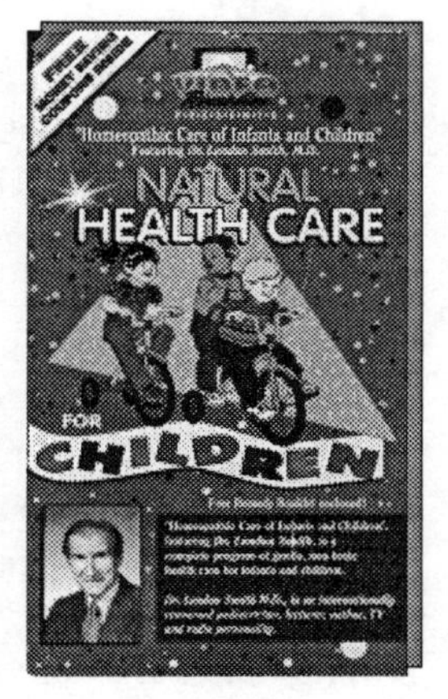

The "Immune Power" Booster

Stuart Berger, M.D., who died in 1994, was a psychiatrist who practiced in New York City as "a specialist in nutritional medicine treating immune disorders, food allergies and obesity." His books included *Dr. Berger's Immune Power Diet, The Southampton Diet, How to Be Your Own Nutritionist, What Your Doctor Didn't Tell You in Medical School,* and *Forever Young: 20 Years Younger in 20 Weeks.* All of these books contain many claims for which there is no basis in reality. Berger also wrote a health advice column for *The New York Post.*

The Southampton Diet's key feature was to eat "happy foods," which contain amino acids that produce "positive neurotransmitters" in the brain, and to avoid "sad foods," which produce "negative neurotransmitters." Dairy products, poultry, fish, eggs, whole grains, leafy greens, and various fruits were in the former category, while sugar, chocolate, lobster, lentils, chick peas, and foods containing choline and lecithin were in the latter. Brain function involves a complex balance of chemicals that work together. The idea that some of the chemicals that transmit impulses between the brain and nerve cells are "positive" and others are "negative" is nonsense.

Dr. Berger's Immune Power Diet published in 1985, became a best seller after Berger appeared on the "Donahue" show; the publisher told *People* magazine that during the next three days more than fifty thousand copies were ordered. Berger said that his system had enabled him to reduce from 420 pounds to 208. (He was 6'-7" tall.) The book claimed that overweight and numerous other health problems are the result of an "immune hypersensitivity response" to common foods, and that "detoxification" and weight loss followed by food supplements can tune and strengthen the immune system. Berger also claimed that cytotoxic testing had provided "superb results" in tracking down the "danger foods" for thousands of his patients. To determine supplement dosage, the results of "IQ Quizzes" for vitamins, minerals, amino acids, lifestyle, stress, and exercise were totaled to get one's "Immune Quotient." The lower your "IQ," the "weaker" your immune system, and the higher the dosage of twenty-three or more supplements you should take.

Kurt Butler has pointed out that many foods identified as "happy" in *The Southampton Diet* are listed in the *Immune Power Diet* among the "Sinister Seven"—foods that "create immune damage in the overwhelming majority of patients" and are closely linked to food binges and excess weight. Neither listing, of course, was correct. The *Harvard Medical School Health Letter* stated that the *Immune Power Diet* was "selling a collection of quack ideas about food allergies that have been around for decades" and "should have been listed in the fiction category." The book's popularity was probably related to public concern about AIDS and the immune system.

What Your Doctor Didn't Learn in Medical School states that one in four Americans suffers from hypothyroidism and that millions more suffer from hidden yeast (Candida) infections, hidden food sensitivities, and other "phantom diseases" that "too often are ignored by our medical practitioners." *How to Be Your Own Nutritionist* contains "Personal Prescriptions" for supplementation by diabetics, dieters, medication users, and fifteen other individual categories. These books, too, are replete with quack ideas.

In 1986, *New York* magazine revealed that many patients had spent thousands of dollars for testing and expensive dietary supplements at Berger's office. In 1990, "Inside Edition" aired two television programs describing what happened when a reporter and a prominent New York allergist had visited Berger complaining of fatigue. Both noted that their contact with him lasted about two minutes, included no physical examination, and culminated with diagnoses of chronic fatigue syndrome and allergy to yeast. The reporter's cost was $845 for the first visit, with an estimated total of about $1,500 through the third visit. A former patient described a similar experience that had cost over $1,000. And a former employee said that Berger ordered his employees to indicate on blood test reports that every patient was allergic to wheat, dairy products, eggs, and yeast. The reporter's visit had been filmed with a hidden camera. Berger obtained a court order stopping "Inside Edition" from showing the tape during the initial program. But two weeks later, after the U.S. Supreme Court sided with the producers, the tape was shown. During the interim, complaints were received from more than a hundred former patients and employees. Berger sued "Inside Edition" for alleged violation of federal wiretapping laws and trespassing on private property, but the case was dismissed by a judge within a year.

The New York City Medical Examiner's office, which reported its autopsy findings, said that Berger weighed 365 pounds at the time he died. The cause of death—at the age of forty—was heart disease, with obesity and cocaine abuse as "significant contributing factors."

The "Progressive Nutritionist"

Shari Lieberman is one of the few dietitians who is solidly aligned with the health-food industry. She is also the only dietitian the American Dietetic Association (ADA) has disciplined for violating its contemporary ethical standards. In 1986, the ADA censured her for failing to adhere to two of its standards of responsibility. In 1987, Dr. Stephen Barrett asked the ADA to determine whether she was still violating the standards. No formal investigation took place, however, because Lieberman resigned her ADA membership after being notified of the complaint. In 1989, new charges were filed, based on advice in her question-and-answer column in the magazine *Better Nutrition and Today's Living*. In 1994, following a lengthy appeals process, the ADA suspended her Registered Dietitian credential for a period of three years for violating Principle 7 of its Code of Ethics, which requires dietetic practice to be "based on scientific principles and current information." When that period is over she may request that her credential may be restored.

Lieberman holds an M.A. degree in clinical nutrition from New York University and acquired a Ph.D. degree in 1993 from The Union Institute, an "alternative" school that is accredited but has questionable academic standards (see section on Gary Null above). Her Ph.D. dissertation, "Functional Neuromuscular Stimulation: A Non-Invasive Approach for Objective Evaluation of Muscle Fatigue and Recovery Characteristics," compared the effect of high-carbohydrate and high-fiber drinks on the performance of paralyzed leg muscles in five men whose spinal cord had been injured. Lieberman is also secretary of the Certification Board for Nutrition Specialists (CBNS), a recently-formed organization that is issuing a "Certified Nutrition Specialist" ("C.N.S.") credential. An accredited degree and professional experience are required, but CBNS's eligibility standards are less rigorous than those of the American Board of Nutrition (described in Chapter 22 of this book).

Lieberman practices what she calls "preventive medicine and progressive nutrition" in New York City. In an interview in the January 1993 issue of *Health Foods Business,* Lieberman said that she counsels about thirty patients per week and recommends "a base line of supplements for just about everyone." She also writes regularly for several magazines, has appeared regularly on a show syndicated by the Home Shopping Network, and has lectured to health-food retailers on how to legally protect themselves while advising customers. Her seminar at the 1992 NNFA convention covered "how you can actually talk with a customer without being arrested." Her main suggestions were: (1) set up a reference library of books and file folders, with a folder for each product ingredient; (2) sponsor lectures by "progressive" nutritionists and other practitioners; and (3) utilize a book of testimonials from satisfied customers.

In 1987, Lieberman advertised in *Whole Life* magazine that she used "the most progressive screening tools," which she identified as hair analysis (to

THE TIME HAS COME FOR NUTRI-TION TO TAKE ITS RIGHTFUL PLACE ALONGSIDE MEDICINE AND OTHER THERAPIES

Nutrition has emerged as an alternative and adjunctive therapy for virtually all areas of health care. Medical research has shown that nutrition is necessary in the prevention and treatment of cancer, heart disease and diabetes. The National Cancer Institute has stated that over 30% of all cancers could be avoided through diet modification and as much as 90% could be prevented if environmental carcinogens are avoided.

Research has demonstrated that excesses of certain nutrients enhance immunity. Nutrition has also been shown to be important in the treatment and prevention of osteoporosis, intestinal and bowel disorders, skin problems, hormonal problems, allergies, hyper-cholesterolemia as well as other related problems. Excesses of certain nutrients have also been shown to be protective against environmental pollutants. Stress - including emotional, environmental, physical, chemical and mental - has a direct impact on our nutritional requirements. Stress lowers our body reserves of vitamins and minerals and at the same time increases our needs.

To OPTIMIZE and INDIVIDUALIZE your nutritional program I use the most progressive non-invasive nutritional screening tools. The tools enable me to create an **OPTIMAL NUTRITIONAL PROGRAM** that allows the body to use its remarkable capacity to heal itself. In addition, I incorporate diet and exercise into your program to make it complete.

Understanding your **OPTIMAL NUTRITIONAL PROGRAM** is as important as the program itself. I spend time explaining all your results in detail so that when I design your program, you will know exactly what you are taking and why. Education is an important part of patient care. It allows patient independence rather than dependence so frequent visits are not necessary.

If you would like more information, please feel free to call.

(212) 529-1297

Ask About my New Weight-Loss Program

The text of Shari Lieberman's ad in 1993 and 1994 issues of *Newlife* magazine. Her Lifeway™ program is described on its label as "the first permanent weight loss system – for women."

assess mineral imbalances and toxic metal accumulation), iridology (the condition of all organs is "mapped" in the iris), saliva testing (saliva is crystallized to determine what herbs an individual needs for the healing process), nutritional blood interpretation (to find "imbalances"), and nutritional kinesiology (muscle-testing to verify "sensitivities and weaknesses"). Then, according to the ad, she recommends "a complete vitamin, mineral, herbal, diet, exercise and cleansing program . . . to allow the body to use its remarkable capacity to heal itself." Dr. Barrett's 1987 complaint to the ADA challenged these practices and several of the supplement recommendations mentioned in *Design Your Own Vitamin and Mineral Program.* Her subsequent ads (example above) have been less detailed.

Lieberman's 1987 book *Design Your Own Vitamin and Mineral Program* was republished in 1990 in a longer version called *The Real Vitamin and Mineral Book.* Both editions state that "you cannot get all the nutrients you need from today's food" and that "the RDAs are the nutritional equivalent of the minimum wage. They are probably good enough to keep you alive, but how good is the quality of that life?" Instead, Lieberman postulates higher "Optimum Daily Allowances (ODAs)" and suggests that "nutrition should be our first line of defense if an illness or condition is not life-threatening." These ideas have no basis in reality.

Regarding patients in her private practice Lieberman wrote:

> They come to me with every variety of problem and needs. Some are specific, such as acne, psoriasis, thinning hair, menstrual problems, blood sugar problems, intestinal disorders, high blood pressure, high cholesterol, an inability to sleep, fatigue, depression, or nervousness. These people turn to me as an adjunct or an alternative to the treatment offered by their physician.

Although some of these conditions are diet-related, most are not, and few provide a reason to take supplements. But Lieberman claims to have found them valuable for dozens of problems, including aging, cataract prevention, kidney stones, depression, asthma, and shingles. She suggests that everyone should take supplements—starting with her ODA values and adding more to cope with emotional stress, enhance immunity, prevent cardiovascular disease, prevent cancer, alleviate skin problems, prevent diabetes, and/or prevent osteoporosis. For sinusitis, bronchitis, allergies, asthma, cancer prevention, and several skin problems, she suggests daily dosages of 50,000 to 100,000 IU of vitamin A. This advice is both inappropriate and unsafe. Her sample worksheet suggests that emotional stress is a reason to take 3,000 to 5,000 mg of vitamin C daily, which is ridiculous. Much of her advice appears to be based on faulty interpretation of research reports.

In January 1994, two weeks after her R.D. credential was suspended, Lieberman was consulted by Zhixin Xu, associate editor of *Nutrition Forum* newsletter. Xu said he was concerned about fatigue and thinning hair, but he also said that he might be getting nervous and sometimes lost his appetite. Based on these symptoms, Lieberman said Xu might have a "marginal problem" with his thyroid gland that hair and saliva tests could corroborate. She advised him to take vitamin C and kelp supplements and to begin an aerobic exercise program.

Two months later Xu returned for his test results. Based on the hair analysis report, he was told that his copper and chromium levels were low, which might cause problems with his cholesterol control, immune response, and blood sugar control. Based on the saliva test (herbal crystallization analysis), Lieberman told Xu there were problems with his circulation, lymphatic/immune system, digestive system, and nervous system. The digestive system, she said, "shows up as a little bit of a problem . . . . related to hair loss. . . . There is something going on hormonally." Lieberman also said that Xu had "the circulation of a sixty-year-old man" and that his liver was "a little on overload," although there was "nothing wrong with it." She prescribed a vitamin/mineral supplement, a chelated copper supplement, and two herbal tinctures: *PRO* (which stands for "prostate reproductive system") and *LYM* ("for the immune and reproductive systems"). During both visits Lieberman said she was a Registered Dietitian and gave Xu printed information and a receipt that bore the initials "R.D." after her name. Hair analysis and herbal crystallization analysis have no practical value for evaluating the body's nutritional status or glandular function (see Chapter 7). In June 1994, the New York State Department of Health ordered the lab that performed Xu's hair analysis to stop accepting and/or testing speciments collected in New York State because it lacked a permit to do so.

Banding Together

Promoters of questionable health and nutrition practices often organize to multiply their effectiveness. How can one tell which groups are reliable and which are not? There is no sure way, but six precautionary questions may help:

1. *Are its ideas inside the scientific mainstream?* Some groups admit that they were formed because their founders felt alienated from the scientific community. One group that made no secret of this was actually called the American Quack Association (see Chapter 12).

2. *Who are its leaders and advisors?* The International Society for

Fluoride Research may sound respectable, but it is actually an antifluoridation group. The International Academy of Preventive Medicine (now called the International Academy of Nutrition and Preventive Medicine) numbered among its leaders Carlton Fredericks, Linus Pauling, Lendon Smith, and other promoters of questionable nutrition practices. The Health Resources Council is an advocacy group founded by Gary Null to promote "alternative" health methods. The Therapeutic Foods Nutrition Council (claimed to be "a panel of leading national experts . . . on the forefront of research") was established by Shari Lieberman "to help educate and enlighten the public about the ever-changing role of diet and nutrition, as it relates to the prevention of, as well as adjuvant therapy for, a variety of health disorders."

3. *What are its membership requirements?* Is scientific expertise required—or just a willingness to pay dues? An organization open to almost anyone may be perfectly respectable (like the American Association for the Advancement of Science), but don't let the fact that an individual belongs to it impress you. The International Academy of Nutritional Consultants and the American Association of Nutritional Consultants issued attractive certificates, but their only requirement for "professional membership" was payment of a $50 fee. Some "institutes" are simply names adopted by an individual or a few individuals who wish to make their work sound more respectable. A few quackery-promoting groups have called subscribers to their magazines "members" in order to appear larger than they actually are.

4. *Does it promote a specific treatment or treatments?* Most such groups should be highly suspect. A century ago, valid new ideas were hard to evaluate and often were rejected by the medical community. But today, effective new treatments are quickly welcomed by scientific practitioners and do not need special groups to promote them. The American College of Advancement in Medicine (formerly called the Association for Chelation Therapy) falls into this category. So do the World Research Association and various other groups that promote questionable cancer therapies; the American Academy of Environmental Medicine (which promotes "clinical ecology"); the American Schizophrenia Association (which promotes megavitamins); and the latter's parent organization, the Huxley Institute for Biosocial Research. And we may add the National Wellness Coalition, whose stated mission is "to promote wellness principles, policies and practices as the key to affordable, effective health care and a healthy prosperous nation." Despite the rhetoric, however, the coalition pays very little attention to proven health methods and promotes a broad spectrum of unscientific approaches. Physicians for Responsible Medicine, headed by animal-rights activist Neal D. Barnard, M.D., promotes strict vegetarianism and a variety of dubious "alternative" treatments.

5. *Does it espouse a version of "freedom of choice" that would abolish government regulation of the health marketplace?* Such "freedom" is nothing more than a ploy to persuade legislators to permit the marketing of quack methods without legal restraints. Several groups with this philosophy are discussed in Chapter 20.

6. *How is it financed?* The Council for Responsible Nutrition, despite its respectable-sounding name, is a Washington, D.C., group that represents manufacturers and distributors of food supplements and other nutritional products. Don't assume, however, that funding by an industry makes an organization unreliable. Reliability should be determined by judging the validity of a group's ideas rather than its funding. The National Dairy Council and the Institute of Food Technologists are highly respected by the scientific community for their accurate publications on nutrition.

The Bottom Line

All of us are exposed daily to many ideas about health, some of which are accurate and some not. Promoters of questionable and unscientific methods are working hard to gain your allegiance. When you are well, unless you are taken in to an extreme degree, what you believe may not matter much. But if you have a health problem—particularly a serious one—misplacing your trust can seriously harm you or others who rely upon your judgment.

18

Further Thoughts on Quackery and the Media

Publicity is obviously a major factor—if not *the* major factor—in the sale of food supplements. Chapter 5 describes how the health-food industry reaches prospective customers through its own channels of communication. This chapter focuses on the spread of misinformation through the general media.

Vitamins in the News

On April 6, 1992, *Time* magazine carried a cover story called "The New Scoop on Vitamins," by Anastasia Toufexis. The cover headline read: "The Real Power of Vitamins: New research shows that they may help fight cancer, heart disease, and the ravages of aging." The article stated:

> More and more scientists are starting to suspect that traditional views of vitamins and minerals are more limited. While researchers may not endorse the expansive claims of hard-core vitamin enthusiasts, evidence suggests that the nutrients play a much more complex role in assuring vitality and optimal health than was previously thought.

A photo of a vitamin-filled soup dish was captioned, "Do you need a soup of supplements? Almost every week brings new hints that vitamins may help you stay healthy longer, especially if you can't stand broccoli and Brussels sprouts." The balance of the article provided a confusing look at research tidbits and speculations garnished by more double-talk and hedged statements.

The National Nutritional Foods Association (NNFA) welcomed the article as "a watershed event for the industry. . . . the most positive public relations tool that the industry has been able to use in years." NNFA sent a copy to every member of Congress as part of the campaign to undercut FDA regulation (see Chapter 20). Multiple copies were distributed to health-food stores to give to customers. Speaking at the 1992 NNFA convention and trade show, Toufexis stated:

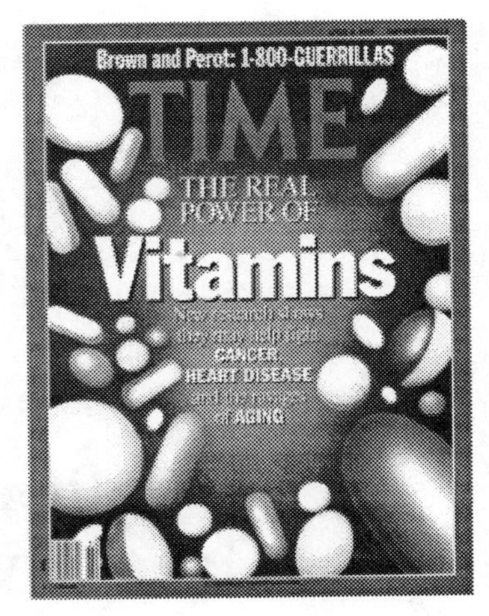

> In fifteen years at *Time,* I have written many health covers. One on the difficulties of losing weight was *Time*'s number-one best-selling issue on the newsstand in 1986. . . . But I have never seen anything like the response to the vitamin cover. It whipped off the sales racks, and we were inundated with requests for copies. There are no more copies. Vitamins is the number-one selling issue so far this year.

During the past few years, similar reports have appeared in many other publications and on many broadcasts. Vitamins are "newsworthy" because *preliminary* research has led to speculations that heart disease and cancer may be preventable by taking supplements. The fact that supplementation may be a waste of money and might do harm—if mentioned at all—has been given little emphasis. Not surprisingly, people are thinking more about vitamins, and vitamin sales, particularly of antioxidants, have risen sharply (see Chapter 8).

Information that will attract a wide audience is considered "newsworthy." It may be new, startling, alarming, or amusing; or it can have any other quality that editors or producers believe will interest the particular audience toward which their efforts are directed. Magical claims about "nutrition" tend to be regarded as more newsworthy than the "unvarnished truths" of nutrition science. The people who make these claims are also regarded as newsworthy.

The "Alternative" Bandwagon

During the past few years, the news media have publicized "alternative" methods in ways that will cause great public confusion. Most reports have contained little critical thinking and have featured the views of proponents and their satisfied clients. Many have lumped approaches (such as biofeedback, hypnosis, and a low-fat diet) that have real value with nonsensical methods (such as homeopathy) and concluded (incorrectly) that "alternatives" are moving into the scientific mainstream. Most have suggested that "alternative" methods have become increasingly popular, even though utilization data have not been compiled for most "alternative" practices. Some commentators have decried the high cost of medical care and suggested (incorrectly) that "alternatives" may prove to be less expensive.

Many reports have exaggerated the significance of the National Institutes of Health (NIH) Office of Alternative Medicine (OAM). *Time*, for example, stated that "the NIH program is supported by an odd alliance of New Age believers and old-school quackbusters. Both sides want to sort out once and for all what works." This statement was absolutely untrue. No "quackbuster"—"old school" or otherwise—"supports" the OAM program or is "allied" with any New Age believer. NIH does not have the resources to "sort out what works," and even if it did, negative test results rarely influence quack beliefs.

The OAM program resulted from a 1991 federal law ordering NIH to foster research into unconventional practices and allocating $2 million per year to do the job. Senator Tom Harkin (D-IA) secured its passage at the urging of former Congressman Berkley Bedell and another promoter of "alternative" cancer methods. In various interviews, Bedell acknowledged that he had undergone unconventional treatment "to replenish nitrogen" for a suspected recurrence of prostate cancer. Two years later, Harkin became convinced that he himself had relieved a severe allergic condition by taking large amounts of bee pollen.

Early in 1992, NIH appointed a twenty-person ad hoc advisory panel that included Bedell and leading advocates of acupuncture, energy medicine, homeopathy, Ayurvedic medicine, and several types of "alternative" cancer therapies. A few qualified researchers were placed on the panel, but they have had little influence over subsequent events. Panel members were considered "professional service contractors" and did not have to file conflict-of-interest statements or promise to refrain from using their advisory status in advertising their products and services. Although several "quackbusters," including us, were interviewed for possible appointment to the panel, we were neither selected nor even notified about the first meeting. As we predicted, many of the panelists have been trumpeting their appointment as evidence that whatever they promote is valid.

Early this year, OAM awarded grants of up to $30,000 to carry out twenty research proposals. We doubt that such studies will yield useful results. Even if they do, however, any benefit is unlikely to outweigh the publicity bonanza given to quack methods. So far, OAM's main achievement has been to serve as a magnet for the news media. We fear that the massive publicity given to vitamins and "alternative" methods has encouraged widespread false beliefs that these modalities have enormous potential value.

Journalistic "Balance"

If you were a reporter, would you try not to arouse false hopes with your reports? Would you try to determine what is true and share this information with your audience? About fifteen years ago, Dr. Stephen Barrett administered a questionnaire to twenty editors and reporters from Eastern Pennsylvania newspapers. One question was:

> Dr. John Banks, President of the National Nutrition Research Association, is the speaker at the local women's club which you often cover. He claims that a certain nutrient has great healing powers not yet sufficiently appreciated by scientists. He does not seem to be far-fetched, but his ideas are completely new to you. Would you be more likely to report this as a straight news event or to evaluate his claims by seeking another opinion?

Fifteen of the twenty said they would report this as a straight news event. Seven out of those fifteen said that even if they consulted a physician who said the claims were utter nonsense, they would still report the event without including any criticism! When questioned further, they said that reporters of news events should report them as they happen, without making judgments. If critics of "Dr. Banks" (a fictitious name) want their say, they should create their own news events to get coverage.

"Nonjudgmental" attitudes of this sort, which are common among reporters, help explain why the sensational claims of fraudulent "nutrition" are expressed so frequently in the media. The foolishness of these claims does not usually make them less newsworthy, and may even make them *more* newsworthy!

Several other factors work against accurate coverage of topics related to health and nutrition:

- Many more people are actively promoting nutrition misinformation than are actively opposing it. The sheer force of numbers works against the truth.
- Time works to quackery's advantage. It is much easier to report a lie as a straight news event than it is to investigate it.
- Some journalists who have been misled by false nutrition ideas cannot write accurate reports.
- Most promoters of nutrition misinformation often are regarded as "underdogs" in a struggle against the "establishment." As such, they tend to be treated much more sympathetically than we believe they

deserve. Most editors insist that articles which attack false ideas be "balanced" so that the apparent "underdog" gets a "fair" hearing. Even science editors who know the health-food industry is selling the public a bill of goods rarely feel a duty to issue effective public warnings.

- Publications that accept ads for food supplements are often unwilling to risk offense to their advertisers. A blatant example of this occurred in 1980 when *Self* magazine published an article by a freelance writer listing money-saving tips from Barrett's college textbook on consumer health. Advice about not wasting money on vitamins was deleted from the writer's manuscript by the magazine's editors.
- Many publications pander to advertisers by publishing articles that promote their products and/or services. This policy is more prevalent among smaller, low-quality magazines and newspapers with small editorial budgets, but many large publications do this also. Health-food publications and some women's magazines are consistent offenders in this category. *Entrepreneur* magazine's manual for health-food retailers advises that when a store opening is going to be advertised in a newspaper, a news release should be given to the ad salesperson "who will make certain it gets into the paper."
- Many publications use sensational claims to generate sales. Tabloid newspapers and women's magazines, for example, frequently carry articles on "quickie" reducing diets or "superfoods." Marilynn Larkin, a freelance writer in New York City, has noted that topic selection is commonly based on sales appeal rather than scientific merit. Even a well-written article may be accompanied by a sensational headline that contradicts the article itself.
- Many editors fear that attacks on nutrition quackery will stir up controversy from readers who regard nutrition as their religion. Worse yet, they may be afraid that attacking the credibility of a promoter will provoke a libel suit.

When a newspaper or magazine prints a questionable nutrition claim, most editors are willing to publish a rebuttal letter that contains accurate information. Few radio and television outlets have equivalent policies.

The Electronic Soapbox

The most influential sources of health and nutrition misinformation are television talk shows and tabloid news programs with huge audiences. The typical talk-show guest has written a popular book, is promoted by a professional public relations firm, and can afford to spend lots of time publicizing his claims because book sales will repay him for the time. Opponents of quackery are rarely in this position. Some opponents are willing to appear on talk shows in their home community and in other cities when they attend professional meetings. But virtually all of them have other professional duties (teaching, research, or patient care) that limit their availability for public appearances. Many talk-show hosts and producers are "true believers" who gobble vitamins and other "supplements" by the handful.

All the major television talk shows have given tremendous publicity to promoters of quackery. Some vitamin pushers have been talk-show guests more than a hundred times within a single year. Critics rarely appear on these shows, and when they do, they are almost always outnumbered by proponents and by members of the audience who give testimonials. The most dangerous example we have seen was Sally Jesse Raphael's 1988 program in which four patients stated that an unconventional method had cured them of cancer when conventional methods had failed. Although a token rebuttal expert was permitted to comment briefly, she could not evaluate these claims because she was unable to investigate them before the show. Subsequent investigation by "Inside Edition" found that three of the four had not been cured and the fourth, who had been treated conventionally, had a good prognosis. "Inside Edition" has great interest in protecting the public against health frauds and quackery and has produced a steady flow of excellent reports.

Among television tabloids, CBS's "60 Minutes" is by far the worst offender. In 1990, for example, it aired a half-hour program called "Poison in Your Mouth," which suggested that mercury-amalgam fillings were dangerous. Although this allegation was false, the broadcast induced many viewers to seek replacement of their fillings with other materials.

In the spring of 1993, "60 Minutes" struck again with a program called "Sharks Don't Get Cancer," narrated by Mike Wallace and focusing on the nonsense of biochemist William I. Lane, Ph.D., author of *Sharks Don't Get Cancer.* Wallace began by calling attention to the book and stating that Lane says that sharks don't get cancer. The program focused on a study in Cuba of twenty-nine "terminal" cancer patients who were given shark-cartilage preparations. Although the program contained many disclaimers, it was clearly promotional. Wallace visited the site of the experiment, filmed several of the patients doing exercise, and reported that most of them felt better several weeks after the treatment had begun. (The fact that "feeling better" does not indicate whether a cancer treatment is effective was not mentioned.) Two American cancer specialists then described the results as intriguing. Charles B. Simone,

M.D., who is philosophically aligned with the health-food industry and treats patients with shark cartilage, said that three of the Cuban patients appeared to have improved. The other cancer specialist, who appeared to be solidly scientific, noted that evaluation was difficult because many of the x-ray films were of poor quality, but he thought that a few tumors had gotten smaller. (The reasons why this might not be significant were not mentioned.) After noting that shark cartilage was sold in health-food stores, Wallace remarked on the inadvisability of "going to the nearest health-food store" and was seconded by Simone, who said it would be foolish to do so unless all else had failed.

Curiously, Wallace neglected to mention two important facts. First, when shark cartilage is taken by mouth, the protein it contains is broken down during digestion so that it does not enter the body intact. Thus even if shark cartilage contained a substance that inhibited tumors, taking it by mouth would not work. Second, like all animals, sharks *do* get cancer. Lane's book actually says so, although it claims that the number is "insignificant." The preface notes that "while *ALMOST No Sharks Get Cancer* might have been a bit more accurate, it would have been a rotten title." The Smithsonian Institute's *Registry of Tumors in Lower Animals* indicates that sharks even get cancers of their cartilage.

About two weeks before the program aired, a leading manufacturer of shark-cartilage capsules telephoned health-food retailers about the program and advised them to stock up on their product. Following the program, other manufacturers began marketing shark-cartilage products and referring to the program in their advertising. The leading distributor of books to health-food stores has advertised *Sharks Don't Get Cancer* with the headline: "As featured on 60 Minutes. Finally, What The World Has Been Waiting For . . . A Major Cancer Breakthrough." Meanwhile, a review by the National Cancer Institute concluded that the data from the Cuban study were scanty and unimpressive.

The effects of a "60 Minutes" plug can last for decades. Its 1980 report, "Doc Willard's Wonder Water," told how John Wesley Willard, Ph.D., a chemistry professor, had mixed water with various chemicals to produce a solution that can help humans, livestock, and plants. The program indicated that no scientific tests had been conducted, but it included testimonials from people who said it worked against emphysema, dandruff, pink eye, and burns. The publicity boosted the demand for *Willard's Water* and other brands of "catalyst-altered water," which typically sell for $2 to $3 per ounce. Despite FDA regulatory action and Willard's death in 1991, these products are still marketed with long lists of unsubstantiated health claims.

In July 1994, NBC aired "Cured! The Secrets of Alternative Healing," a two-hour special misrepresenting "alternative" methods as the "medicine

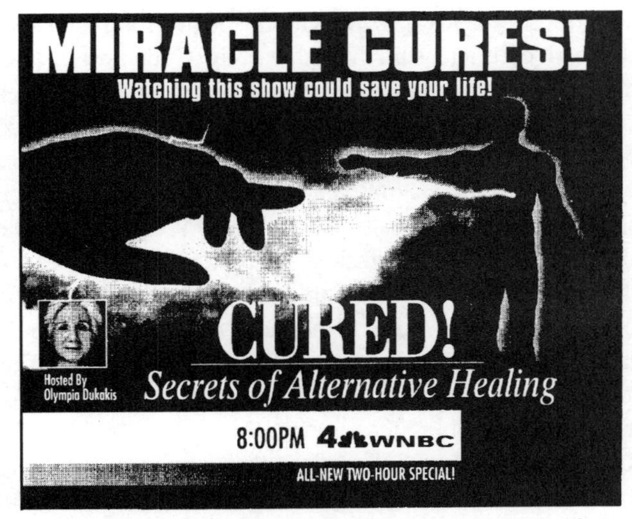

Irresponsible ad in New York City edition of *TV Guide*

of the future." The program featured "reenactments" in which acupuncture, homeopathy, and herbal treatment were portrayed as miraculously effective after scientific care had failed. Comments from responsible critics (including us) were interspersed, but the overall message, pontificated by hostess Olympia Dukakis, was: "Don't place too much faith in doctors. By seeking out alternatives and learning about self-care, you can take control of your health."

Curiously, this program was followed by a segment on NBC's "Dateline," which took a responsible look at the activities of Lucas Boeve, the proprietor of a clinic in the Dominican Republic where patients are treated with ozone gas. Boeve stated that he cured cancer, AIDS, Alzheimer's disease, Parkinson's disease, arthritis and many other diseases, and that he had provided an ozone machine that had cured "Magic" Johnson of AIDS. Unlike the producers of "Cured! The Secrets of Alternative Healing," however, Dateline's staff investigated thoroughly—by checking on all the cancer and AIDS patients on a list of success stories provided by Boeve. Of thirteen cancer patients: two had died; three could not be found; two refused to be interviewed; three were alive but still had cancer; and three said they had been helped, but their doctors said they were probably cancer-free before ozone therapy. Of two AIDS patients, one said he felt well but still was HIV positive, and the other had not been retested for HIV. "In all," a commentator concluded, "not one documented cure on Boeve's own list." In addition, Johnson's representatives said that he had had nothing to do with Boeve (or ozone therapy) and was still infected with the virus.

Nutrition Coverage in Popular Magazines

The American Council on Science and Health (ACSH) has rated nutrition coverage in twenty-two high-circulation magazines between 1990 and 1992. After eight articles from each magazine were chosen randomly, they were retyped in a standard format with the names of authors, magazine titles, and other identifying features removed. Four experts then judged the articles for accuracy, clarity, and validity of recommendations. The highest rating ("best") went to *Cooking Light*, with a score of 91 out of a possible 100 points. Eleven magazines received a "good" rating: *Consumer Reports* (88), *Good Housekeeping* (88), *American Health* (88), *Better Homes and Gardens* (87), *Glamour* (86), *Reader's Digest* (85), *Parents* (85), *Woman's Day* (80), *Prevention* (80), *McCall's* (80), and *Redbook* (80). Nine were rated "fair": *Harper's Bazaar* (77), *Runner's World* (77), *Family Circle* (77), *Self* (76), *Health* (75), *Mademoiselle* (75), *Vogue* (75), *Ladies' Home Journal* (74), and *New Woman* (74). *Cosmopolitan* (62), was judged "poor."

Two magazines not included in ACSH's study deserve special comment. *Shape*, published by Weider Health & Fitness, began publication in 1981. The original editor was Christine MacIntyre, a former college professor trained in exercise physiology. Although the parent company sells dubious nutritional products for athletes (see Chapter 12), MacIntyre was permitted to produce a top-quality magazine. She assembled an expert editorial advisory board that included Dr. Barrett, involved experts in the preparation of articles, published many articles debunking quack concepts, maintained a policy whereby misleading ads seldom got published, and printed a disclaimer that listing as an editorial advisor did not imply endorsement of any products or services advertised in the magazine. *Shape*'s current editor, who took over in 1987 after MacIntyre's accidental death, has not maintained the same editorial standards. Although most articles have been excellent, "alternative" methods have been blatantly promoted and many of the nutrition columns published during the past two years have contained invalid ideas. (A 1993 nutrition column, for example, included recipes for beverages that supposedly could "fuel your immune system," "reduce the harmful effects of stress," and "energize" people in the morning.) When the editor turned down Barrett's suggestions for improvement, he and ACSH president Elizabeth M. Whelan, Sc.D., M.P.H., resigned as advisors.

Longevity magazine began as a newsletter in 1986 and converted to a magazine in 1988. Subtitled "A Practical Guide to the Art and Science of Staying Young," it is part of the Bob Guccione's media conglomerate, which includes *Penthouse* and *Omni*. Although many of *Longevity's* articles are well written and contain standard health-promoting advice, many others promote quackery. About half of its display ads are for questionable supplement products. In October 1993, editor Susan Millar Perry announced that she is "one of the millions of Americans who take vitamins regularly—and their health-preserving potential seriously." She then asked readers to fill out a brief questionnaire about vitamins and mail it to her. Three months later she announced that she had received hundreds of responses from readers, 44 percent of whom said they took between five and ten supplements a day, and 32 percent of whom took eleven or more per day.

Tabloid Newspapers

Tabloid newspapers are another steady source of health misinformation. In 1987, Dr. Barrett analyzed 322 articles on health, nutrition, and psychology appearing during a three-month period in *National Enquirer*, *Globe*, *National*

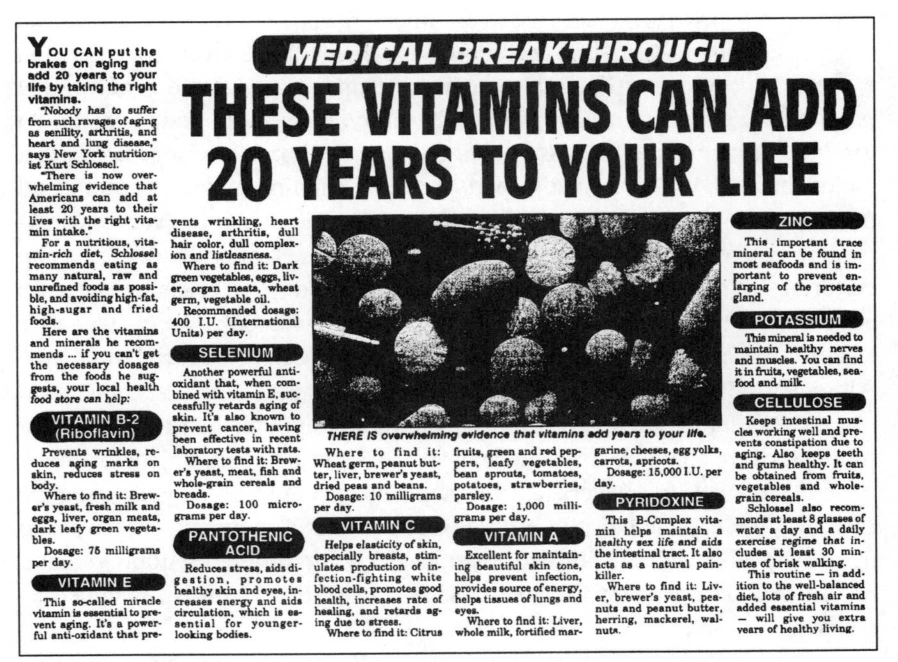

MEDICAL BREAKTHROUGH

THESE VITAMINS CAN ADD 20 YEARS TO YOUR LIFE

YOU CAN put the brakes on aging and add 20 years to your life by taking the right vitamins.

"*Nobody has to suffer* from such ravages of aging as senility, arthritis, and heart and lung disease," says New York nutritionist Kurt Schlossel.

"There is now overwhelming evidence that Americans can add at least 20 years to their lives with the right vitamin intake."

For a nutritious, *vitamin-rich diet*, Schlossel recommends eating as many natural, raw and unrefined foods as possible, and avoiding high-fat, high-sugar and fried foods.

Here are the vitamins and minerals he recommends ... if you can't get the necessary dosages from the foods he suggests, your local health *food store can help:*

VITAMIN B-2 (Riboflavin)

Prevents wrinkles, reduces aging marks on skin, reduces stress on body.

Where to find it: Brewer's yeast, fresh milk and eggs, liver, organ meats, dark leafy green vegetables.

Dosage: 75 milligrams per day.

VITAMIN E

This so-called miracle vitamin is essential to prevent aging. It's a powerful anti-oxidant that prevents wrinkling, heart disease, arthritis, dull hair color, dull complexion and *listlessness*.

Where to find it: Dark green vegetables, eggs, liver, organ meats, wheat germ, vegetable oil.

Recommended dosage: 400 I.U. (International Units) per day.

SELENIUM

Another powerful anti-oxidant that, when combined with vitamin E, successfully retards aging of skin. It's also known to prevent cancer, having been effective in recent laboratory tests with rats.

Where to find it: Brewer's yeast, meat, fish and whole-grain cereals and breads.

Dosage: 100 micrograms per day.

PANTOTHENIC ACID

Reduces stress, aids digestion, promotes healthy skin and eyes, increases energy and aids circulation, which is essential for younger-looking bodies.

Where to find it: Wheat germ, peanut butter, liver, brewer's yeast, dried peas and beans.

Dosage: 10 milligrams per day.

VITAMIN C

Helps elasticity of skin, especially breasts, stimulates production of infection-fighting white blood cells, promotes good health, increases rate of healing, and retards aging due to stress.

Where to find it: Citrus fruits, green and red peppers, leafy vegetables, bean sprouts, tomatoes, potatoes, strawberries, parsley.

Dosage: 1,000 milligrams per day.

VITAMIN A

Excellent for maintaining beautiful skin tone, helps prevent infection, provides source of energy, helps tissues of lungs and eyes.

Where to find it: Liver, whole milk, fortified margarine, cheeses, egg yolks, carrots, apricots.

Dosage: 15,000 I.U. per day.

PYRIDOXINE

This B-Complex vitamin helps maintain a *healthy sex life* and aids the intestinal tract. It also acts as a natural painkiller.

Where to find it: Liver, brewer's yeast, peanuts and peanut butter, herring, mackerel, walnuts.

ZINC

This important trace mineral can be found in most seafoods and is important to prevent enlarging of the prostate gland.

POTASSIUM

This mineral is needed to maintain healthy nerves and muscles. You can find it in fruits, vegetables, seafood and milk.

CELLULOSE

Keeps intestinal muscles working well and prevents constipation due to aging. Also keeps teeth and gums healthy. It can be obtained from fruits, vegetables and whole-grain cereals.

Schlossel also recommends at least 8 glasses of water a day and a daily exercise *regime that* includes at least 30 minutes of brisk walking.

This routine — in addition to the well-balanced diet, lots of fresh air and added essential vitamins — will give you extra years of healthy living.

THERE IS overwhelming evidence that vitamins add years to your life.

This article from the December 24, 1991, *National Examiner* lists the biochemical functions of ten substances present in food, four of which are not vitamins. The article contains no basis for concluding that taking any of the substances in supplement form rather than in food will "add years to your life."

Examiner, Sun, and *Weekly World News* and concluded that only 135 (42 percent) were reliable. Nutrition articles scored especially poorly, because many were based on the views of promoters of nutrition misinformation.

One article in the *National Examiner,* for example, claimed that "a miraculous diet pill will flatten your tummy . . . and you can do it fast without a complicated diet program." The article discussed the Optifast system of weight control, a reputable, medically supervised program. However, the program is not simple, the results are not instant, and the pills involved do not cause weight loss but simply add nutrients to the low-calorie program. "How to Use Vitamins and Minerals to Beat Stress," which appeared in the *National Enquirer,* claimed that "some 50 million Americans may suffer stress and stress-related problems due to vitamin and mineral deficiencies," which is complete nonsense. Articles like these can cause harm by inducing people to waste money on worthless or overblown products.

Advertising "Self-Regulation"

Another factor supporting supplement sales is the advertising of products that are usually not sold through health-food stores. This advertising, done mainly by large pharmaceutical companies, is significant because it reaches the general public and not just "true believers."

A mechanism exists whereby these ads can be challenged if they appear misleading. In 1971, when the FTC was initiating an advertising substantiation program, the National Advertising Review Board (NARB) was formed "to promote higher standards of truth and accuracy in national and regional advertising." Its sponsors were the American Advertising Federation, American Association of Advertising Agencies, Association of National Advertisers, and Council of Better Business Bureaus. The review process is done primarily by the Council's National Advertising Division (NAD), which investigates questionable ads, draws conclusions, and sometimes negotiates settlements. Parties that disagree with NAD's findings can appeal to NARB. If NARB agrees to review the case, it may hold a hearing at which parties to the controversy testify but are not permitted to debate or cross-examine one another.

NAD may initiate action as a result of its own monitoring of advertising, as well as complaints from others. It generally will not consider cases involving: products or companies it does not consider basically legitimate, dietary supplements whose manufacturers are making illegal therapeutic claims, ads that are not distributed nationally, or services by licensed health professionals.

(This means that NAD is very unlikely to consider any of the ads that appear in health-food magazines.) NAD's investigations tend to be slow, and even ads that are discontinued as a result of an inquiry usually have run long enough to achieve their intended purposes.

When NAD accepts a case for "investigation," it asks the advertiser for substantiation, which may then be shown to the complainant for rebuttal. Closed cases are classified in the monthly *NAD Case Report* as "substantiated" or "modified or discontinued." NAD closes about a hundred cases a year. The results in vitamin-related cases have included:

• In 1982, in an ad for *Z-BEC,* A.H. Robins stated that "the B-Complex and C vitamins you take today probably won't do anything for you tomorrow. Because they're water-soluble and are eliminated daily." After NAD investigated, the company agreed that future advertising addressed to people in normal health would not contain claims that the entire day's vitamins must be supplied on a daily basis.

• In 1986, AARP Pharmacy Service pledged to stop recommending *Activitamins* for seniors who "play tennis or golf, or like to bike, jog or walk." AARP also indicated it would discontinue ads suggesting that supplements of "the protector vitamins" (C, E, and beta-carotene) would "ensure added protection against harmful free radicals."

• In 1989, E.R. Squibb & Sons pledged to revise a television commercial for its *Theragran-M*. The commercial, which showed individuals involved in various energetic activities, had stated: "If only you had more energy. This kind of energy comes from eating a balanced diet with vitamin B-complex and biotin—the energy releasers. To be sure you're getting enough energy-releasers take *Theragran-M* high-potency multivitamins. . . . Unleash your energy." In support of these claims, Squibb's attorney provided chapters from nutrition texts explaining how energy refers to the chemical energy locked in foods. However, NAD expressed concern that consumers viewing the commercial would understand "energy" to mean the physical energy that enables people to engage in strenuous activities.

• In 1989, we complained to NAD that the Council for Responsible Nutrition (CRN)'s "Vitamin Gap" ad was misleading (see Chapter 3). Even though the ad contained many errors, NAD's executive director (who believes in "nutrition insurance") concluded that CRN had performed a public service by suggesting that supplements might be helpful. We then appealed to NARB, which held a hearing. NARB's final report expressed concern that readers of the ad "might confuse the mass standards of the RDAs with an individualized measure of efficiency" and urged CRN—if it resumed its advertising campaign—to precisely describe the nature of the "risk" to the individual caused by failure to meet RDAs. Despite this insight, the panel considered the ad "fully substantiated when words are taken in their vernacular, as opposed to their technical, meanings." Among other things, the panel thought it was perfectly OK for an advertiser to characterize stress as "robbing" people of nutrients (even though it does not), or to characterize calcium, iron, fiber, and omega-3 fatty acids as vitamins, even though they are not vitamins.

• In 1986, the Florida Department of Citrus advertised that people who exercised couldn't get enough potassium in their diet and that the potassium in grapefruit juice not only would provide enough, but would "balance sodium levels to regulate blood pressure and fight off fatigue." When NAD investigated, a department spokesperson said that the potassium deficiency claims were based on an opinion survey of athletes conducted by a nutrition consultant plus a study of the effects of intense conditioning in young men undergoing basic military training. In addition, a literature survey was provided as substantiation of the roles of sodium and potassium as nutritional factors in controlling blood pressure. NAD's investigator replied that the data obtained from the studies could not support broadly stated claims and expressed concern that the ad overstated the benefits of drinking normal quantities of grapefruit juice—which it did. The spokesperson informed NAD that the claims had been discontinued and that a new campaign would promote grapefruit as a significant source of potassium when part of a healthy regimen, including proper diet and exercise. However, a subsequent ad stated that grapefruit juice is "high in potassium with no sodium: a combination that, along with proper diet and exercise, can help control blood pressure." This was still misleading because drinking normal quantities of grapefruit juice will not lower blood pressure.

In 1993, the department distributed a booklet containing several pages of misleading information about vitamin C. Among other things, the booklet suggests that vitamin C "may offer remarkable protection against heart disease" and "can help prevent tuberculosis." (The latter claim is attributed to "Dr. Irwin Stone," but does not indicate that Stone's "Ph.D. degree" was from nonaccredited Donsbach University.) The booklet also claims (falsely) that vitamin C must be ingested daily because it cannot be stored in the body. The most remarkable thing about these promotions is not their content but the fact that the Florida Department of Citrus is a government agency.

Lack of Peer Review

Chapter 1 of this book describes how scientists are eager to evaluate each other's theories and experimental techniques and to point out any deficiencies. This process of "peer review" is basic to scientific growth and the establishment of scientific facts. The comparable goal of journalism is (or ought to be) ferreting out the truth. Yet journalists almost never publicly criticize each other's work—particularly when health topics are involved.

While the media seem to feel free to criticize whatever they please, and to demand that all sorts of officials and institutions be accountable, there is no visible accountability within the media itself.

Have you ever seen a letter to the editor from a reporter who charged that his own newspaper or magazine misled the public in an article or advertisement about health? Have you ever heard a radio or TV commentator state that misinformation about health was broadcast on his station? Have you ever seen an editorial in print which charged that a health topic was mishandled by another publication? Have you ever seen an expression of editorial outrage directed against poor reporting or advertising that could cause thousands of unsuspecting people to become victims of quackery? Have you ever encountered a warning that the "miracle" claims found frequently in the tabloid newspapers are not worth the paper they are printed on? Except for *Consumer Reports* and a few other publications listed in Appendix E of this book, there seems to be an unwritten rule that reporters and editors never criticize each other's health-related errors in public.

Another thing we have observed is that major media almost never retract misinformation even when faced with indisputable evidence that they have erred. This point was brought home last year following an uproar over an NBC "Dateline" program in which a General Motors Corporation (GMC) truck exploded in flames after a car crashed into its side. When GMC protested, NBC officials dismissed the protests as unwarranted—until GMC filed suit and announced proof that the truck had been rigged with small rockets that had exploded seconds before the crash. NBC quickly issued an apology, and many media outlets criticized NBC's misconduct.

As far as we know, no comparable retraction or criticism has ever taken place following a botched quackery-related story, even one that was capable of killing someone. There is, however, a tiny ray of sunshine on the horizon. *Forbes MediaCritic*, a quarterly magazine launched in 1993, has demonstrated an interest in healthcare issues and will include quackery-related stories within its scope.

The Problem of Libel

How much risk is involved in criticizing nutrition quackery? The answer depends mainly on how it is done. Critics who understand the law and use common sense have little to fear. One cannot libel an idea. Therefore it is not libelous to attack an idea or to list the characteristic signs of quackery or to say that something is "questionable." One cannot libel a large group of individuals or an entire industry. One can libel an individual (or an organization) by engaging in name-calling. Therefore it is inadvisable to call anyone a name (like "quack") unless you are willing to defend this claim in court. It is legal to mention relevant adverse facts about someone who places himself in the public spotlight by claiming to have expert knowledge. But avoid statements about motivation (such as "He's only in it for the money") because they may be impossible to prove.

Libel suits can be costly to defend, and some health-food promoters are inclined to be litigious. Yet they have filed very few such suits, because the likelihood of winning in court is virtually zero. If an industrywide policy of suing critics just to harass them should arise, two things would likely happen. First, the scientific community would rally to help those being sued. Then the courts would begin to order unsuccessful plaintiffs to pay the costs of defense.

In 1978, the National Nutritional Foods Association (NNFA) and three health-food-store owners sued Fredrick J. Stare, M.D., and Elizabeth M. Whelan, Sc.D., M.P.H., as part of "Operation Counterattack," an NNFA strategy to silence critics. The suit charged that Stare and Whelan had "recklessly, maliciously and knowingly disseminated false and defamatory remarks with respect to plaintiffs and the health food industry."

Nutrition scientists all over America responded to this suit with outrage. It was obvious that plaintiffs could not win the suit in court. Their names hadn't even been mentioned in the publications to which they were objecting. Seeing the suit as a threat to the freedom of expression of all nutrition scientists, nutrition organizations and friends of the defendants raised enough money to pay for the suit's defense.

To prove libel under the laws of New York State (where the suit was filed), it was necessary to show that a defendant used defamatory words against plaintiffs that were untrue and caused measurable damages. The judge, who dismissed the case in 1980, ruled that plaintiffs had met none of these requirements. He also warned that "any further suit by plaintiffs against critics of the health food industry should be scrutinized carefully to determine whether it was brought in good faith." (In other words, if plaintiffs filed another spurious suit, they would be held responsible for defendants' legal bills.)

As far as we know, no critic of nutrition quackery has ever been successfully sued for libel or paid one cent to prevent a threatened suit from being filed. However, critics who were defamed have collected significant amounts of money.

• In 1986, a company controlled by Kurt Donsbach published *The Great Medical Monopoly Wars,* which claimed that the American Medical Association, the FDA, drug companies, and various individuals were conspiring to "destroy the American free-enterprise system in the health care field." The book contained false and defamatory statements about Drs. Victor Herbert and John Renner. This information, plus additional false information, was then promoted by the National Health Federation, the Coalition for Alternatives in Nutrition and Healthcare, and various other parties allied with Donsbach. When they refused to stop and to retract the false statements, Herbert and Renner filed suit. In 1991, Renner settled out of court with Donsbach and two other defendants for $60,000. Renner's suit against the book's author, P. Joseph Lisa, is still pending. Herbert's suit proved to be very complicated and has not yet been resolved.

• In August 1991, *Vegetarian Times* magazine published a lengthy cover story questioning whether "quackbusters" were consumer advocates or "medical McCarthyites." The article contained defamations from Lisa's book and attempted to portray Herbert, Renner, Dr. Barrett, and National Council Against Health Fraud president Dr. William T. Jarvis as closed-minded individuals who were unwilling to consider promising "nutritional" methods. To avoid a lawsuit, *Vegetarian Times* paid a total of $21,000 and published a detailed rebuttal from us in its March 1992 issue.

• In 1992, Herbert, Barrett, and Jarvis were defamed again, this time by Loren Israelson, an attorney affiliated with the health-food industry. During a speech at an industry trade show, he stated that we were "vicious and pathological and would stop at nothing" and that *Vegetarian Times* had published a well-written article criticizing us. The speech was tape-recorded and offered for sale, along with tapes of other talks at the meeting, through an ad in *Natural Foods Merchandiser*. Israelson probably had this in mind when he remarked, "Gee, I sure hope that they aren't listening to the tape." Unfortunately for him (and his insurance company), we did listen to the tape and collected a retraction plus $34,000 in out-of-court settlements.

19

Elaborate Marketing Schemes

The health-food industry is marketing thousands of questionable products intended for the treatment of disease. In most cases, however, the intended purpose is not printed on the product label, where it could render the manufacturer an easy target for government regulators. Instead, as described in Chapter 5, this information is transmitted through other channels of communication that are less obvious or may not be subject to regulation. This chapter illustrates elaborate ways in which three manufacturers transmitted illegal messages about their products. The first used publications and seminars. The second distributed flyers promoting "independent" publications that touted the ingredients in its products. The third emphasized research and public relations but, helped by its distributors, disseminated explicit claims through other channels as well. We also describe how the health-food industry marketed a "dietary supplement" that seriously harmed thousands of people, thus demonstrating why tighter regulation of the health-food industry is needed to protect the public.

"Unlimited Promotional Material"

Enzymatic Therapy, Inc., of Green Bay, Wisconsin, probably holds the record for the quantity and variety of promotional material used to make illegal health claims for its products. Its president, Terence J. Lemerond, also heads Biotherapeutics/Phyto-Pharmica (which markets supplements and botanical extracts to professionals), Bay Natural Foods (a health-food store), and the

Naturalean Wellness Center (next door to the store). His other activities have included a radio talk show and a newspaper column. In the local *Yellow Pages,* his name has been followed by the initials "N.D., B.S., C.N.C."

According to an article distributed by Enzymatic Therapy, Lemerond was inspired to enter the health-food business after solving a weight problem with the help of a friend who operated a health-food store. In 1969, he acquired his own store (now called Bay Natural Foods) and engaged in "nutritional consultation." In January 1981, he and his wife incorporated Enzymatic Therapy. Later that year, in ads in *Natural Foods Merchandiser*, it announced a "money-back guarantee on an extraordinary new system of nutritional health care!"

"The success of our case histories would astound you" the ads continued, "Enzymatic Therapy is a dynamic new concept in nutritional supplement formulas. They are directed straight at the ailments of our modern age. Created by a nutritional counselor from his highly successful practice, these formulas are the results of experience—not conjecture."

The ads listed eleven products: *Acne-Zyme* (to support healthy skin tissue and improve complexion), *Acid-A-Cal* (to improve joint function), *Liv-A-Tox* (to support liver function and detoxification), *Vira-Plex* (strengthens against colds, flu and infection), *Pro-Gest-Ade* (for digesting protein), *Liga-Plex* (supports weak ligaments, tennis elbow), *Nucleo-Pro F* (for female problems), *Nucleo-Pro M* (for male problems), *Artho-Flex* ("joint pain, etc., etc."), *Relax-O-Zyme* ("muscle and nerve relaxant"), and *Hypo-Plex* (weight loss, appetite depressant, and control of high or low blood sugar). Each product had a formula number on its label.

A price list subsequently mailed to retailers contained more specific claims. *Nucleo-Pro M,* for example, was said to be for "prostatitis, impotence, male hormonal problems, fatigue and lack of stamina," while *Nucleo-Pro F* was for "female hormonal problems, impotency, irregular menses, fatigue, menstrual cramps." The mailing also included "Research Bulletin #105: ACNE," a two-page flyer that listed and discussed the ingredients in *Acne-Zyme No. 105.* The flyer didn't mention the product's name but said there was a formula available to meet criteria described in the article. The second page contained a disclaimer: "This material is for educational purposes only and is not meant to diagnose or prescribe. Researched by Siri Khalsa, *Nutrition News,* Pomona, CA . . . Permission to reprint granted to Enzymatic Therapy, Inc."

In 1982, Ms. Khalsa also published a book, *You Can Do Something About Common Ailments.* Enzymatic Therapy is not identified in the book, but most chapters are almost identical to the "Research Bulletins." The appendix lists the formula numbers and ingredients of the company's products, and a footnote states, "If the health food store in your neighborhood cannot accommodate you, please write us and we'll tell you where you can locate the formulas."

At the end of 1984, the company boasted: "No other line of supplements can offer you the service, support, and the profitability that comes from working with Enzymatic Therapy formulas," and it promised to supply "unlimited quantities of bag stuffers and promotional material." By that time, it offered about fifty numbered formulas with corresponding "Research Bulletins." Some of these were still attributed to Ms. Khalsa, but most were "researched by the American Society of Nutritional Research" in Phoenix, Arizona.

These flyers, which had four pages, were intended for distribution to customers. The first page of each contained a box in which retailers could print their store's name and address under the message: "For professional health care, shop at . . ." Retailers also received Enzymatic Therapy's "Professional Price List," which listed "suspected symptoms" for which each of the products were supposedly useful, plus a four-page flyer titled "Restricted for Professional Use only" in which detailed therapeutic claims were made for each product.

In May 1985, following an extensive undercover investigation, *Consumer Reports* magazine published a cover story called "Foods, Drugs, or Frauds?" The report listed Enzymatic Therapy among more than forty companies that were violating federal law by making unapproved drug claims for "supplement" products. About a year later, the FDA issued a regulatory letter ordering Lemerond to stop using the "Research Bulletins" to make "false and misleading" representations for *Renatone, Liv-A-Tox, Vira-Plex, and* other Enzymatic Therapy products. Enzymatic Therapy stopped the Research Bulletins but began publishing "Health Guides," a series of forty-five brightly colored flyers that explained how "our specific nutritional and herbal formulas support and enhance a full range of body functions." Most of the guides described the ingredients in various formulas, the products that contained them, and the body organs or functions they could "support." For example, Guide No. 12, "A Comprehensive Guide to Healthy Kidneys," touted *Renatone No. 184* ("to aid the kidney in its vital roles") and *Arbutin Complex No. 802A* ("diuretic and urinary tract antiseptic"), and *K Com No. 808* ("a general tonic for the urinary system"). "Once your patrons realize the many health benefits of proper nutrition," said a promotional flyer for retailers, "you will have loyal customers for life."

Health Guides were available from Lem's Contract Printing in Green Bay (owned by Lemerond's son Bradley). Retailers could order up to 1,200 per month per store and were encouraged to display them in a special 48-pocket rack

SUPPLEMENT	RECOMMENDATIONS	COMMENTS
MVP Program	See labels.	**Complete nutritional support for healthy circulation.** This program includes four unique supplements.
Oral Nutrient Chelates No. 375	Three to six tablets daily.	**Nutritional support for a healthy flow of blood through the heart and vascular pathways.** This combination of nutrients has also been used in a famous German formula.
Cardio-Tone No. 285C	One or two tablets after each meal.	**Contains natural factors known to contribute nutrition to a healthy heart.** Includes Raw Heart Tissue, Potassium, Magnesium, and Hawthorn Berry Extract.
Vasculex No. 813 P.S.E.	One or two capsules three times daily.	**Herbal support for cardiovascular health.** Unique blend of seven botanical extracts, *including Ginkgo and Hawthorn.*
HI/BP No. 275	One or two tablets *twice daily, morning* and evening.	**Natural support for the body systems *involved in maintaining healthy blood* pressure.** Includes Potassium, Magnesium, Niacinamide, and other factors.
Raw Heart L-Carnitine *Complex No. 401A*	One to three capsules daily with meals.	**Aids the body's natural control of blood sugar, cholesterol, and triglycerides.** Contains L-Carnitine with glandular factors.

Products listed in the section on "heart function" in the 1990 Enzymatic Therapy's "Formulas for Health" booklet.

sold by Enzymatic Therapy. In 1990, Lemerond stated that 500,000 to 750,000 of the guides were being distributed each month and that they were used in his Green Bay store. Later that year, the series was replaced by a single twenty-page booklet, "Formulas for Health: Your Guide to Important Health Topics," which discussed "adrenal stress," "heart function," "liver function," "healthy lungs," and twenty other categories for which products were specified. In 1991, the booklet was expanded to thirty-two pages that covered twenty-nine topics and more than ninety products.

During the early 1980s, Enzymatic Therapy offered to provide retailers with two types of nutritional programs for their customers. The "complete" program included a "Nutritional Appraisal Report" plus a hair analysis; the other program was just the appraisal report. "Each completed analysis will be returned to your customers in care of *your* store," the solicitation said. "Nothing for your store to invest, only profit to be made. . . . Each completed computerized analysis will tell your customers exactly which supplements to take and when to take them. THEY WILL BUY THESE SUPPLEMENTS FROM YOU." (How do you suppose Enzymatic Therapy knew in advance that everyone taking the test would "need" supplements?)

In 1986, Enzymatic Therapy began publishing *Formula for Health,* an eight-page newsletter for retailers which, by 1989, was issued monthly. To boost Enzymatic Therapy's monthly specials, later issues of the newsletter were accompanied by reproducible one-page inserts containing a box for the retailer's business card. The first three specials were products "for a healthy immune system," "for healthy digestion," and "to help you breathe easy."

In January 1989, Enzymatic Therapy began publishing *Health Counselor,* a magazine "designed to help educate your customers on the value of health, and ways to support the body by using nutritional and herbal formulas." Single copies were distributed free-of-charge, but retailers were encouraged to buy multiple copies for distribution or sale to their customers. The magazine contained articles boosting herbal remedies and ads for Enzymatic Therapy products. Many ads contained illegal therapeutic claims. In the first issue, for example, on a page marked "advertisement," several formulas were claimed to "support the heart and entire cardiovascular system" and were "particularly useful for individuals with atherosclerosis (hardening of the arteries)."

Seminars and More

For several years, Enzymatic Therapy invited retailers to attend free "nutritional seminar & sales training" sessions. On March 25, 1990, Ira Milner, R.D., audited one with over a hundred retailers and a few chiropractors. Before the program began, participants were asked to sign a "guarantee" that they were not agents of the FDA or any other consumer protection agency and would not tape the seminar for any government agency to use against Enzymatic Therapy. The statement also represented that the sole purpose for attending was to obtain "educational information." During the seminar, Lemerond showed slides of the products and described how to use them for specific health problems. He stated:

> Our products are specifically designed to nutritionally aid and support the various systems and the functions of the body. . . . The goal of Enzymatic Therapy is to provide you and your customers with the finest nutritional formulas of the highest quality, backed by sound scientific research. . . .
>
> I think we provide some of the best literature in the industry. . . . If you aren't using the literature rack and the literature, I encourage you to do so. It is a tremendous sales tool. It's like having another person

> in your store selling for you without having to pay that person, without having to deal with another clerk. One gentleman told me—he was buying between $600 and $1,000 a month of product a month from us—and he said to me one day, "I've never sold one of your products. . . . I just put the rack in the center of the store and let the people take the literature and they sell themselves."

Another seminar speaker was Michael T. Murray, N.D., who practices naturopathy in Bellevue, Washington, and teaches "therapeutic nutrition" and "botanical medicine" at Bastyr University, a naturopathic school in Seattle. Lemerond described Murray as "one of the finest scientists in the United States in the nutritional field" and said he had formulated or reformulated many Enzymatic Therapy products. The company, which undoubtedly views naturopathy as a marketing channel for its products, has donated at least $15,000 to Bastyr University.

Murray is also a prolific writer. He wrote *The 21st Century Herbal* ("a layman's guide to botanical extracts") and is co-author of the *Encyclopedia of Natural Medicine* (a reference guide for patients) and *A Textbook of Natural Medicine* (a massive collection of information about naturopathic methods). He also edited *Phyto-Pharmica Review* (a newsletter related to the herbal products marketed by Biotherapeutics) and produced "The Health Series" of booklets about herbs and common ailments written for laypersons.

Murray is also president of Vital Communications, of Bellevue, Washington. Near the end of 1989, Vital Communications took over as "sponsor" of the seminars and publisher of both *Health Counselor* and *Phyto-Pharmica Review*. In a letter to retailers early in 1990, Murray stated, "Your customers need help in selecting natural products they use to treat themselves, which is their constitutional right. Can you realize how little time you have to help each and every customer who comes into your store, as well as the legal implications involved with trying to be too helpful? *Health Counselor* magazine will solve those problems for you. . . . With just six issues of this bimonthly magazine in publication, *Health Counselor* already has a circulation of 105,000 per issue." Since bulk orders for *Health Counselor* were still placed through Lem's Contract Printing, it was clear that Enzymatic Therapy was using Murray as a "front"—to create an illusion of distance between the company and many of its claims.

The Health Series was also used to promote Enzymatic Therapy products. A 1990 mailing to health-food stores contained Murray's booklet on irritable bowel syndrome (IBS), an Enzymatic Therapy flyer for products whose ingredients were discussed in the booklet, and a cover letter in which Murray told how he prescribed one of the products to patients and suggested that the booklet could help customers "understand how to handle IBS naturally." The mailing was sent under the bulk permit that Enzymatic Therapy has used for years to mail its catalogs and other publications.

At the seminar Milner attended, Murray discussed herbs and various symptoms and conditions for which he said specific Enzymatic Therapy products should be recommended. Participants also received *The Professional Guide to Nutritional and Herbal Formulas*, a 158-page looseleaf manual "published and distributed by Vital Communications, Dr. Michael Murray, N.D.," which describes Enzymatic Therapy products and more than eighty diseases and conditions they supposedly can help. The manual also contains "protocols" for using various products against AIDS, multiple sclerosis, cancer, arthritis, and other serious health problems.

The third speaker at the seminar Milner attended was Kenneth R. Daub, D.C., of Rockford, Illinois, a chiropractor said to "specialize in circulatory and metabolic diseases." Daub developed *MVP*, a supplement program he said was adapted from the work of Hans Nieper, a German physician. At the seminar, Daub distributed a booklet entitled "Owners Manual for a Healthy Circulatory System," which claims that *MVP* can "help the body nutritionally cleanse itself of the life-threatening plaque in the arteries." He also encouraged attendees to request his videotape, which makes similar claims and contains testimonials from people who say his product was effective against high blood pressure, overweight, numbness of the hand and leg, chest pain, fatigue, and lack of energy. At the time of the seminar, Enzymatic therapy was the exclusive distributor of *MVP*. The slogan "Don't be bypassed, use MVP," appeared in its brochure, on the product label, and on refrigerator magnets distributed at the meeting.

Enzymatic Therapy also utilized S&S Public Relations, Inc., of Northbrook, Illinois, which issued news releases and arranged interviews with Lemerond. Like the Health Guides, the releases made claims that would be illegal on product labels.

By 1990, Enzymatic Therapy was marketing about three hundred

Refrigerator magnet distributed at Enzymatic Therapy seminar. A videotape and booklet distributed at the meeting falsely suggested that *MVP* could relieve blockage of coronary arteries and therefore was an alternative to bypass surgery.

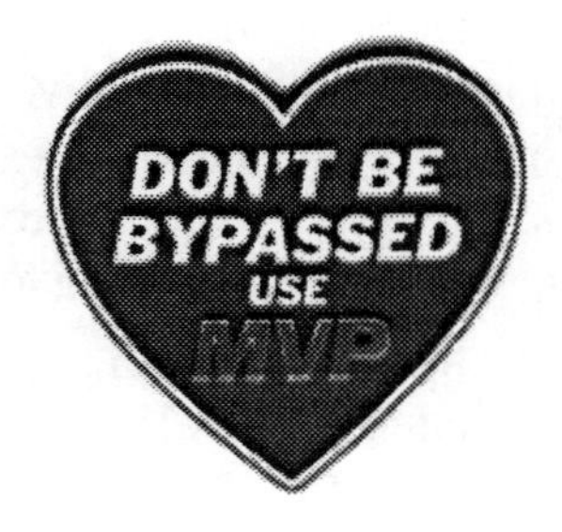

formulas containing vitamins, minerals, herbs, amino acids, and/or glandular tissue, while Biotherapeutics carried about eighty more. Many of these products were intended for the treatment of disease. Rather than seek FDA approval, Lemerond and his associates used subterfuge to "distance" illegal claims from their product labels. Their activities are instructive because they illustrate many of the ways supplement manufacturers communicate the intended uses of their products without putting this information on product labels.

An article in the March 1993 *FDA Consumer* states that the FDA began investigating Enzymatic Therapy in 1985 after receiving complaints from three people who believed they had been harmed by Enzymatic Therapy products. During the next six years, the FDA conducted numerous inspections and ordered Lemerond to stop marketing a few products and to stop distributing violative literature. Although he complied with some of these orders (or said he did), FDA undercover investigations—including attendance at a seminar—found that a pattern of violations persisted. In 1991, the agency finally initiated injunction proceedings against Lemerond, Biotherapeutics, Bay Natural Foods, Lem's Printing, and Lemerond's son Bradley. In November 1992, the FDA obtained a consent decree barring Enzymatic Therapy from marketing products with unproven therapeutic claims. The court order also bars the company from manufacturing or marketing fifty-six listed items unless new promotional material for them is approved by the FDA.

Since the court action, Enzymatic Therapy has initiated a toll-free product information line. If you would like to investigate what its products are for, you can call 1-800-783-2286.

Not-So-Secret Codes

Solaray, Inc., of Ogden, Utah, was founded in 1973 by James L. Beck, whose interest in the health-food industry began after "personal health problems were resolved through natural methods." The company featured herbs and herbal blends until the mid-1980s, when it added "tissue salts" (later referred to as "homeopathic nutrients") to its blends and began marketing new lines of vitamins, minerals, digestive enzymes, "raw glandular concentrates," and various "special formulas"—more than two hundred products altogether. Solaray maintains that its herbal products are superior because they are made from wild herbs. According to Beck:

> Solaray, Inc., firmly believes that cultivated, organically grown herbs are inferior to wild herbs. A wild herb must fight with other plants for nutrients, sun and air. Only the strong plants will survive. On the other

hand, a cultivated herb grows under less stress, allowing diseased or weak herbs to survive.

Solaray's herbal blends are designated by "SP" numbers (SP-1, SP-2, SP-3, and so on). During the early 1980s, the company distributed four-page flyers said to be "a condensed version of Neva Jensen's booklet, *The Herbal Health Guide,* and her cassette course *Herbal Nutrition,* both available exclusively through health food stores." The flyers contained "a few facts about herbs" plus a list of numbered symptoms and ingredients. The numbers corresponded to the "SP" numbers of Solaray's herbal blends. Solaray also distributed a two-page flyer, "Formula Guide excerpt from John Heinerman's book, 'Herbal

Herbal Blends	Table of Contents
1	**Infertility; Impotence and related problems.** Damiana Leaves, Sarsaparilla Root, Saw Palmetto Berries, Siberian Ginseng, Licorice Root, Kelp. Supports #7a, 7c, and 16 (male).
2	**Arthritis; Rheumatism; Bursitis.** Alfalfa, Celery Seed, Burdock Root, Chaparral, Sarsaparilla Root, Comfrey, Kelp, Cayenne, Queen-of-the-Meadow Root. Supports #4 and 11a.
3	**Respiratory Ailments (acts to soothe, tone, and relieve irritation); Hayfever.** Wild Cherry Bark, Pleurisy Root, Slippery Elm Bark, Mullein Leaves, Chickweed, Horehound, Comfrey, Licorice Root, Kelp, Cayenne, Saw Palmetto Berries. Supports #22 and 33.
4	**Skin disorders; Rash; Itch; Psoriasis; General cleansing; Eczema; Acne Vulgaris; Dry and scaly skin.** Dandelion Root, Chaparral, Burdock Root, Licorice Root, Echinacea, Yellow Dock Root, Kelp, Cayenne. Supports #4, 11a, and 13.
5	**To reduce high blood sugar (hyperglycemia); to restore, sustain liver, spleen, kidney, gallbladder and pancreas function.** Dandelion Root, Parsley, Uva-Ursi, Gentian Root, Huckleberry Leaves, Raspberry Leaves, Buchu Leaves, Saw Palmetto Berries, Kelp, Bladderwrack. Supports #19 and 28.
6	**Diuretic; For edema and all edematous conditions; Also a treatment for urinary deficiency and infection.** Parsley, Cornsilk, Uva-Ursi Leaves, Cleavers, Buchu Leaves, Juniper Berries, Kelp, Cayenne, Queen-of-the-Meadow Root. Supports #2, 4, 6, 11a, and 18.
7a	**Female Problems; vaginal and cervical infection, leucorrhea; urinary tract infection.** Goldenseal Root, Witch Hazel Leaves. Comfrey Root, Buchu Leaves, Myrrh Gum, Juniper Berries, Squaw Vine. Supports #6.
7b	**Astringent. To inhibit diarrhea and menorrhagia.** Cranesbill Root, Witch Hazel Leaves, Raspberry Leaves, Uva-Ursi Leaves, Comfrey Root, Shepherd's Purse, Black Haw Bark. Supports #7c and 32.
7c	**Female problems; tonic during pregnancy, delivery, menses, menopause; for pain, cramp, atony, etc.** related to birth, pregnancy, menstruation and menopause. Reduces pain, cramping, uterine atony, and related conditions. Helps maintain hormonal balance. Black Cohosh Root, Licorice Root, Raspberry Leaves, Passion Flower, Comfrey Root, Black Haw Bark, Saw Palmetto Berries, Squaw Vine, Wild Yam Root, Kelp. Tonic for female problems related Supports #1.
8	**Nutritional tonic for the heart.** Hawthorn Berries, Motherwort, Rosemary Leaves, Kelp, Cayenne. Supports #9, 18, and 31.

Portion of "Table of Contents" from the first version "Proven Herbal Blends," a booklet that retailed for $1.50. The number of each blend corresponded to the Solaray product containing the ingredients in the blend.

Dynamics,'" which had a similar setup. Retailers also received a set of two-page "newsletters" by Neva Jensen, each of which was numbered identically to a Solaray product and discussed supposed therapeutic benefits of its ingredients.

A 1984 Solaray brochure for health-food retailers stated:

> Q. What is Solaray's philosophy on labeling their herbal blends SP-1 through SP-35?
> A. Solaray's labels are *professional* and *discreet.* Instead of suggestive labeling, Solaray encourages service, guidance, and informative literature – the things the health foods retailer can best provide. It's clear! Solaray's products are designed for health food stores, not supermarkets. . . .
>
> Q. Does Solaray provide free informative literature?
> A. Yes! Contact us and literature will be sent.

During 1984, Cormorant Books of Lehi, Utah, sent retailers a four-page flyer and a booklet called "Proven Herbal Blends: A Rational Approach to Prevention & Remedy," by Daniel B. Mowrey, Ph.D. The first page urged readers to ask for the booklet at their health-food store; the next two pages reproduced the table of contents, as pictured on the previous page, listing health concerns and ingredients and the "SP" numbers on the bottles of Solaray's herbal blends. A cover letter explained:

> This booklet addressed each product in the SP line separately, explaining in detail what each blend is intended to accomplish. . . .
>
> The accompanying flyer is free to you in whatever quantity you desire. Simply fill out the enclosed Response Card and return it (hopefully with an accompanying order) in the postage paid envelope. We will ensure you will receive a monthly supply of the flyer. In the event you presently carry or intend to carry the Solaray brand herbal blends, you will find this booklet an excellent adjunct to your sales efforts.

In 1985, Cormorant Books sent revised versions of Mowrey's booklet and its promotional flyer, both of which listed the ingredients in Solaray's herbal blends and the conditions for which they were supposedly useful. However, no product numbers were mentioned.

In 1986, a larger and more detailed version of Mowrey's *Proven Herbal Blends* was published by Keats Publishing (copyrighted by Cormorant Books). Although the book mentioned neither Solaray nor its product numbers, the herbs listed for each "health concern" were those in Solaray's products.

During the time that the above documents were distributed, the label of each Solaray herbal blends gave only the following directions: "As a splendid addition to the diet, one or two capsules (as desired) may be taken orally with meals, or with a glass of water." We assume that if the FDA had charged that the flyers were part of Solaray's labeling, the company would have replied that they merely advertised their respective publications. We doubt that a court would have bought such an argument, but as far as we know, the setup went unchallenged. Mowrey has also produced a newsletter called *The Herb Blurb,* which admonishes that its contents are "confidential" and "meant for retailer eyes only."

Food, Drug, or Fraud?

David Horrobin, M.D., Ph.D., has been interested in evening primrose oil (EPO) for more than twenty years. In 1978, after five years of laboratory research, Horrobin and a large company that had been breeding evening primrose plants founded Efamol Ltd. to develop and market EPO. The company maintains its headquarters in Guildford, England, on the outskirts of London, and conducts its basic research at the Efamol Research Institute in Kentville, Nova Scotia.

By the mid-1980s, Efamol's products were being sold in the United States and more than twenty-five other countries. During this period, although Efamol "officially" maintained that its EPO products were foods or "dietary supplements," therapeutic claims for them were disseminated by the company and a succession of American distributors.

In 1984, General Nutrition, Inc., three of its officers, and two of its retail store managers were charged with conspiring to defraud the FDA and violating provisions of the Food, Drug, and Cosmetic Act which require that drug products be approved by the FDA as safe and effective prior to marketing. Court papers in the case alleged:

- Between 1980 and 1981, General Nutrition, its president (Gary Daum), and two vice-presidents conspired to purchase EPO from Efamol Ltd. and to promote and sell it under the name *Gammaprim* for the prevention and treatment of high blood pressure, arthritis, multiple sclerosis, and other ailments.

- In 1980, one of the defendants received a letter from Dr. Horrobin suggesting that Efamol products be marketed without FDA approval. Referring to EPO's supposed beneficial effects, the letter stated, "Obviously you could not advertise Efamol for these purposes but equally obviously there are ways of getting the information across." Subsequent company memos described an elaborate promotional scheme that included newspaper articles, radio talk shows, and publications for use in General Nutrition's retail stores. In addition, oral claims were made by retail employees to prospective customers. FDA investigators posing as customers at various stores in western New York State were told that *Gammaprim* would be better for treatment of high blood pressure than the prescription drugs *Nitrostat* or *Diuril*, and that it was good for arthritis as well.

- By virtue of these claims, *Gammaprim* became a drug within the meaning of the law. However, rather than submitting the product to the FDA for premarket evaluation, defendants sought to disguise it as a food supplement, thereby attempting to defraud the FDA.

In motions to stop the prosecution, the defendants claimed: (1) their right to free speech was being violated, (2) the prosecution was unfair because many other companies making health claims in advertising had not been criminally prosecuted, (3) *Gammaprim* should not be considered a drug because it is not inherently toxic, and (4) the laws under which they were being prosecuted were too vague. In May 1986, these motions were dismissed by a federal judge who noted that the defendants were aware, or should have been aware, that they were breaking the law. A few months later, General Nutrition pled guilty to four counts of misbranding a drug and agreed to pay $10,000 to the government as reimbursement for costs of prosecution. Daum (who was no longer its president) pled guilty to one count of misbranding and was fined $1,000. The remaining charges against other employees were dismissed.

During the early 1980s, Efamol's EPO was marketed in the United States as *Evening Primrose Oil from England*™ by Health From the Sun Products, Inc., of Dover, Massachusetts. The company advertised in trade magazines that EPO was "the biggest sales opportunity since vitamin C . . . . because there is more authoritative medical and nutritional evidence behind Evening Primrose Oil than any other product ever introduced into the health food industry." Horrobin's picture and endorsement of Efamol EPO appeared in this ad with no mention that he was president and managing director of the company that produced it. The ad made no health claims, but retailers who responded were sent multiple copies of customer handouts in which such claims appeared. One was a flyer which claimed that EPO enables weight loss without dieting, slows down the aging process, is effective against PMS, lowers cholesterol as effectively as drugs, lowers blood pressure, can help most people with mild or moderate rheumatoid arthritis, helps hyperactive children, and slows down the progress of multiple sclerosis. Another handout was a magazine article entitled "Evening Primrose Oil—Miracle Worker of the Eighties," written by Horrobin. It stated that half of the people who took 2 to 4 grams of EPO lost weight without a conscious effort to diet and that EPO had significantly improved eczema in adults and children, produced dramatic improvement in women with premenstrual syndrome (PMS), and helped women with painful, lumpy breasts.

In mid-1985, Nature's Way of Springville, Utah, took over as Efamol's exclusive American distributor. Like its predecessor, Nature's Way made few health claims in its magazine ads but transmitted many through other channels. Its May/June 1985 newsletter for retailers, for example, stated that Nature's Way Evening Primrose Oil "assists the body in expelling waste by strengthening the body's immune system, and helping circulation. It is also valuable in fighting skin problems, and helping faulty tear ducts and salivary glands."

The Efamol Corporate Video, distributed in November 1985, contained the following ideas: (1) the company is "pioneering research into natural sources of new medicines," (2) various disorders might be caused by a "metabolic block" in fatty acid metabolism that prevents formation of adequate amounts of prostaglandin, (3) Efamol Ltd. has actively encouraged and coordinated independent research using EPO into a variety of disorders, "including dermatological disease, gynecological problems, and cardiovascular diseases in which possible deficiency of prostaglandins has been implicated," and (4) "Efamol products are currently marketed as foods and dietary supplements and are not licensed for clinical usage other than in approved clinical trials."

In June 1986, Nature's Way announced that it was starting a library of videotapes that retailers could borrow, free of charge, to help train their staff. The first such video contained a lecture Dr. Horrobin gave earlier that year on "The Role of Essential Fatty Acids and Prostaglandins in Health." The lecture was given at a trade show in Anaheim, California, where Horrobin was introduced by Ken Murdock, president of Nature's Way. During the lecture, Horrobin said that although virtually all Americans get abundant amounts of essential fatty acids in their diet, 20 percent "may have flaws in the body" that limit their full use. Thus, he asserted, there occurs a functional deficiency of a metabolite called gamma linolenic acid (GLA), which is needed to produce prostaglandins. Horrobin's solution, of course, was to consume Efamol EPO, which is rich in GLA.

Throughout his lecture, Horrobin stressed that he and his company were deeply committed to research and had generated more than a hundred clinical studies. He said that he was particularly proud of studies with negative results (for weight-reduction, for example) because their existence added credibility to the positive ones. In discussing some of the studies, he showed slides of the dosages used. Thus retailers who attended the lecture, as well as those who viewed the videotape, could tell precisely how to "prescribe" the products to

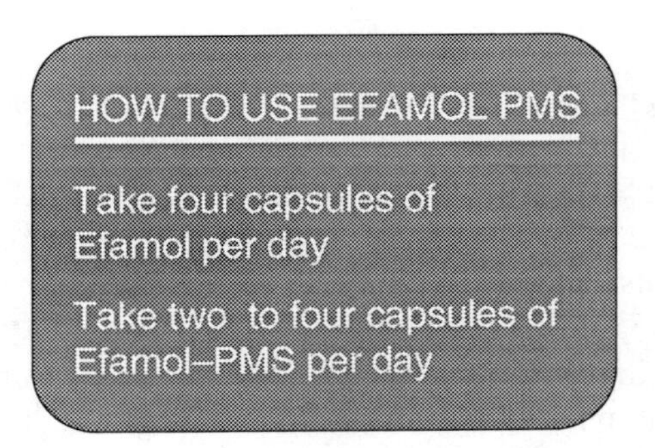

Slide shown to health-food retailers by Efamol president Dr. David Horrobin during a lecture in which he described how clinics were using Efamol products to treat premenstrual syndrome. Consumer literature from Nature's Way suggested starting with four to six capsules of *Efamol PMS* each day for the first two months.

their customers. An undercover investigator who borrowed the tape in 1988 "to show a customer with PMS" was told that ten copies were circulating.

Thus while Efamol and its distributors were marketing EPO as a "dietary supplement," they were also promoting it as a drug. In 1979, the FDA had notified Efamol representatives that EPO could not be imported into the United States unless the company sought and obtained approval by filing an appropriate food additive petition or new drug application. Efamol agreed not to export EPO to the United States, but in 1985 it began shipping it in bulk to California for encapsulation. The capsules would then be shipped to distributors who would market them as dietary supplements through health-food stores or by mail-order. In 1985, the agency issued an Import Alert instructing FDA officials to detain EPO labeled for food use because the agency considered it an unsafe food additive.

In 1988, at the FDA's request, a U.S. marshal seized twenty-one barrels containing EPO and vitamin E, plus quantities of five Efamol products. In 1989, forty-five more barrels of EPO were seized en route to California for encapsulation. In both cases, the FDA charged that Efamol Ltd. was marketing an unapproved food additive. With respect to the products, the FDA also charged that they were unapproved new drugs and misbranded. Federal district judges agreed with the FDA and ordered the seized materials destroyed. Efamol's appeals all the way to the U.S. Supreme Court were unsuccessful.

During these proceedings, Efamol Ltd. was compelled to produce documents which showed how it had spread therapeutic claims through press conferences, news releases, "news bulletins" to distributors, and many other channels of communication. Between 1983 and 1989, the company had issued more than sixty bulletins reporting on EPO research and other developments. Many were accompanied by reprints from scientific journals, newspapers, or magazines. A few were accompanied by a television transcript, booklet, or book. These materials promoted EPO for treating PMS, alcoholism, pregnancy-induced hypertension, atopic eczema, elevated cholesterol levels, hypertension, scleroderma, multiple sclerosis, rheumatoid arthritis, mastalgia (breast pain) and other problems. The bulletins encouraged use of the information for public relations purposes. The company also published and distributed bibliographies of scientific publications relevant to EPO to health-food retailers throughout the United States. Some of the references in these bibliographies were emphasized by highlighted quotes—including some from Dr. Horrobin's papers—which made explicit therapeutic claims for Efamol's EPO. Some of the bulletins included a statement like, "The way in which this information is used must, of course, be consistent with local regulations which generally do not permit direct medical claims in advertisements, etc."

During the same period, dozens of articles in *Bestways Let's Live, Better Nutrition, Today's Living, Total Health, Medical Self-Care,* and other magazines that habitually promote dubious nutrition ideas recommended EPO for PMS and other conditions. Some of these articles mentioned Efamol by name and a few cited Dr. Horrobin's work. Ads for Efamol EPO and/or other EPO products appeared in almost every issue containing an article about evening primrose oil.

The December 1983 issue of the British magazine *She* described a study in which three hundred of its readers took Efamol EPO for premenstrual syndrome. *She*'s article, entitled "The Efamol Verdict," called the results "dramatic" and said that 78 percent showed improvement in depression, 87 percent in irritability, 72 percent in headaches, 75 percent in pain/tenderness, and 71 percent in joint swelling. Soon afterward, an Efamol news bulletin advised: "Perhaps you can organize a similar study in your market. The results to PMS sufferers as well as to sales can only be DRAMATIC."

In October 1985, one bulletin included a "Training Manual," the front cover of which states "strictly for internal use and readership only." Its introduction stated, "If you are to be involved in actually selling Efamol products then you will soon extract the information you require to perform your task efficiently. . . . The manual should be retained of course, for reference purposes for the day when a customer asks that very question you knew the answer to but can't remember." Section 6 of the manual referred readers to several publications that promote the use of Efamol products. The manual stated that one of these publications was "a useful Public Relations tool," while another "considers different medical applications of Efamol."

In March 1987, Efamol Ltd. distributed copies of women's magazine articles reporting that Efamol's EPO had helped its readers with PMS. The accompanying bulletin indicated that the articles "represent another excellent example of the valuable role played by PR in supporting the marketing of Efamol." Another bulletin stated: "Dr. Horrobin has recently written the enclosed review of PMS for a consumer magazine aimed at young mothers in the U.S.A." The article gave specific directions for using *Efamol EPO* for PMS and stated, "For most women, PMS can now be a thing of the past."

Other documents described how Efamol Ltd. had used public relations as a marketing tool. For example, a 1983 bulletin said that the main objective of a news conference held in New York by Dr. Horrobin in 1982 "was to make known as widely as possible the new discovery of the benefits to eczema sufferers of EFAMOL capsules taken orally. Media used: Newspapers, Magazines, Radio, TV, News Agencies." The letter was accompanied by a list of more than one hundred press outlets that carried stories. In August 1983, Efamol Ltd. distributed copies of a *Redbook* magazine article recommending evening primrose oil for PMS. The article described Dr. Horrobin's work and stated that "the usual dosage is six to eight 500-mg capsules daily." Multiple reprints of the *Redbook* article were distributed to health-food retailers throughout the United States by Health From the Sun, described by Efamol Ltd. as the major subdistributor of Efamol in the United States at that time. In October 1985, Efamol Ltd. distributed multiple copies of an article from *Current Therapeutics,* which it said would "be of great value in your PR activities."

In November 1986, Efamol Ltd. distributed an article from Rodale's *Allergy Relief Newsletter* which suggested evening primrose oil for eczema. In a sidebar, Dr. Horrobin advised readers to stick to name brands, such as Efamol or Naudicelle. The company advised its distributors that the article "may be particularly interesting to any local eczema societies you may have."

In March 1987, Efamol Ltd. distributed a news bulletin headlined "American PMS Self-Help Group Publishes Article by Dr. Horrobin." The article stated that "a relatively minor problem of [essential fatty acid] nutrition is the commonest cause of PMS. This can be corrected by lifestyle changes and/or by direct supplementation with GLA in the form of evening primrose oil." The published article was introduced with a note that readers could write directly to Dr. Horrobin "to request reprints of this and other articles describing his research."

In October 1987, Efamol Ltd. distributed an article from a British magazine which stated: "Any misconception that Efamol is a company producing mere dietary supplements and dabbling on the fringe of the medical scene are quickly dispelled by Dr. Horrobin. He has always thought of the

Efamol essential fatty acids as pharmaceuticals, he says, but marketing them originally as nutritional supplements has provided the means to generate cash to fund continuing research." The article also states that product licenses had been applied for in the United Kingdom, Germany, Sweden, Norway, New Zealand, and Canada for the treatment of atopic eczema with an EPO product, while approval for the same product as an over-the-counter supplement for PMS had already been granted in Finland and was pending in France.

Efamol's EPO products were also marketed to health professionals through many channels. In November 1986, Dr. Horrobin sent a memo to Nature's Way suggesting an "Efamol Good Health Program" that would include specified dosages of four EPO products for eczema, diabetes, arthritis, coronary heart disease, high blood pressure, asthma, allergies, psoriasis and PMS. In 1987, Murdock Pharmaceuticals (a Nature's Way subsidiary) distributed much of this information—almost word-for-word—to its physician customers.

A January 1987 memo from Murdock Pharmaceuticals to Dr. Horrobin related how Murdock had exhibited at a convention of the American College of Advancement in Medicine (a group of physicians engaged in such unscientific practices as chelation therapy for atherosclerosis). The memo also mentioned that ads have been placed in *Complementary Medicine* and the *Physicians' Desk Reference for Nonprescription Drugs.* Ads in the Nov./Dec. 1986 and Jan./Feb. 1987 issues of *Complementary Medicine* contained no therapeutic claims but invited doctors to contact Murdock Pharmaceuticals for further information. The earlier ad, shown on the following page, pictured the hands of a doctor writing a prescription for Efamol products.

The listing in the 1986 *Physicians' Desk Reference for Nonprescription Drugs* included dosage and stated: "Indications: For the relief of symptoms of premenstrual syndrome, such as mood changes (anxiety, irritability, nervous tension and depression), water retention (swelling), abdominal bloating, breast pain and tenderness, and fatigue." The same information appeared in the 1987 edition of this book under Murdock Pharmaceuticals instead of Nature's Way.

Murdock's "Efamol PMS Promotion Campaign" included advertisements to pharmacists; letters to physicians, pharmacists and "PMS sufferers"; and a "PMS Symptom and Treatment Chart." The ad to pharmacists (in *California Pharmacist*, Sept. 1987) said *Efamol PMS* was "the primary constituent in a recommended PMS program." The letter to pharmacists mentioned that the product was listed in the *Physicians' Desk Reference for Nonprescription Drugs*.

In May 1987, a Murdock vice-president wrote to the Arthritis Foundation to suggest that the Foundation distribute information that Efamol products are

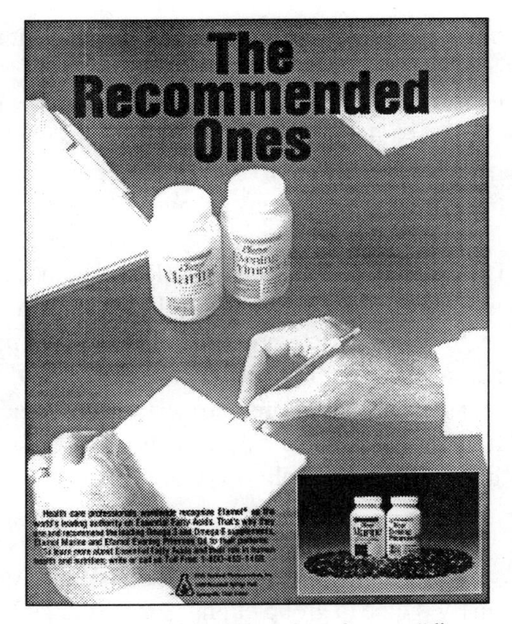

While Nature's Way was marketing Efamol products as "dietary supplements," its professional subsidiary placed this ad for them in *Complementary Medicine*, a magazine "for health care professionals" published by Jeffrey Bland, Ph.D., from 1985 through 1990.

"an alternative in treating arthritis to those who suffer side effects from NSAIDS." (NSAID means nonsteroidal antiinflammatory drug.)

And so on.

During 1988, FDA investigators who visited one pharmacy and several health-food stores were told by a salesperson that EPO was effective for PMS, arthritis, and/or eczema. The investigators were shown magazine articles or other literature containing claims of this type. In 1989, at the FDA's request, Dr. Stephen Barrett reviewed more than a thousand pages of documents and concluded:

> It is clear that Efamol Ltd. has been engaged in a continuous and systematic campaign to establish in the public mind that Efamol EPO is useful against PMS and various other diseases and conditions. It is also clear that any restraint shown in the claims is related to the knowledge that they may be illegal in labeling. . . .
>
> It is self-evident that consumers won't buy products unless they perceive a need for them. It is also obvious that a product claimed to be effective in a troublesome condition (such as PMS) will sell much

> better than one advertised to relieve a supposed deficiency of a chemical (gamma-linoleic acid). . . .
>
> Although Dr. Horrobin has claimed to have done sufficient research to establish that evening primrose oil is safe and effective against PMS and eczema, he has not gained FDA approval for marketing evening primrose oil products as drugs in the United States. Marketing them as "food supplements" is a transparent attempt to evade the food and drug laws.

"Nutrition Roulette"

Was EPO safe and effective for any of its intended purposes? We don't know. Purdue University's Varro E. Tyler, Ph.D., a leading authority on plant medicines, has looked very carefully at Horrobin's writings. In the 1993 edition of *The Honest Herbal,* Tyler states:

> [Horrobin's theories] would be valid only if all of the specified conditions are favorably influenced by additional production in the body of prostaglandin E_1 and if a deficiency of GLA is the single factor responsible for limited prostaglandin production. Both of these factors remain unproven. If they are not true, then [assuming] that evening primrose oil [is effective] in such conditions is somewhat like assuming one's car will run better if the gas tank is completely full instead of half full.
>
> Some clinical evidence exists supporting the possible efficacy of evening primrose oil in the treatment of . . . PMS . . . sore breasts, multiple sclerosis, atopic eczema, various diabetes-associated problems, cardiovascular disease, and several other conditions. . . .
>
> However, the validity of some of the reports has been refuted or at least questioned. An Australian study . . . of evening primrose oil in treating women with moderate PMS concluded that the improvement was solely a placebo effect. . . . Furthermore, there are no data to support the safety of long-term consumption.

Although Tyler has not evaluated the herbal products marketed by Enzymatic Therapy or Solaray, he has written extensively about many of the herbs they are said to contain. *The Honest Herbal* sums up his views with a chart rating the "apparent efficacy" and "probable safety" of more than a hundred herbs and related products. Some appear effective, others do not. Some appear safe, others are known to be toxic. In many cases, however, not enough research has been done to be sure. Tyler also believes (as we note in Chapter 8) that most of the information about herbs transmitted from health-food industry sources to consumers is not reliable.

Throughout *The Vitamin Pushers* we stress that it is illegal and improper to make unsubstantiated health claims for vitamins, minerals, herbs, and the multitude of other products marketed as "dietary supplements." As we note in Chapter 1, "If you can't prove it, you shouldn't sell it." Russian roulette is a stunt in which the player spins the cylinder of a revolver loaded with only one bullet, aims the muzzle at his head, and pulls the trigger. Few people play this "game" because the obvious risk far outweighs any possible benefit. We believe that most of the health-food industry's customers are *unknowingly* engaged in "nutrition roulette" because: (1) the risks involved in taking an ineffective or unproven product exceed the possible benefit, and (2) the health-food industry plays by rules of its own. Its basic philosophy is, "If anything might be good for something—or even if it isn't, but it might sell—put it in a pill and promote the hell out of it."

Now let's see what can be learned from the worst disaster in health-food history.

The "Accident Waiting to Happen"

Since 1980, health claims have been made for L-tryptophan in many books, magazines, booklets, health-food-store flyers, and ads by supplement manufacturers. These sources have recommended it for insomnia, pain, depression, PMS, and overweight, even though it has not been proven safe or effective for any of these purposes. The most flamboyant promotion was an entire book on the subject: *The Pain-Free Tryptophan Diet* (1986) by Robert L. Pollack, Ph.D. Its author suggested that many people have insufficient tryptophan in their diet or have an imbalance involving L-tryptophan that "could be responsible for the extensive physical and emotional suffering that afflicts such a great part of the American population." This idea is utter nonsense.

In 1989, an outbreak of eosinophilia-myalgia syndrome (EMS) occurred among users of L-tryptophan. A hitherto rare and unrecognized disorder, EMS is a debilitating disease characterized by severe muscle and joint pain, weakness, swelling of the arms and legs, fever, skin rash, and an increase of eosinophils (certain white blood cells) in the blood. Over the next year, more than 1,500 cases and twenty-eight deaths were reported to the U.S. Centers for Disease Control and Prevention. The actual toll probably was more than five thousand people, many of whom suffered for years and are still disabled. Some of the victims were children. The outbreak was traced to a manufacturing problem at the plant of Showa Denko K.K., a Japanese company that was the major wholesale supplier. When the link between EMS and L-tryptophan became apparent, the FDA banned its sale.

Examples of Claims Made for L-Tryptophan Products

Manufacturer	Alleged Benefits
AARP Pharmacy Service	Helps minimize the effects of stress, anxiety, depression, and insomnia
Country Life	Aids in mood stabilization and helps counteract nicotine and carbohydrate cravings
Makers of KAL	Increases mental acuity, improves thought processes, improves "thinkability." Large doses (500 to 1,000 mg) are effective in inducing sleep.
Nutrition Headquarters	Also important in the formation of enzymes that can help turn fats into energy
Schiff	Elderly persons suffering from senility problems such as forgetfulness, disorientation, hallucination, depression, argumentativeness, and similar states were relieved when tryptophan was administered. Tryptolyn (a combination of tryptophan and lysine) is more effective than drugs in lowering blood cholesterol.
Vitamin Power	Safe alternative to the synthetically produced sleep aids on the market today

In 1991, FDA officials presented the following account of L-tryptophan's regulatory history at a hearing held by the House of Representatives' Human Resources and Intergovernmental Relations Subcommittee. Until 1973, L-tryptophan and other amino acids were included on a list of food substances that were generally recognized as safe (GRAS) for use as dietary supplements. In 1973, the FDA revoked this GRAS status and stated that they could not be marketed without approval as a food additive. Since approval had not been sought, the agency initiated seizure actions against two manufacturers of L-tryptophan products. The first case was dismissed because L-tryptophan had accidentally been included on a GRAS list published in 1977. The second case was withdrawn before a verdict was rendered, because the FDA believed that the judge was inclined to favor the manufacturer. The FDA also felt constrained by the Proxmire Amendment (1976), which curbed its ability to regulate vitamin dosage (see Chapter 20). Although amino acids were not included under this law, the agency took its passage as a signal that Congress did not want supplement products regulated without serious indications of danger to health. Thus, although the marketing of amino acid supplements was illegal, the FDA did nothing further until the EMS outbreak occurred.

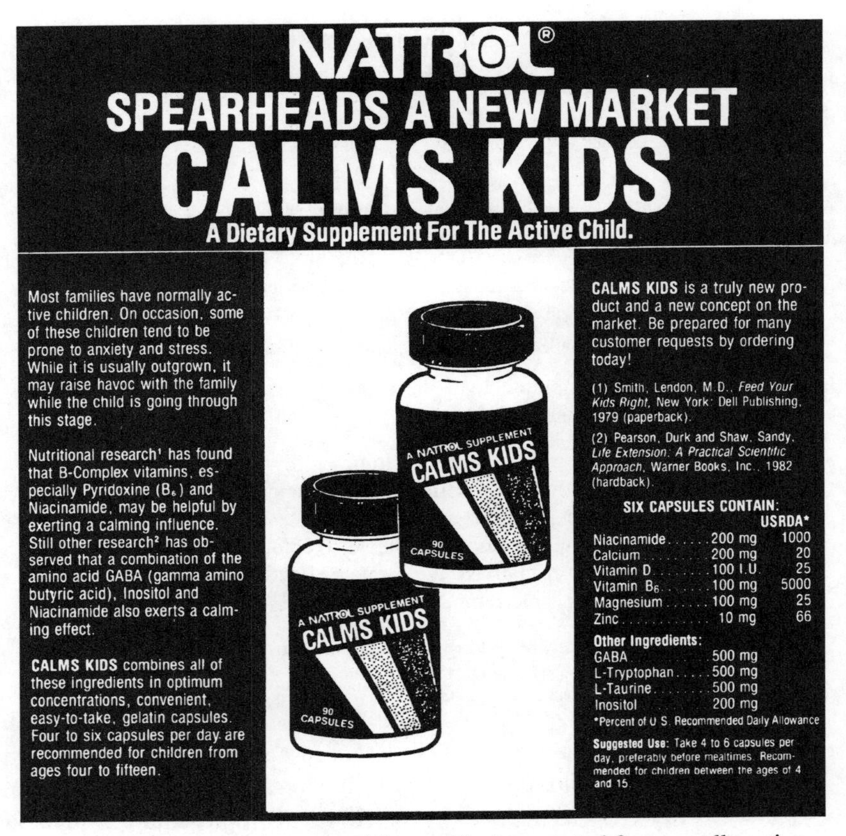

Ad for bogus tryptophan-containing product promoted for normally active children who are "prone to anxiety and stress." Even if the product had worked, do you think normal children should be sedated when they get rambunctious?

During the 1980s, several warnings that L-tryptophan or other amino acids might be dangerous had appeared in scientific and government publications. In 1980, *The New England Journal of Medicine* published a report suggesting that tryptophan might be related to the development of a "scleroderma-like illness." In 1985, an article in *FDA Consumer* discussed L-tryptophan and warned against taking large amounts of any amino acid. In 1986, an FDA policy statement in the *Federal Register* warned that the use of recombinant DNA technology had the potential to lead to new structural features in the product that could affect product safety. And in 1988, the *Annals of Internal Medicine* published a warning letter headlined "The Potential Toxicity of Tryptophan." Meanwhile, of course, the health-food industry marketed L-tryptophan in its usual fashion.

One of the experts who testified at the hearing was Richard J. Wurtman, M.D., professor of neuroscience at M.I.T. and Harvard Medical School, a leading researcher on amino acid metabolism. Wurtman testified that twenty years previously his laboratory discovered that tryptophan levels normally control the production of serotonin, a brain chemical involved in sleep, mood, and appetite. At the time, he thought that tryptophan might become a legitimate drug that could help people sleep, diminish pain, and control mood and appetite.

"Nobody argues about whether tryptophan works," Wurtman continued. "When presented in pure form—which it wasn't in EMS patients—it is an effective compound. . . . I had assumed that pharmaceutical companies might take this discovery and invest the $10 or $20 million, whatever it took then, to do appropriate safety and efficacy studies." Noting that tryptophan might eventually have been approved as a drug, he lamented: "It didn't work out that way. . . . because tryptophan was allowed to be sold as a nutritional supplement. . . . Tryptophan in a bottle is not a nutritional supplement."

Wurtman further explained: In protein, tryptophan comes with twenty-one other amino acids, all of which are needed in order to utilize them and make one's own protein. Pure tryptophan in pills or in a bottle is not natural; the body doesn't handle it the way it handles tryptophan in protein; the body cannot use it to make its own protein. There is not a single person in America who is tryptophan-deficient. Isolated amino-acid deficiencies do not occur. People who have low blood tryptophan levels also have low levels of other essential amino acids as well, because these people are protein-deficient. Giving one amino acid to a protein-deficient person can make matters worse because it means that other amino acids also go down. Thus, in spite of being called a nutritional supplement, bottled tryptophan is a drug because it changes the chemistry of the brain. Since manufacturers did not want to invite FDA regulatory action by openly marketing tryptophan as a drug, they did not list appropriate use, dosage, or contraindications on their labels. Nor was ITS manufacturing process adequately controlled for quality or purity.

"Tryptophan was, in every sense, an accident waiting to happen," Wurtman added. He also described hazards associated with other amino acids still marketed in health-food stores. He believes that marketing of isolated amino acids should not be permitted unless they can meet regulatory standards for prescription drugs.

In response to the EMS epidemic, the FDA commissioned the Federation of American Societies for Experimental Biology (FASEB) to study the safety of amino acids used as dietary supplements. FASEB concluded: (1) single- or multiple-ingredient capsules, tablets, and liquid products are used primarily for pharmacological purposes or enhancement of physiological functions rather than for nutritional purposes; (2) little scientific literature exists on most amino acids ingested for these purposes; (3) no scientific rationale has been presented to justify the taking of amino acid supplements by healthy individuals; (4) safety levels for amino acid supplement use cannot be established at this time; and (5) a systematic approach to safety testing is needed.

We agree with this assessment. Amino acid products should be regulated as prescription drugs.

More Mischief Revealed

When its L-tryptophan was identified as the cause of EMS, Showa Denko realized that it would not only be liable for damages to L-tryptophan victims but would probably be forced to reimburse American manufacturers for whatever costs resulted from legal action. Rather than working at cross-purposes with the manufacturers, Showa Denko agreed to shoulder all the expenses involved. Meanwhile, the American Trial Lawyers Association (ATLA) formed a very efficient suing machine. Twelve attorneys, among whom were some of the country's most talented product-liability specialists, formed a steering committee to gather documents and other information that would be shared with ATLA members who needed them. Although Showa Denko maintained that L-tryptophan was being marketed as a "dietary supplement," documents obtained from Showa Denko indicated otherwise:

• A 1984 memo stated: "If you take a look at each company which constitute the [nutritional supplement] market, they are positioned ambiguously in between medical and food manufactures/distributors. They get around the restrictions on 'Drugs' and sell 'food supplements.'"

• An undated internal memo (shown opposite) contained a long list of other reasons why "semi-healthy people" and "the sick" might purchase L-tryptophan products.

• A 1987 memo concluded that it would be difficult for L-tryptophan to gain government approval as a sleeping pill because "it is difficult to demonstrate the superiority of this drug to [established] drugs, and it cannot be concluded that this drug causes fewer side effects."

• An undated brochure stated that L-tryptophan "has antistress function and minor tranquilizer effect" and had pharmaceutical application as a "sleep inducer" and "antidepressant."

Other documents revealed that in 1988, Showa Denko became aware that its L-tryptophan contained impurities that were unidentified and therefore potentially harmful. The company then began using a new strain of bacteria modified from previous strains by means of biotechnology. (Bacteria were used

Details of L-Trp. Health Food in U.S.A.

How L-Trp Health Food is used in U.S.A., from the literature.

Appeal as Natural Tranquilizer or Anti-Depressant (some sleeping effect)

- Calms down nervous or stressed people
- Revives spirits of depressed people
- Induces sleep

There is no side effect, no addiction, no withdrawal distress. When an excessive amount is taken, it will be naturally excreted out of the system (same as Vitamin C).

Examples of health food application

1) People who don't have appetite in the morning, and who can't sleep well at night
2) Athletes who are feeling stressed before big sporting events[1]
3) Children who are troubled with teenage problems and studies[1]
4) Businessmen who are working on a big project[1]
5) People who are getting nervous with business interviews[1]
6) Students who are cramming before an examination[1]
7) People who have various worries[1]
8) Travelers who are troubled with jet lag[1]
9) People whose biorhythm is disturbed due to the change of an environment[1]
10) Insomnia patient[2]
11) Manic-depressive patient[2]
12) Stressed patient[2]

[1]Semi-healthy people
[2]The sick

Portion of translated internal document indicating that Showa Denko knew that L-tryptophan was being used for pharmacologic purposes in the United States.

to synthesize the L-tryptophan.) Showa Denko did not notify the FDA about the impurities or its modification of the manufacturing process. Nor did the company test the newly made product for safety in humans, even though the FDA had previously cautioned that biotechnologically modified products should be thoroughly tested before public distribution. In fact, instead of increasing filtration to remove the impurities, which would decrease the amount of L-tryptophan produced, Showa Denko continued full-speed production to meet high market demand.

Minneapolis attorney Roger P. Brosnahan, who chaired the steering committee for all plaintiffs who brought cases in federal court, estimates that about two thousand L-tryptophan victims (or their survivors) filed lawsuits or entered negotiations without suing. Most cases have generated little publicity because they were settled out of court with an agreement not to disclose the settlement terms. However, the total amount is known to approximate one billion dollars.

Ethics . . . from the Top

Since General Nutrition Corporation was named as a codefendant in many of the L-tryptophan suits, Brosnahan's steering committee investigated its marketing practices. In August 1992, his partner David L. Suggs deposed General Nutrition Corporation president Jerry D. Horn. After asking whether Horn was familiar with twenty-five government enforcement actions that had been taken against the company between 1969 and 1989, Suggs queried:

Q. Have you developed any written policies regarding ethical matters in marketing your products?
A. Our philosophy is that we'll stay in compliance with the rules for marketing these types of food products. These are food-grade products.
Q. Let me try again. Have you developed any written policy regarding the marketing practices which GNC will or will not engage in?
A. I don't know of any specific policy regarding the marketing of our products.

. . . .

Q. Wouldn't you agree that your company shouldn't sell pills to people to take unless the pills provide some benefit and the pills are safe?
A. The latter part. We shouldn't sell pills that are not safe.
Q. Okay. How about the benefit part?
A. The benefit to each individual is up to them. We don't tell them what kind of groceries to buy in the grocery store.
Q. Well, you weren't selling groceries in your stores, were you?
A. We were selling food. Food products.
Q. People weren't taking your products for food purposes, were they?
A. I would say many of them are. You know, like broccoli. You might buy broccoli in pill form.
Q. Is it your testimony that . . . it's perfectly okay for GNC to put products on its shelves, to sell pills to people if those pills have no benefit? . . .
A. We make the assumption that they make the decision based on some perceived benefit.
Q. Isn't it a fact that . . . whether or not it is going to benefit your body is a question of science and a question of fact?
A. Limited science.
Q. Don't you think that GNC, before it sells pills for people to take, ought to make some evaluation of the science and the facts to . . . determine whether there is in fact some benefit in people taking those pills into their bodies?

A. No. I would say no, we should not. We are not compelled to do that.
Q. So far as you're concerned, and . . . speaking as the chairman of the board of GNC, it's perfectly all right for GNC to sell people pills to take even if those pills have no benefit whatsoever, there's no scientific benefit. Is that correct?
A. That's not what I said.
Q. Well, are you saying, then, that there should be a benefit?
A. The benefit to them is from their perception, their need, their diet, how they're trying to supplement. We don't know each individual's supplement needs to their diet, if any.
Q. So in other words, it's OK for GNC to sell pills for people to take them into their bodies . . . as long as some customer is under the belief or perception that they're going to get some benefit? . . .
A. I'm telling you that it's up to the individual. . . . They make the decision how they want to supplement their diet.

. . . .

Q. Would you agree that your company shouldn't sell pills under the pretext that they're a dietary supplement or that they're food, if in fact they don't have any nutritional value?
A. If they have absolutely no nutritional value, like a placebo or something? Is that your question?
Q. If they have no nutritional value, should you be selling them as dietary supplements or calling them dietary supplements?
A. We shouldn't be selling a product that on the label we don't disclose what is there. If it has no nutritional . . . benefit, why would the customer buy it? I don't understand the question. To my knowledge we sell no products that don't have some nutritional benefit.
Q. In fact, your company sold pills and called them dietary supplements when in fact people were taking them for their drug-like or therapeutic effects. Isn't that right?
A. I don't know that. . . . We make no claims on any of our labels for what the benefits or features of the products are.

. . . .

Q. Would you agree that your company has an obligation to test . . . products before they're sold for human consumption to determine whether they are in fact beneficial?
A. No more than a grocery store does foods coming in. We're a retailer.
Q. You also manufacture products, don't you?
A. We manufacture a portion of our line.
Q. Well, with respect to the products that you manufacture, would you agree that GNC has an obligation to test those products to make sure they are in fact beneficial?

A. You can't test whether an apple a day really keeps the doctor away. There's no way to test that I know of.

. . . .

Q. Drug companies test their products before they're marketed to find out if they're beneficial, don't they?
A. We're not a drug company. . . . I don't know what drug companies do.
Q. You don't know whether drug companies test their products before they put them out on the market—to find out whether they're beneficial? . . .
A. I don't know for sure. It's my understanding that there's an approval process for drugs, yes. . . .
Q. So it's your understanding that the technology for being able to test whether or not something that you take into your mouth that's in pill form is beneficial; correct?
A. I don't know that. . . .
Q. Have you ever heard of things like safety studies or toxicology studies or . . . clinical studies? . . .
A. Some.
Q. And what do those terms relate to?
A. I believe to the drug industry. . . . We're not in the drug business, we're in the food business as defined by the FDA.

Another Questionable Promotion

In the Spring of 1994, the American Medical Association (AMA) launched what it described as its "largest and most comprehensive anti-tobacco and stop-smoking program ever." One part of the campaign is a $69.95 *How-to-Quit*™ kit cosponsored by General Nutrition Centers (GNC) and a division of Orbis Broadcast Group, a communications and public relations company that produces medical programming for cable television. GNC ordered 100,000 kits and paid Orbis $1 million in advance to develop the kit and to cover advertising, in return for the exclusive right to retail it in GNC stores.

The *How-to-Quit*™ kits include a forty-eight-page handbook with a statement in type this size on the inside of its rear cover:

While the American Medical Association ("AMA") does not endorse individual products, it has reviewed the contents of this smoking cessation program for scientific accuracy. Vitamin supplements are not useful aids for smoking cessation. Vitamins will not increase your success in either quitting smoking or remaining nicotine-free over time. Vitamins are NOT a safe substitute for the health benefits of stopping smoking. The AMA's net proceeds from this smoking cessation program will be utilized to promote additional health initiatives.

The kit also contains a videotape, three audiotapes, a diary, a calendar, and other motivational materials—all housed in a 10" x 12" x 1 1/2" plastic album. Investigative reporter David Zimmerman has discovered that the kit has been distributed in two ways. Reporters have received it in its plastic album. In GNC stores, however, the album comes packed inside a cardboard box together with a bottle of multivitamins and a discount coupon for another bottle.

When Zimmerman visited a GNC store in New York City, he was told that the vitamins were especially effective, because vitamins give energy when you are "down" from not smoking. He also learned that the packaging of the vitamins had been negotiated. The AMA's decision to participate in the project was made by officials in its marketing and communications departments after Orbis and GNC had reached an agreement. When officials in the AMA's scientific division learned that vitamins were slated for inclusion within the kit, they succeeded in having the disclaimer inserted in the booklet and the vitamins placed an outer package.

Zimmerman also reported that AMA officials knew that GNC had had some legal difficulties "in the past," but were unaware that trouble was pending. A few weeks after the publicity for the kit began, the FTC announced that GNC had agreed to pay $2.4 million to settle charges of false advertising (described in Chapter 21). Press kits distributed by the AMA's New York press office included one-page descriptions about the creators of the *How-to-Quit*™ program. They also contained a page that described GNC as "the nation's leading provider of health and selfcare products, services and information."

Although the *How-to-Quit*™ program violates no drug laws, its marketing does involve deception. The program supposedly includes a "24-hour toll-free support line." Noting that "sometimes you just need to talk to someone!" the handbook promises "both general and specific advice." However, callers can access only a brief recorded message, after which they are disconnected. Moreover, AMA officials have acknowledged that the *How-to-Quit*™ kit did not undergo clinical testing prior to marketing. The program was designed with the help of experts who believe it will be effective. Evaluation will be done by following purchasers who send in an enclosed registration card or purchase a kit from Orbis by direct mail. The cost of this research will be covered by royalties from sale of the kits.

GNC apparently thought that associating with the AMA would boost its credibility. Orbis and the AMA apparently welcomed GNC's support for what they believed would be a valuable health-promoting program. Whether GNC, Orbis, the AMA, or purchasers of the kit will win or lose in the long run remains to be seen.

Tighter Regulation Is Needed

Marketing a "dietary supplement" with an unsubstantiated health claim is a serious or potentially serious crime. Everybody knows that people who cheat on their income tax can be prosecuted as criminals and wind up in prison. Why has the health-food industry been permitted to cheat on its labels, market worthless products, menace public health, advertise deceptively, and literally get away with murder? The next two chapters address these questions and what we believe should be done.

20

"Vitamin Wars" and Related Mischief

To maximize profits, the health-food industry must minimize government regulation. This chapter describes the activities of trade and "consumer" groups with such a goal. All of these groups have been involved in activities intended to legitimize through politics what they cannot prove through science. Most of their leaders disparage scientific methods of experimentation and treatment.

The National Health Federation, the Foundation for the Advancement of Innovative Medicine, and Citizens for Health are alliances of quackery promoters and followers who engage in lobbying campaigns and many other activities. The Coalition for Alternatives in Nutrition and Healthcare (CANAH) had similar aims, but is now defunct. The People's Medical Society is a "consumer group" that publishes reports and engages in letter-writing campaigns. The National Nutritional Foods Association and the Council for Responsible Nutrition are the supplement industry's major trade associations. The Nutritional Health Alliance is an umbrella group formed to protect the health-food industry from the threat of tighter government regulation. During the past two years, all but CANAH have been engaged in an all-out "war" to reduce regulation of products sold by the health-food industry. Most would also like to abolish regulation of "alternative" practitioners.

An Unhealthy Alliance

The National Health Federation (NHF) is headquartered in Monrovia, California. Its members pay from $36 per year for "regular" membership to a total of $1,000 or more for "perpetual" membership. NHF members receive occasional mailings and a monthly magazine called *Health Freedom News* (formerly called the *NHF Bulletin*). In 1991, it had about 6,600 members.

Since its formation, NHF's stated purpose has been to promote "freedom of choice" by consumers. As expressed for years in its *Bulletin*:

> NHF opposes monopoly and compulsion in things related to health where the safety and welfare of others are not concerned. NHF does not oppose nor approve any specific healing profession or their methods, but it does oppose the efforts of any one group to restrict the freedom of practice of qualified members of another profession, thus attempting to create a monopoly.

At first glance, this credo may seem "democratic" and somehow related to unfair business competition. What NHF really means, however, is that government should not help scientifically based health care to drive questionable methods out of the marketplace. NHF wants anyone who merely *claims* to have an effective treatment or product to be allowed to market it without scientific proof that it works.

NHF promotes unscientific health methods and has little interest in scientifically recognized methods. *Health Freedom News* contains many ads for questionable services and products. Nutritional fads, myths, and gimmicks are mentioned favorably by NHF publications and convention speakers. Worthless cancer treatments, particularly laetrile, have been promoted in the same ways. NHF publications have looked with disfavor on such proven public health measures as pasteurization of milk, immunization, water fluoridation, and food irradiation. Use of nutritional supplements is encouraged by claims that modern food processing depletes our food supply of its nutrients. "Natural" and "organic" products have been promoted with suggestions that our food supply is "poisoned." Chiropractic, naturopathy, and homeopathy are regarded favorably. Books that promote questionable health concepts are given favorable reviews. Antiquackery legislation is condemned. Underlying all these messages are paranoid thoughts that anyone who opposes NHF's ideas is part of a "conspiracy" of government, organized medicine, and big business against the little consumer.

NHF has been very active in the political arena. It presents testimony to regulatory agencies and sponsors legislation aimed at minimizing government interference with the health-food industry. To bolster the influence of its lobbyists, it generates letter-writing campaigns that urge legislators and government officials to support NHF positions. The most notable campaign—described later in this chapter—culminated with passage in 1976 of an amendment to the Food, Drug, and Cosmetic Act that weakened the FDA's ability to police the supplement marketplace.

Not surprisingly, most of NHF's leaders have been economically involved with the issues it has promoted—and at least twenty have been in legal difficulty for such activities. The organization was founded in 1955 by Fred J. Hart, president of the Electronic Medical Foundation, a company that marketed quack devices. In 1954, Hart and his foundation were ordered by a U.S. District Court to stop distributing thirteen devices with false claims that they could diagnose and treat hundreds of diseases and conditions. In 1962, Hart was fined by the court for violating this order. He died in 1976.

Royal S. Lee, D.D.S., a nonpracticing dentist, helped found NHF and served on its board of governors. Lee owned and operated the Vitamin Products Company, which sold food supplements, and the Lee Foundation for Nutritional Research, which distributed literature on nutrition and health. One of the vitamin company's products was *Catalyn,* a patent medicine composed of milk sugar, wheat starch, wheat bran, and other plant material. During the early 1930s, a shipment of *Catalyn* was seized by the FDA and destroyed by court order because it had been marketed with false claims of effectiveness against serious diseases. In 1945, the FDA ordered Lee and his company to discontinue illegal claims for *Catalyn* and other products. In 1956, the Post Office Department charged Lee's foundation with fraudulent promotion of a book called *Diet Prevents Polio.* The foundation agreed to discontinue the challenged claims. In 1962, Lee and the Vitamin Products Company were convicted of misbranding 115 special dietary products by making false claims for the treatment of more than five hundred diseases and conditions. Lee received a one-year suspended prison term and was fined $7,000. Lee died in 1967.

Kurt W. Donsbach, D.C., a protégé of Lee, replaced Fred Hart as NHF's board chairman in 1975 and held that position until 1989. In 1971, after agents of the California Bureau of Food and Drug observed Donsbach telling customers at his health-food store that vitamins, minerals, and/or herbal tea were effective against several serious diseases, he pled guilty to one count of practicing medicine without a license and agreed to cease "nutritional consultation." In the ensuing years, Donsbach has marketed supplement products, issued publications, operated nonaccredited correspondence schools, marketed a bogus "nutrient deficiency" test, and administered dubious treatments at Mexican cancer clinics. (See Chapters 6 and 17 for further details.)

Victor Earl Irons, who was vice chairman of NHF's board of governors for more than twenty years, received a one-year prison sentence in 1957 for misbranding *Vit-Ra-Tox,* a vitamin mixture sold door to door. In 1959, eight products and accompanying literature shipped by V.E. Irons, Inc., were destroyed under a consent decree because the products were promoted with false or misleading claims. Other seized products were ordered destroyed in

1959 and 1960. Irons has claimed that virtually everyone has a "clogged colon," that deposits of fecal material cause "toxins and poisonous gases" to "seep into your blood and poison all your organs and tissues," and that "if every person in this country took 2–3 home colonics a week, 95% of the doctors would have to retire for lack of business." Literature from V.E. Irons, Inc., has stated that "the most important procedure toward regaining your Health is the COMPLETE and THOROUGH cleansing of the colon, no matter what or how long it takes." This was the goal of the "Vit-Ra-Tox Seven Day Cleansing Program," which involved eating no food, drinking a quart or more of water daily, using herbal laxatives and various supplement products, and taking at least one strong black coffee enema each day. Ten years ago, products for this program cost $60, while those for maintenance after the seventh day cost about $100 per month.

Jonathan V. Wright, M.D., who became NHF's board chairman in 1992, is embroiled in disputes with the FDA involving nutritional products that the FDA seized in a much-publicized raid on Wright's clinic and an adjacent pharmacy (see Chapter 17).

Maureen Kennedy Salaman, NHF's current president, hosts a radio talk show and has been very active in promoting questionable cancer remedies. Her 1983 book, *Nutrition: The Cancer Answer,* falsely claims that "the American Cancer Society advocates treating cancer rather than preventing it." In 1984, she was the Populist Party's candidate for Vice President of the United States.

Other NHF board members have included Bernard Jensen, D.C. (see Chapter 7), Terence Lemerond (see Chapter 19), Donald F. Pickett (see Chapter 10), Jack Ritchason, N.D. (see Chapter 10), and Robert Atkins, M.D. (see below and Chapter 17).

CANAH's "Healthcare Rights Amendment"

The most ambitious attempt to destroy health-related consumer protection laws was probably the effort made by the Coalition for Alternatives in Nutrition and Healthcare (CANAH), a nonprofit corporation established in 1984. Its founder, president, and "legislative advocate" was Catherine J. Frompovich, "Ph.D.," who practiced "nutritional consultation" in Richlandtown, Pennsylvania, and operated C.J. Frompovich Publications. Her "Ph.D." was from Columbia Pacific University, a nonaccredited correspondence school. Before she acquired it, her publications described her as "a practicing natural nutritionist who has a Doctor of Science in Diet and Nutrition [and] a Doctor of Naturopathy." At various times, about thirty individuals who practiced or promoted dubious health methods were listed on CANAH's letterhead as advisory board members.

CANAH's activities included support for dubious cancer treatments and opposition to food irradiation, water fluoridation, licensing of nutritionists, and other antiquackery legislation. However, the group's primary goal was enactment of a "Healthcare Rights Amendment" to forbid Congress from restricting "any individual's right to choose and to practice the type of healthcare they shall elect for themselves or their children for the prevention or treatment of any disease, injury, illness or ailment of the body or the mind."

Under current laws, our governing bodies can set licensing standards for health practitioners, institute public health measures, and outlaw remedies that are dangerous or ineffective. CANAH's amendment would have removed all restrictions:

- Government agencies could no longer remove unproven or dangerous remedies from the marketplace so long as a single consumer objects
- Anyone—licensed or not—could engage in any practice labeled "health care" so long as a single consumer wishes it to continue
- Insurance companies might be forced to cover the cost of every practice labeled "health care"
- Courts could not protect children from parents who deny them access to effective health care, even if such neglect will result in their death
- Dangerously psychotic individuals could not be compelled to undergo treatment if anyone objected
- Compulsory immunization would end
- Community water fluoridation would end if a single person in the community objects.

Thus, although promoted in the name of "freedom," CANAH's "Health Care Rights Amendment" would have ended protection of consumers from quackery and health fraud.

Throughout its existence, articles about CANAH's activities and invitations to join it appeared frequently in health-food-industry publications. But in 1990, Frompovich announced that CANAH had been voluntarily dissolved because she could not "continue to work sixteen-hour days for six or seven days a week anymore" as an unpaid volunteer and the group was unable to attract sufficient support to pay her a minimum salary of $20,000 a year. A few weeks before the group ceased operation, Frompovich and a few colleagues presented the Department of Health and Human Services with a plaque and a petition with "close to 100,000 signatures" supporting CANAH's "Healthcare Rights Amendment."

Foundation for the Advancement of Innovative Medicine (FAIM)

FAIM was formed in 1986 and incorporated in 1989 "as a voice for innovative medicine's professionals, physicians, patients, and suppliers." Now headquartered in Suffern, New York, it has about three thousand members. Its professional members, about sixty of whom have been identified in the group's publications, include medical doctors, osteopaths, chiropractors, dentists, psychologists, and social workers, almost all of whom practice in New York or New Jersey.

FAIM defines innovative medicine as "a treatment or therapy of empirical benefit that is yet outside the mainstream of conventional medicine." According to several flyers:

> FAIM's mission is to secure free choice in health care. Our first goal is the development of a membership to serve as both a forum for exchange and a constituency for change. The second goal is to educate both those within the field and the general public as to the benefits and issues of innovative medicine. This activity includes the collection of statistical data with which to advocate our position. The third goal is guaranteed reimbursement for the patients, be it through legislation, litigation or negotiation with state and insurance agencies. And lastly, in laying the groundwork for a climate receptive to medical innovation, we encourage research and development of promising new approaches.

FAIM's quarterly magazine, *Innovation*, has carried articles promoting "alternative" cancer therapies, chelation therapy, homeopathy, shark cartilage for arthritis and for protection against tumor growth, and an oral bacterial preparation for chronic fatigue syndrome. One article describes how to sue insurance companies in small claims court when they deny claims for "complementary" treatment. Other articles blast fluoridation, mercury-amalgam fillings, and sugar (for allegedly causing digestive problems).

FAIM's educational fund (FAIM ED) was incorporated in 1991 "to promote the American health care consumer's access to information and education regarding health care alternatives" and "to support promising research projects that may not currently be the focus of government and private efforts." Each year, FAIM (and/or FAIM ED) sponsors several symposia featuring prominent practitioners and promoters of "alternative" medicine. Exhibitors at these meetings have included marketers of supplements, homeopathic remedies, herbs, and other products that are promoted with questionable claims that would not be legal to place on their labels.

FAIM's current board of trustees is composed of seven medical doctors and one dentist. The board's president—and an FAIM cofounder—is Robert C.

Atkins, M.D., who operates a large clinic, hosts a radio talk show, publishes a newsletter, markets supplement products, and has written several books on his questionable methods (see Chapter 17). FAIM has been lobbying vigorously to persuade the New York State legislature to enact an "Alternative Medical Practice Act" intended to "protect doctors from misconduct actions taken against them for the sole reason that they use alternative or complementary medical treatments." One impetus for this bill was the license revocation proceeding against FAIM board member Warren M. Levin, M.D. (see Chapter 12).

Citizens for Health

Citizens for Health (CFH) describes itself as "a non-profit consumer organization dedicated to promoting good health in America and around the world." It was formed in January 1992 in response to concerns about pending FDA regulations on food labeling. It appears to have grown rapidly, and now has thousands of members and state and local chapters throughout the country. The group's primary activity has been mobilizing opposition to FDA regulation of the supplement marketplace. During 1992, according to a CFH report, the group distributed over 2.25 million brochures related to this issue and raised more than $100,000 for its Jonathan Wright Legal Defense Fund (see Chapter 17). In addition, its members, officers, and staff participated in more than a thousand radio shows. An affiliated professional group, the American Preventive Medical Association (APMA), was launched in the fall of 1992, with more than one hundred doctors from five countries as founding members.

Alexander G. Schauss, the executive director of both CFH and APMA, has promoted questionable theories about diet and behavior for many years. The front cover of his 1981 book *Diet, Crime and Delinquency* identifies him as "an internationally known criminologist" and states that the book is "the first clear guide to correcting behavior through diet which explains how food and environment can promote or prevent crime and delinquency." Schauss is president of the American Institute for Biosocial Research, edits the *International Journal of Biosocial Research*, and is president of Life Sciences Press, all of which share the same post office box in Tacoma, Washington. In 1988, the *Vancouver Sun* published an article titled "Self-claimed nutrition expert faked credentials, probe finds." The article reported that although Schauss was listed as "Dr." or "Ph.D." in the Tacoma city and telephone directories, he did not actually have a doctoral degree. The reporter found that Schauss had registered as a "Ph.D. candidate" at California Coast University, a nonaccredited school in Santa Ana, California, but had not completed his dissertation. For many years, his journal masthead identified him as "Ph.D. (cand.)," or "Ph.D. (c)," which apparently stood for "Ph.D. candidate." He finally acquired his "Ph.D." (in psychology) in December 1992.

Schauss has also been involved with NutriPro, of Foster City, California, which markets a "Personalized Optimal Nutrient Analysis Program." A flyer sent to health-food retailers stated:

> In 1990, NutriPro™ commissioned a team of nutritional scientists at the American Institute for Biosocial Research (A.I.B.R.) to determine the life variables and Optimal Daily Intakes (ODIs). Under the leadership of Dr. Alex Schauss, A.I.B.R. compiled and reviewed over 8,000 published studies on 30 nutrients. Based on this vast body of data, A.I.B.R. developed the NutriPro™ Questionnaire.

The first part of the questionnaire is used to determine an individual's "ODIs," based on "diet, environment, and exercise levels." (One question, however, is "Do you desire to enhance your immunity?") The second part is a three-day food diary. The data are used to generate a computerized report comparing these "ODIs" with the individual's intake of calories, caffeine, and various nutrients. The sample report accompanying the flyer included "ODIs" of 3,036 mg of vitamin C (enough to cause diarrhea), 360 mg of vitamin B_6 (enough to cause nerve damage over a period of months), and excessive amounts of several other vitamins and minerals. NutriPro estimates that selling three programs per day would boost supplement sales by $25,000 per year.

APMA's president is Julian Whitaker, M.D., who practices "preventive medicine" in Newport Beach, California, and publishes *Health & Healing,* a monthly newsletter that promotes a large number of questionable treatments. Whitaker has also designed a high-dosage multivitamin/multimineral supplement offered to his readers for "just" $23.95 for a thirty-day supply. APMA's secretary is Jonathan Wright, M.D., and its treasurer is Jonathan Collin, M.D., publisher of *The Townsend Letter for Doctors*, a forum for "alternative" practitioners. All three and most of APMA's board members practice chelation therapy (see Chapter 12).

People's Medical Society (PMS)

PMS has been engaged in a wide variety of projects that may adversely affect medical practice and consumer protection against quackery. Although some of its aims are laudable, PMS is rooted in deep antagonism to the medical profession and to medical science itself.

PMS was the brainchild of the late Robert Rodale, board chairman of Rodale Press and publisher of *Prevention* magazine. During 1982, he ran a series of editorials criticizing the medical establishment and promising "a grassroots campaign that will turn America's medical system on its head." PMS was officially launched on January 1, 1983, with a large initial loan from Rodale Press, but is now supported by dues payments ($15 per year) from about eighty thousand members. The group's bimonthly newsletter occasionally contains valuable suggestions, but most of its information is slanted to undermine trust in scientific practitioners. Most articles in its newsletters imply that doctors cannot be trusted, and cartoons in every issue ridicule medical care as expensive, unnecessary, dangerous, or impersonal.

From time to time, PMS encourages its members to write to legislators or other government officials. Some campaigns have involved antiquackery legislation (opposed by PMS), funds for organic farming (favored), licensing of nutritionists (opposed), and food irradiation (opposed). At a 1992 hearing for a bill to license "nutritionists" in Pennsylvania, PMS president Charles B. Inlander testified that no such law was needed because "not once . . . have we ever received one single letter or phone call from a consumer asking for protection from an individual or group offering or providing nutritional information."

PMS has published many books, booklets, and special reports. Some contain valuable information, while others promote unscientific methods and/or portray them as equivalent to scientific ones. The PMS booklet *Options in Health Care*, for example, uncritically promotes the theories and practices of acupuncture, acupressure, Chinese medicine, chiropractic, homeopathy, hydrotherapy, metabolic therapy, naturopathy, orthomolecular therapy, psychic healing, and reflexology. PMS's eight-page bulletin on cancer-care options includes promoters of quack cancer methods in its list of sources of information. The bulletin on choosing doctors includes the ridiculous advice that obtaining a health-related degree through a correspondence course "does not in and of itself imply an inferior education." No one can become qualified as a health practitioner through this route, and *all* such programs teach health nonsense.

PMS's forty-eight-page report on high blood pressure contains sound advice but also suggests that practitioners of chiropractic, acupressure, homeopathy, herbal therapy, and megavitamin therapy have much to offer:

> While many of these practitioners can't produce the years of studies and double-blind experimental results that the medical professionals can, they nonetheless provide treatment—often less invasive, less costly, and with fewer side effects than traditional medicine's—that has its adherents and success stories.

(Translation: As long as anyone says that a method works, it is worth considering.)

Another PMS booklet encourages members to start a People's Medical Library in their community. Along with such authoritative references as the *AMA Family Medical Guide, Cecil's Textbook of Medicine, JAMA,* and *The New England Journal of Medicine,* it recommends Rodale Press books on natural healing and natural home remedies and a few other highly questionable publications.

Another PMS booklet, *Deregulating Doctoring,* suggests that medical licensing laws be substantially limited in scope or even repealed. Written by Attorney Lori B. Andrews, vice-chairman of PMS's board of directors, the report suggests that everyone should be free to engage in "such nonhazardous, relatively innocuous activities like advising, giving tips on prevention, making recommendations and offering simple treatments." It recommends that "as a minimum, the definition of the practice of medicine should be restricted so that only inherently dangerous health care activities require a medical license." In other words, state governments should permit any quack whose methods won't kill you on the spot to market them to the public.

PMS also publishes bibliographies on various health topics. Like the People's Medical Library lists, however, these include unscientific publications as well as reputable ones. For example, the bibliography on arthritis includes a book which claims that food allergy is a major cause of arthritis; the cancer bibliography includes a book that boosts macrobiotics; and the diet and nutrition bibliography includes several unscientific books and refers readers to the Academy of Orthomolecular Psychiatry, a Canadian group that promotes megavitamin therapy for mental problems.

Several years ago, *Shape* magazine warned its readers to be wary of any "nutritionist" who touts a degree, certificate, or other credential from any of fifteen nonaccredited schools listed by Dr. Stephen Barrett. PMS's eight-page bulletin, "How to Choose a Nutritionist," contains the list, without mentioning its source, and advises that "other people . . . have found competent, legitimate practitioners with just such credentials." The bulletin also suggests that hair analysis can serve as the basis for nutritional advice. (The correct advice is that hair analysis of nutritional status is the hallmark of a quack.)

PMS's newsletter has referred readers to the Hearing and Tinnitus Help Association (HTHA), whose executive director, Paul Yanick, Jr., claimed to have helped thousands to overcome tinnitus (ringing in the ear) and other hearing and balance disorders through "nutrition" methods. Contributors to HTHA were eligible for a discount on the $200 price of "The Comprehensive Nutrient and Lifestyle Program," which Yanick helped design. According to a flyer distributed by HTHA, this is a computerized analysis that recommends nutrition supplements after analyzing information on dietary and exercise habits; "tissue mineral analysis"; tests on pH, urine, stool, and saliva; and "over 400 questions relating changes that take place in your body when a nutrient becomes deficient."

Publicity materials for one of its books describe PMS as "the largest consumer health organization in America" and state that it is run "by the people" and "for the people." However, its president and board of directors are not elected, and newsletters give no indication that its activities and policies are determined by anyone but Inlander.

Properly directed, consumer groups can accomplish a great deal by educating their members and working constructively to reduce health-care costs and increase consumer protection. In our opinion, the People's Medical Society is doing neither and will do more harm than good in the long run.

National Nutritional Foods Association (NNFA)

NNFA, the health-food industry's largest trade group, represents about 2,500 retailers and 700 manufacturers, distributors, wholesalers, and jobbers. It has a national office in Costa Mesa, California, and regional offices in eight other cities. NNFA traces it origin to the American Health Food Association, which formed in 1936, became the National Health Foods Association in 1937, and merged with the American Dietary Retailers Association in 1970 to become the National Nutritional Foods Association.

NNFA's activities include lobbying, trade shows (see Chapter 5), retailer education (see Chapter 6), legal action (see Chapter 18), and public relations. It publishes a monthly newsletter (*NNFA Today*) and issues frequent "Updates" to inform members about political developments. Its main political strategies during the past few years have been: (1) opposition to state laws that would define the practice of "nutrition" and limit it to people with accredited credentials, and (2) promotion of a federal law that would undermine the FDA's ability to regulate the marketing of dietary supplements. Three of NNFA's twenty-two directors are from companies that have engaged in false advertising described elsewhere in this book (General Nutrition, Nature's Way, and Weider Health & Fitness).

Responsible Nutrition?

The Council for Responsible Nutrition (CRN), located in Washington, D.C., describes itself as "a trade association of the nutritional supplements, ingredients, and other nutritional products industry." Products manufactured by its members are sold in drugstores, supermarkets, convenience outlets, discount chains, and health-food stores, and are also sold directly (person-to-person) and by mail. Its stated purposes are:

> (1) to increase the awareness of the appropriate dietary role for nutritional supplements, ingredients, and other nutritional products by utilizing authoritative and sound scientific, social, and economic information; (2) to enhance the credibility of the nutrition industry message through a proactive communications strategy; (3) to protect and promote the interest of nutritional supplements, ingredients, and other nutritional products industry in the legislative and regulatory arenas; and to promote CRN members' interests through services, activities, and events.

Its bylaws state that "CRN is dedicated to enhancing the health of the U.S. population through responsible nutrition, including the appropriate use of nutritional supplementation." Its activities include lobbying, issuing publications, advertising, interacting with the news media, and sponsoring conferences.

Since 1982, the group's president has been John B. Cordaro, who previously held senior positions with the Food Safety Council, the U.S. Congress Office of Technology Assessment, and the U.S. Department of State's Agency for International Development. He has a B.S. degree in government, economics, and philosophy, and a master's degree in agricultural and nutrition economics. CRN's technical director, who has been with CRN since its founding in 1973, is Annette Dickinson, Ph.D. She received an M.S. degree in food science in 1975 and a Ph.D. in nutritional science in 1992 from the University of Maryland.

CRN has three categories of members. Companies engaged in the manufacture, packaging, or labeling of supplements are eligible for voting membership. Suppliers of services or other support to the supplement industry are eligible for associate membership, while foreign companies or affiliates of voting members can become international correspondents. Dues for voting members are based on annual sales. Currently, there are sixty-two voting members, eight associate members, and four international members. The voting members include Hoffmann-La Roche Inc., Lederle Laboratories, Miles, Inc., Nature's Bounty, Neo-Life Company of America, Nutrilite Products (a division of the Amway Corporation), Rexall Group/Sundown Vitamins, Inc., and Shaklee Corporation, each of which has engaged in questionable promotions mentioned elsewhere in this book. The manufacturing arm of General Nutrition is also a CRN member.

CRN was formed in response to an FDA attempt (described below) to regulate the labeling and dosage of supplement products. Most of CRN's original members were manufacturers from the "health food" side of the supplement industry. But since 1979, membership has broadened to include pharmaceutical and food manufacturers and distributors who are active in the nutritional supplement field. Cordaro estimates that CRN members who are bulk manufacturers supply most of the raw materials used to manufacture vitamin products for the American marketplace and that about half of the vitamin supplements retailed in the United States are manufactured by CRN members.

CRN differs from the other groups discussed in this chapter in that it does not promote false therapeutic claims for supplements. It favors "a new regulatory framework that allows for continued access for safe products [with] truthful and nonmisleading information to allow consumers to make more informed choices."

CRN's code of ethics states that its members "recognize their duty to . . . ensure that consumers are provided with the accurate information they need to make informed choices" and that they "avoid making unsubstantiated or false or misleading claims for their products." In 1985, Cordaro even stated:

> We have turned our back on the extremists in our industry and have disassociated ourselves from those who attempt to make a quick buck through fraudulent products, promises, and practices.

Although few CRN members make unsubstantiated therapeutic claims for their products, several of them—as well as CRN itself—have misrepresented the need for "nutrition insurance" (the supplement industry's backbone). For example:

- For several years, Neo-Life suggested that eating "most packaged foods" was like "putting used motor oil in a new car."
- The 1980 Shaklee Corporation sales manual, which was sold until the end of 1983, stated: "What about your temperament? Are you the emotional type or cool as a cucumber? Stress can cause the body to use up more nutrients faster. Add alcohol, birth control pills, smoking or medications that alter the unique balance in your body achieved by nature's handiwork, and you may need additional nutrients."
- In the mid-1980s, Hoffmann-La Roche advertised widely that, "If your diet, like that of so many people, is coming up short, consider taking Protector Vitamin E . . . an easy, safe and inexpensive way to

ensure added protection." This message was dishonest because vitamin E deficiency on a dietary basis had never been reported in an American adult.

- CRN's 1993 report, *Benefits of Nutritional Supplements,* states that "typical American diets commonly fail to provide levels of nutrient intake that fall short of nutritional goals" and that "for most people, it makes sense to use nutritional supplements regularly than to fail to avail themselves of the potential benefits of supplement use."

In his address to CRN's 1984 annual meeting, Cordaro said:

> I believe that by taking certain actions we can expand the base of the 30 to 40 percent [of the American population] that takes a dietary supplement on a regular basis. Indeed, I believe that by emphasizing our concern with safety first and our belief that our products are useful and needed . . . we will be able to penetrate to the 60 percent of the population not now taking supplements.

In the mid-1980s, CRN cosponsored the distribution of "public-service type announcements" by satellite to about two thousand radio stations. The announcements included the following message from Cordaro:

> A balanced diet could provide all the nutrients that we need. But as a matter of fact, most of us don't eat the right amounts of the right foods all the time. So a vitamin supplement can help us and may also provide other health benefits. For example, some research suggests that large doses of vitamin C may help reduce the frequency and severity of colds and other winter illnesses.

The first sentence of this weasel-worded statement should say "*will* provide." The second sentence is misleading because it isn't necessary to "eat the right amounts of the right foods all the time" in order to be adequately nourished. The third sentence falsely conveys that if someone's diet is faulty, the best way to correct it is with supplements. The final sentence falsely represents that megadoses of vitamin C prevent colds. This simply is untrue (see Chapter 17).

During the late 1980s, CRN became concerned about slumping vitamin sales and sought the reason. After its research suggested that Americans had come to believe they could get all the nutrients they need from food, CRN launched its "Vitamin Gap" ad to persuade them otherwise (see Chapter 3). At a hearing in connection with this ad (see Chapter 18), Dickinson said that everyone should take supplements, not only to avoid deficiency but to obtain optimal amounts. Cordaro and Dickinson recently told Dr. Barrett:

> CRN believes that virtually everyone could benefit from a balanced multivitamin-mineral supplement, and most people could benefit from additional supplements according to need. . . .
>
> CRN is not aware of any particular group which might not benefit from supplements.

In 1987, Barrett tested CRN's code of ethics by filing a complaint about one of its member companies (Natural Organics, Inc., of Farmingdale, New York, marketing under the name Nature's Plus). The complaint involved claims made for eight products in its catalog and product literature. Cordaro responded with a letter to company president Gerald Kessler supporting most of Barrett's allegations. Not long afterward, Cordaro reported that Natural Organics had agreed to incorporate changes he had suggested in its next catalog. Two years later, however, the 1987 catalog was still being distributed and Natural Organics was no longer a CRN member.

The First "Vitamin War"

In 1972, after lengthy study, the FDA proposed that food products be labeled so that ingredients, nutrient content, and other information would be displayed in a standard format. These provisions became regulations with little controversy and remained in effect until recently. But the FDA also proposed that labeling could neither state nor imply that a balanced diet of ordinary foods cannot supply adequate amounts of nutrients

Because this struck at the heart of health-food-industry mythology about "nutrition insurance," the industry responded with lawsuits and a massive letter-writing campaign asking Congress to completely remove FDA jurisdiction over food supplements. This activity was orchestrated by the National Health Federation. Crying "Fight for your freedom to take vitamins!" NHF organized its members and allies into unprecedented political activity. Article after article urging support of the anti-FDA bill appeared in health-food-industry publications and chiropractic journals, and retailers and multilevel companies urged their customers to join the fray. The issue also triggered the formation of the Council for Responsible Nutrition to represent the political interests of major supplement manufacturers. At a Congressional hearing, several representatives reported that they had received more mail about vitamins than about Watergate. Mail favoring NHF's bill was so heavy that some people who wrote against the bill learned that their letters were not read but simply counted as favorable to it!

In 1976, as a result of this pressure, Congress passed the Proxmire Amendment to the Food, Drug, and Cosmetic Act. Though not as restrictive as NHF's original proposal, this prevents the FDA from regulating food supplements unless they are inherently dangerous or are marketed with illegal therapeutic claims. One FDA Commissioner called the amendment "a charlatan's dream." But the impact on the FDA was greater than the wording of the law itself. The apparent political power of the health-food industry made many FDA officials wonder how far the agency could go in regulating supplement promotions that remained illegal. For more than ten years, the agency virtually ignored the supplement industry.

Today's FDA Commissioner, David Kessler, M.D., J.D., who assumed office in 1991, appears to have no such fears. Under his leadership, the FDA has greatly increased the scope and vigor of its enforcement activities. In a recent interview he said:

> Our goal is . . . to ensure compliance with the law. Our laws and regulations are on the books. Once you have laws and regulations, you have to enforce them.
>
> I take the statute very seriously. The law prohibits false and misleading claims on labels. We had a reputation as a paper tiger. Sure it was a shift in policy and we caught industry by surprise. Only when we started taking action did people begin to understand what we meant by enforcement.

"Do-or-Die Time"

In 1990, a few months before Commissioner Kessler was appointed, Congress responded to public pressure for clearer nutrition information on food labels by passing the Nutritional Labeling and Education Act (NLEA), which required the FDA to adopt sweeping new regulations. Shortly before the NLEA was passed, Senator Orrin Hatch (R–UT) engineered an amendment calling for special consideration of dietary supplements and "other similar substances" such as various seed oils, enzymes, amino acids, and herbal tinctures—products the industry calls "supplements" but are actually intended for treating disease. The industry hoped that the standards for supplements would be more lenient than those for foods.

In 1991, after Kessler appointed a Dietary Supplement Task Force, the supplement industry became alarmed that the task force would recommend banning many of its products. In February 1992, about thirty industry leaders attended an "emergency meeting." The participants included manufacturers, retailers, trade association leaders, lobbyists, industry advisors, and editors of industry trade and consumer publications.

"What we heard was that it was do or die time," said the March editorial in *Health Foods Business*. "The enormity of the situation shocked those present into creating a New World Order for our industry. . . . The issues facing the industry in the next few months are a result of converging movements in Congress and in the Food and Drug Administration that by coincidence or design are gathering momentum, much like a tornado about to strike."

The supplement industry had good reason to be worried. If the "tornado" had struck, the industry's freedom to mislead the public would be sharply curtailed. Two bills, then pending in Congress, would have greatly strengthened our government's ability to combat health frauds. One would have increased the FDA's enforcement powers as well as penalties for violating the Food, Drug, and Cosmetic Act. The other would have amended the Federal Trade Commission Act to make it illegal to advertise nutritional or therapeutic claims that would not be permissible on product labels. But the industry was even more nervous about the FDA's pending regulations for product labeling.

The meeting resulted in formation of the Nutritional Health Alliance (NHA) to enable all segments of the supplement industry to coordinate their efforts. NHA's president is Gerald Kessler, president of Nature's Plus, a company that has illegally marketed more than twenty products (see Chapters 8 and 11). Within weeks, NHA launched a massive letter-writing campaign and began raising large sums of money.

NHA's Legislative Agenda

In December 1992, bolstered by a flood of letters to Congress, Senator Hatch gained passage of the Dietary Supplement Act of 1992, which prevented the FDA from issuing new regulations for supplements until the end of 1993. In April 1993, Hatch and Representative Bill Richardson (D-NM) introduced bills titled the Dietary Supplement and Health Education Act of 1993. Hatch's version defined "dietary supplements" as vitamins, minerals, herbs, amino acids, and other substances intended "to supplement the diet by increasing the total dietary intake." (This definition covers everything the health-food industry would like to call a supplement.) The bill would also (1) prevent the FDA from classifying such products as drugs or food additives, regulating their dosage, or making them available only by prescription; (2) permit manufacturers to make therapeutic claims based on flimsy evidence; and (3) stall most FDA regulatory actions by permitting manufacturers who receive a warning letter to protest to the Department of Health and Human Services or seek court review. Richardson's version was similar but not quite so restrictive. Passage of either bill would severely weaken the FDA's ability to protect consumers from fraudulently marketed "nutrition" products. *The New York Times* has called these bills "The 1993 Snake Oil Protection Act."

The Dietary Supplement and Health Education Act would also establish an NIH Office of Dietary Supplements, whose duties would include coordinating and promoting research on "the benefits of dietary supplements in maintaining health and preventing chronic disease and other health-related conditions" and advising the FDA on dietary supplement issues. Establishment of the NIH Office of Alternative Medicine has been trumpeted by "alternative" proponents as "government and scientific recognition" of their methods (see Chapter 18). An NIH office for supplements would undoubtedly be abused in the same way by supplement promoters.

NHA's Disinformation Campaign

To support its legislative agenda, NHA generated mail from health-food manufacturers, retailers, and distributors, as well as from health-food-store shoppers, customers of mail-order companies, multilevel distributors, "natural health" practitioners, and bodybuilding and fitness enthusiasts who use supplements. The campaign's leaders want legislators to believe that the outpouring of mail represents a "grassroots" effort by consumers who wish to preserve "freedom of choice." Most of the mail, however, has been generated by people who profit from the sale of supplements or who were misled by those who profit.

To mobilize its troops, NHA harped on two themes: (1) if sellers don't act, most of them will be put out of business; and (2) if consumers don't protest, the FDA will take away their right to buy vitamins. To fire up sellers, NHA advertised in trade publications:

> Every health food store is under immediate threat of siege. Congress wants to give the FDA police powers so they can seize products without notification and use heavy fines and court penalties to close you down. The FDA wants to destroy your supplement business by making many items prescription only. The FDA wants to make it illegal to sell the majority of your best selling products. . . . If current FDA and Congressional actions are passed and enforced, the nutritional supplements industry as we know it will vanish within the next 12–18 months—and most health food stores will be out of business.

To fire up consumers, NHA and many allies portrayed the FDA as a Gestapo-like agency and urged them to "write to Congress today or kiss your

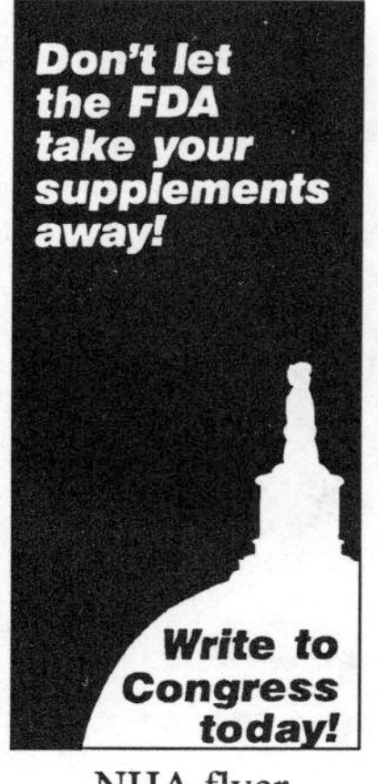

Don't let
the FDA
take your
supplements
away!
Write to
Congress
today!
NHA flyer

vitamins goodbye!" NHA also claimed—without substantiation—that "if FDA has its way, you will have to go to a doctor for prescriptions for many supplements and then pay $80 for a supplement which presently costs $10 at a health food store." Many stores set up a "political action center" with sample letters and stationery that customers could use for writing their own. (NHA even advised retailers to offer a 5 percent discount every time a customer brings in an additional personally written letter to send.) Some stores held a "blackout day," displayed empty shelves, or conducted other publicity stunts to reinforce this type of message. Virtually every publication philosophically aligned with the health-food industry published articles and editorials urging readers to write their legislators on this issue. Several groups organized fax campaigns as well.

Another stimulus was a videotaped sixty-second public service announcement intended to dramatize government interference with people's freedom to take vitamins. The video begins by depicting a SWAT team, guns drawn, raiding a private home to arrest the owner (played by Mel Gibson), who is located in the kitchen holding a bottle of vitamin C. "It's only vitamins," Gibson protests as he is handcuffed, "vitamin C, you know, like in oranges." During the "arrest," viewers were told:

> The federal government is actually considering classifying most vitamins and other supplements as drugs. The FDA has already conducted raids on doctors' offices and health food stores. Could raids on individuals be next? Protect your right to vitamins. Call Congress now.

The scenario, of course, is as fictitious as the claims that the supplement industry makes for most of its products. The FDA is not out to destroy the supplement industry. It merely wants honest labeling.

In a speech from the Senate floor, Hatch stated that the FDA had "repeatedly attempted to impose unnecessarily stringent standards that would leave many if not most supplement companies with no practical choice but to close their doors." As a result, he claimed, "consumers are left uninformed and the nation pays millions of dollars for health care that could have been saved through disease prevention."

Hatch's idea that FDA regulation would leave consumers uninformed is ludicrous. Strict labeling regulations would not stop the industry from communicating through talk shows, books, health-food magazines and newsletters, public relation firms, oral claims by retailers, and other channels. The idea that

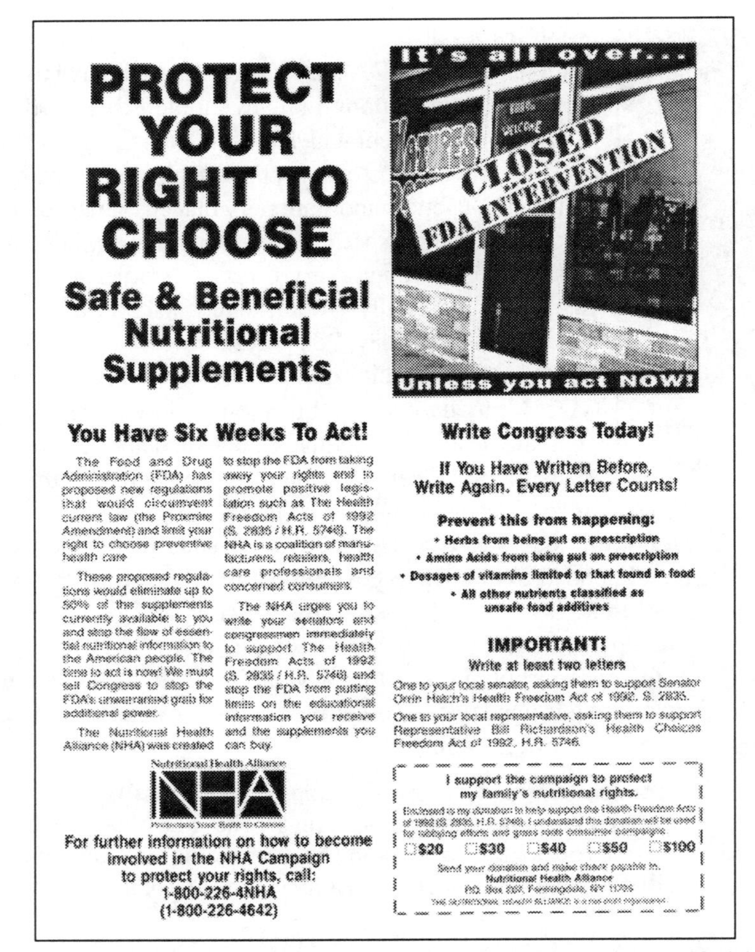

Ad warning that proposed FDA regulations would "eliminate up to half of the supplements currently available to you and stop the flow of nutrition information to the American people." Neither assertion was true.

supplement-industry strategies would lower health-care costs is even more ridiculous. Some vitamin pushers recommend a sound diet that is low in fat and high in fiber, but others recommend diets that are unbalanced or nutritionally inadequate. Although some people can benefit from taking supplements, others can be harmed; and virtually everyone connected with the industry recommends supplements unnecessarily and/or inappropriately.

The public does need protection, not from the FDA, but from those who exploit misinformation and false hope. The Hatch/Richardson bills would not protect consumers but would make it easier for them to be exploited. Bruce

Silverglade, director of legal affairs for the Center for Science in the Public Interest (CSPI), emphasized this point when he testified against the bills at a hearing held in 1993 by the Senate Committee on Labor and Human Resources. If the bill were passed, Silverglade warned, "manufacturers could hype products on the basis of preliminary, shaky, and inconclusive evidence that would preclude consumers from making an informed choice." That, of course, is precisely what the health-food industry wants.

NHA's campaign has generated hundreds of thousands of communications to Congress and has inspired a majority of both houses to sign as cosponsors. In May 1994, the Senate committee released an amended version of Hatch's bill for a full Senate vote after Hatch pledged to make two modifications: (1) for two years, supplements could not be marketed with health claims unless there is "significant scientific agreement" on their truthfulness; and (2) during this period, a seven-person commission appointed by the President would develop recommendations on how supplements should be regulated.

The substitute bill is now called the Dietary Supplement Health and Education Act of 1994. As this book goes to press, it is not clear whether it will become law during the current session of Congress. But it is clear that any such bill would have disastrous consequences for the American public.

More Mischief

In May 1994, Senator Thomas Daschle (D–SD) introduced the "Access to Medical Treatment Act," which would permit licensed practitioners to administer unproven treatments that are within their scope of practice and meet certain conditions. The most important of these are:

- Someone requests it in writing.
- The practitioner states the nature of the treatment, reasonably foreseeable side effects, and results of such treatment by the practitioner and others. [Since *written* disclosure is not required, proving what a practitioner actually says might be impossible.]
- The practitioner warns that the treatment "has not yet been approved or certified by the Federal Government and any individual who uses [it] does so at his or her own risk."
- There is no evidence that the treatment itself is a danger to the individual. [Testing for safety *before* administering the treatment would not be required as it is now.]

According to the May 1994 *Citizens For Health Report,* the driving force behind Daschle's bill was Berkley Bedell, the former Congressman who persuaded Senator Tom Harkin to seek passage of the law that led to establishment of NIH's Office of Alternative Medicine (see Chapter 18). The *Report* stated that CFH and "numerous other non-profit groups" had helped Bedell prepare the bill for introduction and that Harkin would also be a key player in the final push for passage of Hatch's bill. NNFA plans to hold a $100-per-person reception for Harkin at its July 1994 convention and has promised that all attendees can have their photo taken with the senator.

Current federal laws make it illegal to market unproven methods across state lines. Dashle's bill would enable any food, drug, or device to be introduced into interstate commerce as long as it is intended for treatment under his bill's "safeguards." Thus while Hatch's bill would free the health-food industry to market countless numbers of quack products, Daschle's bill would enable licensed practitioners to prescribe them without fear of federal interference—all in the name of "health freedom."

The Real Issue

During the past century, scientists have developed methods for determining what approaches are effective in preventing and treating disease. At the same time, laws have been passed to protect the public from methods that are ineffective or promoted with misinformation. The health-food industry is battling to weaken these laws. With Senator Hatch as its leading standard-bearer, the industry is striving to gain through politics what it cannot achieve through science. Its massive disinformation campaign alleges that "consumer freedom" is at stake and that consumers need protection from the FDA. Nothing could be further from the truth!

During the past twenty years, we have collected advertisements and product literature containing false, misleading, and unsubstantiated claims for thousands of products sold through health-food stores, multilevel (person-to-person) companies, and the offices of unscientific practitioners. Every one of these documents is evidence of violation of federal and state criminal laws. We have also collected hundreds of reports and other documents related to government regulation of supplement manufacturers.

Having observed the health-food industry for many years, we consider it a form of organized crime. What its leaders really want is the freedom to mislead consumers without government interference. The real issue facing Congress is whether promoters of quackery should be permitted to cheat the public. Our answer is *no!*

21

How Much Can the Law Protect You?

Anastasia Toufexis, who wrote *Time* magazine's April 6, 1992, cover story, "The Real Power of Vitamins," has a low opinion of the supplement industry. Three months after the article appeared, she spoke at the National Nutritional Foods Association's annual convention in Nashville, Tennessee:

> You've seen the articles in *The New York Times* and elsewhere over the last six months or a year. Now, does this mark a new day in how the press views the vitamin supplement industry or the nutritional supplement industry? Are we going to be friends? Nope, afraid not. For many journalists the industry still has a lousy reputation, ranking just above the tobacco industry, and no group could possibly sink lower in health writers' estimation than the tobacco group.

Ms. Toufexis was talking about credibility and ethics. To remain profitable, the supplement industry must convince people that (1) dangerous products are safe, (2) useless products are useful, (3) unnecessary products are essential for good health, (4) adverse scientific findings should be ignored, and (5) doctors can't be trusted.

Some of the industry's lies are protected by the doctrines of freedom of speech and freedom of the press. It is perfectly legal to tell a lie in a publication or on a talk show as long as you are not selling the product at the same time. It is not legal to make false claims on the label of a product, in an advertisement, or during a direct sale; but prosecution of law violators is limited. This chapter discusses how the laws work and what can be done to strengthen them. Let's begin by examining the impact of regulation on America's largest health-food-store chain: General Nutrition.

"Golden Opportunity"

General Nutrition Corporation (GNC) was founded in 1935 as a small store in Pittsburgh called Lackzoom, which sold only vitamins and minerals. By 1941, there were six such stores in Pittsburgh. The company began mail-order sales in 1947 and adopted the General Nutrition Center name (also abbreviated GNC) in 1959. By 1963, there were twelve GNC stores outside of the Pittsburgh area. The number of stores grew steadily to a peak of about 1,300 company-owned stores in 1985 with total income of about $400 million. Legal troubles and declining sales caused the company to close about three hundred stores between 1985 and 1987, but a franchising program plus improved sales enabled it to expand again. The mail-order division was sold to Nature's Bounty in 1989.

Today the parent corporation is called General Nutrition Companies, Inc. (GNCI) and is listed on the NASDAQ Stock Market. GNCI's 1993 annual report states that on February 5, 1994, there were 1,044 company-owned stores with total sales of $429 million, plus 509 franchised outlets, which tend to have

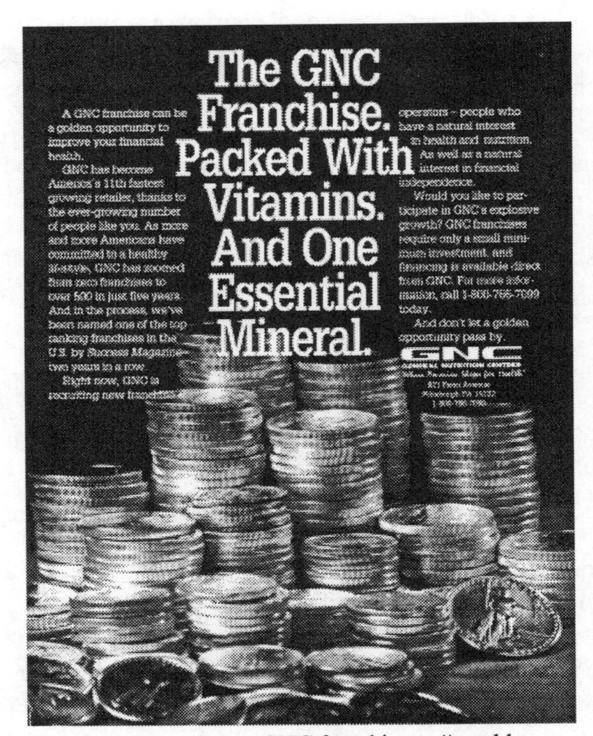

This ad describes a GNC franchise as "a golden opportunity to improve your financial health."

higher sales volumes than company-owned units. The report also states that GNCI operates the largest supplement manufacturing facility in the United States, with 1993 sales of $46.6 million. The report predicted that 350 more GNC retail outlets would be opened during 1994.

"Unconscionable Advertising"

General Nutrition has been the target of numerous government regulatory actions. In 1969, the FTC brought false advertising charges regarding claims for *Geri-Gen* ("therapeutic tonic") and *Hemotrex.* The case was settled by a consent decree in which GNC was prohibited from advertising that such products may be useful in preventing or relieving tiredness, listlessness, or "run-down" feelings. In 1973, a supply of vitamin C/bioflavonoid tablets was seized and destroyed under a consent agreement after the FDA charged that their labeling made false and misleading nutritional claims. In 1980, the FDA seized a powdered-milk product touted as a cure for arthritis and the Postal Service stopped false representations for *Model-Etts,* an alleged reducing aid. In 1981, the FDA brought action against GNC for claiming that lysine cured genital herpes. In 1982, the Postal Service charged that advertising for *Advantage Starch Block* contained false representations that the product blocked the absorption of calories from starch-containing foods. A false representation order was obtained, and the California Department of Health issued an embargo.

During 1984, the Postal Service charged GNC with making false representations for thirteen products: *Risk Modifier* (a nutrient mixture claimed to decrease cancer risk); *Life Expander Choline Chloride* (claimed to improve memory); *Mental Acuity Formula* (supposedly able to prevent or retard memory loss due to aging); *Life Expander Fat Fighter* (containing DHEA, claimed to cause weight loss without dietary modification); *Challenge Maximum Body Builder* (claimed to have special muscle-building properties); *L-Glutamine* tablets (claimed to "keep you mentally and emotionally in balance"); *Lipotropic Fat Fighter* tablets (a nutrient mixture that supposedly could reduce body fat); *Spirulina* (which supposedly will "turn off your brain's appetite control center"); the *24-Hour Diet Plan* and the *Practical Diet Plan* (both "guaranteed" to produce weight loss of "up to 10 pounds in two weeks"); *Life Expander Growth Hormone Releaser* (claimed to cause weight loss without dieting); *Herbal Diet Formula* (supposedly capable, by itself, of causing weight loss); and *Inches Be Gone* (a body-wrapping cream claimed to reduce any area where you want to lose inches). The complaints were settled with a consent agreement.

In 1984, the FTC charged GNC with making deceptive claims that its *Healthy Greens* might help people prevent cancer. GNC's ads suggested that the product, which was composed of dehydrated vegetables and a few vitamins, was based on findings of the 1982 National Academy of Sciences report on diet and cancer. The report had concluded that the incidence of cancer was lower among people whose diet was rich in certain vegetables. Although the report recommended against supplementation with the nutrients in these foods, GNC and a few other manufacturers pretended otherwise. In 1986, Administrative Law Judge Montgomery K. Hyun concluded:

> GNC's unconscionable, false and misleading advertising found in this case is not an isolated incident but in fact is a part of a continuing pattern. . . . GNC's false and deceptive advertising in this case may be seen as an indication of GNC's propensity to employ false and misleading advertisements.

In 1984, as noted in Chapter 19, the FDA initiated a criminal prosecution, charging that GNC, three of its officers, and two retail store managers had illegally conspired to promote and sell an evening primrose oil product with claims that it was effective against high blood pressure, arthritis, multiple sclerosis and other diseases. In 1986, the company pled guilty to four counts of misbranding a drug, and its former president, Gary Daum, pled guilty to one misbranding count. The company agreed to pay $10,000 to the government as reimbursement for costs of prosecution, and Daum was sentenced to pay a $1,000 fine.

In 1985, GNC recalled *Appetite Control Factor with CCK* and *Life Expander Fat Fighter* after the FDA warned that claims made for the product made it an unapproved new drug.

In 1989, the Pennsylvania Department of Health obtained a consent agreement regarding a Helsinki formula hair treatment. GNC had marketed this with false claims that it was a proven treatment for thinning hair and that its vitamin supplement contained "those special nutrients that have been proven helpful in an overall hair-care regimen." During the same year, the 1984 FTC complaint was settled by a consent agreement in which GNC agreed to donate $600,000 for nutrition research and was prohibited from making any claim for any company-produced product that cannot be substantiated by scientific evidence.

In 1994, GNCI settled yet another FTC complaint charging that the company had violated previous orders against false and unsubstantiated claims. This time forty-two products were involved, most of them related to other manufacturers' products marketed though GNC stores from 1989 through 1993. The products included fifteen alleged weight-control products, eighteen alleged "ergogenic aids," five bogus hair-loss preventers, two alleged antifatigue products, and two purported disease-related products. GNCI also agreed to pay a civil penalty of $2.4 million. One of the antifatigue products, *Sublingual B Total,* was said to be effective against tiredness, listlessness, "depleted" feeling, "run-down" feeling, and easy fatiguability. Believe it or not, an ad suggesting that people who feel "sluggish" use this product was still being televised a month after the settlement agreement was signed!

These government actions only tell part of the story. GNC and/or its retailers have engaged in countless illegal acts—from false advertising to practicing medicine without a license— that did not trigger government action. In Chapter 19, we report how GNC president Jerry Horn said the company was not "compelled" to determine whether the products it sells are safe or beneficial. It remains to be seen whether the recent FTC action will persuade GNC to stop breaking the law or whether the company will merely regard it as a minor cost of doing business. GNC also contributed several hundred thousand dollars to the Council for Responsible Nutrition's dubious "Vitamin Gap" campaign (see Chapter 3).

Now let's examine how the law works.

The Legal Lineup

Three federal agencies and various state and local agencies can act against false claims made by sellers of food supplements. The Postal Service has jurisdiction over products sold by mail. It has a vigorous program but is hampered by loopholes in its law. The Federal Trade Commission (FTC) can regulate the advertising of nonprescription products and health-related services. It has a powerful law but insufficient manpower. The Food and Drug Administration (FDA) presides over the labeling of products marketed with therapeutic claims. It has a powerful law but is not using it to full advantage. In addition, as noted in Chapter 20, the FDA has been under political siege for the past two years. Some overlapping of jurisdiction exists. All three of these agencies could take action against someone who advertises a vitamin product with illegal health-related claims and sells it by mail.

State enforcement activities are administered by the state attorney general, local district attorneys, and state licensing boards. State laws and their enforcement priority vary considerably from state to state. Courts also play an important role in regulating quackery and health frauds.

Most people overestimate the extent to which laws can protect our society against quackery and health frauds. As should be apparent from this book, the amount of wrongdoing exceeds the resources of law enforcement agencies and the courts. The health-food industry has found that crime pays. So don't assume that because a "supplement" product is marketed, it is legitimate.

FTC Regulation

The FTC has jurisdiction over advertising of foods, nonprescription drugs, cosmetics, and devices that are sold or advertised in interstate commerce. Section 12 of the FTC Act allows the government to attack false advertising that could injure consumers as well as competitors. In determining what is false, what is left out may be considered as well as what is said.

The FTC has broad powers to investigate complaints. If it concludes that the law has been violated, it may attempt to obtain voluntary compliance by entering into a consent order with the violator. Signers of a consent order need not admit that they have violated the law, but they must agree to stop the practices described in an accompanying complaint. If a consent agreement cannot be reached, the FTC can issue an administrative complaint or—if a problem is considered serious enough—seek a court order (injunction) to stop the improper practices.

When an administrative complaint is disputed, an administrative law judge holds a formal hearing similar to a court trial. If the judge finds that the law has been violated, a cease-and-desist order or other appropriate relief can be issued. Initial decisions by administrative law judges can be appealed to the five-member commission, which acts like a court of appeal. Respondents who are dissatisfied with the commission's decision can appeal their case through the federal court system. FTC actions often result in restitution to consumers and/or a financial penalty against the advertiser.

Cease-and-desist orders set forth findings and prohibit respondents from engaging in practices determined to be illegal. When final, these orders act as permanent injunctions. Penalties for violating consent agreements or cease-and-desist orders can be very heavy—including corrective advertising and fines of up to $10,000 per day for continued violations.

When the FTC believes that a problem affects an entire industry, it may promulgate an industry guide or trade regulation rule. Guides are interpretive statements without the force of law; rules represent the conclusions of the commission about what is unlawful. Before guides and rules are established, interested parties are given opportunity to comment. Once a rule is established, the commission can take enforcement action without lengthy explanations about why a particular ad is unfair or deceptive. A reference to the rule is enough. In health matters, problems are almost always handled on a case-by-case basis rather than through rulemaking. During the mid-1970s, the FTC considered regulating advertising claims for testimonials, protein supplements, and "health," "organic," and "natural" foods. Considerable discussion took place, but no rule was established.

The FTC's activities are reported in the weekly *FTC News Notes* and an annual report, both of which are available free of charge to interested parties.

Although the FTC has a very effective law, the agency can handle only a small percentage of the violations it detects. The situation could be greatly improved if Congress passed a law enabling state attorneys general to enter federal court so that the results of their regulatory actions would apply nationwide.

Postal Regulation

The Postal Service has jurisdiction over situations where the mail is used to transfer money for products or services. Postal inspectors look for misleading advertisements in magazines and newspapers and on radio or television. They also receive complaints from the public and from other government agencies. From the thousands of complaints it receives each year, the Postal Service selects those that it feels are most significant—particularly cases that might generate a large amount of mail or pose physical danger to the public.

Title 39, Section 3005, of the United States Code can be used to block promoters of misleading schemes from receiving money through the mail. If sufficient health hazard or economic detriment exists, an immediate court order to impound mail may be sought under Section 3007 of the Code. Title 18, Section 1341, provides for criminal prosecution. The maximum penalties are five years in prison and a fine for each instance proved. The 1984 Criminal Fines Enhancement Act allows fines of up to $100,000 (or $250,000 if death results) per offense for up to two offenses. Under Section 1341, intent to deceive must be proved—a task which can be difficult and time-consuming. Section 1341 is seldom used in health-related cases.

The Postal Service does not usually assert jurisdiction when companies solicit only credit card orders by telephone and deliver through private carriers such as United Parcel Service. However, the Justice Department may seek an injunction under Section 1345, which allows federal district courts to enjoin acts of mail and wire fraud.

Most mail-order health schemes attempt to exploit people's fear of being unattractive. Their promoters are usually "hit-and-run" artists who hope to make a profit before the Postal Service stops their false ads. Common products include "miracle weight-loss" plans, fitness and bodybuilding products, spot-reducing devices (claimed to reduce specific parts of the body), anti-aging products, and supposed sex aids. When a scheme is detected, postal inspectors can file a complaint or seek an agreement with the perpetrator. When a complaint is contested, a hearing is held by an administrative law judge. If the evidence is sufficient, this judge will issue a False Representation Order (FRO) enabling the Postal Service to block and return money sent through the mail in response to the misleading ads. Although the order can be appealed to the courts, very few companies do this. Each voluntary agreement and FRO is accompanied by a cease-and-desist order that forbids both the challenged acts and similar acts. Under the Mail Order Consumer Protection Amendments of 1983, if this order is violated, the agency can seek a civil penalty in federal court of up to $10,000 per day for each violation.

Criminal cases, consent agreements, and FROs are noted in the quarterly *Law Enforcement Report,* which is issued free of charge to interested media and consumer protection agencies. Cases of false advertising of health-related products are almost always handled with voluntary agreements or FROs, which impose no financial penalty. The agency's effectiveness would be greatly increased by passage of a law enabling it to generate financial penalties larger than the amount of money collected by the perpetrator of a fraudulent scheme. It would also help if laws were passed to make it simple for the Postal Service to initiate criminal prosecution in cases where health products are involved. Current mail-fraud laws require that intent to deceive be proven, which is difficult to do if a perpetrator professes a sincere belief in his product. As noted above, the Food, Drug, and Cosmetic Act has no such requirement.

Postal officials have said that their agency has been hampered by unwillingness on the part of the Justice Department to handle more of their cases. If this is true, the law should be changed so that Postal Service attorneys can pursue cases in federal court when the Justice Department refuses.

It would also help to pass laws discouraging publishers of magazines and newspapers from accepting ads for bogus health-related products sold by mail. Almost all such ads are misleading.

In 1977, Dr. Stephen Barrett headed a Pennsylvania Medical Society Committee on Quackery study that screened mail-order ads in five hundred nationally circulated magazines. One fourth were found to contain health advertisements. (Health-food and fitness magazines were excluded.) *Out of 150 products, not one appeared to be capable of living up to its advertised claims.*

In 1985, the FDA conducted a one-month survey of advertisements for health products in American newspapers and magazines. The survey found 435 questionable ads, 249 of them for weight-loss products (mostly diet pills). Gross deceptions appeared in ads for waist wraps, vibrating belts, and sauna suits advertised to help lose weight. There were eighty-nine ads for hair-restoration schemes, forty-two for products and forty-seven for "clinics." Wrinkle removers were also common. Other ads found in the survey included products for hemorrhoids, varicose veins, and indigestion, "rear end" kits for shaping, pills for the "ultimate orgasm," and cheap, quick ways to treat arthritis, heart disease, alcoholism, depression, and high blood pressure.

In 1991, Dr. Barrett reported on his study of magazines, tabloid newspapers, direct-mail catalogs, television infomercials, multilevel companies, and other channels through which health-related mail-order products are marketed. The study included a survey of one issue each of 463 magazines circulated during the summer of 1990. Dubious ads appeared in fifty-six out of 423 (13 percent) general audience magazines and twenty-three out of forty (58 percent) health and fitness magazines. In the general magazines, about fifty companies advertised about seventy dubious products. In health-food publications, fifteen companies advertised twenty-four dubious products. In fitness and bodybuilding magazines, twenty-six companies advertised more than sixty products. All but one product (a sweat-reducing device) were misrepresented. Tabloid newspapers (*Globe, National Examiner, Sun, National Enquirer,* and *Weekly World News),* which were surveyed for several months, contained between five and ten misleading ads per issue. Curiously, the company with the largest total number of false ads in its many publications was Macfadden Holdings, Inc., the corporate descendent of food faddist Bernarr Macfadden (see Chapter 17).

Is there any reason our society should permit this level of fraud? Why should newspaper and magazine publishers be permitted to line their pockets with profits from misleading ads? Many publishers are already doing an effective job of screening out solicitations for bogus products. The rest should be forced to set standards for screening ads and to forfeit any money they collect for permitting easily detectable frauds to be advertised. A new federal law or an FTC trade regulation rule could accomplish this. Publishers could also be required to report fraudulent ads they turn down. This information might help law-enforcement agencies stop the ads from appearing elsewhere.

FDA Regulation

The FDA traces its roots to just after the turn of this century, when consumers needed all the protection they could get. Patent medicines, which were worthless but not always harmless, were widely promoted with cure-all claims. The country was plagued by unsanitary conditions in meat-packing plants. Harmful chemicals were being added to foods, and labels rarely told what their products contained.

The Pure Food and Drug Act, passed in 1906, has been strengthened by many subsequent amendments and related acts. Together, these various laws are concerned with assuring the safety and effectiveness of all products intended for use in the diagnosis, prevention, and treatment of disease. The 1938 Food, Drug, and Cosmetic Act bans false and misleading statements from the labeling of foods, drugs, medical devices, and cosmetics. Drugs must have their active ingredients listed and be proven safe before marketing. The Kefauver-Harris Drug Amendments, passed in 1962 in the wake of the Thalidomide tragedy, require that drugs must also be proven effective before marketing. Other amendments extend this requirement to devices.

Under the law, "labeling" is not limited to what is on a product's container. It also includes claims made by any written or graphic matter which explains a product's use and is physically or contextually connected with its sale. Thus promotional material used to sell a product or to explain its use can be construed as labeling whether it is used before or after a sale.

The FDA's jurisdiction covers all intended uses of a product, whether they are contained in labeling or not. Section 502(f)(1) of the Food, Drug, and Cosmetic Act requires that all drugs and devices bear adequate directions for all intended uses, whether promotion is done by oral claims, advertising, or otherwise.

If the FDA determines that a product is a "new drug," it must have FDA approval for movement in interstate commerce. Violation of this provision can lead to seizure of the product and a court injunction against its sale. To be classified as a "new drug," a product does not actually have to be new; it can also be a familiar substance proposed for a therapeutic use that is "not generally recognized by experts as safe and effective." For example, a claim that a vitamin concoction "can relieve arthritis" would make the concoction a new drug with respect to that claim. The product would also be misbranded because—since it doesn't work—it is impossible to provide adequate directions to achieve the intended effect. (A product is misbranded if its labeling lacks required information or contains false or misleading information.)

Marketing a drug that unapproved or misbranded is a criminal offense. A first offender may be imprisoned for up to one year. Any subsequent offense is a felony punishable by up to three years in prison. Because misbranding and marketing an unapproved new product are separate offenses, a repeat offender could be sentenced to as much as six years in jail. The 1984 Criminal Fines Enhancement Act amended all federal criminal laws to allow fines of up to $100,000 (or $250,000 if death results) per offense for up to two offenses. To obtain a conviction, intent to mislead need not be proven. Even a single shipment of one product is sufficient grounds for conviction.

When products are marketed improperly, the FDA may issue a warning letter specifying the violations and demanding to know how the problem will be corrected. If a warning is ignored, or if the FDA decides to begin with more forceful action, the agency can initiate court proceedings for a seizure, injunction, or criminal prosecution. If an injunction is violated, the court has considerable discretion in determining the punishment and can order imprisonment or a large fine. The FDA has concentrated its efforts against health frauds on products that are inherently unsafe or are illegally marketed for the treatment of serious diseases. Worthless yet harmless articles promoted to improve health, athletic ability, or appearance—which the agency classifies as "economic frauds"—have been given little regulatory attention.

We believe it would be helpful if the FDA banned large numbers of products that serve no useful purpose. Homeopathic products, for example, should be removed from the marketplace unless they are proven safe and effective for their intended purpose. (In August 1994, we petitioned the FDA to hold homeopathic remedies to the same standards as other drugs.) Over-the-counter sales of single- and multiple-ingredient amino acid products should be banned because such products are really drugs in disguise and have no rational use as dietary supplements. Herbal products should be more tightly regulated.

Examples of FDA regulatory actions are reported in the weekly *FDA Enforcement Report* and monthly magazine *FDA Consumer,* both of which are available by subscription. *FDA Consumer* is an excellent magazine, written for the public, which covers food, nutrition, drugs, devices, common ailments, scientific health care, health and nutrition ripoffs, and government enforcement actions. Free reprints of many articles are available on request.

Many observers believe that FDA enforcement would be much more effective if it emphasized criminal prosecution rather than civil action. If this were done, wrongdoers might hesitate to commit acts that could land them in jail. A few years ago the FDA created an Office of Criminal Investigations and increased the number of agents doing undercover criminal investigation. However, it is not yet apparent how much priority the new program will give to quackery-related products.

Civil action, which carries no financial penalty, stops some schemes but does not usually prevent them from being profitable. This problem could be remedied by a law enabling the FDA to generate large civil penalties. As noted in Chapter 20, the current vitamin war was triggered in part by the introduction of a bill of this type.

FDA officials have said that their agency has been hampered by unwillingness of the Justice Department to handle criminal prosecutions. If this is true, the law should be changed so that FDA attorneys can prosecute in federal court when the Justice Department won't do so.

FDA Commissioner David Kessler, M.D., J.D., who assumed office in 1990, is by far the most effective leader the FDA has had in modern times. Under his direction, agency function has been streamlined and enforcement activities have increased greatly. He has gone after nutrition quackery with vigor. The health-food industry is very alarmed about this and is pressing for legislation that would greatly hamper regulation of dietary supplements.

State and Local Regulation

State efforts against health frauds and quackery are carried out under licensing and consumer protection laws. The grounds for disciplinary action and the effectiveness in policing the marketplace vary considerably from state to state and from one agency to another.

State licensing boards can take action against practitioners who appear to be unfit or who engage in various quack or unethical practices. Some physicians and dentists have been disciplined for departing from accepted standards of scientific care, but actions of this type are not common—and may take years to complete. Proponents of "alternative" methods have persuaded a few states to amend their medical practice acts so that physicians cannot be disciplined merely because they depart from scientific medical standards—and federal legislation with a similar effect has been considered.

The situation is even worse where clinical standards are minimal or nonexistent. State boards that regulate chiropractors, acupuncturists, naturopaths, and homeopaths appear to be doing little or nothing to protect the public from unscientific and unethical practices. State licensing boards only discipline a small percentage of licensed practitioners who routinely make "fad" diagnoses, prescribe huge doses of vitamins, or use hair analysis, muscle testing, or other bogus tests as a basis for recommending food supplements. These practitioners cause physical and/or financial harm, and their offices are centers of misinformation. We think all of them should have their licenses revoked. Insurance companies could play an important role in this process by reporting the activities of unscientific practitioners and dubious laboratories to state licensing boards.

State attorneys general and local district attorneys may have jurisdiction in cases that involve false advertising, theft by deception, practicing without a license, and various other types of consumer fraud. States also have laws that regulate the manufacture and marketing of drug products within their borders. Many of these parallel the Federal Food, Drug, and Cosmetic Act. Again, both the nature of the laws and the vigor with which they are enforced vary considerably from state to state.

Some states have special laws that can be used to combat the abuses described in this book. California has strict rules regulating cancer treatment products, with the burden of proof of efficacy and safety being placed on the producer of the substance. Approval of the State Department of Public Health must be obtained to sell, prescribe, or administer a drug or device for the diagnosis or treatment of cancer. Texas has a law enabling its Department of Health to embargo the sale of improperly marketed drug products, including "dietary supplements" marketed with health claims. A Florida law forbids the advertising, labeling, or commercial distribution of any product lacking FDA approval and represented to have an effect on any of a long list of health problems. A few states prohibit people from advertising that they have degrees from nonaccredited schools. About half the states have provisions regulating nutritionists. Some make it illegal for unqualified persons to call themselves dietitians or nutritionists, while others define nutrition practice and who is eligible to do it. In states that regulate nutrition practice, health-food retailers are still permitted to give limited advice about diet and the use of their products, but are not permitted to do nutritional assessment or counseling. New York City has a law enabling its Department of Consumer Affairs to combat false advertising. On the negative side, a few states have legalized certain quack practices and may even regard them as tourist attractions.

As noted in Chapter 5, most health-food retailers are willing to recommend products to customers who ask what they should take for a health problem. Although "diagnosis" and "treatment" are illegal without a professional license, agencies in most states ignore such activities in health-food stores. Perhaps if more people who realize they have been victimized were to complain about it, law enforcement authorities would take the situation more seriously.

In most cases where state or local authorities stop a dubious promotion, the action will not stop the promotion in other states. To address this problem, state attorneys general have begun to team up for multistate actions and their national organization has formed a health-care task force that will deal with frauds. The FDA is helping to coordinate this effort. We believe that special attention should be given to multilevel companies that are making unsubstantiated health claims for their products (see Chapter 10).

Victim Redress

Many cases are known in which excess vitamins or minerals have harmed people. How many preachers of nutrition gospel have ever mentioned this fact on a radio or television talk show? This deception by omission should be prosecuted as negligence chargeable not only to the huckster, but also to the talk-show host and sponsoring network. It seems possible that "reckless endangerment" laws could be revised or interpreted to include endangerment of public health by promotion of dangerous nutritional practices. We also wonder whether the more dangerous misrepresentations by quacks could be enjoined as a public nuisance. Perhaps a public-spirited prosecutor will try these approaches someday. If the First Amendment does not protect smut speech and writings that are alleged to injure mental health, why should it protect misleading "nutrition" claims that can be proven harmful to physical health? It is not legal to shout "Fire!" in a crowded theater where no fire exists. Do you think other misinformation that can kill people deserves protection under our First Amendment?

Under our civil laws, it should be possible for a private citizen to recover substantial damages if harmed by reliance upon misinformation purveyed by a self-appointed "nutrition expert." The citizen would need to establish that the "expert" has a duty not to mislead. A licensed physician who recommends a remedy has a duty to use care in selecting it and to warn of complications. A patient harmed because a doctor fails to do either of these things can sue for malpractice. Is it too much to expect that unlicensed promoters of quackery can be held responsible for the harm they do?

A California case has created a precedent that can be cited by anyone who has been harmed by following the advice of a nutrition quack when given in a broadcast. In *Weirum vs. RKO General, Inc.,* the Supreme Court of California upheld a jury verdict of $300,000 against a radio station. The station had offered a cash prize to the first person who could locate a traveling disc jockey. Two teenagers spotted the disc jockey and tried to follow him to a contest stopping point. During the pursuit, one of the cars was forced off the road, killing its driver. The jury found that the broadcast had created a foreseeable risk to motorists because its contest conditions could stimulate accidents. Many radio and television stations which broadcast nutrition quackery have been put on notice by scientists that they are creating an unreasonable risk of harm. Such stations might have serious difficulty defending themselves against suits by injured listeners. So might publishers who ignore warnings about quacky books.

We know of five suits that have been brought against authors and/or publishers of books that contained irresponsible nutrition advice. None of these cases reached a jury that could decide on its merits. Chapter 17 describes three out-of-court settlements brought by parents whose children were harmed during the 1970s by advice in Adelle Davis's book *Let's Have Healthy*

Children. Another suit was brought against the publisher of a diet book by the administrator of the estate of a woman who allegedly died in 1977 after following the book's advice. This case was dismissed by a judge, and the dismissal was upheld by a state court of appeals. The appeals court reasoned that publishers are protected by the First Amendment right to freedom of the press and that a book could not be considered a defective product under the state's tort laws. Another suit, brought against the author and publisher of *The 8-Week Cholesterol Cure*, was settled out of court for an undisclosed sum. The author, Robert E. Kowalski, had recommended megadoses of niacin without making it clear that lack of close medical supervision would be hazardous. Dr. Barrett, who served as an expert witness, believes that the plaintiff would have prevailed if this case had gone to trial.

The law with respect to supplement products is much clearer. Many cases have been won by victims (or their survivors) who charged that a supplement or herbal product was unsafe or was negligently or improperly prescribed. The National Council Against Health Fraud's task force on victim redress offers help to people who have been seriously harmed by a quack practice.

The Role of the Court System

Our court system also plays an important role in regulating nutrition-related quackery, because judges and sometimes juries must decide how to interpret the laws and penalize lawbreakers. Several types of situations undermine efforts to control quackery:

- Court delays often work to the advantage of lawbreakers, especially in the appeals process. Companies under fire from the FDA, for example, may be permitted to continue selling bogus products until all appeals have been exhausted. Practitioners facing revocation of their license often remain in practice for many years while appealing their case through the courts.
- In some cases, courts have ordered insurance companies to pay for dubious treatment. In others, courts have refused to order parents to see to it that their children receive reliable treatment; several deaths have been reported among children with cancer whose parents discontinued or failed to utilize conventional treatment.
- In quackery-related cases where criminal convictions are obtained, sentencing tends to be light.

Greater Accountability Would Help

Consumer protection would probably be improved if the FTC, FDA, Postal Service, and state regulatory agencies were forced to be more accountable. As far as we know, none of them has ever revealed meaningful statistics about the number of health frauds they have detected and what percentage they have acted against. Statistics of this type would enable legislators and the public to see the magnitude of the problem and what might be done about it.

We believe that all agencies charged with protecting the public from health frauds and quackery should be required to make meaningful data available on what they are doing about them. This could be accomplished by maintaining a list of prosecutions, both in progress and completed, that is accessible year-round through each agency's public information office and is published at least once a year in a report to Congress (or, in the case of state agencies, to the state legislature). The report should include tabulations of the number of health-related complaints received, the number judged valid, and the number subjected to regulatory action. The agencies should also be required to recommend improvements in the law that might enable them to work more effectively.

To encourage the reporting of health frauds, a share of any penalties assessed could be given to the complainant and/or nonprofit groups involved in fighting health frauds. To promote public awareness, the records of out-of-court settlements involving health frauds should not be sealed unless a court determines that the public interest would be served by doing so.

Caution Is Needed!

Quite frankly, we are not optimistic that any of the consumer protection measures we recommend in this chapter will be carried out in the United States in the foreseeable future. In fact, an opposite trend is apparent. Although quackery is increasing, too many government officials do not see it as a serious problem that deserves priority.

This book should enable you to recognize which sources of nutrition information are not reliable. Ultimately, your best protection will be your own good sense. If the vast majority of American physicians wouldn't use a particular product or service or recommend it to their loved ones, you shouldn't either. A reasonable level of caution plus guidance from reliable sources should protect you from being victimized.

22

Where to Get Reliable Nutrition Advice

In most professions, educational standards are controlled by licensing laws that protect the public. But in nutrition, anyone who so chooses can declare himself (or herself) an "expert." We have already discussed the training (or lack of it) of phonies. This chapter tells how real experts are trained and how you can get reliable advice. It also tells where to complain about questionable products and promotions.

If you have a question about nutrition, the most convenient person to ask is probably your own physician. Doctors are often accused of not knowing much about nutrition. This charge usually comes from food faddists and vitamin pushers who would like everyone to believe that they are the experts while physicians are nutrition illiterates. It also comes from patients who are disappointed when their doctors correctly inform them that "supernutrition" is not the key to "superhealth" and that "some is good" does not mean "more is better." Nutrition, after all, is part of medicine, not a substitute for it.

Most physicians know what nutrients can and cannot do and can tell the difference between nutrition truths and quack nonsense. A doctor who is unable or too busy to answer questions you have about meal planning can refer you to a qualified professional—usually a registered dietitian.

Respectable Credentials

Many accredited universities offer nutrition courses based on scientific principles and taught by qualified instructors. A bachelor's degree requires four years of full-time study which qualify a graduate for entry-level positions in dietetics or food service, often in a hospital. A masters degree in nutrition, which can widen career opportunities and improve chances for advancement, requires two more years of full-time study beyond the undergraduate level. People who wish to become nutrition researchers usually pursue a Ph.D. in biochemistry. This requires a minimum of two years of additional study plus a thesis based on original laboratory research. Those wishing to concentrate on teaching or educational research usually seek the degrees of Ph.D. or Ed.D. in nutrition education. A nutrition education dissertation will be less oriented toward laboratory research than one in science, but must still provide an original contribution to the field of nutrition education. With few exceptions, a nutrition-related degree from an accredited university signifies a broad background in nutrition science and a thorough grasp of nutritional concepts.

In addition to an academic degree, most legitimate nutritionists seek professional certification. There are two professional associations that are restricted to qualified nutrition scientists. Active membership in the American Institute of Nutrition (AIN) is open to respected scientists who have published meritorious original research on some aspect of nutrition, who are presently working in the field, and who are sponsored by two AIN members. Nominees are considered by a membership committee, a council of officers, and the membership. The clinical arm of AIN is the American Society for Clinical Nutrition (ASCN), which has similar requirements but specifies clinical research. All ASCN members are also members of AIN, and about 70 percent of them are physicians. These requirements, plus an enforceable code of professional responsibility, make it highly unlikely that a promoter of quackery will become (or remain) a member of either of these organizations.

Nutritionists at the doctoral level may also seek certification by the American Board of Nutrition as specialists in clinical nutrition (M.D.s only) or human nutrition sciences (M.D.s and Ph.D.s). To obtain this credential, they must pass both written and oral examinations on a wide range of topics, including deficiency diseases, toxicity of excess vitamins, metabolism, food-drug interactions, therapeutic diets, and the significance of the Recommended Dietary Allowances. Currently there are about three hundred board-certified nutrition specialists in the United States., Most are affiliated with medical schools and hospitals, where they conduct clinical research and offer consultation to primary-care physicians.

Registered dietitians (R.D.s) are specially trained to translate nutrition research into healthful, tasty diets. Compared to physicians, they usually know less about basic biochemistry, physiology and metabolism, but more about the nutrient content of specific foods. The R.D. certification is available to bachelor- and master-level nutrition graduates as well as to holders of a Ph.D., degree. To qualify, they must have appropriate professional experience and pass a comprehensive written test covering all aspects of nutrition and food-service management. To maintain their credential, they must also participate regularly in continuing-education programs approved by the American Dietetic Association (ADA). Most of the country's 55,000 active R.D.s work in hospitals. Typically, they counsel patients and conduct classes for pregnant women, heart and kidney patients, diabetics, and other persons with special dietary needs. Dietitians are also employed by community agencies such as geriatric, day care, and drug/alcohol abuse centers. Some dietitians do research. Others engage in private practice where they counsel physician-referred clients. The ADA also has a certification process for advanced-level practitioners and for specialists in renal (kidney), pediatric, and metabolic nutrition.

About half of the states have licensing or certification for dietitians and/or nutritionists. While holding such a credential is a positive sign, in some states the standards are not high enough to prevent unqualified individuals from becoming licensed.

How to Write for Help

Many organizations evaluate and publish accurate information about nutrition. Some serve and communicate primarily with health and nutrition professionals, while others communicate primarily with the public. Should you write to any of them for information, keep in mind that the individual who receives your letter is likely to be extremely busy. You will be most likely to get a helpful response if you do the following:

- Type your letter to assure legibility. Make sure your return address is on the letter as well as the envelope, and include your telephone number.
- Ask your question as specifically as possible.
- Tell something about yourself and why you need the information. Indicate briefly what you already know or have read.
- Enclose a stamped, self-addressed envelope large enough to accommodate what might be sent.
- If writing to a voluntary organization, consider making a small donation if you can afford one.

Government Agencies

The Food and Drug Administration will answer inquiries and offers a variety of educational materials about nutrition and nutritional quackery. Its consumer affairs offices in more than twenty-five major cities can furnish speakers for interested groups. The FDA is also interested in receiving complaints about food-supplement products marketed with false claims or inadequate directions for use. Its address is 5600 Fishers Lane, Rockville, MD 20857.

• The Postal Service can act against products sold through the mails with false claims. From time to time, it issues publications about detecting frauds. Complaints about questionable mail-order promotions should be sent to the Fraud Division, Chief U.S. Postal Inspector, Washington, DC 20260.

• The Federal Trade Commission has jurisdiction over advertising which is false or misleading. It issues brochures on consumer strategy, a few of which discuss health and nutrition issues. Complaints about false ads should be addressed to the FTC Bureau of Consumer Protection, Washington, DC 20580.

• The U.S. Department of Agriculture, which developed the concept of basic food groups so important to the teaching of sound nutrition, can answer questions and provide literature on nutrition and diet. Its Food and Nutrition Information Center, located at the National Agricultural Library, Beltsville, MD 20705, can be reached by calling 301-504-5414. The USDA Meat and Poultry Hotline, which answers questions about food safety, can be reached at 800-535-4555.

• The Agriculture Extension Service of each land-grant university can answer questions about nutrition. Home economists at USDA county cooperative extension services can answer questions about food preparation. Your local telephone directory (blue pages) can tell you if your community has either of these two services available.

• The Department of Health and Human Services (DHHS) has several nutrition services. Its Administration on Children, Youth and Families (ACYF) administers the Head Start Program and develops nutrition education materials and services for parents of low-income families. The address of its central office is P.O. Box 1182, Washington, DC 20013. Contact with local Head Start programs can be made through local school systems. DHHS's Administration on Aging provides services to persons age sixty or older. Its national and regional offices provide publications and other information. They also make referrals to state and local offices that provide group meals, home-delivered meals, and nutrition education. The national office is located at 330 Independence Ave., S.W., Washington, DC 20201. Additional publications are available from the Health Services Administration of the U.S. Public Health Service,

Washington, DC 20201, and the U.S. Government Printing Office, Pueblo, CO 81009.

• The National Health Information Clearinghouse, P.O. Box 1133, Washington, DC 20013, can refer callers to sources of information on its list. Caution: Although most of its sources are reputable, the list includes a few groups involved in unscientific nutrition practices.

• The National Institute for Dental Research, the National Institute for Allergy and Infectious Diseases, the National Cancer Institute, the National Institute of Arthritis, Metabolism and Digestive Diseases, and the National Institute of Child Health and Human Development, all have educational material about nutrition as it applies to their areas of interest. Their address is 9000 Rockville Pike, Bethesda, MD 20892.

• State health departments and some local health departments can be excellent sources of information about nutrition.

Scientific and Professional Organizations

• The American Academy of Allergy and Immunology issues position papers related to food allergies and to questionable methods of diagnosis and treatment. Its address is 611 E. Wells St., Milwaukee, WI 53202.

• The American Institute of Nutrition and the American Society for Clinical Nutrition, both mentioned above, are located at 9650 Rockville Pike, Bethesda, MD 20814. ASCN publishes the *American Journal of Clinical Nutrition*, the most widely respected clinical nutrition journal.

• The American Dietetic Association has a variety of publications and will answer questions. Its address is 216 W. Jackson Blvd., Chicago, IL 60606. State and local dietetic associations are usually eager to be helpful. Dial-A-Dietitian services are available in a number of cities.

• The American Dental Association's Office of Public Information can answer questions about nutrition that pertain to dental health. Its address is 211 E. Chicago Ave., Chicago, IL 60611.

• The American Medical Association publishes reports on responsible and questionable practices through its Council on Scientific Affairs and other channels. Its address is 515 N. State St., Chicago, IL 60610. The AMA has published an excellent book on "alternative" methods, but it does not investigate them on a regular basis (see final section of this chapter).

• The Institute of Food Technologists issues scientific summaries and position papers on topics related to food processing. Its address is 221 N. LaSalle St., Chicago, IL 60601. IFT also has food-science communicators available for media interviews in more than forty cities.

• The International Life Sciences Institute publishes monographs and books related to various nutrition topics. Its address is 1126 16th St., N.W., Washington, DC 20036.

• The National Center for Nutrition and Dietetics, an affiliate of the American Dietetic Association, maintains a toll-free hotline to answer questions about nutrition and make referrals to registered dietitians. Its number is 800-366-1655.

• Many accredited colleges and medical schools with nutrition departments are excellent sources of information.

Voluntary Agencies

Many voluntary agencies provide reliable information about nutrition and quack practices related to their areas of special interest. Most notable are:

- American Cancer Society, 1599 Clifton Road, N.E., Atlanta, GA 30329
- American Diabetes Association, 1660 Duke St., Alexandria, VA 22314
- American Heart Association, 7370 Greenville Ave., Dallas, TX 75231
- Arthritis Foundation, 1314 Spring St., N.W., Atlanta, GA 30309
- Asthma and Allergy Foundation of America, 1125 15th St., N.W., Washington, DC 20005
- Juvenile Diabetes Foundation, 432 Park Ave. S., New York, NY 10016
- National Multiple Sclerosis Society, 204 E. 42nd St., New York, NY 10017

Consumer Protection Organizations

• The American Council on Science and Health (ACSH) has a special interest in chemical and nutritional issues in our lives. Membership, open to anyone, costs $50/year. Several times a year, ACSH publishes reports based upon thorough review of current scientific evidence on particular topics. It also publishes a quarterly magazine (*Priorities*) and maintains a speakers bureau. Its address is 1995 Broadway, New York, NY 10023.

• Better Business Bureaus located in many cities can sometimes provide information about products sold with nutrition or health claims. The Council of Better Business Bureaus's national office is located at 1515 Wilson Blvd., Arlington, VA 22209. The National Advertising Division occasionally exerts pressure on companies that cannot justify questionable claims made in national advertising (see Chapter 18). Its address is 845 3rd Ave., New York, NY 10017.

• Consumer Health Information Research Institute (CHIRI), operated by

John H. Renner, M.D., answers questions related to health frauds and quackery. Its address is 300 Pinkhill Road, Independence, MO 64057 (telephone 816-753-8850).

• The National Council Against Health Fraud (NCAHF), Inc., investigates questionable methods, publishes a bimonthly newsletter and occasional position papers, conducts seminars, and maintains a speakers bureau. Information about NCAHF membership, which costs $20 to $30/year, can be obtained by writing to William T. Jarvis, Ph.D., P.O. Box 1276, Loma Linda, CA 92354, or phoning 909-824-4690. The council also maintains a Task Force on Victim Redress, which provides information and legal guidance to people who have been seriously harmed by quackery or health fraud. It is chaired by Dr. Stephen Barrett, who can be contacted at P.O. Box 1747, Allentown, PA 18105 (telephone 610-437-1795).

The table on the following page indicates where you can complain or seek help for a problem related to quackery or health fraud. Where more than one regulatory agency appears to have jurisdiction, complain to each one,

A Special Plea to the American Medical Association

Quackery proponents often portray the American Medical Association (AMA) as their major enemy. The fact is, however, that the primary political concerns of both the AMA and the majority of its members are excessive paperwork and government intrusion into medical practices.

The AMA is still the leading publisher of scientific health information. For many years, it maintained a Committee on Quackery and a fully-staffed Department of Investigation that monitored and reported on many questionable practices in the health-care marketplace. In 1975, however, these activities were abolished—along with many others—when the AMA underwent a financial crisis. Since that time, it has issued a few quackery-related reports through its Council on Scientific Affairs and its Diagnostic and Therapeutic Technology Assessment (DATTA) process. The *Journal of the American Medical Association* also provides valuable but infrequent reports. The AMA's *Reader's Guide to "Alternative" Health Methods*, co-authored by Dr. Barrett and published in 1993, is the most comprehensive reference book on quackery-related literature ever published.

Although these activities are laudable, the AMA: (1) has no official position on the majority of "alternative" health practices, (2) does not have a single spokesperson who is well informed in these matters and authorized to deal with inquiries from journalists, and (3) has no mechanism through which it can monitor the marketplace and develop a plan for dealing with health frauds and quackery. Nor do its primary news outlets (*American Medical News* and American Medical Television) keep physicians informed about the serious problems we describe in this book.

We believe that the AMA has the intellectual and financial resources to correct this situation—and that it should do so. In 1993, at Barrett's urging, the Pennsylvania Medical Society passed a resolution urging the AMA to: (1)

Where to Complain or Seek Help

Problem	Agencies to Contact
False advertising	FTC Bureau of Consumer Protection Regional FTC office National Advertising Division, Council of Better Business Bureaus Editor or station manager of media outlet where ad appeared
Product marketed with false or misleading claims	National or regional FDA office State attorney general State health department Local Better Business Bureau Congressional representatives
Bogus mail-order promotion	Chief Postal Inspector, U.S. Postal Service Regional Postal Inspector State attorney general Editor or station manager of media outlet where ad appeared
Improper treatment by licensed practitioner	Local or state professional society (if practitioner is a member) Local hospital (if practitioner is a staff member) State professional licensing board National Council Against Health Fraud Task Force on Victim Redress
Improper treatment by unlicensed individual	Local district attorney State attorney general National Council Against Health Fraud Task Force on Victim Redress
Advice needed about questionable product or service	National Council Against Health Fraud Consumer Health Information Research Institute Local, state, or national professional or voluntary health groups

establish a Committee on "Alternative" Health Methods, whose functions would be to gather, interpret, and disseminate accurate information; (2) identify and/or develop expert spokespersons who can speak publicly about these methods; and (3) invite physicians from a broad spectrum of health organizations and regulatory agencies to participate on the committee. However, the AMA House of Delegates did not adopt the resolution, citing concerns about cost and the belief that the Council on Scientific Affairs was involved in this area. The council's staff then drafted a position paper on "alternative" methods, but the council quietly mothballed it.

We don't know how much the balance of power would be shifted toward science and consumer protection if the AMA became more involved in the war against quackery. But we'd sure like to find out!

23

How You Can Avoid Getting Quacked

Most people think of themselves as hard to fool. Few people consider themselves vulnerable to quackery. Yet quackery is thriving. This chapter summarizes our advice on how to avoid becoming its victim.

• *The key point is to stay away from tricksters.* Don't make the mistake of thinking you can read an unreliable publication, visit a health-food store, or consult an "alternative" practitioner and sort out any legitimate ideas from the rest. Nobody can do this with 100 percent certainty. Note the signs of quackery identified in Chapters 2 and 3 of this book. If you encounter them, head elsewhere for your advice. Appendix E lists reliable publications.

• *Remember that quackery seldom looks outlandish.* Its promoters often use scientific terms and quote (or misquote) from scientific references. Some actually have reputable scientific training but have gone astray.

• *Ignore anyone who maintains that most diseases are caused by faulty nutrition or can be remedied by taking supplements.* Although some diseases are related to diet, most are not. Moreover, in most cases where diet actually is a factor in a person's health problem, the solution is not to take vitamins but to alter the diet.

• *Be wary of fad diagnoses.* Some practitioners seem to specialize in the diagnosis and treatment of problems considered rare or even nonexistent by responsible practitioners. Years ago, hypothyroidism and adrenal insufficiency were in vogue. Today's "fad" diagnoses are "environmental illness" (also called "multiple chemical sensitivity"), "candidiasis hypersensitivity," "parasites," "Wilson's syndrome," and "mercury-amalgam toxicity." Chronic fatigue syndrome, while not rare, is also being overdiagnosed by unscientific practitioners. Be wary, too, of anyone who says that food allergies can cause hyperactive behavior or a myriad of health problems. Claims of this type are being made by bogus nutritionists, "clinical ecologists," and various other "alternative" practitioners. These subjects are discussed in Chapters 7 and 12.

• *Don't take action based solely on an anecdote or testimonial.* If someone claims to have been helped by an unconventional remedy, ask yourself and possibly your doctor whether there might be another explanation. Even if someone actually was helped by an offbeat method, you can't tell how many others who did the same thing were not helped. Nor can one person's experience enable you (or them) to distinguish between cause-and-effect and coincidence. Moreover, some anecdotes and testimonials are complete fabrications.

• *Be skeptical of talk-show guests and hosts who discuss nutrition.* The number of individuals promoting quackery through the airwaves greatly exceeds the number opposing it. Don't assume that anybody screens talk-show guests (or hosts) to see whether their opinions are well founded. The primary interest of most hosts and producers is to increase the size of their viewing or listening audience so they can attract more advertising dollars.

• *Be wary of products and practices described as "natural," "nontoxic," "holistic," "complementary," and/or "alternative."* These are the buzzwords of the quack.

• *Avoid multilevel organizations like the plague.* We've looked closely at more than forty of them. In every case, the income opportunity was exaggerated and the health-related products were either useless, overpriced, and/or inappropriate for self-medication. Nor are the people who distribute multilevel products qualified to give health advice.

• *Don't read magazines that are loaded with ads for supplement products.* We refer to these as "health-food magazines" because they deliberately promote the ingredients in the products advertised. The number of supplement ads is a rough indicator of the quality of a magazine's contents. The more ads, the worse the editorial contents. Reliable publications attract few supplement ads, and the best publications won't run them.

• *Don't buy "nutrition insurance" unless you need it.* Most people who eat a variety of foods get all the nutrients they need from their diet. If you think your diet may be deficient, analyze it by recording what you eat for several days and comparing the number of portions of food in the various food groups with those recommended in Appendix A of this book. If you don't feel comfortable doing this yourself, ask a registered dietitian or physician to help you. If you have a shortfall, try to correct it by adjusting your diet. If this is impossible and you conclude that you need a supplement, use the suggestions at the end of Chapter 3 to guide your purchase.

• *Don't play nutrition roulette!* The health-food industry markets more than twenty thousand "supplement" products. Most are worthless, and some are dangerous. The few that are useful (such as niacin for cholesterol control) are not appropriate for self-medication but should be taken under responsible medical supervision. And remember that health-food stores are centers of misinformation.

• *Don't join the "supplement-of-the-month club."* It seems that hardly a month goes by without some new "supplement" concoction being marketed. Some are based on misinterpretation of preliminary experimental findings. Some are just the result of the manufacturer's wild imagination. The likelihood of a "breakthrough" product emerging from within the health-food industry is approximately zero. If you are tempted to buy its latest fad, ask your doctor instead.

• *Never patronize a practitioner who prescribes vitamins to most patients or who sells vitamins in his/her office.* One of the surest signs of quackery is the selling of vitamins in one's practice. Avoid any practitioner—licensed or not—who does this. Scientific practitioners do not sell vitamins. Unscientific practitioners often do—at two to three times their cost. The most common offenders in this regard are chiropractors and bogus "nutritionists." You should also be wary of physicians who give B_{12} shots to large numbers of patients. Periodic B_{12} injections are appropriate when intestinal absorption of this vitamin is impaired—as happens in pernicious anemia. But some doctors prescribe them for fatigue and many other conditions for which there is no objective benefit.

• *Don't buy homeopathic remedies.* Remember that they are not approved by the FDA but merely tolerated. They have no proven effectiveness, and few have even been tested.

• *Remember that very few herbs have practical value.* Herbs are promoted primarily through literature based on hearsay, folklore, and tradition. As medical science developed, it became apparent that most herbs did not deserve good reputations, and most that did were replaced by synthetic compounds that are more effective. Many herbs contain hundreds or even thousands of chemicals that have not been completely cataloged. While some may turn out to be useful, others could well prove toxic. With safe and effective treatment available, treatment with herbs rarely makes sense. Moreover, many of the conditions for which herbs are recommended are not suitable for self-treatment.

• *Ignore diets or diet products promised to make you lose more than a pound or two per week.* While crash diets can provide faster initial weight loss, they may also lack important nutrients, may injure health, and do not help people learn to readjust their long-range eating habits. Most nutritionists recommend a low-calorie, low-fat, balanced diet plus an exercise program, with a weight-loss goal of one to one and a half pounds a week. For most people, successful weight-control requires a lifelong commitment to a change in lifestyle, eating habits, and dietary practices. No matter how much weight you want to lose, modest goals and a slow course will maximize the possibility of both losing the weight and keeping it off. Many people who go on a crash diet gain back more than the amount lost during the crash.

• *Never buy a "nutritional" product by mail because of claims you read about it in an ad.* During the past twenty-five years, neither of us has encountered a product of this type that was legitimate. The most common ones are "miracle" diet pills, all of which are fakes. Others include vitamins and/or other substances promised to relieve your arthritis, make you look younger, thicken your hair, extend your life, increase your energy, or make you a better athlete. No mail-order pill can do any of these things. Most are harmless but some are not, and all are a waste of money.

• *Remember that no single test can determine the body's nutritional state.* Genuine nutrition assessments include a dietary history and a physical examination to look for signs of malnutrition. Most people who require such assessments are seriously (and obviously) ill. When a hair analysis, blood chemistry profile, "allergy" test, muscle test, eye examination, or questionnaire is used as the basis for recommending dietary supplements, you can be sure the recommendation is inappropriate.

• *Don't buy "special" vitamins or a "water-purifier" over the phone.* If you receive a call or a piece of mail announcing that you have won a prize, don't bother responding. Offers like this are invariably "boiler room" scams whose participants ply their trade at a telephone bank set up for the purpose of conning people. State attorneys general have received complaints about hundreds of scams whose victims were told that to collect the "prize" they must spend hundreds of dollars for some item. Such prizes are virtually worthless, the purchased items are grossly overpriced, and the "money back guarantee" is an empty promise. Many people who fall for these schemes receive nothing at all.

• *Don't fall for paranoid accusations.* Unscientific practitioners typically claim that the medical profession, drug companies, and the government are conspiring to suppress whatever method they espouse. No evidence to support such a theory has ever been demonstrated. It also flies in the face of logic to believe that large numbers of people would oppose the development of treatment methods that might someday help themselves or their loved ones.

• *Follow a healthy lifestyle.* To protect your health, do what really matters: (1) don't use tobacco products, (2) eat a balanced diet, (3) maintain a reasonable weight, (4) exercise appropriately, (5) don't abuse alcohol, (6) wear a safety belt while driving, and (7) have in your home at least one smoke detector whose signal can arouse you from sleep.

• *Maintain a reasonable level of skepticism.* Don't jump on the bandwagon and try a nutrition-related product just because you hear about it on a broadcast or in a newspaper, magazine, or book. The news media often report preliminary research findings without placing them in proper perspective. Their favorite during the past two years has been "antioxidants" (see Chapter 8). If a news report tempts you, check it out with a trustworthy health professional.

• *Use the services of a reliable primary physician.* The best way to take advantage of modern medical science is to establish a relationship with a doctor you can trust—preferably before you become ill. Your best bet is a board-certified family practitioner or internist affiliated with a teaching hospital. A trustworthy physician can steer you toward high-quality medical care and away from frauds and quackery. Have periodic physical and laboratory examinations as recommended by your doctor and keep your immunizations up-to-date.

• *Don't let desperation cloud your judgment.* If you feel that your doctor isn't doing enough to help you, or if you have been told that your condition is incurable and don't wish to accept this fate without a struggle, don't stray from scientific health care in a desperate attempt to find a solution. Instead, discuss your feelings with your doctor and consider a consultation with someone whom the medical community considers to be a leading expert. Many people have published stories about how they found a "cure" after doctors said they had no hope of recovery from a serious illness. Among the many cases we have been able to check, not one such story proved true.

• *Support stronger consumer protection laws.* Although quackery will never be driven completely from the marketplace, it can be diminished by stronger laws and more vigorous enforcement.

A Brief "Success" Story

Some years ago, a reader of an antiquackery book sent the following letter:

> Gentlemen: I've just finished reading "The Health Robbers" and found it to be quite an eye-opener. I've been interested in nutrition for the past three years or so, spurred on by chronic fatigue and encouraging friends. Naturally, I've been ingesting food supplements by the handful, reading *Prevention* and related books, worrying about "harmful" things in my family's diet, and getting all kinds of static from my kids. Recently I determined to try to find out what is the right course to pursue, nutritionally, for my family and me, and yours was the first book I came across in the library relative to my search. I believe what

> it says and have experienced a definite sense of release after reading it. Yesterday I put all my vitamin bottles away and I don't mind telling you it was scary! (Is this whole movement based on fear?)

It certainly is. Nutrition misinformation is deeply ingrained in our society. But if you have the courage to live in the real world, this book can help you find it.

A Final Comment

This book was written to protect you from being victimized by vitamin pushers. We hope it will also arouse you to take action. If you have been helped by this book, please do the following:

- Recommend it to others.
- Urge your local school and public libraries to obtain copies.
- Ask the editors of publications to which you subscribe to review the book.
- Ask local talk-show hosts to invite us, or other people who talk responsibly about nutrition, to be guests on their programs. Responsible scientists can be obtained through the American Institute of Nutrition, American Society for Clinical Nutrition, American Council on Science and Health, American Dietetic Association, Institute of Food Technologists, National Council Against Health Fraud, and other organizations and agencies listed in Chapter 22 of this book.
- Report questionable health matters to appropriate federal agencies, to your Congressional representatives, and to us. Chapter 22 tells where to complain.
- Remember that NCAHF's Task Force on Victim Redress offers a free medicolegal analysis to determine whether victims of quackery have grounds for legal action.
- Keep up-to-date on nutrition quackery by joining the National Council Against Health Fraud and subscribing to *Nutrition Forum* (described in Appendix E).

Remember, in matters of health there should be no tolerance for deception. Your effort in opposing quackery may save many people from being hurt—and may even save a life!

Appendix A

Guidelines for Healthful Eating

These guidelines, developed by the United States Departments of Agriculture and Health and Human Services and presented here in modified form, describe the kinds and amounts of foods that make up a nutritious diet. They let you make the choices to fit your eating style and needs.

The first section of this guide provides seven guidelines for a healthful diet—advice for healthy Americans two years of age or more. By following these guidelines, you can promote good health and reduce your chances of getting certain diseases. These guidelines are the best, most up-to-date advice from responsible nutrition scientists and are the basis of Federal nutrition policy.

The second section divides commonly eaten foods into five groups according to the nutritional contributions they make. By following it, you'll be choosing foods adequate in all nutrients and appropriate in calorie content.

More complete discussions of these guidelines are available in "Nutrition and Your Health: Dietary Guidelines for Americans" (HG-232) and "USDA's Food Guide Pyramid" (HG-249). Both booklets can be obtained from Consumer Information Center, P.O. Box 100, Pueblo, CO 81002.

General Guidelines

1. *Eat a variety of foods* to get the energy, protein, vitamins, minerals, fatty acids, phytochemicals, and fiber you need for good health.

2. *Maintain healthy weight* to reduce your chances of having high blood

pressure, heart disease, a stroke, certain cancers, and the most common type of diabetes.

3. *Choose a diet low in fat, saturated fat, and cholesterol* to reduce your risk of heart attack and certain types of cancer. Because fat contains over twice the calories of an equal amount of carbohydrates or protein, a diet low in fat can help you maintain a healthy weight. Have your blood cholesterol tested and interpreted by a physician, and adjust your diet accordingly

4. *Choose a diet with plenty of vegetables, fruits, and grain products* which provide needed vitamins, minerals, fiber, complex carbohydrates, and phytochemicals, and can help you lower your intake of fat.

5. *Use sugars in moderation.* A diet high in sugars may have too many calories and too few nutrients and contribute to tooth decay. However, most people who meet the guidelines for numbers of servings and overall fat content do not have to worry about how much sugar they consume.

6. *Use salt and high-sodium foods in moderation* to help reduce your risk of high blood pressure.

7. *If you drink alcoholic beverages, do so in moderation.* Alcoholic beverages supply calories, but few or no nutrients. Drinking alcohol is also the cause of many health problems and accidents and can lead to addiction.

Daily Food Guide

The Food Guide Pyramid in Chapter 1 emphasizes foods from five food groups. Each of these groups provides some, but not all, of the nutrients people need. For good health it is advisable to consume foods from all of the groups. A sixth category—fats, oils, and sweets—is represented by the small tip of the pyramid. Foods in this category provide calories and little else and should be used sparingly by most people.

How many servings per day from each food group?

The recommended number of servings depends on how many calories you need, which in turn depends on your age, sex, size, and how active you are. Almost everyone should have at least the lowest number of servings in the ranges, except when a reliably diagnosed genetic disorder dictates otherwise.

The following calorie level suggestions are based on recommendations of the National Academy of Sciences and on calorie intakes reported by people in national food-consumption surveys.

For adults and teens

1600 calories is about right for many sedentary women and some older adults.
2200 calories is about right for most children, teenage girls, active women, and many sedentary men. Women who are pregnant or breastfeeding may need somewhat more.
2800 calories is about right for teenage boys, many active men, and some very active women.

For young children

It is hard to know how much food children need to grow normally. If you're unsure, check with your doctor. Preschool children need the same variety of foods as older family members do, but may need less than 1,600 calories. For fewer calories, they can eat smaller servings. However, it is important that they have the equivalent of two cups of milk a day.

For you

The table below tells how many servings you need for your calorie level. For example, if you are an active woman who needs about 2,200 calories a day, nine servings of bread, cereals, rice, or pasta would be right for you. You'd also want to eat about six ounces of meat or alternates per day. If you are between calorie categories, estimate servings. For example, some less active women may need only two thousand calories to maintain a healthy weight. At that calorie level, eight servings of bread would be about right.

Number of Daily Portions from Each Food Group for People Who Consume 1600, 2200 or 2,800 Calories per Day

Calorie Level	1600	2200	2,800
Bread Group Servings	6	9	11
Vegetable Group Servings	3	4	5
Fruit Group Servings	2	3	4
Meat Group (Ounces)	2–3	2–3	2–3
Milk Group Servings*	5	6	7

*Women who are pregnant or breastfeeding, teenagers, and young adults to age twenty-four need three servings.

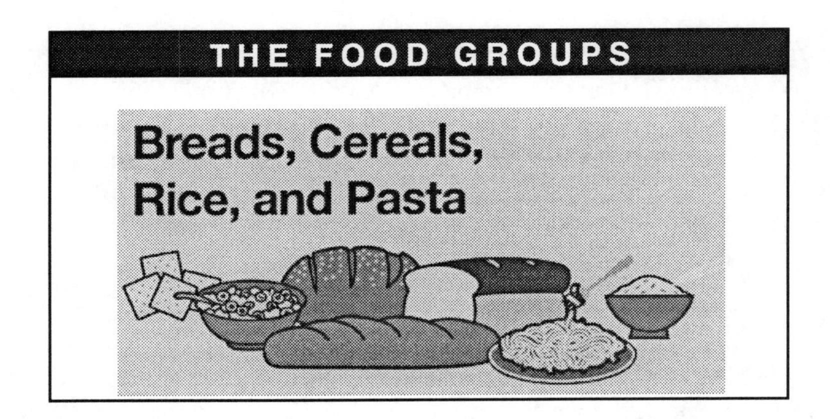

These foods provide complex carbohydrates (starches), which are an important source of energy, especially in low-fat diets. They also provide vitamins, minerals, and fiber. The Food Guide Pyramid suggests six to eleven servings of these foods a day.

What counts as a serving?

- 1 slice of bread
- 1 ounce of ready-to-eat cereal
- $^{1}/_{2}$ cup of cooked cereal, rice, or pasta

Aren't starchy foods fattening?

No. It's what you add to these foods or cook with them that adds most of the calories. For example: margarine or butter on bread, cream or cheese sauces on pasta, and the sugar and fat used with the flour in making cookies.

Selection tips

- To get the fiber you need, choose several servings a day of foods made from whole grains, such as whole-wheat bread and whole-grain cereals.
- Choose most often foods that are made with little fat or sugars. These include bread, English muffins, rice, and pasta.
- Baked goods made from flour, such as cakes, cookies, croissants, and pastries, count as part of this food group, but they are high in fat and sugars.
- Go easy on the fat and sugars you add as spreads, seasonings, or toppings.
- When preparing pasta, stuffing, and sauce from packaged mixes, use only half the butter or margarine suggested; if milk or cream is called for, use low-fat milk.

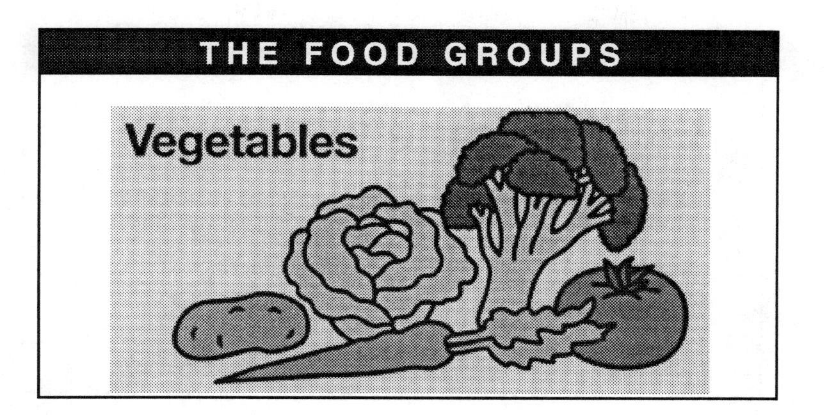

Vegetables provide vitamins, such as vitamins A and C, and folate, and minerals, such as iron and magnesium. They are naturally low in fat and also provide fiber. The Food Guide Pyramid suggests three to five servings of these foods a day.

What counts as a serving?

- 1 cup of raw leafy vegetables
- 1/2 cup of other vegetables, cooked or chopped raw
- 3/4 cup of vegetable juice

Selection tips

- Different types of vegetables provide different nutrients. For variety eat:
  dark-green leafy vegetables (spinach, romaine lettuce, broccoli)
  deep-yellow vegetables (carrots, sweet potatoes)
  starchy vegetables (potatoes, corn, peas)
  legumes (navy, pinto, and kidney beans, chickpeas)
  other vegetables (lettuce, tomatoes, onions, green beans).
- Include dark-green leafy vegetables and legumes several times a week—they are especially good sources of vitamins and minerals. Legumes also provide protein and can be used in place of meat (but contain no vitamin B_{12}).
- Go easy on the fat you add to vegetables at the table or during cooking. Added spreads or toppings, such as butter, mayonnaise, and salad dressing, count as fat.
- Use low-fat salad dressing.

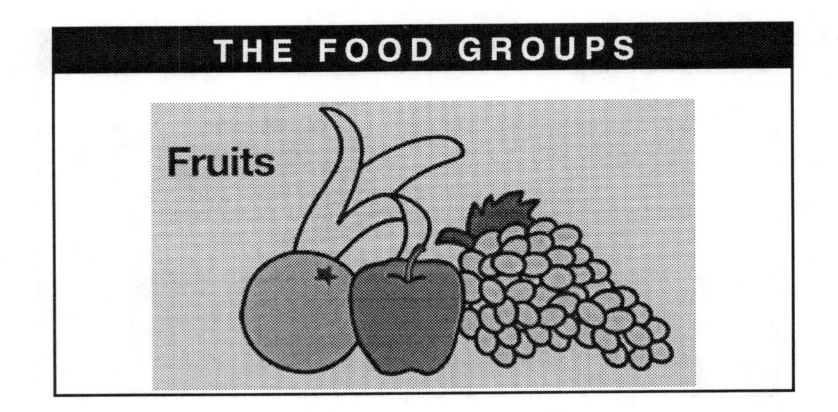

Fruits and fruit juices provide important amounts of vitamins A and C and potassium. They are low in fat and sodium. The Food Guide Pyramid suggests two to four servings of fruits a day.

What counts as a serving?

- 1 medium apple, banana, or orange
- 1/2 cup of chopped, cooked, or canned fruit
- 3/4 cup of fruit juice

Selection tips:

- Choose fresh fruits, fruit juices, and frozen, canned, or dried fruit. Pass up fruit canned or frozen in heavy syrups and sweetened fruit juices unless you have calories to spare.
- Eat whole fruits often. They are higher in fiber than fruit juices.
- Have citrus fruits, melons, and berries regularly. They are rich in vitamin C.
- Count only 100 percent fruit juice as fruit. Punches, "ades," and most fruit drinks contain only a little juice and lots of added sugars. The new food labels must disclose the percentage of juice in these fruit beverages. Grape and orange sodas don't count as fruit juice.

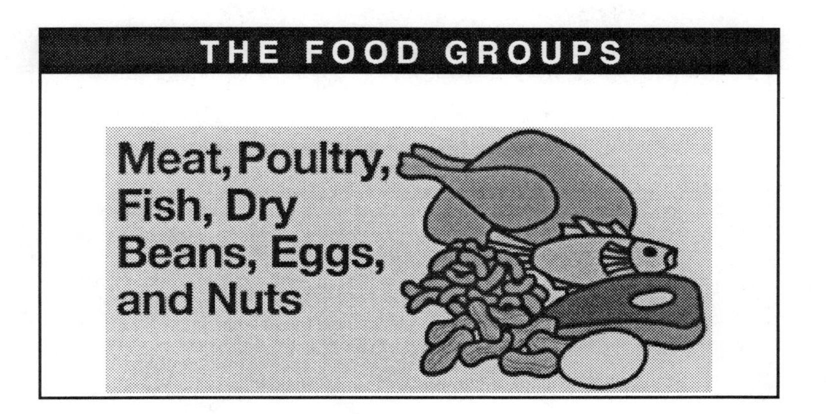

Meat, poultry, and fish supply protein, B vitamins, iron, and zinc. The other foods in this group—dry beans, eggs, and nuts—are similar to meats in providing protein and most vitamins and minerals. The Food Guide Pyramid suggests two to three servings each day of foods from this group. The total amount of these servings should be the equivalent of five to seven ounces of cooked lean meat, poultry, or fish per day.

What counts as a serving?

- Count 2 to 3 ounces of cooked lean meat, poultry, or fish as a serving. A 3-ounce piece of meat is about the size of an average hamburger, or the amount of meat on a medium chicken breast half.
- For other foods in this group, count 1/2 cup of cooked dry beans, 1 egg, or 2 tablespoons of peanut butter as 1 ounce of meat (about 1/3 serving).
- Counting to see if you have an equivalent of 5 to 7 ounces of cooked lean meat a day is tricky. Portion sizes vary with the type of food and meal. For example, 6 ounces might come from: 1 egg (count as 1 oz. of lean meat) for breakfast, 2 ounces of sliced turkey in a sandwich at lunch, and a 3-ounce cooked lean hamburger for dinner.

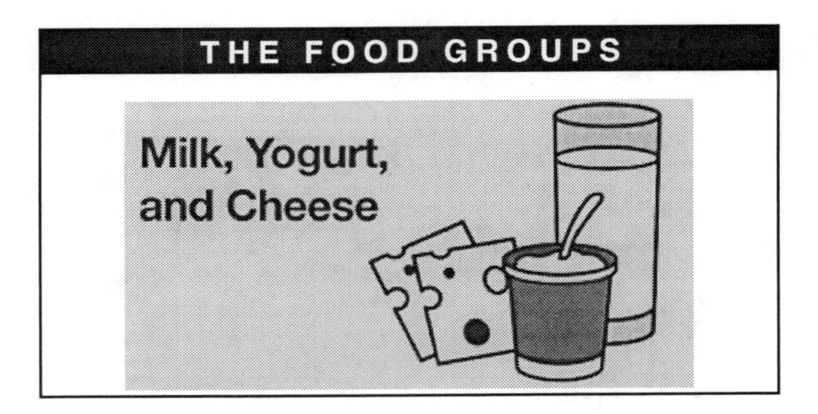

Milk products provide protein, vitamins, and minerals. Milk, yogurt, and cheese are the best sources of calcium. The Food Guide Pyramid suggests two to three servings of milk, yogurt, and cheese a day—two for most people, and three for women who are pregnant or breastfeeding, teenagers, and young adults to age twenty-four.

What counts as a serving?

- 1 cup of milk or yogurt
- $1^1/2$ ounces of natural cheese
- 2 ounces of process cheese

Selection tips

- Choose skim milk and nonfat yogurt often. They are lowest in fat. One and a half to 2 ounces of cheese and 8 ounces of yogurt count as a serving from this group because they supply the same amount of calcium as one cup of milk.
- Cottage cheese is lower in calcium than most cheeses. One cup of cottage cheese counts as only $^1/2$ serving of milk.
- Go easy on high-fat cheese and ice cream. They can add a lot of fat (especially saturated fat) to your diet.
- Choose "part skim" or low-fat cheeses when available and lower-fat milk desserts, like ice milk or frozen yogurt.

Appendix B

The New Food Labels

In 1993, the FDA and the U.S. Department of Agriculture published final regulations providing for consistent, scientifically based labeling for almost all processed foods. These rules, intended to provide more meaningful information about the nutritional value of foods, constitute the most extensive food labeling reform in the country's history. The FDA estimates that about 90 percent of processed food will carry nutrition information. In addition, uniform point-of-purchase nutrition information will accompany many fresh foods, such as fruits, vegetables, raw fish, meat, and poultry. Although this is voluntary, it will be mandated if voluntary compliance is found to be insufficient.

Modern nutrition labeling began in 1974 when the two agencies established voluntary rules and began requiring nutrition information on labels of products that contain added nutrients or that carry nutrition claims. Other than requiring sodium and permitting potassium to be added to the voluntarily listed components, the rules remained essentially unchanged until recently.

Reference Values

The new rules provide a basic format for the nutrition panel ("Nutrition Facts"), which expresses nutrient contents as "% Daily Value." Daily Values combine the information from two sets of reference values—Daily Reference Values (DRVs) and Reference Daily Intakes (RDIs)—neither of which appears on the labels themselves.

The DRVs cover fat, carbohydrate, protein, and fiber, for which no set of standards previously existed. For labeling purposes, 2,000 calories has been established as the reference for calculating percent Daily Values. Where space permits, labels will include information in which selected daily values for both a 2,000- and a 2,500-calorie diet are listed; and manufacturers are permitted to list daily values for other calorie levels. Regardless of calorie level, the DRVs are based on a diet containing 60 percent carbohydrate, 10 percent protein, 30 percent fat (including 10 percent saturated fat), and 11.5 grams of fiber per 1,000 calories. The DRVs for cholesterol, sodium, and potassium remain the same regardless of calorie level.

The RDIs will replace the U.S. RDAs (U.S. Recommended Daily Allowances), which were introduced in 1973 as reference values for vitamins, minerals, and protein in the labeling of foods and drugs. The U.S. RDAs and current RDIs are based on the 1968 Recommended Dietary Allowances (RDAs) set by the National Research Council. The main reason for the change in terminology is to avoid confusion due to the similarity of the terms "RDA" and "U.S. RDA." A second reason is that most of the U.S. RDAs are higher than necessary for most people. Except for protein, however, the actual values will remain the same for the near future.

Sample Label

Serving sizes are intended to reflect the amounts that people actually eat.

The nutrients required on the nutrition panel are those considered most important to the health of today's consumers, most of whom need to worry about getting too much of certain items (such as fat) rather than too few (as was the case years ago with certain vitamins and minerals).

Fats, carbohydrates, and proteins are the nutrients that provide energy (calories).

Nutrition Facts

Serving Size 1/2 cup (114g)
Servings Per Container 4

Amount Per Serving

Calories 260 Calories from Fat 120

	% Daily Value*
Total Fat 13g	**20%**
Saturated Fat 5g	**25%**
Cholesterol 30mg	**10%**
Sodium 660mg	**28%**
Total Carbohydrate 31g	**11%**
Dietary Fiber 0g	**0%**
Sugars 5g	
Protein 5g	

Vitamin A 4% • Vitamin C 2%
Calcium 15% • Iron 4%

* Percent Daily Values are based on a 2,000 calorie diet. Your daily values may be higher or lower depending on your calorie needs:

	Calories:	2,000	2,500
Total Fat	Less than	65g	80g
Sat Fat	Less than	20g	25g
Cholesterol	Less than	300mg	300mg
Sodium	Less than	2,400mg	2,400mg
Total Carbohydrate		300g	375g
Dietary Fiber		25g	30g

Calories per gram:
Fat 9 • Carbohydrate 4 • Protein 4

% Daily Value shows how a food fits into the overall daily diet. Some daily values are maximums, as with fat, while others are minimums, as with carbohydrates.

The Daily Values are based on daily diets of 2,000 and 2,500 calories. Individuals should adjust these values to fit their own calorie intake. (Moderately active people consume about fifteen calories per day for each pound of body weight.)

The FDA would like the RDIs to be based mainly on the 1989 RDAs, which are more appropriate than their 1968 predecessors. In 1991, it proposed the following values, many of which are lower than their corresponding U.S. RDAs:

Nutrient	***RDI***	***U.S. RDA***
Vitamin A (International Units)*	3,300	5,000
Vitamin C (milligrams)	60	60
Calcium (milligrams)	900	1,000
Iron (milligrams)	12	18
Vitamin D (International units)*	360	400
Vitamin E (International units)*	27	30
Vitamin K (micrograms)	65	
Thiamin (milligrams)	1.2	1.5
Riboflavin (milligrams)	1.4	1.7
Niacin (milligrams)	16	20
Vitamin B_6 (milligrams)	1.5	2.0
Folate (micrograms)	180	400
Vitamin B_{12} (micrograms)	2.0	6.0
Biotin (micrograms)	60	
Pantothenic acid (milligrams)	5.5	10
Phosphorus (milligrams)	900	1,000
Magnesium (milligrams)	300	400
Zinc (milligrams)	13	15
Iodine (micrograms)	150	150
Selenium (micrograms)	55	
Copper (milligrams)	2.0	2.0
Manganese (milligrams)	3.5	
Fluoride (milligrams)	2.5	
Chromium (micrograms)	120	
Molybdenum (micrograms)	150	
Chloride (milligrams)	3,150	

* The U.S. RDAs for vitamins A, D, and E are expressed in International Units (IU). Their RDIs utilize different units of measurement. To facilitate comparison, we have converted them into International Units.

If the proposed RDIs were implemented, the percentages of vitamins and minerals on most food labels would generally be higher than they are now. This is a good idea because the RDIs are closer than the U.S. RDAs to most people's actual requirements. However, the supplement industry is concerned that lower

RDIs will decrease supplement sales by increasing people's knowledge that the foods they consume contain adequate amounts of nutrients. The industry's protest campaign (described in Chapter 20) has delayed implementation of new values. Meanwhile, FDA is working with the National Academy of Sciences to review the appropriateness of these numbers.

Appendix C

Supplements and "Health Foods"

The following is a list of commonly promoted "supplements," "health foods," and other products sold in health-food stores. Those marked with an asterisk (*) can cause health difficulties as noted.

Acidophilus: *Lactobacillus acidophilus* is a bacterial organism that ferments the sugars present in milk and milk products such as yogurt. Acidophilus supplements are claimed to aid digestion and promote the health of the digestive tract. This is impractical because oral doses of the bacteria may not survive the acidic environment of the stomach. Acidophilus preparations such as sweet acidophilus milk can be useful to persons who have difficulty digesting lactose (a condition called lactose intolerance). These products are produced by adding acid-tolerant strains of acidophilus bacteria to milk. Those surviving passage into the intestine will produce lactase and also digest the milk's lactose. However, individuals with lactose intolerance should have guidance from a physician, and use of lactase enzyme without the bacteria may be preferable.

Activated charcoal: Supplements labeled "activated organic charcoal" are usually said to be made from natural organic peat moss. Charcoal supposedly absorbs intestinal gases and "serves as a powerful detoxicant" that combats "gas" and "makes you feel intestinally clean." However, this product is of little value and can add to gastrointestinal distress by interfering with the action of digestive enzymes.

***Alfalfa:** Although advocates of alfalfa suggest that it contains certain nutrients that more common plant foods do not, alfalfa actually has less nutritional value than most of the more popular vegetables such as broccoli, carrots, and spinach.

Claims have also been made that alfalfa contains all of the essential amino acids, but this is untrue. Alfalfa tea contains saponins, which can adversely affect digestion and respiration. Alfalfa contains L-canavanine, a toxic amino acid that can bring out latent immune disorders, particularly hemolytic anemia, lupus erythematosus, and rheumatoid arthritis.

***Aloe vera:** Unsubstantiated claims are made that aloe vera products can cure or alleviate colitis, bursitis, asthma, glaucoma, hemorrhoids, boils, arthritis, intestinal problems, acne, poison ivy, anemia, tuberculosis, cancer, diabetes, depression, multiple sclerosis, stretch marks, varicose veins, and even blindness. Aloe skin creams or gels are probably harmless; and even though it will not reverse the aging process, topical aloe may exert some skin softening and moisturizing effects. However, aloe juice acts as a laxative and can cause gastrointestinal upset. Veterinarians use it as a laxative for horses.

Amino acids: Various amino acids have been claimed to suppress appetite, relieve insomnia, depression, and pain, and help build muscles and improve athletic performance. There is scant support for these claims, and very little is known about the safety of supplementation with individual amino acids (see Chapter 19). The FDA Dietary Supplements Task Force has recommended that capsules and tablets of individual amino acids be regulated as drugs.

Bach Flower Remedies: A homeopathic offshoot consisting of thirty-eight products claimed to cure illness by alleviating underlying emotional stresses (see Chapter 9). There is no scientific evidence to support this theory.

***Bee pollen:** Bee pollen is claimed to be a "perfect food," but it contains no nutrients that are not present in conventional foods. It is also touted as an aid to athletic performance, although actual tests on swimmers and runners have shown no benefit. In susceptible individuals, bee pollen can cause anaphylactic shock, a life-threatening allergic reaction in which swelling of the throat can cause suffocation.

Beta-carotene: Beta carotene is a pigmented component of plant foods that the body converts into vitamin A. Although diets rich in carotene-containing foods are associated with a lower incidence of cancer, the reason for this association is unknown and probably involves other phytochemicals rather than beta-carotene. Beta-carotene supplementation may lower the incidence of heart disease, but a definitive answer may not be known for many years (see discussion of antioxidants in Chapter 8).

Bioflavonoids: Bioflavonoids are promoted as essential for good health. They are claimed to aid in resistance to colds and the flu. Scientific tests have shown this claim to be false. Bioflavonoids have never been found to be useful in humans for the treatment of any condition. Bioflavonoids are sometimes referred to as "vitamin P," but they are neither vitamins nor essential for humans.

Blackstrap molasses: Blackstrap molasses is the dark, less-refined form of molasses. It is less sweet than other syrups and has a distinctive flavor. It is touted as a "wonder food" that can restore hair color and cure anemia. Blackstrap molasses is simply another form of sugar. It cannot reverse the graying of hair. It does contain significant amounts of iron; consuming a few tablespoons of molasses at regular intervals can contribute significantly to iron intake. This could be good for people whose diet otherwise contains insufficient iron to meet their needs, but could be bad for certain others whose diet already contains enough (see Chapter 1). For this reason, iron supplementation should not be done without competent medical advice.

***Bone meal:** Powdered bone is claimed to be a rich source of calcium. Actually, its calcium is poorly absorbed. FDA scientists have found that many bone meal samples contained high levels of lead, a toxic mineral.

Boron: The mineral boron is falsely claimed to be a "supernutrient." It is promoted as an "ergogenic aid," aphrodisiac, and arthritis remedy. Adequate amounts of boron are readily available from food. There is no reliable evidence that supplements can increase lean body mass or strength in humans.

Brewer's yeast: A yeast is used to ferment carbohydrate in making beer. It is a source of protein and several of the B vitamins, but it is certainly no miracle food and has no value for anyone eating an average American diet.

Carob: Carob beans have been cultivated in Mediterranean countries since ancient times. Carob is now used in dog biscuits, as a flavoring agent in chewing tobacco, and as a chocolate substitute in candy and snack foods. It is lower in fat than chocolate and is caffeine-free, but it is similar in caloric content and does not taste like real chocolate. Claims of wondrous health benefits associated with carob intake are false.

"Catalyst-altered water": Water claimed to have been altered by adding special submicroscopic particles of silicone, which form a network of molecules that makes the water more "bioactive." There is no reason to believe that this water has any healing properties or is significantly different from normal drinking water (see Willard's Water in Chapter 18).

***Chaparral:** An herb, used in teas, capsules, and tablets, purported to delay aging, cleanse the blood, and treat cancer. In 1993, the FDA warned consumers not to use it because it contains a chemical that can cause serious liver and kidney damage. Most manufacturers have voluntarily stopped marketing chaparral-containing products.

***Chelated minerals:** Chelate means "to bind." Minerals in chelated supplements usually are bound to an amino acid, which may increase the efficiency with which they are absorbed from the intestines and excreted through the kidneys. When chelation increases absorption, it equally increases excretion, so there is no net gain. Individuals with a medically diagnosed need for mineral supplements should not take chelated forms, which are more expensive and not effective.

Chlorophyll: The pigment responsible for the green color of plants. It "traps" the energy from sunlight, enabling the plant to synthesize carbohydrates. Claims that chlorophyll is effective against many diseases and reduces odors are not substantiated. It can kill certain types of bacteria, but is too weak to be of practical use as an antibiotic. Chlorophyll is sometimes said to be equivalent to the "blood of plants," but it is not.

Choline: Not essential in the diets of humans, choline is in many foods. Thus, even if one did require a dietary source, supplements would be unnecessary. Although research is being conducted concerning choline compounds in the treatment of certain brain disorders, use of supplements will not improve memory, protect the liver, or "counter the aging process" as claimed by faddists.

Chromium picolinate: A chromium-containing dietary supplement patented by Gary W. Evans, Ph.D., and claimed to help shed fat and increase muscle mass. Independent research does not support these claims. (Patenting laws do nor require proof that claims made for health products are valid.)

Cider vinegar: Vinegar made from apples, touted as a cure-all, often in conjunction with honey. Cider vinegar is claimed to "keep the body in balance," thin the blood, cause weight loss, and aid in digestion—none of which is true. Like the supermarket variety, cider vinegar is an acceptable condiment (flavoring agent), but the myths surrounding its use should be ignored.

***Coenzyme Q_{10}:** Coenzyme Q_{10} is a substance produced in the body. Preliminary evidence suggests that, under some circumstances, it may help keep atherosclerotic plaque from forming by acting as an antioxidant in blood lipid particles. But there is no evidence that coenzyme Q_{10} supplements (which are destroyed by the digestive process) prevent aging or even increase coenzyme Q_{10} levels in body tissues. Supplementing with coenzyme Q_{10} may be dangerous for some people.

Cold-pressed oils: Most vegetable oils are filtered to remove impurities and have antioxidant preservatives added to prevent rapid spoilage. "Cold-pressed" oils undergo a different type of processing. Two types are available: crude, which is dark and still contains sediment and plant solids; and the lighter, filtered version which is more like regular oils. Neither has any health advantage over oils processed by the usual methods. According to *Consumer Reports*, cold pressing takes place between 140°F and 475°F—which is certainly not "cold."

Dehydroepiandrosterone (DHEA): "DHEA pills" have been promoted with false claims that they have antiaging properties and can cause effortless weight loss. In experiments with certain strains of mice, DHEA has blocked tumors and prevented weight gain. Scientists have speculated that declining levels of this adrenal hormone after young adulthood play a role in aging. However, significant dosages can cause unwanted hair growth, liver enlargement, and other adverse effects that make its use impractical. During the mid-1980s, several "DHEA" products marketed through health-food stores were found to contain little or no DHEA. In 1985, the FDA ordered manufacturers to stop marketing DHEA products as weight-loss aids.

Desiccated liver: Dried liver in pill or powder form contains a number of nutrients. However, it has no advantage over cooked liver and is more expensive.

***Desiccated thyroid:** Dried thyroid gland from a pig or cow is available as a prescription drug for treating hypothyroidism (low thyroid function), but responsible physicians rarely prescribe it because its hormonal content can vary from batch to batch; synthetic hormone pills are more reliable. Desiccated thyroid is also an ingredient in some products sold in health-food stores. Dietary supplements containing glandular substances are supposed to be processed so that they contain no active hormone. However, cases have been reported of individuals who ingested toxic amounts of thyroid hormone while self-medicating with such products.

Dibencozide: An "ergogenic aid" claimed to increase appetite, muscle growth, and athletic performance. These claims are not supported by published scientific studies.

***DMSO (dimethyl sulfoxide):** A solvent, similar to turpentine, promoted for arthritis relief. In a sterile form it is available as a prescription drug for treating a rare bladder condition called interstitial cystitis. There are no controlled studies showing that DMSO is safe and effective for arthritis. When applied to body surfaces it is rapidly absorbed and, if contaminated, can carry toxic substances into the body. DMSO can be dangerous if used in an enema, as recommended by some promoters.

***Dolomite:** Dolomite, mined from rocks, contains calcium and magnesium, but in a poorly absorbable form. Lead, arsenic, mercury, and other contaminants have been found in dolomite samples in amounts ample enough to cause nerve damage and other health problems.

Enzymes (oral): Many products containing enzymes are marketed with claims that they can enhance body processes. Enzymes are proteins that act as catalysts in the body. Enzymes present in food are treated in the digestive tract the same way as any other protein: acid in the stomach and other digestive chemicals reduce them to smaller constituents that are no longer enzymes by the time they are absorbed into the body. The tiny amounts of amino acids oral enzymes provide make no significant nutritional contribution. Pancreatic enzymes have some legitimate medical uses in diseases that cause decreased secretion of pancreatic enzymes into the intestine, but these conditions are not appropriate for self-diagnosis or self-treatment.

Evening primrose oil: It is possible that EPO is effective against a few conditions (see Chapter 19). However, it has not been proven safe for long-term use and it is illegal in the United States to market EPO with health claims. The FDA has seized some quantities of the oil, but EPO products are still marketed.

Fertile eggs: These eggs supposedly have been fertilized by a rooster, while the supermarket varieties have not. Fertilized eggs tend to spoil faster and cost more. Faddists claim that fertilized eggs come from hens that are happier, better adjusted, and more "alive." Nutritionally, however, they are equivalent. Some faddists claim that brown eggs are nutritionally superior to white eggs. However, egg color is hereditary and has nothing to do with nutrient composition.

Fish-oil capsules: Epidemiologic research has found that Eskimos and others whose diet is rich in certain fatty acids have less heart disease than other Americans or Europeans. Other research has found that supplements of omega-3 fatty acids (found in fish oils) can help lower blood cholesterol levels and inhibit clotting, which means they may be useful in preventing atherosclerotic heart disease but harmful in promoting hemorrhage. However, it is not known what dosage is appropriate or whether long-range use is safe or effective. Most authorities believe it is unwise to self-medicate with fish-oil capsules; they should be used only by individuals at high risk for heart disease who are under close medical supervision. However, eating fish once or twice a week is probably beneficial. The FDA has ordered manufacturers to stop making claims that fish-oil capsules are effective against various diseases.

Gamma-oryzanol: An "ergogenic aid" claimed to release growth hormone and stimulate muscle growth. These claims are not supported by published scientific studies.

***Garlic:** Raw garlic and garlic-oil capsules are claimed to "purify the blood," reduce high blood pressure, and prevent cancer, heart disease, and a variety of other ailments. Some studies have found that people given daily garlic or garlic extract had lowered their blood cholesterol levels. The *Harvard Health Letter* cautions that any evidence of benefit is preliminary and that garlic can produce bad breath, heartburn, and flatulence and can inhibit blood clotting.

***Germanium:** "Organic germanium" is touted as a "miracle drug" for a wide range of health problems. Proponents claim that cancer, heart disease, mental deficiency, and many other problems are due to an "oxygen deficiency" that organic germanium can eradicate. There is no scientific evidence to support these claims. A few germanium products have been tested for antitumor activity, but no practical application has been found. Although many health-food stores sell germanium products, it is illegal to market them with therapeutic claims. The FDA has banned importation of germanium products intended for human consumption and has seized germanium products from several U.S. manufacturers. Germanium supplements have caused irreversible kidney damage and death.

***Gerovital (GH3):** A substance falsely claimed to have "anti-aging" or "rejuvenating" properties. GH3 has been claimed to prevent or relieve arthritis, arteriosclerosis, angina pectoris, and other heart conditions, neuritis, deafness, Parkinson's disease, depression, senile psychosis, and impotence. It is also claimed to stimulate hair growth, restore pigments to gray hair, and tighten and smooth skin. The main ingredient in GH3 is procaine, a substance used for local anesthesia. Although many uncontrolled studies describe benefits from the use of GH3, controlled trials using procaine have failed to demonstrate any. Low blood pressure, breathing difficulty, and convulsions have been reported among users.

Ginkgo biloba: Evidence exists that ginkgo can improve cerebral blood flow, particularly in geriatric patients. However, there is no evidence that it can reverse the aging process or prolong life, as some proponents claim. Since no manufacturer has obtained FDA approval for ginkgo products, it is not legal to market them with health claims in the United States.

***Ginseng:** Ginseng herb is being promoted as a healthy tonic, stimulant, aphrodisiac, and cure-all. There is little or no scientific evidence to support these claims. Some studies have found that many "ginseng" products contained little or no ginseng; other products can produce symptoms resembling estrogen or other steroid poisoning. The FDA requires that any product containing whole, ground, or powdered ginseng must be labeled for use only in tea.

Glandular extracts: These products, sold as "food supplements," are claimed to cure diseases by augmenting glandular function in the body. Actually they contain no hormones and therefore can exert no pharmacologic effect upon the body. If they did produce such an effect, they would be dangerous for self-medication.

Glutamic acid: Health-food promoters claim that a variety of substances can increase memory power; one is glutamic acid, the principal amino acid metabolized by the brain. Although scientists are studying the relationship between memory and the intake of certain amino acids, using supplements with the hope of improving brain function is at best premature and has been harmful. If one's diet is reasonably well balanced, there is no reason to add any amino acid supplement with the hope of improving memory.

***Goat milk:** The milk of goats has been touted as a highly nutritious substitute for cow milk; it actually is no more nutritious than cow milk. The late Paavo Airola, naturopath and author of several books advocating questionable nutrition practices, claimed that goat milk contains special factors effective against arthritis and cancer. This is untrue. Like nonpasteurized milk from any animal, goat milk can carry diseases (see "raw milk," below).

Granola: Granola is the common term used to describe various cereals and candy bars composed largely of oats plus other grains, fruits, seeds, and nuts. Touted as "natural" and rich in nutrients, granola products tend to be high in sugar (usually brown sugar and/or honey), fats (from vegetable oils, nuts, seeds, and coconut), and calories.

Green-lipped mussel: Green-lipped mussel, harvested in New Zealand and made into supplement capsules, has been marketed by several American companies. Claims that it is effective against arthritis are not supported by scientific studies. During the mid-1980s, FDA action stopped a major manufacturer from marketing green-lipped mussel as an arthritis remedy. However, similar products are still marketed as "mucopolysaccharides" (see Chapter 8).

Guarana: An herb that contains a significant amount of caffeine.

Gymnema sylvestre: An herb claimed to decrease the craving for sweets and to inhibit absorption of sugar by the digestive tract, thereby causing weight loss. Although chewing the plant's leaves can prevent the taste sensation of sweetness, there is no reliable evidence that the chemicals they contain can block sugar absorption or produce weight loss.

Honey: Although honey is portrayed as more nutritious than table sugar, there is little nutritional difference between the two. Honey is a crude form of mixed sugars, mainly fructose and glucose, with a small amount of sucrose and only trace amounts of micronutrients. Table sugar is pure sucrose, whose molecules consist of equal parts of fructose and glucose. Being sticky, however, honey is more likely to contribute to tooth decay. It is also more expensive than table sugar. Honey's intense sweetness is due to the free fructose it contains.

Inositol: Contrary to popular claims, supplements of inositol will not alleviate baldness, reduce blood cholesterol levels, or aid weight loss. Inositol is not a B vitamin, and the body can manufacture all the inositol it needs. Even if it were a vitamin, supplements would be unnecessary because it is readily available in our food supply.

***Kelp:** A seaweed common in the Japanese diet. Tablets of kelp are prepared from dried seaweed and promoted in health-food stores as a weight-reduction aid, a rich source of iodide, an energy booster, and a "natural" cure for certain ailments, including goiter. Kelp is high in iodide, a mineral needed to prevent goiter. However, iodized salt furnishes an adequate supply of this mineral to our diet at a fraction of the cost of kelp. Excess iodide can be detrimental to health.

Lecithin: Lecithin is manufactured by the liver and present in many foods, including soybeans, whole grains, and egg yolks. Claims that lecithin supplements can dissolve blood cholesterol, rid the blood stream of undesirable fats, cure arthritis, improve brain power, and aid in weight reduction are unsupported by scientific evidence.

***Ma huang:** An herb that contains ephedrine, a decongestant and nervous-system stimulant. Ephedrine can raise blood pressure and therefore is hazardous to individuals with high blood pressure. Products containing ma huang are marketed as weight-loss aids even though they have not been proven safe and effective for this purpose. Some entrepreneurs are selling ephedrine/caffeine combinations as stimulants. Serious illnesses and deaths have been reported among users of these products.

Octacosanol: Raw wheat germ is claimed to contain an active ingredient called "octacosanol." This substance, present in many plant oils, is not essential in the human diet. Claims that it improves stamina and endurance, reduces blood cholesterol, and helps reproduction are unsubstantiated.

PABA (para-aminobenzoic acid): A vitamin for bacteria, but not for humans. It is claimed that dosages taken orally can prevent or reverse the graying of hair, but no scientific evidence exists to support this claim.

Papain: An enzyme, present in papaya extract, that is promoted as a digestive aid, cure for gum disease, and weight-reduction aid. When taken by mouth, papain is rapidly destroyed in the digestive tract. Its only significant use is as a meat tenderizer; it can be added to meats before they are consumed and while the enzyme is still chemically active.

***Pau d'arco:** An herbal product, sold through health-food stores and by mail, said to be an ancient Inca Indian remedy prepared from the inner bark of various evergreen trees native to the West Indies and Central and South America. Proponents claim pau d'arco tea is "a powerful tonic and blood builder" and is effective against cancer, diabetes, rheumatism, cystitis, prostatitis, bronchitis, gastritis, ulcers, liver ailments, asthma, gonorrhea, ringworm, and even hernias. The barks contain lapachol, a chemical recognized as an antitumor agent. However, human studies have found that as soon as significant blood levels are attained, side effects were severe enough to require that the drug be stopped. Laboratory studies have demonstrated that lapachol also possesses antibiotic, antimalarial, and antischistosomal properties, but scientific studies have not been done in humans because of its toxicity.

***Propolis (bee glue"):** A resinous material bees collect and use to fill cracks in their hives. It has mild antibacterial properties but has not been scientifically demonstrated to have practical use as a medication. Skin inflammation has occurred among users of cosmetics containing propolis, and mouth ulcers have been reported following the use of propolis-containing lozenges.

***Protein supplements:** Protein powders, tablets, and liquids have been falsely advertised as strength-promoting and especially important to athletes. The RDA for protein is easily obtained by eating a well-balanced diet. Supplements provide no additional benefit and, in large amounts, can cause nutritional imbalances and kidney problems.

***Raw milk:** Nonpasteurized milk. Public health authorities advocate pasteurization to destroy any disease-producing bacteria that may be present. Health faddists claim that it destroys essential nutrients. Although about 10 percent of the heat-sensitive vitamins (vitamin C and thiamin) are destroyed in the pasteurizing process, milk is not a significant source of these nutrients. On the other hand, contaminated raw milk can be a source of harmful bacteria, such as those that cause undulant fever, dysentery, and tuberculosis. "Certified" milk is unpasteurized milk with a bacteria count below a specified standard, but it still can contain significant numbers of disease-producing organisms. In 1987, the FDA ordered that milk and milk products in final package form for human consumption in interstate commerce be pasteurized. The sale of raw milk has been banned in about half the states, but is still legal in California, which contains the largest source.

***RNA/DNA:** Supplements of these genetic materials are claimed to rejuvenate old cells, improve memory, and prevent skin wrinkling. When taken orally, they are inactivated by the digestive process. Even if they could be absorbed and reach the cells, they would not work because human cells utilize human nucleic acids, not those from lower animals. If RNA from yeasts or sardines could actually work in people, it would turn them into yeasts or sardines. Ingesting large amounts can raise blood uric acid levels, which can cause problems.

Royal jelly: Food for queen bees. Claimed to increase endurance, it has been recommended for athletes. It is also advertised as rich in calcium pantothenate (claimed to be "vitamin B_5"), a supposed antioxidant-antistress nutrient also used in "miracle" skin creams and hair tonics. These claims are unsubstantiated.

Rutin: A chemical related to the bioflavonoids. Rutin is not a vitamin for humans. It is illegal for supplement labels to carry nutritional claims for rutin, but this substance is often included in multivitamins by sellers who wish to create the impression that their product is "more complete."

Sea salt: Proponents of sea salt claim that it is unrefined and therefore more nutritious than ordinary salt, but actually it is refined to remove impurities. Sea salt contains as much sodium as table salt, but table salt can have the advantage of being iodized with the correct dose. "Seawater concentrates" have been marketed with claims that they can cure cancer, diabetes, and a whole host of other diseases. These claims are both false and illegal.

Spirulina: A blue-green alga, some species of which have been used as a dietary staple in several parts of the world. Spirulina is similar to soybeans in nutrient content. It contains protein of fair quality plus some other nutrients, but nothing that cannot be obtained much less expensively from conventional foods. Despite claims by proponents, spirulina has no value as a weight-reduction aid or as a remedy for any disease. Law enforcement agencies and courts have ordered several multilevel companies to stop making illegal therapeutic claims for spirulina products, but others continue to do so (see Chapter 10). Some products sold as "spirulina" have contained no spirulina, and some have been found to be contaminated with insect parts. Claims that spirulina products contain vitamin B_{12} have also been shown to be false.

Sprouts: Sprouts add bulk to sandwiches and salads and provide various textures and flavors, depending on the type of seed from which they are sprouted. Their nutrient content depends mainly on the species used. The nutritional value of sprouts has been exaggerated. They contain modest amounts of vitamin C, but certainly no "life force," as enthusiasts have claimed.

Superoxide dismutase (SOD): An enzyme promoted as an "antioxidant" that supposedly protects body tissues against environmental contaminants, heart disease, cancer, and arthritis. The body has its own supply of functioning antioxidants, including various enzymes and vitamins C and E. SOD taken orally is digested in the gastrointestinal tract and not absorbed intact.

Tissue salts: A set of twelve highly diluted mineral substances claimed to be effective against a wide variety of diseases and conditions (see Chapter 2). Their use is based on the absurd notion that mineral deficiency is the basic cause of disease. Many are so dilute that they could not correct a mineral deficiency even if one were present .

***"Vitamin B_{15}":** "Vitamin B_{15}," also referred to as "pangamate," "pangamic acid," and "Russian Formula," is a name that has been used to promote various chemicals and products, none of which is a vitamin. "Pangamic acid" was patented in 1949 by Ernst T. Krebs, Sr., and his son, Ernst, Jr., the developers of laetrile. "B_{15}" has been fraudulently claimed to purify the air, provide the body with instant oxygen, slow down the aging process, and be effective against cancer, heart disease, alcoholism, diabetes, glaucoma, allergies, and schizophrenia. However, "B_{15}" products offer no health benefit and have contained ingredients that could cause cancer and have other adverse effects. The FDA has banned the sale of several such products, but similar ones are still marketed.

***Wheat bran:** A fiber of wheat grain, bran is composed mainly of cellulose, an insoluble fiber. It is effective against constipation, but so are whole grains, fruits, and vegetables in the diet. The claim that wheat bran can lower cholesterol is untrue. Excessive intake of bran can cause bloating and diarrhea and has produced intestinal obstruction requiring surgery.

Wheat germ: Wheat germ is a source of protein, several B vitamins, vitamin E, some minerals, and fiber. It is neither a cure-all nor a dietary essential. It is amply provided in whole wheat products. As a supplement, it is relatively high in calories and cost.

Wheat grass juice: A juice, made from sprouted wheat berries, said to be high in chlorophyll and claimed to "cleanse" the body, neutralize toxins, slow the aging process, and prevent cancer. Its principal proponent, the late Ann Wigmore, attributed these supposed benefits to enzymes in the plant that supplement the body's enzymes when ingested. These claims are nonsense.

Yogurt: Yogurt is a fermented milk product that is nutritionally equivalent to the whole or low-fat milk from which it is made. It is a good source of calcium, riboflavin, and other nutrients—as are all milk products—but it is not a "perfect" food with magical antiaging properties, as it is sometimes claimed.

Appendix D

One Hundred Companies That Have Marketed Illegally

During the past ten years, hundreds of companies have marketed "dietary supplement," herbal, and/or homeopathic products with unsubstantiated claims and/or misleading advertising. "Unsubstantiated" means not generally recognized by experts as both safe and effective for its intended purpose—the standard of scientific proof upon which government regulation is based.

Based on our analysis of product literature, advertisements, government documents, and other materials, we believe that each company listed below has illegally marketed at least one product by doing one or more of the following:

- Made an unsubstantiated claim that a product was effective for preventing or treating a disease. The claim appeared in literature or other material distributed by manufacturers or authorized distributors. Such a product would be an unapproved "new" drug.
- Failed to provide adequate directions for a product's intended use, as construed from the product's name, product literature, or communication through other channels. Such a product would be misbranded.
- Made a false, misleading, or unsubstantiated statement in an advertisement.

This appendix is not a complete list but merely reflects documents we have in our files. Most of the companies we list have illegally promoted more than one product. A few have marketed over a hundred, and many of the promotions involve more claims than are specified. Some companies are no longer in business.

Companies that have been subjected to federal regulatory action during the past ten years are designated by the abbreviation for the agency initiating the action: [FDA] = Food and Drug Administration, [FTC] = Federal Trade Commission, and [USPS] = U.S. Postal Service. Companies subjected to state action are designated by the abbreviation of the state(s) involved, e.g., [CA], [NY], [PA], [TX]. Those cited for deceptive trade practices by the New York City Department of Consumer Affairs are designated [NYC]. The regulatory activity may have involved products or claims other than the ones mentioned here. Many of the claims have been discontinued due to enforcement actions or other pressures. Companies marked with an asterisk (*) are discussed elsewhere in this book; the relevant pages are listed in the index.

***AARP Pharmacy Service**, Alexandria, Virginia, during the mid-1980s, marketed an L-tryptophan product with a false representation that tryptophan "helps to minimize the effects of stress, anxiety, depression and insomnia on the body."

Active Marketing Concepts, Carmel, Indiana, has falsely stated that its bee-pollen product contained sixteen vitamins and would increase energy and stamina, reduce stress, increase immunity, and rejuvenate glandular activity.

Advanced Medical Nutrition, Inc., Hayward, California, has inappropriately claimed that its *Candida-Pak* "helps overcome yeast infections." A component of the program, *Basic Preventive,* is falsely described as containing "optimum levels of more than 30 nutrients."

Alacer Corporation, Irvine, California, was cited by New York City Department of Consumer Affairs for marketing *E-mergen-C*, a multivitamin/mineral drink featuring vitamin C, whose package claimed that the AIDS virus "can be successfully inhibited in its action with approximately 12 grams of vitamin C daily." [NYC]

***Alliance USA**, Richardson, Texas, has marketed Nature's Nutrition™ *Formula One* with a flyer claiming that one of its ingredients (kola nut) is "thought to strengthen the heart" and another ingredient (bladderwrack) "helps normalize the thyroid gland." [TX]

Alta Health Products, Pasadena, California, has solicited retailers with literature containing unsubstantiated claims that its pau d'arco product is effective against cancer, diabetes, asthma, and many other diseases.

***American Image Marketing**, Nampa, Idaho, has falsely claimed that *Dr. Willard's Catalyst Altered Water* "acts as a 'normalizer' on all living things that are not in their normal state." The company has also made unsubstantiated claims for *Barley Green* and other products. [FDA]

***Amway Corporation**, Ada, Michigan, has distributed video- and audiotaped sales aids that exaggerate the likelihood that individual diets are lacking in essential nutrients.

Arkopharma, Inc., Fairfield, New Jersey, was ordered by the FDA to stop making unsubstantiated claims for *Arko-Skin, Ark-Menopause, Arko-Rheuma, Arko-Flu, Arko-Aging, Arko-Bone,* and several other products. [FDA]

***The Atkins Center for Complementary Medicine**, New York City, has made unsubstantiated claims for *Acute Infection Formula, Cardiovascular Formula, Anti-Fatigue Formula, Anti-Arthritic Formula, Heart Rhythm Formula, Antidepressant Formula*, and other supplement products.

***Barth's**, Westbury, New York, has marketed *Eye-Vites, Nutri-Mem, Ear-Vites, Nutri-Arth, Hair Repair, Bio-Disk, All-Day Maxi-Stress, Imunoplex* and other products that could not do what their name suggested. [FDA]

***Bee-Alive, Inc.**, Valley Cottage, New York, has made unsubstantiated claims that its royal jelly products were effective in preventing a large number of health problems. [FDA]

Bio-Botanica, Inc., Hauppauge, New York, was ordered by the FDA to stop claiming that Nature's Answer brand *Homeopathic Herpes Creme* could relieve "skin eruptions caused by Herpes viruses." [FDA]

Bioenergy, Inc., Boulder, Colorado, has solicited orders for coenzyme Q_{10} by mailing order forms accompanied by flyers, booklets, and/or testimonials containing unsubstantiated claims for them.

***Biological Homeopathic Industries, Inc.**, Albuquerque, New Mexico, has made unsubstantiated claims that its products are effective for a large number of diseases and conditions. [FDA]

Biosource, Santa Barbara, California, has marketed *Longevity Pack, Brain Power Pack, Heart of Health Pack,* and *Immuno-T*, none of which has been proven to do what its name suggests.

Bricker Laboratories, Valley Center, California, has made unsubstantiated claims that *GH*™ *Growth* can increase muscle size, increase ability to burn off fats, and increase immune protection. The "immune" claim is related to "thymus substance," an ingredient which the company suggests makes up for cessation of thymus gland function that occurs at puberty.

Cartilage Technologies, Inc., Port Chester, New York, was ordered by the FDA to stop making unsubstantiated claims that its *Cartilade* (shark cartilage) capsules were effective against symptoms of arthritis, psoriasis, and other inflammatory conditions, and that they could block or impede progression of many other abnormal conditions. [FDA]

***CC Pollen Company**, Phoenix, Arizona, has falsely represented that its bee-pollen products could produce weight loss, permanently alleviate allergies, reverse the aging process, and cure, prevent, or alleviate impotence or sexual dysfunction. Has also falsely asserted that bee-pollen products are an effective antibiotic for human use and cannot result in an allergic reaction.[FTC]

***Cell Tech, Inc.**, Klamath Falls, Oregon, has falsely stated that some of the ingredients in its Super Blue-Green algae products "aid the brain and nervous system in functioning more efficiently." This statement was misleading because the tiny amount found in the products would have no significant effect in a person eating a normal diet. Also stated falsely that "chlorophyll is vital for the body's assimilation of amino acids and for syntheses of enzymes."

Center for Interior Services, Inc., New Berlin, Wisconsin, has made unsubstantiated claims that Jaydee's *Nail Food*, a protein/vitamin/mineral drink mix, "builds strong, healthy fingernails nature's way, from the inside out."

Country Life, Hauppauge, New York, has marketed *Thyro-Max Support* ("a nutritional aid for the health of the thyroid gland") and *ReSurge* ("the bedtime regenerative supplement for stress reduction, muscle relaxation, tissue repair and increased respiratory capacity").

Dash Nutritional Products, Tuscaloosa, Alabama, has made unsubstantiated claims that *Russian Formula DMG* "improves your training and endurance," *Smilax Gold* "enhances your body's testosterone levels without the harmful side effects of steroids," and *GTF Muscle Fuel* "enhances the release of growth hormone."

Dr. Leonard's Healthcare Products, Brooklyn, New York, has carried false representations in its mail-order catalogs for supplements from several manufacturers. Ethical Nutrients' *Thyro-Vital*, for example, has been suggested as a way of preventing or remedying chronic fatigue. Quantum, Inc.'s *Day Trim* and *Night Trim* amino acid formulas have been falsely represented as a "round the clock weight-loss program." Energy Factors, Inc.'s *Heart-Ex* has been falsely claimed to "prevent cholesterol build-up in your arteries."

Earthrise Company, San Raphael, California, has been ordered by the FDA to stop making unsubstantiated claims for *Imun-N-Sure Colds & Flu Formula* and *Step Ahead PMS Nutritional Supplement Plus Spirulina.* [FDA]

***Ecomer, Inc.**, Perkasie, Pennsylvania, has been ordered by the FDA to stop making claims that *Exsativa* can increase muscle strength, endurance time, and performance, and that taking Ecomer's shark liver oil product would help ensure that the body has enough alkylglycerols to make white blood cells. [FDA]

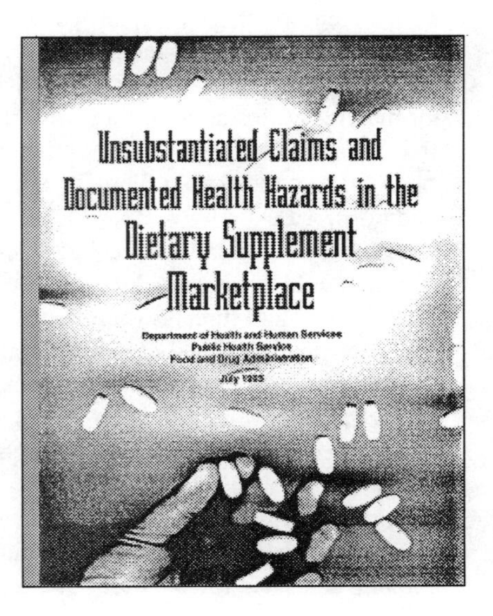

This 110-page report, presented by FDA Commissioner David Kessler at a Congressional hearing in July 1993, lists more than four hundred "dietary supplement" products that had been marketed with unsubstantiated health claims. The report also lists FDA regulatory actions taken since November 1990 against 188 products that had been marketed with claims related to serious diseases.

Edom Laboratories, Deer Park, New York, has made unsubstantiated claims for many amino acid products, including *His* (a "raw glandular" product claimed to restore male potency and increase male sexual response) and *Hers* (an analogous product that "may help women reach their sexual potential"). Both products contained 125 mg of niacin, enough to produce flushing, which Edom's catalog falsely claimed to be "the same flushing effect described by Masters and Johnson." [FDA]

***Efamol, Ltd.**, Guildford, England, and its American distributors have used elaborate means to promote evening primrose oil products for therapeutic purposes that lack FDA approval. [FDA]

En Garde Health Products, Van Nuys, California, is marketing *B12/Folic Acid Boost* with false claims that it is "anti stress, reduces irritability," is "calming and energizing," and is a "nervous system tonic." The company also markets *Zinc Boost* (with magnesium and vitamin B_6) with false claims that it "helps the body cope with stress, aids healing, helps fertility, increases stamina, strengthens cell membranes, and reduces evidences of aging, such as graying of the hair." Both are liquid products administered by taking two drops under the tongue.

***Enrich International**, Pleasant Grove, Utah, has marketed many products with unsubstantiated claims and used a bogus questionnaire to determine which body systems supposedly need nutritional help. [FDA]

***Enzymatic Therapy, Inc.**, Green Bay, Wisconsin, has made unsubstantiated therapeutic claims for scores of products. [FDA]

***Futurebiotics**, Brattleboro, Vermont, has made unsubstantiated health claims for *Dilovasic, Livercare, Maximum Immune Support, Stressaway, TrymTone 1200, Ultraglan,* and other products. [FDA].

***General Nutrition**, Pittsburgh, Pennsylvania, has made false or misleading claims for scores of supplement products. [FDA] [FTC] [USPS] [CA] [PA]

Golden Pride/Rawleigh, West Palm Beach, Florida, markets a Formulas for Health™ line that includes Formula #9, an aloe vera drink falsely claimed to "cleanse the body of toxins" and "help relieve other internal and intestinal disorders." BeforeGolden Pride merged with Rawleigh, its newspaper carried testimonial letters stating that various products had cured the writer of serious ailments. The FDA has ordered the company to stop making unsubstantiated claims for another formula. [FDA]

Great American Health & Nutrition, Fullerton, California, has marketed *Burn Off,* an amino acid product falsely claimed to "stimulate growth hormone" and "speed up the body's digestive system so that the body's excess fat is more quickly disseminated, giving it less time to become a permanent resident."

Great Earth International, Inc., Santa Ana, California, has falsely claimed that three of its products would enable users to lose weight, build muscle, burn fat, promote healing, protect against mental and physical stress, and/or strengthen the immune system. The company has also made unsubstantiated claims for vitamin E ("helps dissolve existing clots . . . making the heart a more efficient pump"), *Yeasterol* ("to control . . . Candida albicans, a troublesome yeast"), *Lowestrol* ("may not only counter the build-up of cholesterol deposits, but may also appear to reduce the blood's tendency to clot"), *Elavita Formula DP* ("gives the body and brain the special nutrients it needs" for alertness, memory, motivation, learning, sex drive, and positive emotions), *Nutrimmune* ("shown to boost the body's defense system"), *Thymosin* ("Boosts the body's resistance to disease!"), and *Rejuvacell* ("Anti-aging . . . retards hair loss . . . lowers blood pressure, improves sexual function . . . reduces cholesterol"). [FTC] [CA]

Green Foods Corporation, Carson, California, was ordered by the FDA to stop stating that its *Green Magma* is "necessary to activate immune system cells" and has eliminated a long list of diseases and conditions. [FDA]

***Health Center for Healthy Living**, Naples, Florida, markets scores of herbal products that have not been proven to be safe or effective for their intended purposes. [FDA]

Health Concerns, Alameda, California, has made unsubstantiated claims that *Astra Essence* "promotes longevity useful in our society where many may show signs of premature aging or kidney deficiency from fast-paced lifestyles."

***Health From The Sun Products, Inc.**, Dover, Massachusetts, has made unsubstantiated claims that *Sanhelios Juniper Caps* "keep the blood clean and free of impurities" and that *Royal Jelly* could act as a "tonic to the nervous system."

The Heritage Store, Virginia Beach, Virginia, markets several tonics (based on the notions of Edgar Cayce) with unsubstantiated health claims. *Optikade®*, for example, is said to have "a stimulating and cleansing effect on the digestion and circulation, thereby improving the eyesight," and *De-Tense* is claimed to be "an herbal detoxifier and eliminant" recommended in a Cayce "reading" for an individual with high blood pressure.

Highland Laboratories, Inc., Mt. Angel, Oregon, was ordered by the FDA to stop claiming that ten products were appropriate for a large number of diseases and conditions. One product was *GeOxy 132*, a germanium product that was falsely claimed to strengthen the immune system, and control and reverse chronic allergies, arthritis, hepatitis, cancer, leukemia, cataracts, cardiovascular disease, asthma, and heavy metal poisoning. [FDA]

***L&H Vitamins**, Long Island City, New York, has falsely advertised that *Enduraplex* (which contained octacosanol) "improves stamina and endurance, reduces heart stress, and quickens reaction time"; that *Sugar Block* (which contained *Gymnema sylvestre*) blocks the absorption of sugar calories; and that *K Complex* helps prevent stress from damaging health, enhances body's resistance levels, strengthens organs, increases physical and mental energy, improves the heart and circulation, and fights chronic fatigue and weakness. [NY]

***L&S Research**, Lakewood, New Jersey, has made false and unsubstantiated claims that several Cybergenics products would help users to build muscle, lose weight, or lower blood cholesterol. [FTC] [NYC]

***Lederle Laboratories**, Wayne, New Jersey, has suggested in its ads that emotional stress and ordinary physical stress cause depletion of water-soluble vitamins and that *Stresstabs* might reduce the effects of psychological stress. [NY]

Life Enthusiast Co-op, Federal Way, Washington, was ordered by the FDA to stop suggesting that *Excela* powder is effective against heart failure, failing eyesight, multiple sclerosis, memory loss, gum disease, and many other health problems. [FDA]

***Life Extension Foundation**, Hollywood, Florida, has marketed *Cognitex 2* with unsubstantiated claims that "it's the most scientific formula ever designed as aid to memory & mental function." [FDA]

***Light Force**, Santa Cruz, California, has marketed spirulina products with unsubstantiated claims that they can suppress appetite, boost immunity, and increase energy. Company sales materials claim that spirulina is a "superfood" and "works to cleanse and detoxify the body." Its magazine has carried reports about users who lost weight or recovered from arthritis, cancer, multiple sclerosis and serious injuries while taking Light Force products.

***Makers of KAL**, Woodland Hills, California, has claimed that supplemental L-tryptophan supplements can increase mental acuity, "improve thought processes," and "increase thinkability."

***Meditrend International**, San Diego, California, has falsely claimed that applying a homeopathic solution to a spot-bandage placed at an "acupuncture point" on the wrist would generate a "bioelectrical message" to the brain's appetite-control center, thereby enabling the user to control appetite. [FDA] [PA]

***Michael's Health Products**, San Antonio, Texas, has made unsubstantiated therapeutic claims for a large number of products. [TX]

***Miles, Inc.**, Elkhart, Indiana, has falsely advertised that extra vitamins are needed to cope with the ordinary stresses of living. [FTC] [CA] [NY] [TX]

Multiway Associates, Batesville, Arkansas, has made many unsubstantiated claims for supplement and herbal products. *ReVital* was falsely claimed to be an anti-aging product. *Combat* was falsely claimed to provide "nutritional immune support." *STN-Pancreas* was falsely claimed to "nutritionally support the pancreas," implying that the product would prevent or alleviate hypoglycemia and diabetes. In 1985, the FDA ordered Multiway to stop misrepresenting another formula as an "oral chelation" product that would improve circulatory function. [FDA]

***Nat-rul Health Products**, Chestnut Ridge, New York, has marketed many products with unsubstantiated claims stated in ads and/or implied in product names. During the mid-1980s, these included *Cardio-Endurance* ("to help maintain fitness"), *Superb Nails* ("feed your nails from within"), *Hair-Vites*, *Mega-Stress*, *Maximum Virility*, *Arthri-Ade*, *Life Prolonger*, and *Maximum Memory* ("may aid your thinking and memory processes").

Natrol, Inc., Chatsworth, California, was ordered by the FDA to stop making unsubstantiated claims that four of its products could strengthen the immune system, normalize blood cholesterol, and prevent several serious illnesses. [FDA]

***Nature Food Centres**, Wilmington, Massachusetts, has made unsubstantiated claims in mail-order catalogs that lecithin helps prevent kidney problems, dissolve cholesterol deposits, fight against atherosclerosis, decrease insulin needs for diabetics, and revive sluggish brain cells.

Nature-All Formulas, Inc., Orem, Utah, was ordered by the FDA to stop claiming that *Colostrum Tablets* can furnish nutrition support for a weakened or impaired immune system. [FDA]

Nature's Best, Inc., Springfield, Missouri, was ordered by the FDA to stop claiming that six herbal products would exert various preventive and therapeutic effects. [FDA]

***Nature's Bounty**, Bohemia, New York, has marketed *Ener-B* (B_{12} product administered through the nose) with false claims that B_{12} is "difficult to absorb." (The small percentage of people who can't absorb B_{12} can develop pernicious anemia, a life-threatening illness that should have medical attention.) Mail-order catalogs have made unsubstantiated claims for several dozen products. [USPS].

Nature's Herbs, Orem, Utah, has advertised that its *Yeastop* would help "maintain control over yeast 'overgrowth' (*Candida albicans).*" The same ad, however, said that the product was "not designed for the treatment of any illness or infection." [FDA]

***Nature's Plus**, Farmingdale, New York, has marketed at least twenty products with false or unsubstantiated claims. It has claimed that its coenzyme Q_{10} was "a nutritional breakthrough in the quest for life and longevity" and that its germanium product was "known to have miraculous effects on human health, energy and vitality." The company has also marketed *Imune•Gard* to "help revitalize your body's natural defenses against disease!"

***Nature's Sunshine Products**, Inc., Spanish Fork, Utah, markets many herbal products with unsubstantiated claims that they nourish, strengthen, or support body organs and systems. [FDA]

***Nature's Way**, Springville, Utah, has made unsubstantiated claims that *Cantrol* is effective in controlling yeast infections and that various combinations of ordinary symptoms are a sign that someone has a yeast problem. [FDA] [FTC]

***Neo-Life Company of America**, Fremont, California, has marketed products with false claims that they can help the body restore nutrients "robbed" by such stresses as "worry, overwork, deadlines, or just daily problems."

Nova Nutritional Products, Inc., Inglewood, California, has falsely claimed: (1) the typical diet is deficient in enzymes because they are destroyed by cooking; (2) this causes incomplete digestion; (3) that causes partially digested fats to accumulate in arteries and lymphatic systems; and (4) raw foods or the company's enzyme-containing supplements would correct this problem.

***Nu Skin International**, Provo, Utah, has made unsubstantiated claims that products could prevent hair loss or remove wrinkles. [FDA] [FTC]

Nutri-Cell, Inc., Orange, California, has marketed *Nutri-Cell De-Oxy-Flo* with unsubstantiated claims that the nutrients it contains are effective against coronary atherosclerosis.

Nutri-Cology, Inc., San Leandro, California, has advertised that its *Pro-Oxygen* contains "vitamin 'O' - the most important of them all!" and that "most of us do not consume sufficient oxygen in our day-to-day life." The ad was for an "organic germanium" product "believed to be a key active principle in many natural healing substances." [FDA]

Nutrition 21, San Diego, California, makes unsubstantiated claims that daily use of chromium picolinate, which it manufactures and sells to other companies, will cause people to "lose the fat; keep the muscle."

Nutrition for Life, Houston, Texas, falsely claims that its Bio Enhanced Water "helps to eliminate body toxins as it balances the body's pH chemistry." The company's distributor kit includes a book containing more than twenty pages of testimonials "experienced while using 'Bio' type Catalyst Water." The kit also includes an audiotape in which optometrist Alex Duarte (introduced as "one of the most noted authors, lecturers, and nutritionists in all of America") makes unsubstantiated health claims for shark cartilage, an "oral chelation" product, and other Nutrition for Life products. Duarte also advised listeners who wanted more information to read his book *Eat Smart, Stay Healthy.*

Nutrition Headquarters, Inc., Carbondale, Illinois, was ordered by the FDA to stop claiming that *Atherex* was useful for treating or preventing coronary artery disease, angina pectoris, and other circulatory problems. [FDA]

Nutritional Life Support Systems, San Diego, California, was cited by the New York City Department of Consumer Affairs for engaging in a deceptive trade practice by marketing *Pro-Immune Anti-Oxidant* herbal capsules without a required disclaimer that the product had not been proven to be effective against the AIDS virus. [NYC]

Nuva International, Inc., Cincinnati, Ohio, has falsely claimed that its spirulina product could "turn off the brain's hunger center"; falsely claimed that its "anti-stress" formula would provide "optimum protection against stress-related effects"; and falsely implied that the product could help protect against "stress-related illnesses such as ulcer, hypertension, colon disease, cardiovascular disease, arthritis, and others."

Padma Marketing Corporation, Berkeley, California, has marketed *Padma 28* herbal formula accompanied by leaflets stating that it was "more effective for treating circulatory disorders than any pharmaceutical drug!" [FDA]

Parrillo Performance, Cincinnati, Ohio, has claimed that *CapTri Liquid* would decrease cholesterol absorption and reduce blood cholesterol level. [FDA]

The Pierson Company, Norwalk, California, has falsely advertised that "Simply by matching blood type (A,B,O or AB) to the *Meta*-Type™weight loss program, you can minimize potential allergic reactions, keep your fat-burning system at peak performance and break the weight gain cycle. A specialized supplement works with the diet to provide nutritional support to those parts of your system that are the weakest."

Rainbow Light Nutritional Systems, Santa Cruz, California, has falsely claimed that its Foundation Enzyme™ products are "the missing link to radiant health" and that "enzyme deficiencies are America's number one nutritional problem and are responsible for more dis-ease than all other nutritional shortages combined." The products have included: *Detox-Zyme* (to "help the body rid itself of toxicity"), *Aller-*

Zyme (guaranteed to eliminate allergies and sensitivities within fourteen days), and *Trim-Zyme* ("to facilitate weight control" by helping the body "more efficiently digest and metabolize fats").

*__Rexall Showcase International__, Ft. Lauderdale, Florida, makes unsubstantiated claims for several homeopathic products.

*__Rockland Corporation__, Tulsa, Oklahoma, has been ordered to stop selling *Body Toddy* with unsubstantiated claims that it was effective against aging, cancer, diabetes, cataracts, high blood pressure, thyroid deficiencies, stroke, heart attack, high cholesterol, depression, loss of memory, and many other problems. The product—touted to "supercharge your immune system"—was claimed to be a liquid concentrate of pure natural minerals that come from a "natural deposit phenomenon of prehistoric vegetable and plant matter." [FDA] [CA]

*__Schiff Bio-Food Products__, Moonachie, New Jersey, during the late 1980s, promoted "ergogenic aids" claimed to counter stress, increase endurance, and provide "unsurpassed body building and energizing fuels." Its other products have included *Yeas•Trol,* a vitamin/mineral/herbal program "for women concerned about yeast infections," *Tryptolyn* (a combination of tryptophan and lysine said to be "more effective than drugs in lowering blood cholesterol"), and a germanium product marketed with claims that "researchers are publishing studies extolling . . . its importance to the human body as an energizer and immune stimulant."

*__Seroyal Brands, Inc.__, Concord, California, in 1987, published a *Bioregulation Therapy Guide* containing sixty-eight pages of recommendations and dosage schedules for using Seroyal "nutritionals" for more than a hundred diseases and conditions.

*__Sharper Image Corporation__, San Francisco, California, has made unsubstantiated claims that regular use of *Oxy-Energizer* would improve stamina and endurance. [FTC]

*__Solaray, Inc.__, Ogden, Utah, has engaged in an elaborate scheme to convey unsubstantiated claims for many of its products.

*__Solgar Company__, Lynbrook, New York, has falsely represented that its *Joggers* multivitamin/mineral tablets are "rich in anti-stress vitamins" and would "insure maximum efficiency of the body chemistry while developing aerobic exercise capability."

Source Naturals, Santa Cruz, California, has falsely advertised that *Life Defense* was "the first comprehensive immune defense supplement" and that *Imu-T Boost* represented "a dramatic breakthrough inspired by research on cold sores."

*__Squibb, E.R. & Sons__, Princeton, New Jersey, has falsely advertised that its *Theragran Stress Formula* would help relieve stress resulting from "the complications of everyday life" and that biotin is difficult to obtain in an average diet. [NY]

Standard Homeopathic Co., Los Angeles, California, has marketed *Hyland's Cell Salts* with unsubstantiated claims that they can "relieve deficiency symptoms" and "boost the energy in your cells."

*__Sunrider International__, Torrance, California, markets herbal products with unsubstantiated claims that they can help "regenerate" the body and support, nourish, strengthen, enhance, and/or stimulate various organs or body functions. Sunrider and its distributors have also disseminated testimonials that products were effective against arthritis, ulcers, high blood pressure, emphysema, pancreatitis, and other serious conditions. [FDA] [CA]

***Swanson Health Products**, Fargo, North Dakota, has illegally marketed *Heart Food* and *Cardiolife* (claimed to prevent heart attacks), *Cata Rx* (promoted as a cure for cataracts), *Gymnema Sylvestre* (claimed to block absorption of sugar into the body), *Willard's Water* (promoted as an infection fighter), and *Co-Enzyme* Q_{10} and *Acidophilus* (promoted as digestive aids). [FDA]

***Twin Laboratories**, Ronkonkoma, New York, has been cited by the New York City Department of Consumer Affairs for engaging in a deceptive trade practice by marketing a multivitamin/mineral product called *Immune Protectors* without a required disclaimer that the product had not been proven to be effective against the AIDS virus. [NYC]

***Unipro, Inc.**, Fremont, California, has marketed amino acid products with many unsubstantiated claims, including: (1) No one can take too many amino acids because "your digestive system would regurgitate them"; and (2) *Endorphomin* "minimizes feeling of depression" and exerts "a positive and significant influence on an athlete's feeling of well-being, reward and euphoria" because it "delivers inhibitors and precursors of the opioid peptides, catecholamines and the brain neurotransmitter serotonin."

***United Sciences of America**, Carrollton, Texas, marketed products with unsubstantiated claims that they could prevent many serious diseases. [FDA] [CA] [NY] [TX]

Vibrant Life, Burbank, California, has falsely claimed that *Liqui-Trim* (an amino acid combination) and *Tri Amino Acids* release growth hormone, which would help weight control and "boost" the immune system.

Vital Corporation, Las Vegas, Nevada, and a leading distributor have falsely promoted *By-Pass*, "a homeopathic oral chelation product," as effective for improving circulation.

The Vitamin Healthcenters, a health-food-store chain headquartered in Marleton, New Jersey, has made unsubstantiated claims for *Amino Hair,* a high-potency formula claimed to reverse male pattern baldness, and *Immuno-C,* which was promoted as helpful against arthritis, AIDS, flu, atherosclerosis, and cancer. [PA]

***The Vitamin Shoppe**, North Bergen, New Jersey, was ordered by the FDA to stop making unsubstantiated claims that *Sun Chlorella* would strengthen the immune system, reduce cholesterol levels, lower high blood pressure, and stimulate tissue repair and healing. [FDA] [NY]

Wakunaga of America Co., Ltd., Torrance, California, has made unsubstantiated claims that *Kyolic Super Formula 103* "helps strengthen the body's immunological system" and is "the ideal supplement for cardio-vascular problems."

***Weider Health & Fitness**, Woodland Hills, California, has marketed many "ergogenic aids" that will not do what their names suggest. [FTC]

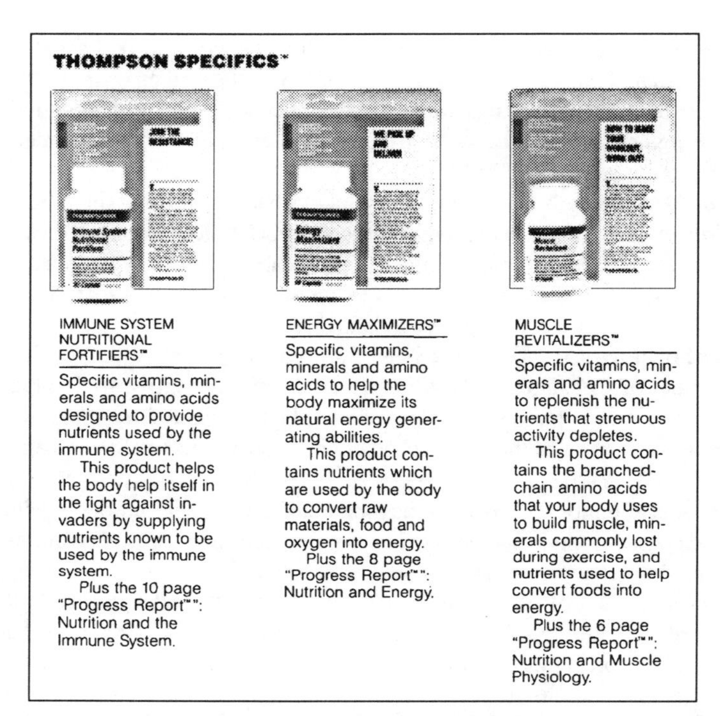

Portion of ad in *Natural Foods Merchandiser* for the William T. Thompson Company's "Informational Packaging™ system," which was prominently advertised to retailers for several months in 1987. Each package consisted of a bottle and a booklet encased in plastic. The products are no longer marketed. Thompson's operating assets were acquired in 1990 by Rexall Sundown, Inc.

***William. T. Thompson Company**, Carson, California, during the late 1980s, marketed an "informational packaging system" in which twelve products were packaged with "progress reports" explaining their rationale (see illustration above). Most of the reports contained misleading statements. The one accompanying *Energy Maximizers,* for example, falsely stated that bee pollen would "help your body maximize its energy-generating potential."

Yerba Prima Botanicals, Ashland, Oregon, has made unsubstantiated claims that its "Internal Cleansing Program" (composed of herbs, psyllium husks, and an externally applied cream) can assist the body in "eliminating a lifetime's accumulation of impurities" and "keep toxins and metabolic waste from building up."

Appendix E

Recommended Reading

The following publications can help you deepen and keep current your knowledge of health information and misinformation. Most of the books can be obtained from bookstores, either directly or by special order. Out-of-print books not available at your local public library may be obtainable through interlibrary loan. Back issues of newsletters and magazines may be available at libraries or from the publisher.

Basic and Practical Nutrition

C. Cook-Fuller and S. Barrett (eds.). *Nutrition 93/94.* Guilford, Conn.: Dushkin Publishing, 1993. A sourcebook containing more than sixty well-written articles from magazines, newsletters, and journals. Updated about once a year.

The Food Guide Pyramid (HG–252). Hyattsville, Md.: U.S. Department of Agriculture Human Nutrition Information Service, 1992. Booklet on implementing the U.S. Dietary Guidelines. Available from the Consumer Information Center, Pueblo, CO 81009.

S.T. Herbst. *Food Lover's Companion.* Hauppauge, N.Y.: Barron's Educational Series, Inc., 1990. Comprehensive definitions of over three thousand food, wine, and culinary terms.

S. Gershoff and C. Whitney. *The Tufts University Guide to Total Nutrition.* New York: Harper Collins, 1992. Basic nutrition information for consumers.

V. Herbert and G.J. Subak-Sharpe (eds.). *Total Nutrition: The Only Guide You'll Ever Need.* New York: St. Martin's Press, 1994. A comprehensive sourcebook by a team of experts from the Mount Sinai School of Medicine.

G. Hodgkin. *Diet Manual, Including a Vegetarian Meal Plan, Seventh Edition.* Loma Linda, Calif: Seventh-day Adventist Dietetic Association, P.O. Box 75, Loma Linda, CA 92354. Provides up-to-date guidance on scientifically-based vegetarian meal planning.

P. Kwiterovich. *Beyond Cholesterol.* Baltimore: The Johns Hopkins University Press, 1989. Discussion of the relationship between diet and cardiovascular disease and how to lower dietary fat content.

Nutrition and Your Health: Dietary Guidelines for Americans (HG 232). Washington, D.C.: U.S. Departments of Agriculture and Health and Human Services, 1985. Booklet about dietary balance. Available from the Consumer Information Center, Pueblo, CO 81009.

E. Satter. *How to Get Your Kid to Eat . . . But Not Too Much.* Palo Alto, Calif.: Bull Publishing, 1987. Information and advice on influencing healthful eating behavior.

A. Simopoulos, V. Herbert, and Beverly Jacobson. *Genetic Nutrition: Designing a Diet Based on Your Family Medical History.* New York: Macmillan Publishing Co., 1993. Explains how to take hereditary factors into account while following a healthful diet based on the USDA Food Guide Pyramid.

F.J. Stare, V. Aronson, and S. Barrett. *Your Guide to Good Nutrition.* Amherst, N.Y.: Prometheus Books, 1991. A discussion of dietary balance and avoidance of nutrition fads and frauds.

E. Tribole. *Eating on the Run.* Champaign, Ill.: Life Enhancement Publications, 1987. Handbook of convenient low-fat eating strategies for busy people.

Contemporary Quackery

Arthritis Foundation. *Unproven Remedies Resource Manual.* Atlanta: Arthritis Foundation, 1991. Comprehensive discussion of unproven treatment methods.

S. Barrett and W.T. Jarvis (eds.). *The Health Robbers: A Close Look at Quackery in America.* Amherst, N.Y.: Prometheus Books, 1993. A comprehensive exposé of health frauds and quackery.

S. Barrett and the editors of Consumer Reports. *Health Schemes, Scams, and Frauds.* Yonkers, N.Y.: Consumer Reports Books, 1990. Overview of common forms of quackery, including updated versions of several articles previously published in *Consumer Reports.*

S. Barrett and B.R. Cassileth (eds.). *Dubious Cancer Treatment: A Report on "Alternative" Methods and the Practitioners Who Use Them.* Tampa, Fla.: American Cancer Society, Florida Division, 1991.

A. Bender. *Health or Hoax: The Truth about Health Foods and Diets.* Amherst, N.Y.: Prometheus Books, 1986. An analysis of the health-food industry and many of its products.

L. Bennion. *Hypoglycemia: Fact or Fad?* New York: Crown Publishers, 1985. A lucid analysis of the fad diagnosis versus the real disease.

K. Butler. *A Consumer's Guide to "Alternative" Medicine.* Amherst, N.Y.: Prometheus Books, 1992. Hard-hitting exposé that includes original research by the author.

H. Cornacchia and S. Barrett. *Consumer Health: A Guide to Intelligent Decisions, Fifth Edition.* St. Louis: Mosby Year Book, 1993. A referenced textbook covering all aspects of health care.

R.P. Doyle. *The Medical Wars.* New York: William Morrow and Co., 1983. A lucid analysis of the scientific method and its application to sixteen medical controversies.

F. Fernandez-Madrid. *Treating Arthritis: Medicine, Myth, and Magic.* New York: Plenum Press, 1989. Combines a fascinating history of arthritis quackery with insights about modern treatment.

J. Fried. *Vitamin Politics.* Amherst, N.Y.: Prometheus Books, 1984. A classic investigation of megavitamin therapy and its proponents.

V. Herbert and S. Barrett. *Vitamins and "Health" Foods: The Great American Hustle.* Philadelphia: George F. Stickley Co., 1981. An investigative exposé of the health-food industry.

P. Huber. *Galileo's Revenge: Junk Science in the Courtroom.* New York: Basic Books, 1991. Describes how professional "expert" witnesses have been permitted to bolster unfounded health claims in liability suits.

C. Marshall. *Vitamins and Minerals: Help or Harm?* Philadelphia: J.B. Lippincott Co., 1985. A comprehensive look at the sources, functions, benefits, dangers, and controversial aspects of vitamins and minerals.

J.P. Payne et al. *Alternative Therapy.* London: British Medical Association, 1986. A detailed report on "alternative" therapies and how they can be scientifically evaluated.

J. Raso. *Mystical Diets.* Amherst, N.Y.: Prometheus Books, 1993. A fascinating exploration of food cults, their gurus, and offbeat nutrition practices.

______ *"Alternative" Healthcare: A Comprehensive Guide.* Amherst, N.Y.: Prometheus Books, 1994. An exploration of unscientific physical, mental, and spiritual approaches to health and health care.

J. Renner. *Health Smarts.* Kansas City, Mo.: HealthFacts Publishing, Inc., 1990. Brief essays on consumer strategies, dubious products, and quack practices.

W.A. Sibley. *Therapeutic Claims in Multiple Sclerosis.* New York: Demos Publications, 1992. An evaluation of more than one hundred methods that indicates which are promising and which appear worthless.

D. Stalker and C. Glymour (eds.). *Examining Holistic Medicine.* Amherst, N.Y.: Prometheus Books, 1985. A devastating exposé of "holistic" propaganda and practices.

F.J. Stare and E.M. Whelan. *Panic in the Pantry.* Amherst, N.Y.: Prometheus Books, 1992. An analysis of facts and fallacies related to the safety of America's food supply.

V. Tyler. *The Honest Herbal, Third Edition.* Binghamton, N.Y.: Haworth Press, 1993. A referenced evaluation of more than one hundred herbs and related substances.

E.M. Whelan. *Toxic Terror: The Truth behind the Cancer Scares.* Amherst, N.Y.: Prometheus Books, 1993. An exposé of false claims that Americans are seriously endangered by chemicals in food, air, water, and other elements of our environment.

C.A. Wulf, K.A. Hughes, K.G. Smith, and M.W. Easley. *Abuse of the Scientific*

Literature in an Antifluoridation Pamphlet. Columbus, Ohio: American Oral Health Institute, 1985, 1988. A detailed refutation of claims made by antifluoridationist John Yiamouyiannis, Ph.D.

J. Yetiv. *Popular Nutritional Practices: A Scientific Appraisal.* San Carlos, Calif.: Popular Medicine Press, 1986. A referenced analysis of more than one hundred nutrition topics of current concern.

J.F. Zwicky, A.W. Hafner, S. Barrett, and W.T. Jarvis. *Reader's Guide to "Alternative" Health Methods.* Chicago: American Medical Association, 1993. An analysis of more than 1,000 reports on unproven, disproven, controversial, fraudulent, quack, and/or otherwise questionable approaches to solving health problems.

History of Quackery

R. Deutsch. *The New Nuts Among the Berries.* Palo Alto, Calif.: Bull Publishing Co., 1977. How nutrition nonsense captured America.

M. Fishbein. *Fads and Quackery in Healing.* New York: Blue Ribbon Books, 1932. A comprehensive analysis of healing cults and "various other peculiar notions in the health field."

N. Gevitz (ed.). *Other Healers: Unorthodox Medicine in America.* Baltimore: The Johns Hopkins University Press, 1988. Essays on homeopathy, chiropractic, Christian Science, divine healing, folk medicine, osteopathy, the botanical movement, and the water-cure movement.

J. Roth. *Health Purifiers and Their Enemies.* New York: Prodist, 1977. A sociological overview of the "natural health" movement and its critics.

J.H. Young. *American Health Quackery.* Princeton, N.J.: Princeton University Press, 1992. A collection of essays dealing with many aspects of quackery.

______ *The Medical Messiahs.* Princeton, N.J.: Princeton University Press, 1992. A social history of health quackery in twentieth-century America.

Weight Control

L.J. Bennion, E.L. Berman, and J.M. Ferguson. *Straight Talk about Weight Control.* Yonkers, N.Y.: Consumer Reports Books, 1991. A comprehensive look at the current state of knowledge on weight control.

L. Lamb. *The Weighting Game.* Secaucus, N.J.: Lyle Stuart, Inc., 1988. A useful reference for health professionals and serious dieters interested in the why's and how's of weight loss.

G. Mirkin. *Getting Thin.* Boston: Little Brown, 1983. Practical discussion of weight-control facts and fads.

F.J. Stare and E. M. Whelan. *The Harvard Square Diet.* Amherst, N.Y.: Prometheus Books, 1987. A straightforward approach to dietary and behavioral modification.

Congressional Hearings

R.J. Durbin et al. *Dietary Supplements.* Appropriations Subcommittee on Agriculture, Rural Development, Food And Drug Administration, and Related Agencies, House Committee on Appropriations, October 18, 1993.

P. Mink et al. *FDA's Regulation of the Dietary Supplement L-Tryptophan.* Human Resources and Intergovernmental Relations Subcommittee, House Committee on Government Operations, July 18, 1991.

C. Pepper et al. *Quackery: A $10 Billion Scandal.* Subcommittee on Health and Long-Term Care of the Senate Select Committee on Aging, May 31, 1984.

W.V. Roth et al. *Weight Reduction Products and Plans.* Permanent Subcommittee on Investigations, Senate Committee on Governmental Affairs, May 14 and 15, 1985.

H.A. Waxman et al. *Regulation of Dietary Supplements.* Subcommittee on Health and the Environment, House Committee on Energy and Commerce, July 29, 1993.

R. Wyden et al. *Deception and Fraud in the Diet Industry.* Subcommittee on Regulation, Business Opportunities, and Energy, House Committee on Small Business, March 26 and May 7, 1990.

Government and Government-Sponsored Reports

S.A. Anderson and D.J. Raiten (eds.). *Safety of Amino Acids Used As Dietary Supplements.* Bethesda, Md.: Federation of American Societies for Experimental Biology, 1992. Examines the marketing, research status, and safety of amino acids supplements.

G. J. Dykstra et al. *Dietary Supplements Task Force Final Report.* Rockville, Md.: Food and Drug Administration, 1992. Recommendations for labeling of dietary supplements and related products.

C.E. Edwards et al. *Report of the Advisory Committee of the Food and Drug Administration.* Washington, D.C.: U.S. Dept. of Health and Human Services, 1991. Summarizes FDA difficulties in carrying out its mission and how its resources might be used more effectively.

FDA Staff. *Unsubstantiated Claims and Documented Health Hazards in the Dietary Supplement Marketplace.* Rockville, Md.: Food and Drug Administration, 1993. A 110-page report on unsubstantiated claims by health-food retailers and manufacturers and hazardous ingredients in supplement and herbal products. Available for $18 from LVCAHF, Inc., P.O. Box 1747, Allentown, PA 18105.

Federal Food, Drug, and Cosmetic Act, as Amended, and Related Laws. Washington, D.C.: U.S. Government Printing Office, 1990 (GPO Stock #017-012-00347-8). Complete text of the Food, Drug, and Cosmetic Act, including amendments through October 1989, available for $7.50 from U.S. Government Printing Office, Supt. of Documents, Washington, D.C. 20402.

Food and Drug Administration. *A Study of Health Practices and Opinions.* Springfield,

Va.: National Technical Information Service, U.S. Dept of Commerce, 1972 (Publication #210978). Classic study illustrating why people are vulnerable to quackery.

Food and Drug Administration. *Food Labeling; General Requirements, Final and Proposed Rule*. Federal Register 59(2):349–437, January 4, 1994. Most recent version of the FDA's proposed regulations for the labeling of dietary supplements.

H. Gelband et al. *Unconventional Cancer Treatments.* Washington, D.C.: U.S. Government Printing Office, 1990. A comprehensive report from the Office of Technology Assessment.

Louis Harris and Associates. *Health, Information and the Use of Questionable Treatments: A Study of the American Public.* Rockville, Md.: Food and Drug Administration, 1987. Results of an FDA-sponsored survey of 1,514 adults to determine their health status, beliefs about treatment, and use of unscientific treatment for arthritis, cancer, and other health problems.

C.W. Keller. *Report of the Presiding Officer on Proposed Trade Regulation Rule Regarding Advertising and Labeling of Protein Supplements.* Washington, D.C.: Federal Trade Commission, June 15, 1978. Reports the findings of an FTC official who investigated claims related to the marketing and use of protein supplements.

C. Pepper et al. *Quackery, A $10 Billion Scandal.* Washington, DC: U.S. Government Printing Office, May 31, 1984. Report of a four-year Congressional investigation of health frauds and quackery.

Use of Bovine Somatotropin (BST) in the United States: Its Potential Effects. Washington, D.C.: Executive Branch of the Federal Government, 1994. Report on the safety and economic significance of BST, a hormone that can increase milk production.

F.E. Young et al. *Review of Fluoride Benefits and Risks.* Washington, D.C.: U.S. Dept. of Health and Human Services, 1991. Report of an expert panel that reviewed the safety and benefits of water fluoridation.

Nutrition Reference Books for Professionals

M.L. Brown (ed.). *Present Knowledge in Nutrition, Sixth Edition.* Washington, D.C.: International Life Sciences Institute–Nutrition Foundation, 1990. Scientific summaries of fifty-nine topics in basic and clinical nutrition.

Committee on Diet and Health, National Research Council. *Diet and Health.* Washington, D.C.: National Academy Press, 1989. Comprehensive discussion of the relationships between dietary factors and the incidence of chronic disease.

Food and Nutrition Board, National Research Council. *Recommended Dietary Allowances, Tenth Edition.* Washington, D.C.: National Academy Press, 1989. Current version of the RDAs, based on the work of the 1985 Committee on Dietary Allowances.

R.C. Frank and H.B. Irving. *The Directory of Food and Nutrition Information.* Phoenix: Oryx Press, 1992. Provides detailed description of information available from more than one thousand sources. Includes a few that are unreliable.

H. A. Guthrie, M.F. Picciano, and A. Scott. *Human Nutrition.* St. Louis: Mosby Year Book, 1995. Basic nutrition textbook.

C.E. Koop. *The Surgeon General's Report on Nutrition and Health.* Washington, D.C.: U.S. Dept. of Health and Human Services, 1988 (GPO Stock #017-001-00465). Comprehensive discussion of the relationships between dietary factors and the incidence of chronic disease.

L.K. Mahan and M. Arlin. *Kraus's Food, Nutrition & Diet Therapy, Eighth Edition.* Philadelphia: W.B. Saunders Co., 1992. Comprehensive resource book on clinical nutrition for professionals.

J.A.T. Pennington. *Bowes & Church's Food Values of Portions Commonly Used, Sixteenth Edition.* Philadelphia: J.B. Lippincott Co., 1994. Authoritative data on the nutrient composition of 8,500 generic and brand-name foods

N.L. Pennington and C.W. Baker (eds.). *Sugar: A User's Guide to Sucrose.* New York: Van Nostrand Reinhold, 1990. Comprehensive discussion of the history, sources, production, and utilization of sugar.

M.E. Shils, J.A. Olson, and M. Shike (eds.). *Modern Nutrition in Health and Disease, Eighth Edition.* Philadelphia: Lea & Febiger, 1994. The most comprehensive nutrition textbook for professionals.

F.S. Sizer and E.N. Whitney. *Nutrition Concepts and Controversies, Sixth Edition.* Eagan, Mich.: West Publishing Co., 1994. Analyzes basic issues confronting consumers.

Newsletters

Consumer Reports on Health, Box 36356, Boulder, CO 80322. Presents detailed reports on health strategies, with occasional reports on quackery.

Diet Busine$$ Bulletin, 181 S. Franklin Ave., Suite 608, Valley Stream, N.Y., 11580. Quarterly report on hard-to-get information about the products, services, and economics of the commercial weight-loss industry.

Harvard Health Letter, P.O. Box 420300, Palm Coast, FL 32142. Features superb analyses of controversial issues, particularly those involving recent research.

Johns Hopkins Medical Letter, Health after 50, P.O. Box 420179, Palm Coast, FL 32142. Solid information on basic health strategies.

Lahey Clinic Health Letter, P.O. Box 541, Burlington, MA 01805. Solid information on basic health strategies.

Lawrence Review of Natural Products, Facts and Comparisons, 111 West Port Plaza, Suite 423, St. Louis, MO 63146. Authoritative monthly monographs on herbs and other naturally occurring products.

Mayo Clinic Health Letter, P.O. Box 53889, Boulder, CO 80322. Solid, practical information with occasional reports on quackery.

Mirkin Report, Box 6608, Silver Spring, MD 20916. Excellent summaries of news on fitness, nutrition, and health.

NCAHF Newsletter, P.O. Box 1276, Loma Linda, CA 92354. Covers a wide variety of events related to quackery and health frauds.

Nutrition Forum, P.O. Box 747924, Rego Park, NY 11374. Features in-depth reports and undercover investigations related to quackery and health frauds.

Probe, Box 1321, Cathedral Station, New York, NY 10025. David Zimmerman's investigative newsletter on science, media, policy, and health.

Tufts University Diet and Nutrition Letter, P.O. Box 57857, Boulder, CO 80322. Solid, practical information, with occasional reports related to quackery.

Magazines

Consumer Reports, P.O. Box 53029, Boulder, CO 80322. Covers a moderate number of topics related to health and nutrition.

FDA Consumer, Superintendent of Documents, P.O. Box 371954, Pittsburgh, PA 15250. Covers nutrition, food safety, drugs, and other medical topics.

Healthy Weight Journal, Route 2, Box 905, Hettinger, ND 58639. Covers research, frauds, and other topics related to weight control. (Formerly called *Obesity & Health.)*

Priorities, American Council on Science and Health, 1995 Broadway, New York, NY 10023. Focuses on controversies involving lifestyle, environmental chemicals, and quackery.

Skeptical Inquirer, P.O. Box 703, Buffalo, NY 14226. Features critical analyses of "paranormal" claims. Plans to include a regular column on health-related issues.

Index